Taijiquan Master Reference

An Anthology

Volume 1

COMPILED BY
MICHAEL A. DEMARCO, M.A.

VIA MEDIA PUBLISHING | ARTICLES FROM THE JOURNAL OF ASIAN MARTIAL ARTS

Disclaimer

Please note that the author and publisher of this book are not responsible in any manner whatsoever for any injury that may result from practicing the techniques and/or following the instructions given herein. Participation in martial arts activities can be dangerous and can lead to serious injury. The material presented in this book is intended for reference only, and the reader assumes all risks associated with attempting to perform any of the activities described herein. Before attempting any of the physical activities described in this book, the reader should consult a physician for advice regarding their individual suitability for performing such activity.

All Rights Reserved

No part of this publication, including illustrations, may be reproduced or utilized in any form or by any means, electronic or mechanical, including photocopying, recording, or by any information storage and retrieval system (beyond that copying permitted by sections 107 and 108 of the US Copyright Law and except by reviewers for the public press), without written permission from Via Media Publishing Company.

Warning: Any unauthorized act in relation to a copyright work may result in both a civil claim for damages and criminal prosecution.

Copyright © 2025
by Via Media Publishing Company
941 Calle Mejia #822
Santa Fe, NM 87501 USA

Book and cover design
by Via Media Publishing Company

ISBN 979-8-9922430-0-0

www.viamediapublishing.com

Dedication

To all those who have contributed to the
Journal of Asian Martial Arts (1992–2016)
providing articles of high academic standards
that will continue to inspire research and practice.

Table of Contents

Preface ix

- The Origin and Evolution of Taijiquan 1
  Michael A. DeMarco, M.A.

- A Brief Description of Chen Style Master Du Yuze 23
  Wong Jiaxiang; Michael DeMarco M.A., Trans.

- The Presence of the Eyes in the Action of Taijiquan 32
  Sophia Delza

- The Daoist Origins of the Chinese Martial Arts 41
  Charles Holcombe, Ph.D.

- Taijiquan: Learning How to Learn 57
  Linda Lehrhaupt, Ph.D.

- Thoughts on the Classic of Taijiquan 65
  Carol M. Derrickson, M.A.

- The Development of Zheng Manqing Taijiquan in Malaysia 77
  Nigel Sutton, M.A.

- An Encounter with Chen Xiaowang:
  The Continuing Development of Chen Style Taijiquan 93
  Dietmar Stubenbaum

- The Necessity for Softness in Taijiquan 103
  Michael A. DeMarco, M.A.

- Zheng Manqing and Taijiquan: A Clarification of Role 115
  Robert W. Smith, M.A.

- Principles and Practices in Taijiquan 132
  Peter Lim Tian Tek

- Inner Circle Taiji Training Exercise 142
  Stuart Kohler, M.A.

- Remembering Zheng Manqing: Some Sketches from His Life 150
  Robert W. Smith, M.A.

- In Search of a Unified Dao: Zheng Manqing's Life
  and Contribution to Taijiquan 165
  Barbara Davis, M.A.

- The Luoshu as Taiji Boxing's Secret Inner-Sanctum Training Method ... 192
  Bradford Tyrey and Marcus Brinkman

- The Combative Elements of Yang Taijiquan 198
  Peter Lim Tian Tek

- Breathing in Taiji and Other Fighting Arts 210
  Robert W. Smith, M.A.

- Chen Weiming, Zheng Manqing, and the 277
  Difference Between Strength and Intrinsic Energy
  Robert W. Smith, M.A.
- Dalü and Some Tigers 290
  Robert W. Smith, M.A.
- Taijiquan as an Experiential Way for Discovering Daoism 301
  Michael A. DeMarco, M.A.
- Internal Training: The Foundation for Chen Taiji's 312
  Fighting Skills and Health Promotion
  Adam Wallace
- Immortality in Chinese Thought and Its Influence 341
  on Taijiquan and Qigong
  Arieh Lev Breslow, M.A.
- Chen and Yang Taiji Converge in Hangzhou City 358
  Donald Mainfort, M.A.
- Body-Mind Connections in Chen Xin's 372
  Illustrated Explanation of Chen Style Taijiquan
  Miriam O'Connor, M.A.
- Yang Taiji Practice Through the Eyes of Western 383
  Medical Health Guidelines
  Michael A. DeMarco, M.A.
- The Nature of Rooting in Taijiquan: A Survey 397
  Stuart Kohler, M.A.
- The Pedagogy of Taijiquan in the University Setting 406
  Andy Peck, M.S. Ed.
- Reviving the Daoist Roots of Internal Martial Arts 412
  Mark Hawthorne
- The Nurturing Ways of Chen Taiji: An Interview with Yang Yang 422
  Michael A. DeMarco, M.A. and A. Edwin Matthews
- Taiji's Chen Village Under the Influence of Chen Xiaoxing 452
  Stephan Berwick, M.A.
- Chen Xiaowang on Learning, Practicing, and Teaching Chen Taiji 462
  Stephan Berwick, M.A.
- An Introduction to Seizing Techniques in Chen Style Taijiquan 466
  Yaron Seidman, L.Ac.
- Comparison of Yang Style Taijiquan's Large and Medium Frame Forms 473
  Joel Stein, M.S.

Sources of Original Publication 482

Index 484

Preface

Via Media Publishing was founded in 1992 in order to produce the peer reviewed quarterly *Journal of Asian Martial Arts* (1992–2012)—the first publication of its kind to focus on martial traditions in an academic format. Many of the authors were scholar–practitioners, who utilized their unique talents to present articles from various specializations, such as Asian Studies, kinesiology, history, anthropology, philosophy, and physical education.

Those who were serious about this field subscribed to the journal to read articles noted for their high academic and aesthetic standards. Most were in the United States, Canada, and Europe, but also in other areas of the world. These naturally included martial art schools and individual practitioners. There was a strong base among university and public libraries too.

As founder of Via Media, I've decided to assemble this anthology of articles relating to taijiquan. There are over three hundred million taiji practitioners worldwide, drawn to the art mainly for health maintenance and it therapeutic value. Researchers can benefit from this handy anthology, particularly for the information and analyses presented, including the rich bibliographic listings. Taiji practitioners will also gain insights to benefit their own practice, be it for health and/or self-defense.

Note that page numbering is consecutive from Volume 1 through Volume 2. The index covers both volumes.

Included in both volumes are sixty-four articles, the same number of hexagrams in the *Book of Changes* (*Yijing*). In addition to 735 illustrations, there are glossaries, maps, charts, and bibliographies. *Taijiquan* is the term representing the general category of study, but taijiquan can be subdivided into its branches, from the original Chen Family Style to the highly popular Yang Family Style. Other lineages are presented, such as the Wu and Sun systems.

The variety of material in this anthology reflects in-depth scholarly research and the experience of master practitioners. It will be a valuable source taijiquan enthusiasts for future decades. By making this book available to individuals and libraries, we hope this rare material will greatly contribute to further research in this field and inspire many to learn taijiquan with aspirations to mastery.

Michael DeMarco

Michael DeMarco, Publisher
Santa Fe, NM, January 2025

• 1 •

The Origin and Evolution of Taijiquan
by Michael A. DeMarco, M.A.

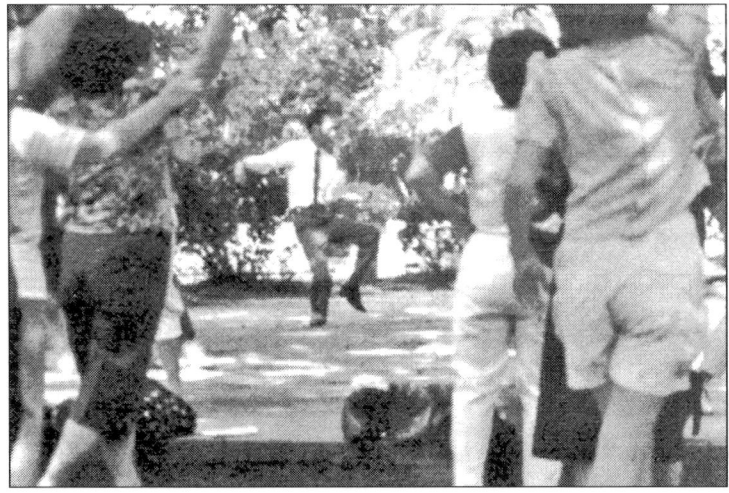

Taijiquan enthusiasts arrive in Taipei's 2/28 Peace Park before sunrise, benefiting from their practice in an atmosphere of fresh air and tranquility. Later in the morning, disco-style exercisers arrive to gyrate in beat with blaring disco music. Photo by M. DeMarco.

**I am not one who was born in the possession of knowledge.
I am one who is fond of antiquity, and earnest in seeking it there.**
– *Confucian Analects,* 7: 19

History, according to the Chinese tradition, is not to be understood as a passage of time toward a perfect human state. On the contrary, it is seen as a regression away from a splendid "Golden Age" when their ancestors lived in a utopian state more than four thousand years ago. All things wise and good were believed to have existed during this period. It represented a period which held secrets for proper living, supreme health and happiness. Even for the martial arts, what is deemed most worthy is held to be the creation of sagacious warriors of antiquity.

The Chinese fanatical respect for antiquity presents some formidable barriers for any student of their culture. It was a common practice for many Chinese writers to falsely assign their works to an earlier time to gain greater respect and fame for their works. Sometimes, besides placing their works in an earlier period, writers would credit a work as being "brushed" (they did not use pens yet!) by an earlier figure of prestige. Oftentimes the work would be anonymous, not dated, not punctuated, and filled with incomprehensible symbolic jargon. This certainly occurred in martial art literature as well. Trying to trace the origin of a boxing system can cause a researcher to perform a wonderful assortment of kicks and punches simply out of academic frustration!

Taijiquan, as part of the cultural history of China, is encrusted in a confusing maze of facts and fiction. This is a reality which needs constant attention in studying the history of any martial art. The following theories on the origin of taijiquan show how myth and legend are blended within the Chinese cultural heritage. Fortunately, with a critical eye for reliable data, we can present a sound overview regarding the evolution of taijiquan.

Theories of Early Dynastic Origin

One theory states that taijiquan originated during the end of the Liang dynasty (502–557 CE) and the beginning of the Chen dynasty (557–589 CE). These dynasties had their capital at Nanjing in present-day Jiangsu Province on the Yangtze River.

Another theory holds that the creation of taijiquan came slightly later, during the Tang dynasty (618–907 CE). The Tang capital is situated in present-day Shaanxi Province. Then called Changan, the great city is now referred to as Xi'an. It is the place where the famed life-sized terra cotta warriors, which marked the grave site of China's First Emperor of Qin, were recently unearthed.

In placing the origin of taijiquan at such early periods, the two theories stated above lack solid verification. These seem to be attempts to place the time of origin to an early era simply for added prestige. If these theories were accepted, a period in the history of taijiquan representing hundreds of years would be left vacant.

There is no doubt that many boxing schools existed during these early dynastic times, but their connection to the creation of taijiquan remains a remote root of the evolutionary tree of boxing. Taijiquan clearly comes into being as a later branch in the development of martial arts.

Zhang Sanfeng as Possible Inventor

Many of today's taijiquan teachers will state that their art is derived from the system of Zhang Sanfeng. According to popular belief, he was a famous Daoist living on Mount Wudang in Hebei Province, a master of internal alchemy, and a boxer of the highest grade. Because of his fame, he was invited to the Imperial court by three different Emperors. Although he never did appear after numerous attempts to find him, he was canonized in 1459 by the Emperor Yingzong. There is a shrine in Beijing dedicated to "the Immortal Sanfeng" in the well-known White Cloud Monastery of the Quanzhen Daoist sect.

Most writings describe Zhang Sanfeng, alias Junbao, as an extraordinarily tall, bearded figure, with large eyes. His feats of magic included riding through the air on a crane, and he could be at different places at the same time. It is even believed that after he died in the 1390's, he miraculously came back to life once again.

All these accounts regarding Zhang Sanfeng serve to add an aura of semi-religious awe for the god-like creator of taijiquan. There are Zhang Sanfeng spirit-medium cults in China, particularly in the province of Sichuan. Nonetheless, in official bibliographies there is no mention of him even practicing taijiquan. Perhaps the most scholarly article in the English language on this subject was written by respected sinologist Anna Seidel, who states:

> His biographies and legends lack even the faintest allusion to his being a boxing master . . . . We know next to nothing about [Zhang] Sanfeng's historical existence and his thought. (484)

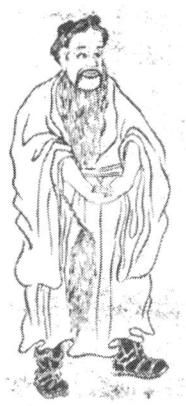

Zhang Sanfeng. Ink rubbing of the legendary founder of taijiquan.

Once faced with the facts, the story of Zhang Sanfeng turns into a symbolic legend which represents the unknown influences that have contributed to the birth of taijiquan. As the patron of this style, the Daoist Zhang Sanfeng parallels the role Bodhidharma plays as the Buddhist patron of the Shaolin boxing school. The Daoist sanctuary on Mount Wudang was dedicated to the God of War named Chen Wu. This god was of supreme importance in war-ridden China during the Ming dynasty (1368–1644). Despite the contradicting facts, many continue to believe that it was this god who revealed the art of taijiquan to Zhang Sanfeng in a dream.

The technique of attributing the origin of taijiquan to Zhang Sanfeng is just one illustration of the Chinese use of antedating. In so doing, taijiquan is given the respect of antiquity and the sacredness of a paranormal manifestation. Zhang represents an ideal boxing master with supernormal abilities. Believed to have lived for at least two centuries, he is often credited with creating the most efficient boxing system known.

Zhang Sanfeng's story fits in well with the popular beliefs prevalent during the Ming dynasty. The thought of the time was influenced by Daoism, particularly the beliefs in immortals and esoteric techniques for self-cultivation. Through all the uncertainty, we eventually arrive at a point in time when taijiquan is taught and practiced. It is beyond all doubt that taijiquan was practiced in a Henan village more than 200 years ago. In this small commune, known as Chenjiagou, it is still practiced today. The known masters living there give no mention of Zhang Sanfeng as part of the taijiquan tradition but present their own theory of origin.

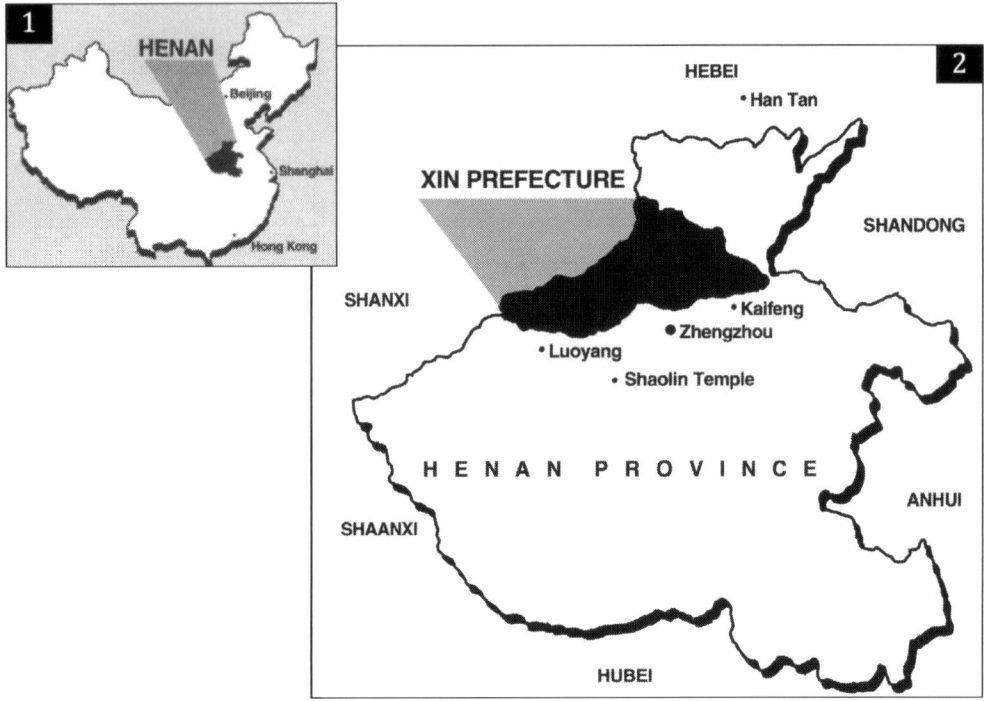

(1) Peoples Republic of China showing the central location of Henan Province.
(2) Above: Location of Xin Prefecture and adjoining provinces around Henan.
(3) Details of western Xin Prefecture. For the area outlined in the slanted square below, compare with following Space Shuttle photo.

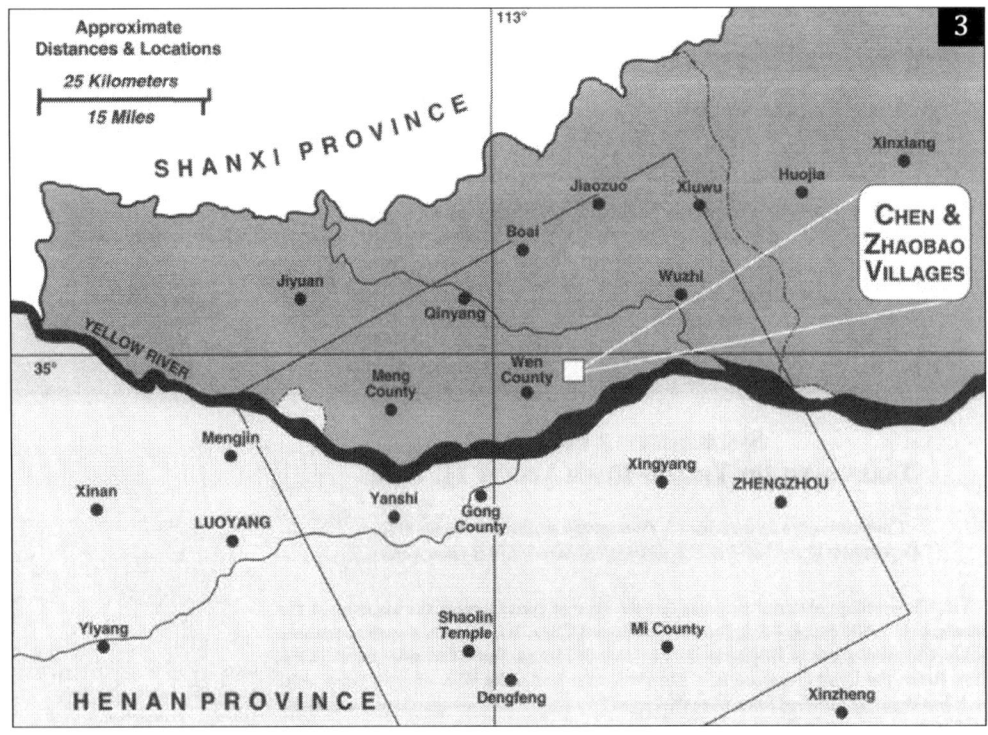

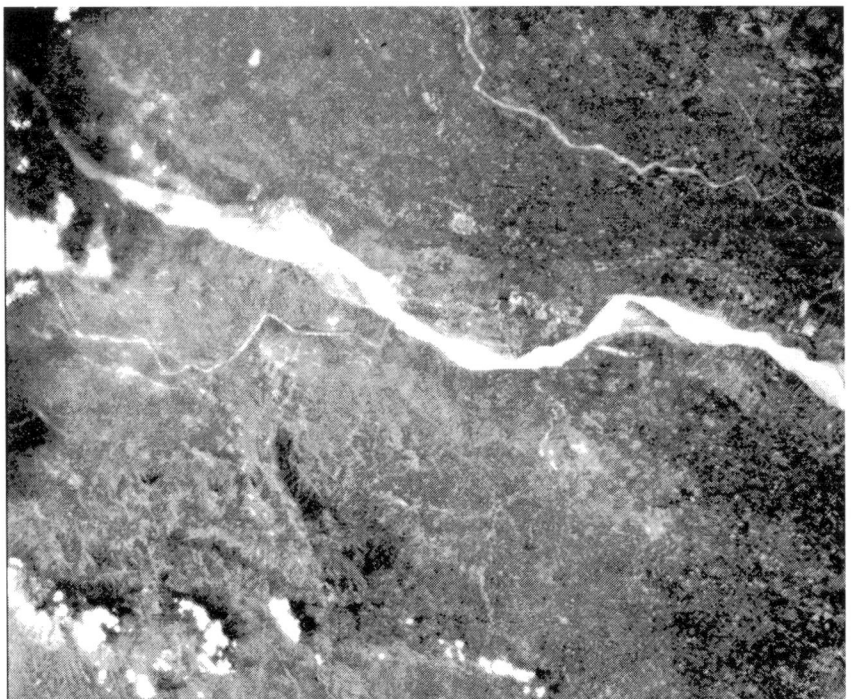

Space shuttle photo taken over the Yellow River
Compare with map on page 4. Photograph available from the U.S. Department of the Interior, U.S. Geological Survey EROS Data Center. The Chen Village obtained its name for the sake of convenience: the majority of the approximately 1,800 people living there are surnamed Chen. It is actually a small commune, roughly 400 miles south of Beijing in the province of Henan. Just a few miles north of the Yellow River, the Chen commune is in Xin Prefecture under the Wen administrative unit. This is less than one hundred miles from the city of Luoyang, which was previously a dynastic capital and a great cultural center.

Origination at Chen Village

For those who have not been swayed by the emotional attraction of placing the origination of taijiquan in either the early dynastic periods or at the time of Zhang Sanfeng, the theory that it originated in the Chen Village seems a more likely alternative. Here we find an exact location, verified dates, known boxing masters, and a clearly applicable historic setting for its origin.

The Chen Village plays a unique role along with Henan province in China's historical development. In the most remote times, this area spawned one of China's earliest Stone Age cultures. By the 11th century, Luoyang was one of two metropolitan areas with a population of over one million people. Because of its riches, the area was often subject to barbaric invasions as well as internal rebellion.

In contrast to the external threats, internal problems were usually caused by peasant dissatisfaction resulting from natural and political disasters. The rapid increase in population during the later dynasties placed greater burdens on the

Henan people. They had to face floods and food shortages, as well as exploitation by those holding political power. By 1600, about half of the provincial lands had been given to friends and relatives of the Imperial house as gifts or rewards. This abusive practice uprooted many peasants from their land.

The social structure of the Chen clan illustrates many features prominent among other small communes attempting to solve similar problems. One result of the insecure political situation during the Ming/Qing dynasties is that small groups of related people would bind themselves together into their own social unit. They organized themselves around a village leader and set up a communal system which would provide for their every need. Their major concern was focused on having sufficient amounts of food and water. But in a time of incessant warfare, rebellion and banditry, knowledge of the martial arts became a necessity for the protection of one's farm, home and family.

It is not surprising that the Shaolin Monastery, like the Chen Village, is located in Henan Province. The monastery is about fifty miles southeast of the former capital of Luoyang. Other clans became noted for their own styles of boxing, but the Shaolin Temple and the Chen clan became the most famous for their superior systems. The monastery was also a social unit which had need of protecting its agricultural lands and religious art treasures. Likewise, the Chen Village formed its own small protective group within society. In doing so, it placed emphasis on developing a martial art useful for the defense of its inhabitants against any outsiders, regardless of their boxing system.

Numerous theories have been stated which attempt to tie the Chen Village in with the creation of taijiquan. By trying to find the earliest point in time when taijiquan was formed, we are presented with the scantiest of facts. One figure we find with substantial documentation is Wang Zongyue.

Wang Zongyue was a native of Shanxi, the province just north of Henan. It is said that he introduced a new form of boxing to the people of Chenjiagou when he stopped for a while in the village during his travels. This was said to have occurred during Emperor Qianlong's reign (1736–1795). A schoolteacher by profession, Wang was a learned man, credited with linking the original thirteen postures into a continuous sequence. In so doing, he applied the Daoist philosophy and concepts of yin/yang to the new style. One book, the *Taijiquan Lun*, is reputedly his work. In it is found the first mention of taijiquan as the formal name given to this system.

Wang Zong from Shaanxi Province is often confused with Wang Zongyue from Shanxi. The former is believed to be a disciple of the legendary Zhang Sanfeng. Because of the similarity of names and as an attempt to push the taijiquan lineage back further in time, Wang Zongyue is sometimes said to have learned his art from Zhang Sanfeng. Wang, living during a much later period, could not have been a student of Zhang.

Regardless of the confusion surrounding Wang Zongyue, there is little doubt about his influence at Chenjiagou. Since the village was already famed for its boxing, there is the greatest probability that a synthesis of styles took place. This seems to be the case because Wang only affected a Chen Style that had been previously developed.

Although Wang Zongyue is credited with the first mention of the name taijiquan, we are primarily concerned with the evolution of the boxing form itself. Formerly it was known as *Changquan*, or Long Fist. By tracing the style prevalent at Chenjiagou during the time when Wang Zongyue was visiting, we find that a particular style had already been in existence there for several years.

Chen Wangting, alias Zouting, is credited as the true founder of the Chen Style taijiquan. It is estimated that he lived from 1597 to 1664 and was a garrison commander in the Wen County where the Chen Village is located. A military man, Chen absorbed many noted styles during his travels. Later he created his own style.

According to significant historical data and fables, Chen Wangting has received recognition as the true inventor of taijiquan and the "push-hands" exercises. Adopting and modifying movements from many martial art styles, plus tempering these movements with his own wisdom, he created the Chen system. Chen's new syncretic forms were to be performed in a fashion compatible with the then prevalent theories of Daoism.

Chen Wangting was the ninth-generation heir of the Chen family, which was to carry on his unique boxing style to the present day. About 95% of the villagers living there today practice at least one of the forms originally taught by Chen himself. But this Chen Style, originally so secretive, has moved outward from its place of origin with the passing of years. Until roughly one hundred years ago, taijiquan was largely practiced only in Henan province. Since then, it has swept to the four quarters of China and then into overseas areas where Chinese have immigrated.

Although it is the more modern Yang Style that is popular throughout the world, the Chen Style is also making its move into other areas outside of China proper. But this is on a much less noticeable scale, for the Chen Style of taijiquan was always a rare style, even in China. It was a style reserved only for a select few. For this reason, the Chen Style is a relatively uncommon martial art system whose exceptional traits are know more from hearsay than from actual experience.

Masters and Evolution

In tracing the lineage of taijiquan, we can take an analytical approach by starting with the present-day masters and work our way back through time. By doing this, we amass an overpowering list of teachers and students. Many of the teachers are mediocre, to mention nothing of the students. There are only a few teachers of major significance. These are the masters who have truly developed the art of taijiquan.

The following chronology illustrates just how the various styles emerged from the original in light of the historic setting. It also presents the preservation of the Chen Style through the direct lineage.

There is a confusing array of taijiquan styles including the Yang, Chen, Woo,

Hao, Sun and Wu. Plus, there are additional distinguishing adjectives such as the new, old, big frame, simplified, small frame, and an assortment of newly imagined styles. Like a substitute for a Chinese "water torture," we are supposed to bear the burden of figuring out how all these styles are related. As an additional hindrance, many of the names are found presented only in the Chinese rendering.

Chen Wangting

In a temple at Chenjiagou there is a painting of Chen Wangting, honoring him as the founder of the system. It is logical that the founder would not be a "Zhang" as Zhang Sanfeng, or a "Wang" as Wang Zongyue. As a rule, Chen Wangting's system was to be handed down only to descendants of the Chen family. While his original forms have largely been preserved through direct lineage, variations have occurred with time, some becoming separate styles.

The Chen Style has been carried on through private instruction, passing from teacher to student over the past two centuries. This style was rarely presented in public. Literature regarding the subject has likewise been scanty. It was a highly secretive art form, requiring oral instructions from a master.

Today, the seclusive tradition which surrounds the Chen Style has apparently changed. People may think that because there is some literature and demonstrations of Chen Taijiquan that it is now openly presented to the public. Upon closer examination, what was written is found to present only a limited view of the system as a whole. Visual presentations usually consist of the basic form which, impressive in itself, is only an introduction to other sets.

Chen Wangting, previous to developing his own style, was influenced by a general Qi Jiguang, who reputedly designed a routine consisting of 32 movements which he synthesized from sixteen boxing styles. Chen, in turn, combined 29 of these movements with others and used them to form a total of seven different routines. Five of these were rudimentary, from which one remains as a standard routine for junior students.

Movements in the first routine are practiced with the feet leading the hands. The second routine is characterized with hand movements leading. Another noted feature is that there is a greater percentage of harder movements in the second routine. A later development, a third routine, attempts to perfectly blend the hard and soft movements in harmonious physical orchestration.

The style that Chen Wangting created was a physical embodiment of Daoist philosophy, particularly the concept of yin/yang. His system is a harmonious blending of hard/soft, fast/slow, passive and active. Within the yin there is potential yang, and vice versa. One of the Chen routines is called *paochui*, or the "cannon fist." This term describes the intrinsic power present in Chen Wangting's system. The cannonball sitting in a stationary barrel becomes an active, hard-hitting projectile due to the explosive power inherent in its design. Chen Wangting developed such a system for his martial art, always potent with power.

Compared to all other styles of taijiquan, the Chen Style is also the most strenuous to practice. It includes very difficult leg work, utilizing squats, leaps and various kicks. Often there are changes in tempo. Movements include a circling and twisting of the waist known for producing "cork-screw strength" and "twisting energy." A hand strike, for example, actually starts from the heels allowing energy to move through the legs, waist, torso, shoulders, arms, and then into the hands. The end result is a blow stemming from the whole body, not just muscular power from one arm.

There are many features common to all taijiquan styles. However, a distinguishing feature of the Chen Style is its unique employment of physical laws to ensure maximum power for boxing. This is illustrated, for example, in the perfect alignment of the index finger to the elbow. The hand and arm form a straight line. Whether the hand formation is open or closed, the wrist should not be bent in any way. This plum line straightness is paramount in the Chen Style's use of the hands and can also be seen in the upright posture of the spine. It provides maximum power and safety from possible injury which could otherwise result during combat.

Regarding footwork, there is also a difference from other styles. In the posture called "rooster stands on one leg," for example, the foot of the raised leg points directly forwards with the sole parallel to the ground. This movement differs from the Yang Style where the toe points downwards. This simple variance is utilized for additional power as when used for a knee strike to an opponent's mid-section.

The examples above show some of the unique features embodied in Chen Taijiquan. These movements include a large spectrum of fighting techniques: numerous open and closed hand strikes, qinna holds, jumping kicks, kicking from low postures, throws, and a wide assortment of blocks. During each set, special attention is given to one's technique, including the duration of the routine, strength developed, changes in rhythm and use of breathing.

Chen Wangting's system of taijiquan has been preserved through direct lineage from his time to the present day. In order to distinguish his original style from later branches of taijiquan, it is simply referred to as *laojia*, or the "old frame" system. A few other major schools which branched out from this direct lineage will be discussed later.

The Chen Lineage

The next major figure of the *laojia* is Chen Changxing (1771–1853). He was the 14th generation grandmaster who lived in Chenjiagou and was directly descended from the founder. Because of his upright posture and revered character, he was referred to as "Mr. Name Board" (comparing him to a board which listed ancestors names, an object of great respect). Chen Changxing is also remembered as the teacher of Yang Luchan, who later founded the now popular style associated with his family name. Although this new-found branch began at this time, the mainstream of laojia continued in its own familial succession.

We can see how selective laojia masters are by observing the style's lineage. Chen Changxing was the direct descendant of the founder. He, in turn, as the 14th generation grandmaster, passed his knowledge on to his son, Chen Gengyun. This 15th generation grandmaster served as a military guard for the gentry class in Shandong Province. He became well-known for providing security for the Chinese upperclass, while his name became a symbol of law and order. The law was enforced through his superior martial prowess, or simply through the fear of it.

The son of Chen Gengyun, who became the 16th generation Grandmaster, was Chen Yanxi. Following in his father's footsteps was no easy task. Chen Gengyun was held in such prominence that a monument was dedicated to him along a Shandong road that was used to transport the rich cargo he protected for the gentry. The governor of the province, upon seeing this monument, decided to seek out Chen Gengyun to ask him to teach his children the old Chen Style. Since Chen Gengyun had already died a few years previous, Chen Yanxi was commissioned for the task.

One significant aspect of Chen Yanxi giving instruction to the children of Shandong's governor is that the governor was to become a famous figure in China's history. His name was Yuan Shikai, a political-military man having great influence in the events which were to shape China's future.

Yuan was a pivot in the power struggles in the Beijing capital. He was the leading military figure in north China who at one time declared himself Emperor and also became the President of the new republic. Yuan met Chen during the final days of the Qing dynasty. In this period of tragic disunity, China was plagued by revolutions, rebellions, and foreign intervention. Shortly after the Boxer Rebellion of 1900, warlords carved up the land in proportion to their own military strength and political cunning.

The significance of Yuan Shikai's asking Chen Yanxi to teach his family reinforces the belief that the laojia Chen Style had gained a reputation as the most fearsome of all fighting systems. The Chen family name was already legend in places far distant from Henan Province.

There is another interesting note regarding a student of Chen Yanxi named Du Yuze (1896–1990). Du was the son of Du Yueh, the leading official in charge of the Henan country where the Chen Village is located. Du, originally from Boai city located north of Chenjiagou, later moved to Taiwan. From among his list of students, he selected a few to become his adopted "sons" to carry on his inherited taijiquan tradition. More details regarding Du's life can be found in a booklet written by his "number one adopted son," Wang Jiaxiang, dedicated to Master Du for his 82nd birthday.

Next in the family lineage was Chen Fake (1887–1957), the son of Chen Yanxi. Chen Fake, the 17th generation grandmaster, went to Beijing in 1920 on personal business. There he became the first master of the Chen system to teach publicly. It was noticed, however, that he had changed the content and way of practicing the routines. It is most probable that his instruction to university classes differed from what he presented in private.

In Beijing, Chen Fake was often confronted with challenges from noted masters of various styles. Although he himself was a gentleman of great self-control, in instances of persistent antagonism, the fierceness of his system would prove overwhelming once unleashed. Defeated masters, such as Xu Yusheng, would acknowledge Chen Fake's superiority and sometimes humble themselves enough to become his students. Chen could defend himself with ease but refrained from hurting his opponents.

Chen Fake's public teachings have continued in their changed form under such teachers as Tian Xiuchen and Kan Guixiang in Beijing. The laojia system has been retained hereditarily. Chen Zhaoquai inherited the system, becoming the 18th generation grandmaster. He was Chen Fake's second son who carried on the tradition until his death in May, 1981.

The current grandmaster and, therefore, the 19th in order is Chen Xiaowang. As the grandson of Chen Fake, he is the living embodiment of the Laojia system. He recently developed a simplified Chen exercise comprised of 38 forms which is gaining popularity in the People's Republic of China. The present Chen Style influence has also reached the United States. A student under Chen Zhaoquai, Gene (Ching Hong) Chen, presently teaches in San Francisco. Gene Chen is the Chairman of the Chen Taijiquan Association of America.

From the taijiquan mainstream, representing the Chen lineage beginning with Chen Wangting, a clear picture can be drawn which illustrates where other styles emerged. In addition to the Laojia Chen system, the *xinjia*, or "new frame" system is among the earliest variants.

The Xinjia, Wu, Hao, and Sun Styles

Chen Yuben and Chen Yuheng were twins who inherited taiji from the founder Chen Wangting. Chen Yuben is credited with changing the laojia forms to make a "new family" system, or *xinjia*, composed of 83 forms. Yuben passed this new style on to his son, Chen Zhungshen (1809–1871). A long list of students followed this teaching, most bearing the Chen family name. This style, although differing from the laojia, made the Chen Style more available to the public. Chen Ziming and Chen Chunyuan were the leading figures of the xinjia until the middle of this century.

Another student of Chen Yuben was Chen Qingping (1795–1868), who created a style characterized by small movements largely derived from xinjia. It is referred to as *xiao* (small) *jia*, or *Zaobaojia*, Zaobao being the village where Chen Qingping lived. Because a great portion of his students did not bear the Chen surname, we find later styles of taijiquan classified under other surnames.

Immediately after Chen Qingping comes a series of newly formed schools. The founders of these schools modified the taijiquan as taught by their teachers, re-naming their new methods according to their own surnames. The list of innovators includes Wu Yuxiang, Hao Weizheng and Sun Lutang.

Wu Yuxiang (1812–1880) was from a village in the southern part of Hebei Province, Hantan Prefecture. The founder of the Yang Style, Yang Luchan, was also from this village. A wealthy store owner, Wu Yuxiang had employed Yang as an assistant. He also hired Chen Changxing to teach his sons the Chen Style. Wu was fortunate to have studied the laojia style from Chen Changxing and the xinjia by Chen Qingping before his own Wu Style took shape.

The brother of Wu Yuxiang was Wu Chengching, a magistrate in central Henan Province, who reportedly found a rare treatise on taijiquan in a salt store and purchased it for his brother. The author was believed to be Wang Zongyue, the martial art practitioner said to have visited Chenjiagou in the mid-18th century. Wu Yuxiang himself wrote at least five articles regarding the practice of taijiquan.

Some of the Chen Style can be seen within the Wu system, incorporating energetic movements such as a forward jump kick executed while slapping one's toes. Wu taught Li Yiyu (1883–1932), who was his sister's son. Another student of his was Hao Weizheng (1849–1920). Actually, derived from the Wu school, the Hao Style takes its name from Hao Weizheng who popularized this particular branch of taijiquan. Hao Yuehju, Hao Weizheng's son, carried on this tradition but deleted some of the more strenuous movements derived from the Chen Style.

Born in Baoding, Hebei Province, Sun Lutang (1861–1932) was a student of Hao Weizheng. Sun's style required much flexibility and was fairly fast paced, reminiscent of the Chen system. For some time, Sun lived in Beijing. Approaching 70 years of age, he was made Chairman of the Jiangsu Province Boxing Association. The Sun Style is also known as the *huobujia*, or the "lively pace" style.

Thus, the major schools of taijiquan classified under the surnames Wu, Hao and Sun were all derived from the xinjia Chen system as founded by Chen Yuben. In addition to this branch, two other styles have been recognized as major schools: the Yang and a Wu Style which is not affiliated with the school of Wu Yuxiang. Within the overall evolutionary development of taijiquan, these schools emerge under special conditions which fostered their unique characteristics and popularity among the masses.

The Yang School Lineage and Branches

Why is the Yang Style the most popular of taijiquan styles? Because of its superior fighting techniques? Greater health benefits?... Many such questions are answered with the understanding of who the style's founder was, how he gained his knowledge, and how he passed on this knowledge.

Yang Luchan (1799–1872), also known as Yang Fukui, was a native of Hebei Province, Hantan Prefecture, Yunglienxien administrative unit. Here, the founder of the Wu Style, herbalist Wu Yuxiang, also lived. As mentioned previously, Yang worked for Wu, and it was through this connection that Yang had the opportunity to learn the Chen Style. Yang's relative, Li Pokui, also was employed here.

Yang began to learn taijiquan by practicing the movements he secretly observed while Chen Changxing taught Wu's sons. The discovery of Yang's ability to learn taijiquan so well by simply watching the lessons encouraged Chen to accept him as a student. Yang was a natural. Under the tutelage of Master Chen, Yang became a master in his own right. It is believed that Yang spent a total of 18 years at Chenjiagou. In later years, Yang went to the capital city of Beijing where he soon earned the nickname "Unbeatable Yang." This was due to Yang's defeating numerous famed boxers. Some stories say that after 18 masters had challenged him, Yang remained "untouchable."

When he went to Beijing, Yang gave public instruction in the art of taijiquan. But it must be remembered the style he taught was not the same as those systems he himself learned. Beijing was the capital of China, which during the Qing dynasty was ruled by the Manchus, not the Chinese themselves! The Manchurian Royalty, upon hearing of the famed boxer, asked for instruction. Yang taught Manchus and others, although he did not include the fast, powerful movements associated with his studies of the old Chen system. He concentrated only on the yin movements, which were slow and soft. In so doing, he created a new style which helped taijiquan become known for its therapeutic benefits.

Although what Yang taught publicly was largely health oriented, his private teachings must have included his philosophy and techniques for self-defense. After all, he did teach the emperor's guards! It would be hard to imagine such warriors wasting their time on a martial art without effective fighting techniques.

Proof that Yang Luchan had passed on a formidable fighting art is exemplified in the lives of his sons, Yang Jianhou (c.1839–1917) and Yang Banhou (c.1837–1892). When Jianhou was 80 years old, he was attacked from all sides by nine men. All nine were ineffective against Jianhou's defense. Each attacker was knocked away by a smooth series of blows and ward offs.

When Yang Banhou's reputation also began to spread, he was challenged by a well-known boxer named Liu. Hundreds, perhaps thousands, came to view the event. During their encounter, Liu grabbed Banhao's arm, but his grip was easily countered, resulting in Liu's defeat. Yang Luchan complimented his son's success in combat but explained that he had not yet reached the true artistic pinnacle of taijiquan. After all, Banhao's shirt sleeve was slightly torn in the contest.

Before Yang Luchan's sons became so formidable, they were forced into practice day and night under an almost reclusive spirit. Failures in learning their boxing lessons resulted in brow beatings at their father's hands. The psychological pressure was overwhelming for the sons. Banhao once tried to scale the family courtyard wall to freedom but failed. His brother, Jianhou, was unsuccessful in a suicide attempt.

Compulsory studies alone did not make the Yang brothers superior boxers. Upon the death of their father, many friends, family members, and students gathered at Yang Luchan's graveside. A senior student with extraordinary boxing skills proclaimed himself the only worthy heir of the Yang Style Taijiquan. Chen Xiufeng had reason to claim this honor. First, he was no doubt better skilled than either of the Yang brothers. He was noted for possessing great internal energies for defeating any opponent, even without making physical contact. An example of this power is illustrated by his lifting a heavy wooden chair with the "sticking energy" of his palm. This formidable reputation served to intimidate the Yang brothers.

Yang Banhou and Yang Jianhou were inspired to study in earnest, with the help of their father's secret manuals. Afterwards, Jianhou was said to have attained the ability to levitate. So sensitive became his control over inner energy that a swallow could not take flight from his open palm. Such feats were not performed for amusement only. These abilities illustrate requirements for executing boxing techniques at the ultimate level of proficiency. Thus, both had finally reached a proficiency in the martial arts that their father had originally wished.

Chen Xiufeng later conceded the title back to the Yang brothers. He himself continued teaching in the Yencheng district of Henan Province. Mild-mannered Yang Jianhou attracted many students. His irritable brother, Banhou, chose only a small number of disciples. Because of this, his teachings eventually became extinct.

There are some interesting aspects of Yang Banhou's following. Being taught by his father and a little by Wu Yuxiang, the found of the Wu Style, Banhou passed on his acquired knowledge to a select few. One of his students was a farmer named Chang Qingling. Another Banhou student was a Manchurian whose Chinese name was Wu Quanyou (1834–1902). He was a dedicated student. After mastering the teachings of Banhou, Quanyou carefully imparted what he had learned to his son Wu Jianquan (1870–1942).

Wu Jianquan perfected the teachings of his father. His way of practicing taijiquan became known as the Wu Style. Sometimes his style and that of Wu Yuxiang's are differentiated by rendering their names into "Wu" and "Woo." In Chinese, both characters are written differently. For anyone who can read the Chinese, the names are easily distinguished. Wu Jianquan took his method to Shanghai. Later this Wu Style also became popular in Hong Kong and Singapore.

A student of Wu Jianquan became very well known, not particlarly for his martial art skills, but for his political standing. His name was Chu Minyi. Chu was the brother-in-law of Wang Qingwei, once President of China's Nationalist Government. Chu himself was ambassador to Japan after 1937.

Wu Jianquan's son-in-law, Ma Yuehliang, is likewise a teacher of the Wu Style. In Shanghai, Master Ma taught Sophia Delza, who taught in New York city at her own studio as well as at the United Nations. She wrote one of the first books in English dealing with taijiquan.

The above lineage stemming from Yang Banhou is only one branch of Yang Luchan's original style. The founder had other disciples. His student, Wu Hoqing, is said to have written a book of taijiquan but ascribed it to the earlier figure Wang Zongyue. Forging Wang's name on the taijiquan treatise helped make the book more popular.

Another student of Yang Luchan was Wang Lanting. Although Wang died at an early age, he possessed such great skills that he was a source of pride for his teacher. A student of Wang Lanting, Li Pinfu, illustrates the effectiveness of Wang's teachings. Li was once challenged by a qigong specialist. As his antagonist spoke, Li remained calm, petting a pet dog that he was holding in his arms. The impatient challenger darted forward only to be easily rebuffed by Li, who tenderly held onto his pet during the short scuffle.

The most influential line to descend from Yang Luchan was to pass on to his younger son, Yang Jianhou (1839–1917). Of pleasing disposition, Jienhou attracted many students. He was very proficient with weapons as well as the open-hand techniques. Two of his sons studied with him: Yang Shaohou (1862–1929) and Yang Chengfu (1883–1936).

Shaohou, the eldest son, began his study of taijiquan at the early age of seven. He learned much from his uncle Yang Banhou. In later years Shaohou became a superb boxer, but because of his rough manner most disciples studied with him for only a short time. According to rumor, he killed some of his opponents in boxing matches. The most important aspects of his art, characterized by small, compact movements, were imparted to very few. As a result, Yang Shaohou's style of taijiquan is very rare. He committed suicide in Nanjing in 1929, leaving only one son, Yang Chensheng.

Yang Jianhou had a second son, Chaohou, who died young and, therefore, did not perpetuate the Yang Style. The third son on the other hand, Yang Chengfu, had great influence. He systematized the style into the form so familiar today: natural postures utilizing steady, slow, expansive movements, executed with tensionless ease. Yang was never defeated even though most of his skill was self-taught. Beginning studies at age twenty, he was not very interested in taijiquan while his father lived. A genius in his own right, we can only imagine what accomplishments Yang Chengfu would have made if he had studied more diligently with his father.

The Yang Style was spread by Yang Chengfu from Beijing where he taught, to other areas of China, including Nanjing, Shanghai, Guangzhou and Hong Kong. Of Yang's four sons, it is Yang Zhenduo (born 1926, in Yongnian County, Hebei) who inherited the family system. Zhenduo has been very active in furthering interest in the art in China. He has also traveled overseas to share his special insights and knowledge. However, it is due to Yang Chengfu's senior disciples that the art was dispersed throughout the world. Part of his work includes a treatise on taijiquan called *Yang's Ten Important Points*.

Among the many students of Yang Chengfu are such well-known masters as Dong Yingjie (1888–1960) and Zheng Manqing (1900–1975). The first mentioned studied under Yang for close to twenty years, beginning at age seventeen. Dong taught in Hong Kong and his son, Dong Huling, taught in Hawaii.

It was in 1941 that taijiquan was first formally introduced in the United States under the instruction of Choy Hokpeng (1886–1957). Choy was also a student of Yang Chengfu. He started an institute in San Francisco which eventually had branches in Los Angeles and New York. His son, Choy Kamman, remains teaching in San Francisco. Another Yang Chengfu student also had great impact in the United States: Mr. Zheng Manqing.

CHART I: Old Chen Style Lineage

Others? ⋯ Qi Jiguang (1528-1587) Designed a routine consisting of 32 movements synthesized from 16 boxing styles.

Chen Wangting (1597-1644) Founder. c. 9th generation of Chen Pu clan. Designed seven different routines from 29 of the 32-movement routine learned from General Qi. One remains as the standard "Old Family Set" comprised of 74 forms.

- Chen Yuben (see Chart II)
- Chen Yuheng (see Chart II)
- Chen Bingqi
- Chen Pinjen

Chen Pingwang

Wang Zongyue (1736-1795) From Shanxi Province. Visited the Chen Village.

Chen Changxing 14th generation (1771-1853) Nicknamed "Mr. Name Board." First routine is the oldest form known; basis of later developments.

- Chen Hochai → Chen Hsi
- Li Pokui — Chen Wutian
- Yang Luchan (see Charts III and IV) — Chen Wuchang

Chen Gengyun 15th generation (died age 79). Son of Chen Changxing.

Chen Yanxi 16th generation (died age 81). Son of Chen Gengyun.

- Du Yuze 17th generation. (see Chart II) → Wang Jiaxiang, Tu Zongren, Li Haochen, Tsao Delin

Chen Fake 17th generation (1887-1957). Great grandson of Chen Changxing. Went to Beijiing in 1928. First to teach publicly.

- Chen Zhaopi Chen Fake's nephew.
- Gu Liuxin (1909-1990)
- Tien Xiuchen (died 1984).
- Chen Zhaoxu eldest son of Chen Fake. → Chen Xiaoxing younger brother of Chen Xiaowang.
- Feng Zhiqiang (b. 1926).
- Li Jianhua
- Pan Wingchou
- Many other students.

Chen Zhoquai 18th generation. Second son of Chen Fake.

- Feng Dabiao
- Zhang Chundong
- Chen Chinghong
- Ma Hong

Chen Xiaowang 18th generation (born 1946). Eldest son of Chen Zhaoxu. Main representative of the Chen Family Taijiquan. Developed a simplified 38-movement set.

CHART II: New Chen Style Lineage & Others

Chen Yuben & Chen Yuheng — Chen Fengchang
Created the
"New Style."
　　　　　　　　　　　Chen Jishen ——— Chen Sen
　　　　　　　　　　　(1809-1865)
　　　　　　　　　　　Chen Sande ——— Chen Chungli
　　　　　　　　　　　Chen Baoshen
　　　　　　　　　　　Chen Tingdong　　Chen Miao
　　　　　　　　　　　Chen Zhongshen — Chen Tong
　　　　　　　　　　　(c. 1809-1871).　　Chen Fuyuan
　　　　　　　　　　　Son of Chen Yuben. Liu Changchuan
　　　　　　　　　　　　　　　　　　　Chen Xing ——— Chen Chunyuan
　　　　　　　　　　　　　　　　　　　(1849-1929)　　(?-1949)
　　　　　　　　　　　　　　　　　　　Grand-nephew　Chen Ziming
Chen Qingping (1795-1868) — Chang Ishan　　　of Chen Yuben. (?-1951)
Nephew of Chen Yuben.　Chang Kai　　　　Chen Kuei Chen —
Created Zhaobao Style.　Ho Chaoyuan　　Zhongshen's son.
　　　　　　　　　　　Li Jingyen　　　　Li Jingyen ——— Chen Mingbiao
　　　　　　　　　　　First studied under　　　　　　　(Chen Yenxi's
　　　　　　　　　　　Chen Zhongshe,　　　　　　　　nephew)
　　　　　　　　　　　then under Chen
　　　　　　　　　　　Qingping.
　　　　　　　　　　　　　　　　　　　　　　　　　Du Yuze
　　　　　　　　　　　　　　　　　　　　　　　　　(see Chart I)

　　　　　　　　　　　Other Styles:　ZHAOBAO
Wu Yuxiang　　　　　　　　　　　WU
(1812-1880) From Yongnian　　　　　　LI
County. Created Wu Style　　　　　　 HAO
from the Old Chen Style he　　　　　　&
learned from Yang Luchan　　　　　　SUN
(c. 1851) and the New Chen
Style he later learned from
Chen Qingping (c. 1852).

Li Yilu
(1832-1892) Nephew of Wu
Yuxiang. Created the Li Style.

Hao Weizheng ———————— Ma Tongwen
(1849-1920) Created　　　　Li Xiangyuan
the Hao style.　　　　　　 Hao Yueru (1877- — Hsu Chen
　　　　　　　　　　　　　 1935) Son of Hao　Hao Xiaoju
　　　　　　　　　　　　　 Weizheng. Deleted　Grandson of
　　　　　　　　　　　　　 energetic jumps　Hao Weizheng.
　　　　　　　　　　　　　 from the set.

Sun Lutang ——————— Sun Chienyun
(1861-1932). Blended Wu　Sun Cunshou
Style with xingyi and baqua　Cheng Huaixien — Chang Shihjung
styles to create the Sun Style.　From Hebei.　　(Tainan)

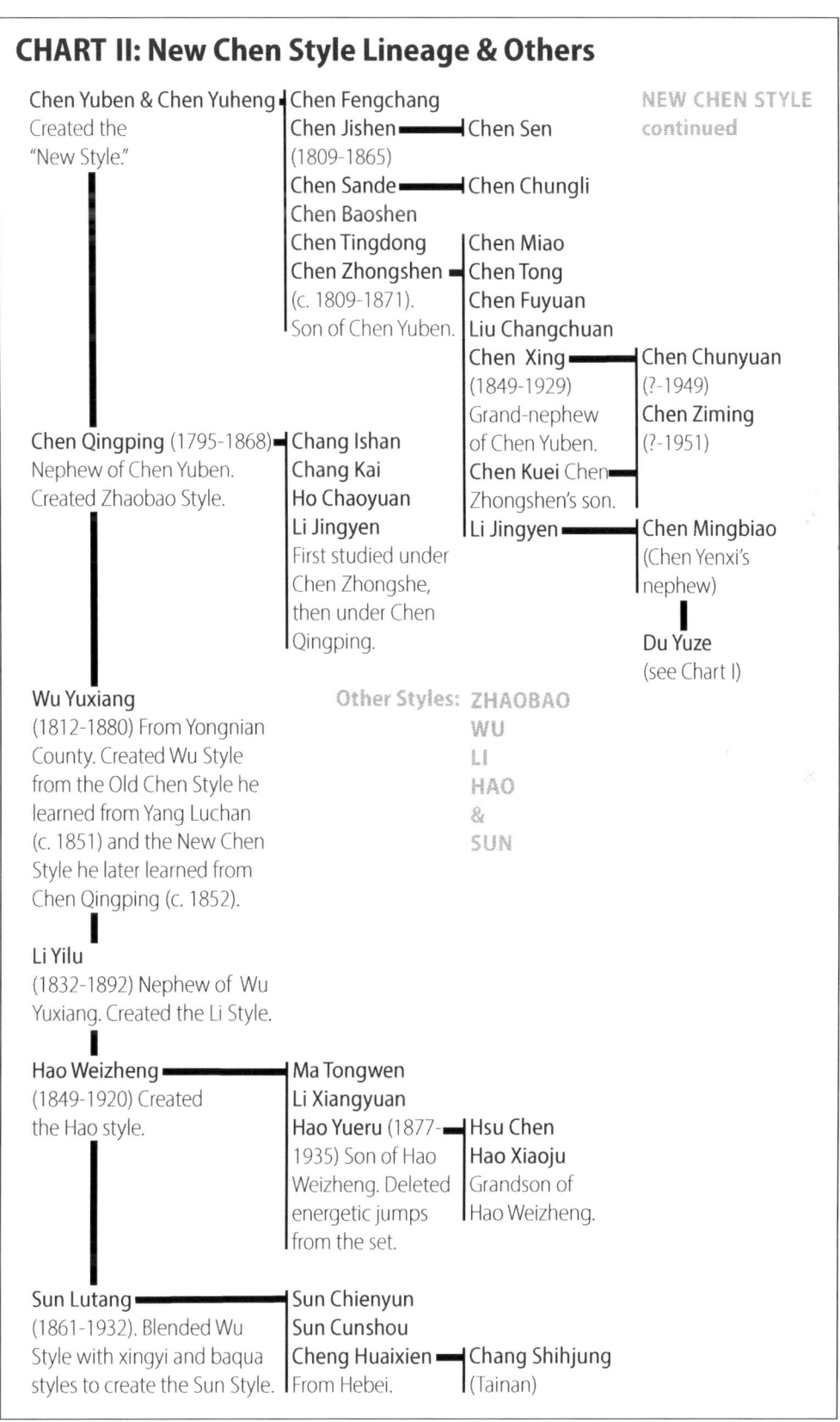

CHART III: Yang Style Lineage

Yang Luchan (1799-1872). Native of Yongnian County, Hebei; taught in Beijig. Nicknamed "Yang the Invincible." Modified the Old Chen Style to better suit goals of health. Founder of the Yang Style.

- Chen Hsiufeng
- Wu Hoqing
- Li Ruidong
- Wang Lanting — Li Pinfu
- Wan Chun (Manchu Nobles' Athletic Camp)
- Ling Shan (Manchu Nobles' Athletic Camp)
- Wu Yuxiang (1812-1880). (see Chart II)
- Quan You (see Chart IV)
- Yang Banhou (1837-1892). Second son of Yang Luchan. (see Chart IV)

Yang Jianhou (1839-1917). Third son of Yang Luchan. Further modified the form from his father into the "middle style".

- Chi De
- Xu Yusheng (1879-1945)
- Yang Chaoyuan
- Yang Shaohou (1862-1929) — Yang Chensheng; Tian Shaoxian
- First son of Yang Jienhou.

Yang Chengfu (1883-1936). Third son of Yang Jienhou. Great influence in spreading the art to many parts of China. Standardized the form of taijiquan with graceful, extended movements, known as the "Big Style." It became the most popular style.

- Dong Yingjie Studied under Yang Chengfu. — Jasmine Dong (Hong Kong). Daughter of Dong Yingjie. Dong Huling (Hawaii). Son of Dong Yingjie. Li Huangtse (Shanghai) Huang Wenshan (Los Angeles)
- Fu Zhongwen Nephew of Yang Chengfu.
- Yang Shouchung (Hong Kong). (b. 1909). Eldest son of Yang Chengfu.
- Yang Zhenji (Handan, Hebei). Second son of Yang Chengfu.
- Yang Zhenguo (Handan, Hebei). Fourth son of Yang Chengfu.
- Chen Weiming — Liang Chingyu (Hong Kong). Chief disciple of Chen Weiming.
- Li Yahsuan
- Wu Huichun (?-1937).
- Wan Lating (died young).
- Choy Hok-peng (1886-1957). — Choy Kamman
- Zheng Manqing (1900-1975). — Liang Tungtsai (born 1900). William C.C. Chen Chang Chihkang Shi Shufeng Huang Shenghsien (Singapore). Many other students.
- Many other students.

Yang Zhenduo (Taiyua, Hebei). Third son of Yang Chengfu, born in 1926. Most of training was under his brothers, Shaouchung and Zhenji.

- Yang Jun (Taiyua, Hebei). Grandson of Yang Zhenduo.

CHART IV: Yang and Wu Style Lineages

Yang Luchan ⎯⎯⎯⎯ **Yang Jianhou**
(1799-1872). Native of Yongnian County, Hebei; taught in Beijing. Nicknamed "Yang the Invincible." Modified the Old Chen Style to better suit goals of health. Founder of the Yang Style.

(1839-1917). Third son of Yang Luchan. Further modified the form from his father into the "Middle Style." (see Chart III)

Yang Banhou ⎯⎯⎯⎯ Chen Xiuieng
(1837-1892). Second son of Yang Luchan. (see Chart III).

Ling Shan (Beijing)
Wan Ch'un
Zhang Qingling ⎯⎯⎯⎯ **Wang Yennien** (Taipei)
Yang Zhaopeng
Wang Jiaoyu (Beijing) ⎯⎯⎯⎯ **Kuo Lienying** (1895-?) San Francisco.

Chiang Yunchung

Quan You ⎯⎯⎯⎯ Wang Maozhai ⎯⎯⎯⎯ Yang Yuting
(1834-1902) Manchu Nobles' Athletic Camp. Also studied under Yang Luchan.

Liu Fengshan

Wang Peisheng (Beijing)

Wu Jianquan ⎯⎯⎯⎯ Wu Cuchen
(1870-1942) Son of Quan You. Founder of the Wu Style that is second in popularity to the Yang Style. Often distinguished from Wu Yuxiang's Wu Style by the spelling Woo.

Wang Junsheng
Chu Mini Brother-in-law of Wang Qingwei, political leader.
Ma Yuehliang (Shanghai) ⎯⎯⎯⎯ **Ma Jiongpou**
Son-in-law of Wu Jianquan.

Son of Ma Yuehliang. (Shanghai)
Sophia Delza (New York)

Sun Rezhi
⋮

Early in his career, Zheng Manqing was a professor living in Beijing. He began the study of taijiquan under Yang Chengfu's guidance to better his health which had deteriorated from tuberculosis. The taijiquan practice had a miraculous effect on his condition. As a result, his dedication to the art became a total commitment. After attaining a high level of boxing skills, Zheng traveled about China accepting and defeating a long line of challengers. On one occasion, while traveling through Sichuan Province, his talents were tested by a Daoist boxer surnamed Zou. Zheng was quickly defeated. This incident inspired Zheng to accept tutelage from this learned master. Zheng then altered some of the Yang Style postures accordingly and his skill increased. As his techniques were perfected, his power became awesome.

Later, Zheng taught in Hunan, Taiwan and then in New York. Many of his students became noted masters of which the best known are living in Taiwan or in the United States. William C.C. Chen is one such student, now master, who originally came to New York with Zheng. Shi Shufeng, another senior student, chose to remain in Taiwan. At times, both Chen and Shi would illustrate their physical powers by letting students strike them anywhere on their bodies. Each time neither would suffer any ill effect.

Like many other sickly persons, Liang Dongcai (aka. T.T. Liang) sought Zheng Manqing's teachings with hopes that taijiquan would cure a physical ailment. In his case, it was a liver ailment. That was in 1950. Born in 1900, Liang continues to teach to this day.

Zheng Manqing had many other students that became well qualified instructors throughout the world. Zheng himself has stated that although the martial arts on mainland China have deteriorated to some degree during this century, there are still quite a few masters left to carry on their boxing traditions. Zheng believed that one of his own students, Zhang Zhigang, is among the most skilled of instructors on the mainland.

Today, taijiquan is truly international with representatives of various branches throughout the world. There remains a rich field of study for those interested in the extent of this influence. Hopefully future research will present in detail the state of this art as it exists in countries wherever it is represented.

References — Books

Chen, Y. (1947). *T'ai Chi Ch'uan – Its effects and practical applications*. Translated by Kuo-shui Chang. Shanghai: Kelly and Walsh, Ltd.

Chen, X. (1987). *Chen style 38 ways taijiquan*. [In Chinese] Hong Kong: Ke Science Popularization Publishing Co., Guangzhou Division.

Cheng, M. and R. W. Smith. (1973). *T'ai chi*. Rutland, VT: Charles E. Tuttle Co.

Delza, S. (1985). *Tai chi ch'uan: Body and mind in harmony*. Albany: State University of New York Press, revised edition.

Draeger, D. and R. Smith (1974). *Asian fighting arts*. New York: Berkeley Medallion Books.

Gu, L. (1986). *Pao chuei: Chen style taijiquan*, 2nd Routine. [In Chinese] Hong Kong: Hai Feng Publishing Co.

Gu, L., with Z. Feng, D. Feng and X. Chen (1984). *Chen style taijiquan*. Hong Kong: Hai Feng Publishing Co., with Beijing: Zhaohua Publishing House.

Horwitz, T., and S. Kimmelman with H. Lui (1976). *Tai chi ch'uan: The technique of power*. Chicago: Chicago Review Press.

Huang, W. (1979). *Fundamentals of tai chi ch'uan*. Hong Kong: South Sky Book Co.

Jou, T. (1981). *The tao of tai-chi chuan – Way to rejuvenation*. Warwick, NY: Tai Chi Foundation.

Liang, T. (1977). *T'ai chi ch'uan for health and self-defense – Philosophy and practice*. New York: Vintage Books.

Lo, B., M. Inn, R. Amacker and S. Foe (1979). *The essence of t'ai chi ch'uan – The literary tradition*. Richmond, CA: North Atlantic Books.

Luo, H. and D. Gu (1988). *Taijiquan: Principles and training*. [In Chinese] Guandong High Level Education Publication Co.

Shen Jiajen, editor et al. (n.d.). *Chen family taijiquan*. [In Chinese] Hong Kong: Hsin Wen Bookstore Publishing Co.

Smith, R. (1974). *Chinese boxing – Masters and methods*. Tokyo: Kodansha International, Ltd.

Soong, T. (1983). *Secret Chen family taijiquan introduction*. [In Chinese] I Chuen Bookstore, Taipei.

Su, K. (1974). *Subtleties of the Chen style old form of taijiquan*. [In Chinese] Taipei: Hua-lien Hua-lien Publishing Co.

Wile, D. (1983). *T'ai-chi touchstones – Yang family secret transmissions*. Brooklyn, NY: Sweet Ch'i Press.

Yang, J. (1986). *Advanced Yang style tai chi chuan, Vol. I*, Boston: Yang's Martial Arts Academy.

References — Articles

Bu, X., "Birthplace of taijiquan boxing," In Land Where Martial Arts Began (6), Beijing: *China Reconstructs* (1983), p. 26–30.

Chen, G. "Chen style tai chi: The 'real' tai chi chuan?" *Inside Kung-Fu*, Vol. 9, No. 11 (Nov 1982), p. 73–76.

Chen, G. with T. Chan and R. Judice. "Power without pride: The ethical grandmaster of Chen tai thi," *Inside Kung-Fu*, Vol. 2, No.7 (July 1984), p. 63–65.

Hefter, L. (June 1982). "Chen style tai chi chuan," *Inside Kung-Fu*, Vol. 9, No. 6, p. 36–41.

Kan, G. (June 1982). "A brief history of Chen style tai chi chuan," Anthony Chan and Diana Hong, translators. *Inside Kung-Fu*, Vol. 9, No. 6, p. 41.

Meehan, J. (August 1984). "The combat secrets of Chen tai chi," *Inside Kung-Fu*, Vol. 11, No. 8, p. 69–73.

Miller, R. (April 1982). "Chen style tai chi," *Black Belt*, Vol. 20, No. 4, p. 46–48.

Seidel, A. (1970). "A taoist immortal of the Ming dynasty: Chang San-feng," In *Self and Society in Ming Thought*, W. T. deBary, editor. New York: Columbia University Press, p. 483–531.

Stubenbaum, D. (May 1990). "Chen tai chi chuan: Innerer kreis der geheimnisse," [In German] *Karate Budo Journal*, No. 5, p. 54–56.

• 2 •

A Brief Description of Chen Style Master Du Yuze
by Wong Jiaxiang
Introduction and translation by Michael A DeMarco

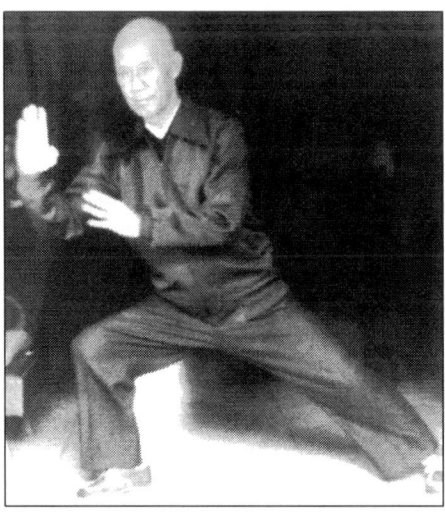

17th Generation Chen Style Master Du Yuze.
Photograph, provided by Tu Zongren, taken in
Du's Taipei living room during the mid-1970's.

Introduction

The following translation is an excerpt from Master Du Yuze's *Eighty-Second Birthday Commemorative Book*, originally written by Wang Jiaxiang. I have chosen to translate part of this booklet for a few reasons. One reason was to commemorate the 94th birthday Master Du had in 1989.

Regardless of age, Master Du was certainly a unique figure in the world of martial arts. Boxing instructors of various styles acknowledge Du Yuze's unique mastery of the Chen system, believing it to be a national treasure. Instructor Adam Hsu, now teaching in the San Francisco area, compared many Chen Styles while in China in 1986. Hsu, previously from Taiwan, wrote in a correspondence that "Du's Chen Style is indeed a national treasure. Even in Chen Village, the birthplace of taijiquan, you find almost no one teaching Chen Style like this."

Along with Du Yuze's unique place in the lineage of Chen Style masters, his personal history is likewise quite interesting. Master Du began his martial art training at an early age partly because of his father's high social standing as a government official. During the later years of the Qing dynasty (1644–1911), when the political and social conditions were not stable, such a position necessitated the need for bodyguards. The Du family lived under constant guard and visitors to their home were limited to close friends, those who had business with Du's father, or hired instructors.

Because of the above conditions, young Du Yuze was able to study with two great teachers: Masters Chen Yanxi and Chen Mingbiao. Under their guidance he learned both the old form (*laojia*) and new form (*xinjia*) sets of the Chen system. Oddly enough, because of the strict household formalities, Master Du never met Chen Fake, the son of Chen Yanxi. Incidently, Chen Fake created the new form, based on the two routines of *laojia* (the second known as cannon fist, or *paochui*).

A word regarding Wang Jiaxiang will help explain his interest and insights in writing the *Commemorative Book*. Mr. Wang, along with Mr. Tu Zongren, Mr. Li Houcheng and Mr. Cao Delin represent the four formal students who have performed the traditional ceremony of kowtowing to Master Du. As a result, they were accepted as "sons" within the Chen Taijiquan family and are numbered as "sons" in that order. This continues the lineage of Chen Yanxi, since Du Yuze was one of his accepted "sons." Mr. Wang Jiaxiang is now nearly seventy years old and continues to teach in the southern Taiwan city of Tainan.

The following translation of his "Brief Description of Master Du Yuze" I hope will provide interesting details in the tradition of a boxing master. Hopefully it will also indicate the deep feeling and dedication necessary to transform the movements into a perfected art form. Those who have been fortunate enough to fall under the tutelage and inspiration of respected Master Du have also accepted the responsibility to pass on the learning in like manner.

Except where noted, the accompanying photographs were taken at Master Du's home on June 8, 1989, while the "sons" of Mr. Tu Zongren were there to receive some additional instruction. Master Du, carefully watching every movement of the students, spoke in a strong clear voice (in Chinese, English or German!) to make critical remarks. When words were of no use, he stood to demonstrate. His gongfu was certainly impressive as was his kind personality which radiated the wisdom of his years. This combination of gentleman and master made Du Yuze an indubitably rare form of dragon.

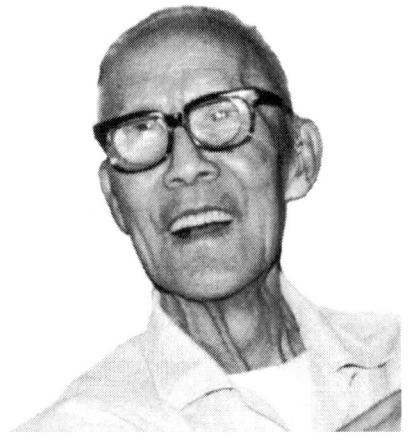

Du Yuze (age 94).
Photo taken June 8, 1989, at his home in Taipei.

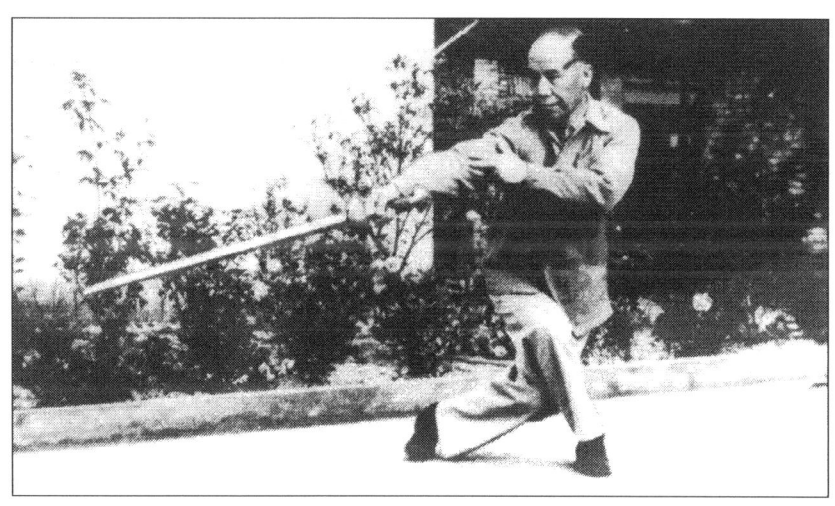

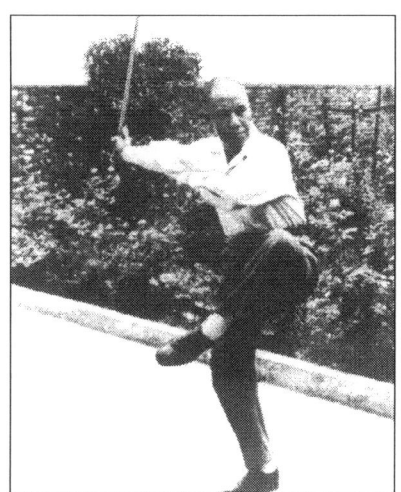
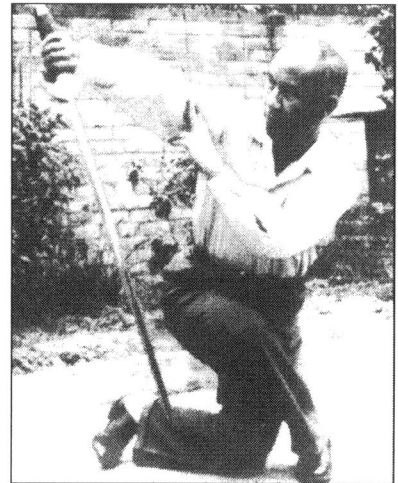

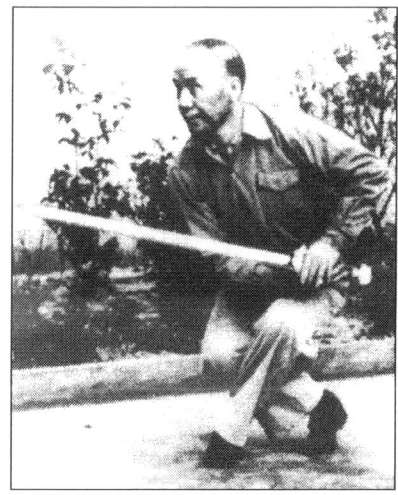
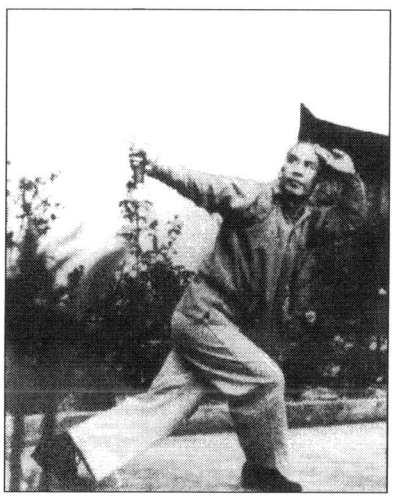

Sword practice. Photos, provided by Wong Jiaxiang,
show Du Yuze in the years prior to his move to Taiwan.

Translation*

Master Du Yuze, whose secondary given name is Du Qimin, was from Henan Province, Boai prefecture. He was born in the twenty-third year of the Qing dynasty's Emperor Guangxu; in other words, fifteen years before the 1911 founding of the Chinese Republic, between 5:00 and 7:00 p.m.

Now he is more than eighty-two years old and still practices taijiquan regularly. This practice includes golden buddha pounds pestle, 1,000 pounds fall, shake foundation and kick twice, concealed-hand strike, strike towards groin, stop opponent with one heel (left and right), swing foot to double target, steps, vertical movements, jumps, leaps... He practices every kind of movement, clearly and crisply, placing all in good order. The result is a boxing borne on the wind. At the same time, he has achieved great strength and the briskness of sound health. Because Master Du does not give up this practice, he has remained at his prime. Ah! If one can do all taiji's profound functions, it is possible to make great progress!

In the eighth year of the Chinese Republican period, when the country was finally stabilized (following great political unrest), Du Yuze attended college to study mechanical engineering. Following his studies, he performed engineering duties in the region of northern China. Afterwards, he came to Taiwan and was employed as an engineering specialist and worked secondarily as a factory manager. Passing through these years in this way was a rewarding experience.

Master Du was originally from Henan, Boai prefecture. Chenjiagou, located in Wen prefecture, is less than seventeen miles away. In the late Qing dynasty, these same areas formed part of what was then the district of Huaiqing prefecture. This rural area had a close-knit society where everybody knew everyone else who lived there.

When he was eighteen years old, Du Yuze kowtowed to Master Chen Yanxi as part of his formal acceptance as a student. Chen Yanxi was the famed sixteenth generation master of the Chen Style and grandson of Chen Changxing. Chen Yanxi taught Du Yuze the *laojia* (old form) Chen family system.

The father of Du Yuze was named Du Yomei. Thirty years before the Qing Emperor Guangxu (reign lasted from 1875 to 1908), Du Yomei had the rare fortune of passing the Jinshi Examination (national civil service examination held at the capital) and was awarded the eleventh degree, the second most outstanding rank that could be received from the Hanlin Academy (government examination office). Du Yomei went abroad to study in Japan during the early Republican years (1912–1949). While in government service, he also traveled to the provinces of Guandong and Guanxi.

Du Yomei asked Chen Yanxi's nephew, Chen Mingbiao, to be his bodyguard, plus his family's personal boxing teacher. He did so because Chen Mingbiao was an expert in archery, the spear and other aspects of the martial arts, including the *xinjia* (new frame) Chen family taiji and *paochui* (cannon fist). Consequently, Du Yuze was able to study the xinjia and paochui styles under his tutelage.

The movements of the Chen Village style of taijiquan are organized in a series, bound together as by a strong silk thread. To elaborate further, the movements are alternating manifestations of fast and slow, varying degrees of hard and soft as well as varying degrees of empty and substantial.

How to execute these principles in their highest degree is a precious secret not easily shown to others, particularly in an agricultural society whose people must work so much while they study. Therefore, the transmission of this knowledge has not been broad. In Taiwan, those who have received training in Chen Style taijiquan are as rare as the mythical phoenix or unicorn. In the past, anyone who could perform the Chen Style learned it, like Master Du, during the Qing dynasty. Because of Master Du's deep commitment to this boxing art, he feels a great obligation to preserve what he learned. He repeatedly made appeals to others in Taiwan to follow this path. Master Du, desiring not to neglect this duty to pass on his knowledge, teaches as much as possible by demonstration, so later generations can advance accordingly.

At present, taijiquan is flourishing as a fruit from its roots in Chenjiagou, the village in Wen prefecture of Henan province. And yet, just how to do the Chen Style taijiquan remains a secret. In addition, the excessive secrecy that surrounds it has placed the art on the verge of extinction. The sixteenth generation Master Chen Pinsan, by giving his total attention for thirteen years, collected, structured, organized and eventually published what he could find regarding taijiquan, including pictures, diagrams and stories.

In the preface at the beginning of this book is a remark that Master Du shares with the respected taijiquan elders: "Indications show that efforts are being made to examine and cultivate the principles of yin and yang in equal fashion." This is being done to incorporate the theory of the epigram into the performance of taijiquan and thus bring the art to its full realization. But to research, study and acquire this special skill requires guidance.

Together with our upcoming generations, we all must share the responsibility of seeing that Chen taijiquan can continue to flourish forever without interruption.

Taiwan, Sixty-Third Year of the Republic of China (1974).
Chrysanthemum Month (ninth lunar month).

Respectfully your student,

Wang Jiaxiang

---

* For clarification, the translator has placed additional information within parentheses. Any imperfections in this translation are solely due to the limited linguistic skills of the translator.

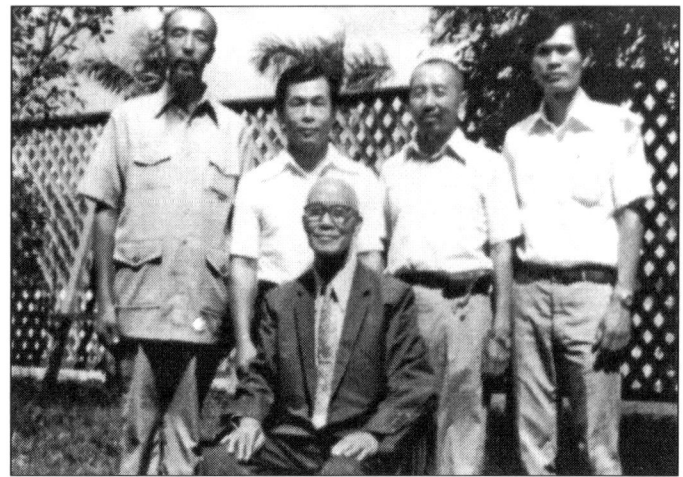 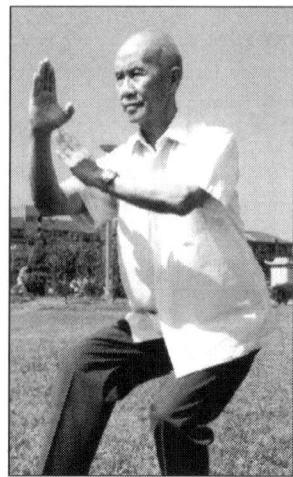

Left: Master Du's adopted sons (*tudi*), standing behind him for a photograph taken on his 80th birthday. Although he instructed other students, only these four were selected to be "sons," thus inheriting the most significant details of his teachings. Standing, left to right: Wang Jiaxiang 王嘉祥, Li Houcheng 李後成, Cao Delin 曹德鄰, Tu Zongren 涂宗仁. Photo provided by Tu Zongren.
Right: On the grounds of Sun Yatsen Memorial Hall, near his home, Du Yuze posed for photos. He was nearly 80 years old at the time. Photo provided by Chong Jiensiong.

Below: Du Yuze demonstrating applications. Master Du removes his shirt to more freely demonstrate movements. Here he shows some defensive blocks, grabs and counter strikes while stressing the application of each according to the yin/yang principles of taiji. Even at 94 years of age, Master Du did not hesitate to stand in to perform movements when talk alone was insufficient. Many of the profound aspects of taijiquan are beyond words. Photos by M. DeMarco.

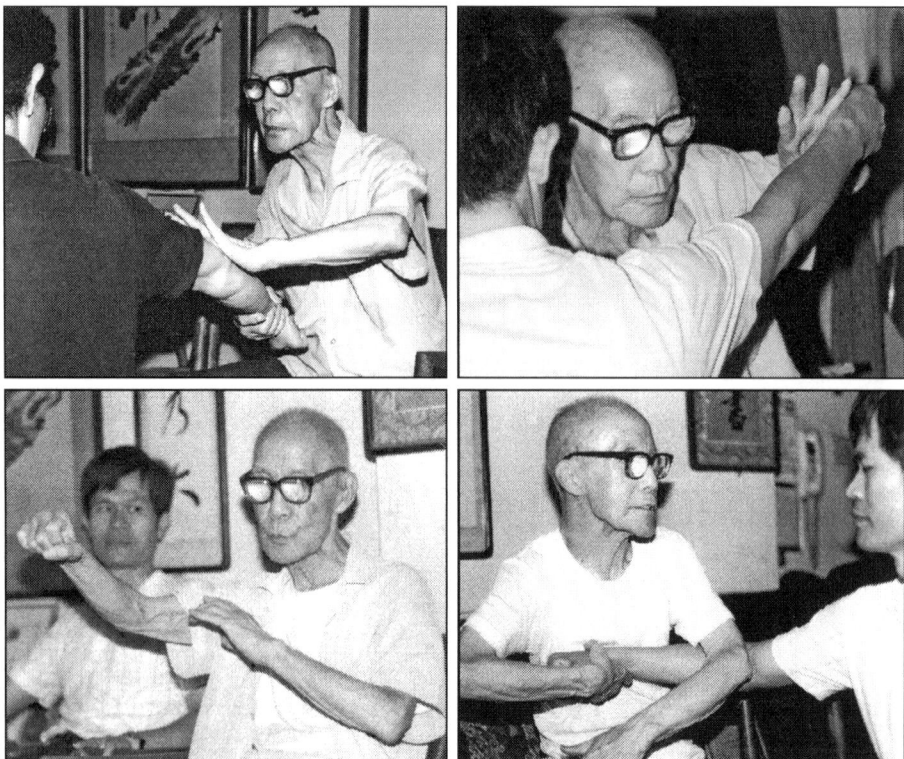

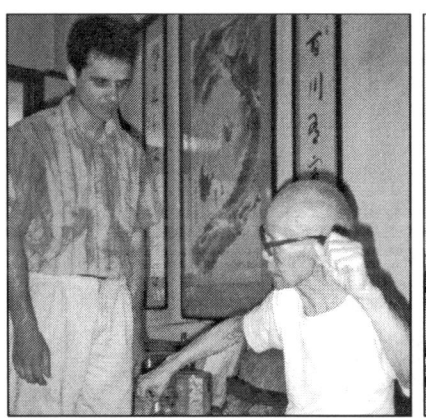 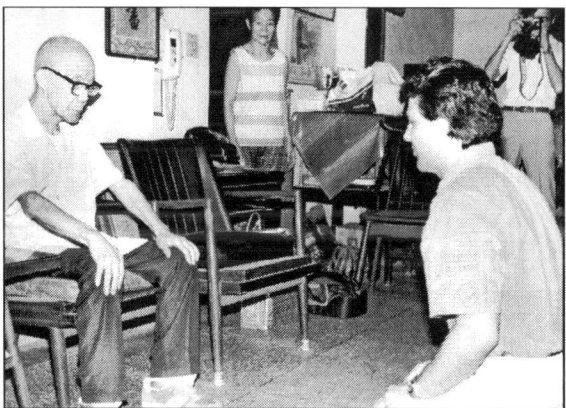

Above, left: Dietmar Stubenbaum receives precious advice from Master Du. After students performed techniques, Du would analyze each movement, usually mixing Daoist theory with varied martial applications. He lamented that many martial arts are losing aspects of their rich heritage. According to him, it was after the introduction of firearms that teachings became more limited in scope. Right: Some photos accompanying this text were taken the day Dietmar Stubenbaum, Michael DeMarco, and Huang Shichuan partook in the ritual for discipleship. Here DeMarco kowtows three times in front of Master Du as part of the ritual. Photos by M. DeMarco.

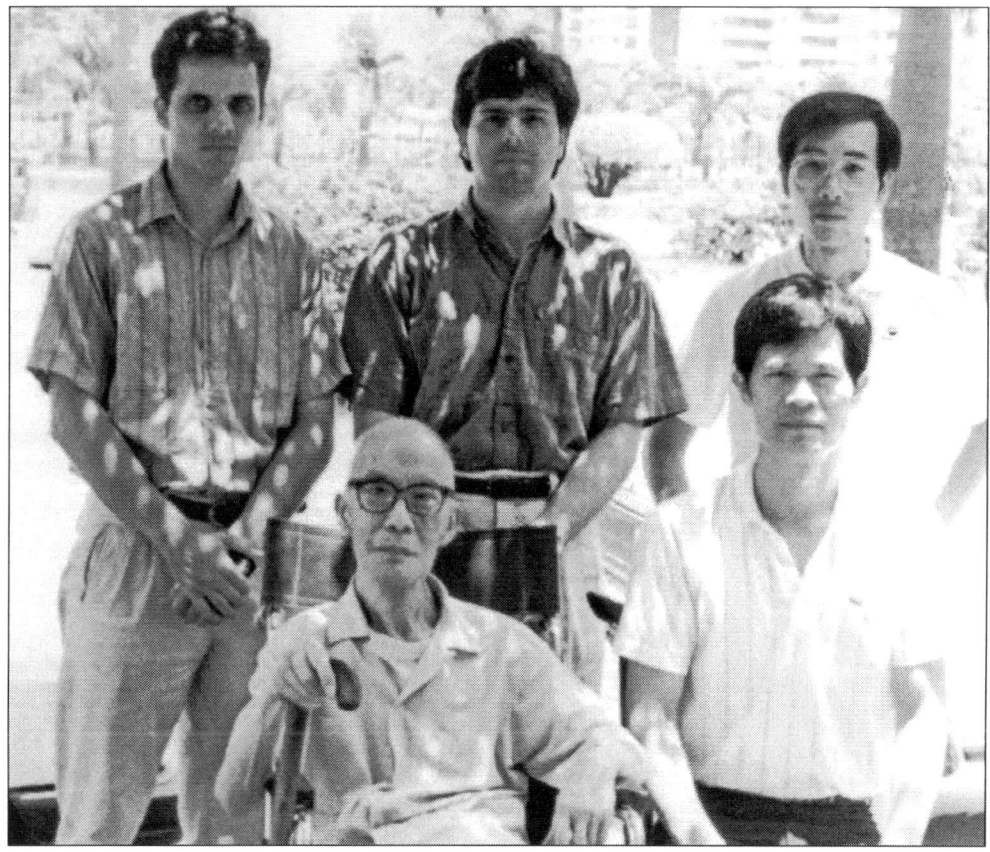

Du's taiji family extends: At center is Master Du with Tu Zongren to his left.
Back row, left to right: Dietmar Stubenbaum, Michael DeMarco, and Huang Shichuan.

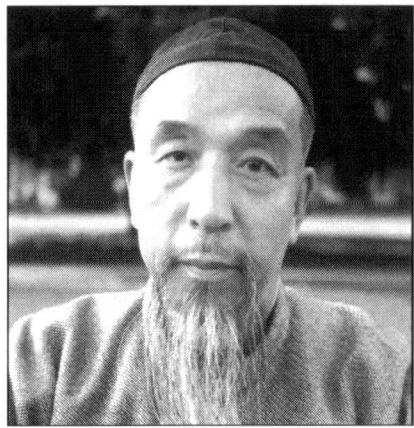 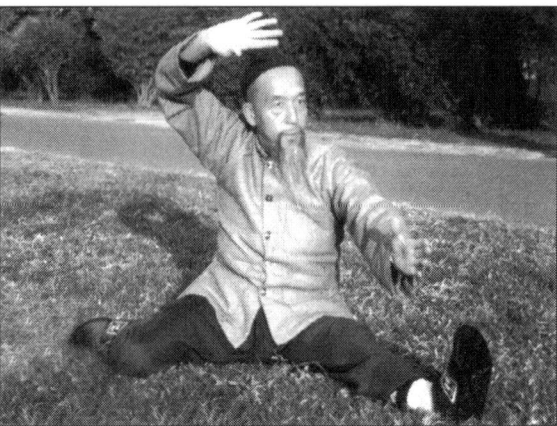

Master Wang Jiaxiang 王嘉祥
Above left: Now a major representative of the eighteenth generation Chen taijiquan masters, Wang is one of the most knowledgeable practitioners of the style living today. Originally from the far northeastern province of Heilungjiang, he now resides in Tainan city, Taiwan. Above right: Mr. Wong practicing a movement from the first routine in which the performer "drops and branches," springing back up immediately into the next movement. Photos provided by Wong Jiaxiang.

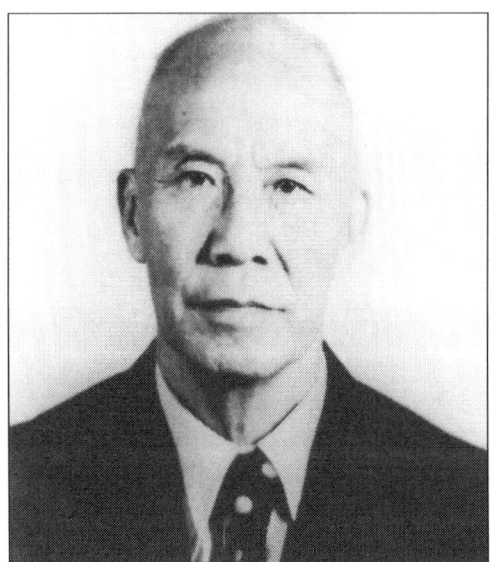 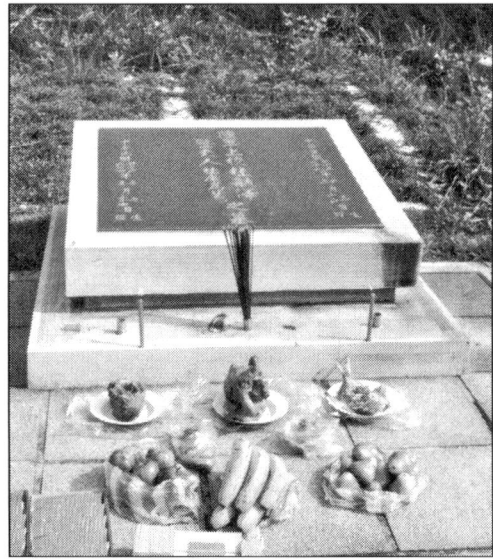

Passing of Grandmaster Du.
On March 16, 1990, Du Yuze peacefully passed away
in Taipei Veteran's Hospital at 10:30 a.m.

ABRIDGED LINEAGE CHART

Chen Yanxi (陳延熙) **& Chen Mingbiao** (陳名標)

Du Yuze (杜毓澤)
17th generation (1886–1990).
From Baoi, Henan; approximately 17 miles from Chen Village.

18th generation disciples according to seniority from left to right:

Wang Jiaxiang	**Tu Zongren**	**Li Houcheng**	**Cao Delin**
b. 1925	b. 1944	b. 1936 – d. 1984	b. 1925
lives in Tainan.	lives in Taipei.	lived in Taipei.	Lives in Chiyi.

19th generation disciples according to seniority from top to bottom:

Lee Chengchong b. 1946 Lives in Chongli.	Michael A. DeMarco b. 1953 Lives in Erie, PA., USA.	Li Yincun b. 1972 in Taipei. Li Houcheng's son.	Suan Shufeng b. 1953 Female disciple Lives in Chiyi.
Tsai Yingchien b. 1947 Lives in Kaohsiung.	Huang Shirchuan b. 1952 Lives in Taipei.		
Ho Hongtsai b. 1952 Lives in Pingtong.	Dietmar Stubenbaum b. 1962 Lives in Friedrichshafen, Germany.		
Lin Chongpor b. 1954 Lives in Taipei.	Lin Shirchien b. 1951 Lives in Taipei.		
Chang Chourjinn b. 1954 Lives in Chiayi.	You Jindi b. 1952 Lives in Taipei.		
Chong Khensiong b. 1956 Lives in Tainan.			
Chou Mingfa b. 1958; Lives in Tainan.			
Chiang Dingfung b. 1961. Lives in Tainan.			
Hwang Shiang b. 1963. Lives in Tainan.			

• 3 •

The Presence of the Eyes in the Action of Taijiquan
by Sophia Delza

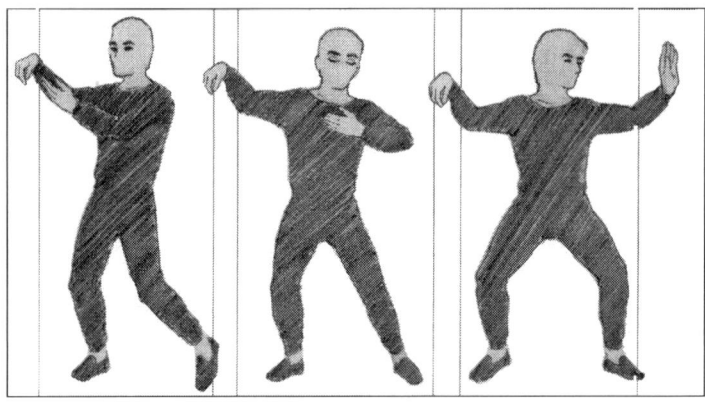

Photos by Lisa Leviki. Drawings by Ray Copper.

In taking the basic position at the start of taijiquan, the stance, torso, spine, shoulder, hand and head positions should be given particular attention. So should the eyes. That we lose track of them during the action, especially in the early learning process, is readily "forgivable." The subtlety of the eye-muscle movement and the necessity of the mind's presence behind the eye-action need not be emphasized until that time when the taijiquan player is prepared, physically and mentally, to experience many of the subtler aspects of the exercise: the smooth balance of the continuous motion, the physiological correctness of the forms, the space-tempo relationships, awareness of stillness in action, as well as the ability to function "intrinsically," i.e., without false effort. An unmistakable look will itself develop when one feels the harmony of what is being done. Eyes will be alert, calm, knowing and poised.

I have, in various essays, given thought to the various structural elements of taijiquan from the point of view of physiology and philosophy. I have closely examined the subtleties in taijiquan's weaving forms and patterns; I have pictured the ever moving yin-yang elements in "The Life of the Hand."¹ Now I venture to analyze more or less scientifically what happens in and to the eyes in a physical way during the active variations of movement.

Just as the physical body acquires a spirit in doing taijiquan, so the eyes (or the mind's eye) become and remain alert, peaceful and contained. The eyes can never be vacuous in taijiquan, nor will they portray anxiety or worry even while one is trying to remember and coordinate, though the eyes can, as we know, radiate any emotion: from hate to love plus all the emotions in between. The spirit of the movement in taijiquan seeps through the whole physical being. Therefore, the eyes—regardless of the physical changes occurring—will feel light, secure, and impersonal. All of this is brought about naturally, not solely by emotional means, but through one's complete physical being.

The regulation of eye movements is as clearly organized in the structure of taijiquan as is the play of every part of the body—large or small—contributing to physical and mental harmony.

The eyes seem to be so quietly set and unmoving during the activity that they are oftentimes outside of one's notice—both the performer's and the observer's. Should the eyes, however, shift randomly or dartingly, the overall impression would be one of nervousness, uncertainty or restlessness.

Eye movements are unnoticed not because there is so much to do and/or observe in the ever-changing patterns of the exercise, but because they are focusing quietly and being instinctively controlled by the smooth consistency required of all taijiquan movement changes.

The word "eyes," as used here, refers to all aspects of their physical composition—eyelids, eyeballs and the muscles (which control the eye's ability to focus far or near, upward, downward, sideways or obliquely)—as well as emotions which can affect their appearance.

In the action of taijiquan, all motion is intrinsically balanced, where form creates the continual variations of yin-yang dynamics, where extremes of tension are never required or permitted, and so it is with the use of the eyes, which respond intrinsically to the necessity of the movement at the moment. Superfluous effort of any kind is not needed to regulate or stimulate the eyes, nor is it ever part of the action of the eyes, such as lowering the eye to look straight down at the body nor raising the lids to see far upward at a 180-degree angle. Both movements are extreme.

Eye muscles are gently manipulated, always in basic slow tempo, adjusted to move or not to move with the body, responding to form, pattern, space and direction, unless otherwise directed by the requirement of the position of the body and head. (This is explained later.) As indicated, the eyes behave in an organically instinctive and intrinsic way, in accord with the nature of taijiquan, which is termed a "soft-intrinsic" system of activating the body for physical, emotional and mental well-being.

The eyes are the cottage of the spirit.
– Chinese proverb

It is more difficult to experience the "soft-intrinsic" variation in the play of than it is, obviously, to feel the dynamic changes in the constantly manipulated body forms. Just as physical action is not animated by an extrinsic force, so the eyes similarly maintain a calm, "impersonal" and therefore natural ease. When frowning, peering, straining, and otherwise expressing strong emotions do not disrupt intrinsic integrity and equilibrium, then the total being can achieve, through taijiquan's harmonious principles, health and superior awareness.

The Basic Eye Position

The way the head is always held (with a few exceptions) affects the basic eye position. The head must be held erect, upright, so that the crown of the head is directed upward vertically as if attached by a "silken cord to the heavens." The chin, therefore, is not pressed inward toward the neck, nor is it tilted upward. The shoulders are low and relaxed, and the neck light. The mouth remains closed with the tip of the tongue lightly resting against the upper palate. With this perfect carriage of the head, the eyes will experience subtle muscular activity but outwardly will appear unchanged.

The overall eye position from which the dynamic variations occur is determined by the way the lids are held or moved. The gaze, in the basic eye position, is lowered to a 45-degree angle. (When the eyes are wide open and look directly forward, the gaze is at a 90-degree angle.) The eyes, with the gaze at a 45-degree angle, can see out at a long diagonal, downward path and come to rest on the ground approximately ten or twelve feet from where one is poised. Eye muscles will feel light and untaxed. They are in a "neutral" position.

The eyes maintain a gaze of 45-degrees 90% of the time during the exercise. We know that without effort the ears hear. So too, the eyes can see without any effort.

FEATURES OF EYE-BEHAVIOR*

*All explanations and illustrations are based on the Wu system of taijiquan.

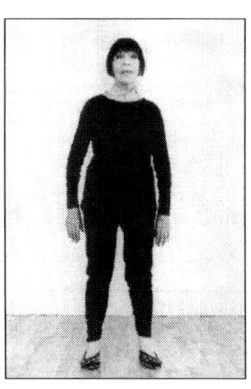 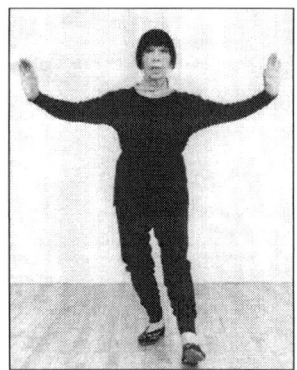

Left: The basic eye position as illustrated in the beginning form of taijiquan.

Right: Following the taiji beginning form, the body shifts its weight right and the knees bend. The eyes continue looking out on a long diagonal path with the gaze at a 45° angle.

I. The Quiet Unmoving Eyes: when eyelids, eyeballs and muscles are not activated and remain downward in the basic 45-degree gazing position.

a) In a position where the body does not move out of place during a series of arm/leg movements, the eyes will be "fixed," looking downward at a 45-degree angle, focusing on an unspecific area on the ground. This is "pure" stillness of the quiet eye.
b) When the knees bend and the figure remains in the same space, the eyes do not change, but simply see a different area, slightly nearer than when the legs are straight. This, too, is "pure" stillness of the eyes.
c) When the entire figure turns, let us say, to the right side, if the body level remains the same, the eyes will simply see another area, without any eye-muscle movement. The gaze is quietly set and remains lowered 45 degrees during the movement.
d) When the movement is such that the entire figure moves forward or backward, as in brush-knee-twist (walking-step form), the eyes do not stir. One sees different areas on the ground farther forward as one advances, farther backward as one retreats. The path of vision remains still.

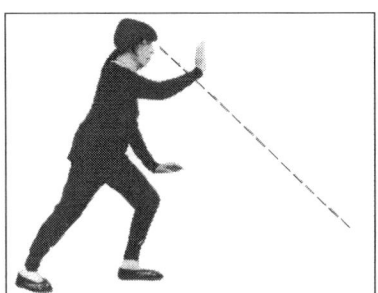

Brush knee, twist step form. The eyes see out on a long diagonal path and the gaze is at a 45⁰ angle. Note: Between the stages of stillness are moments of eye activity necessary when executing the different forms.

The above illustrations emphasize the fact that the eyes and the unchanging muscles have remained still, quiet, and light. Such conscious control helps to create calmness.

II. The Quiet Moving Eyes: muscles react with changes in body positions.
   a) In the hand strums the lute form, a hand moves into the basic line of vision, thus "forcing" an eye-muscle reaction. In the following illustration, the figure has taken a walking stance, with the right arm placed outward shoulder high. The eyes are free to gaze along the basic 45-degree path. The figure then sits back into an empty step form, at the same time bringing the right hand to center, in front of the nose and chin, blocking the line of vision. The eyes are then "forced" to see the tops of the fingers; this activates the eye-muscles. When the hand is removed, the eyes refocus. But "interference" in the line of vision automatically activates the muscles to become tense.

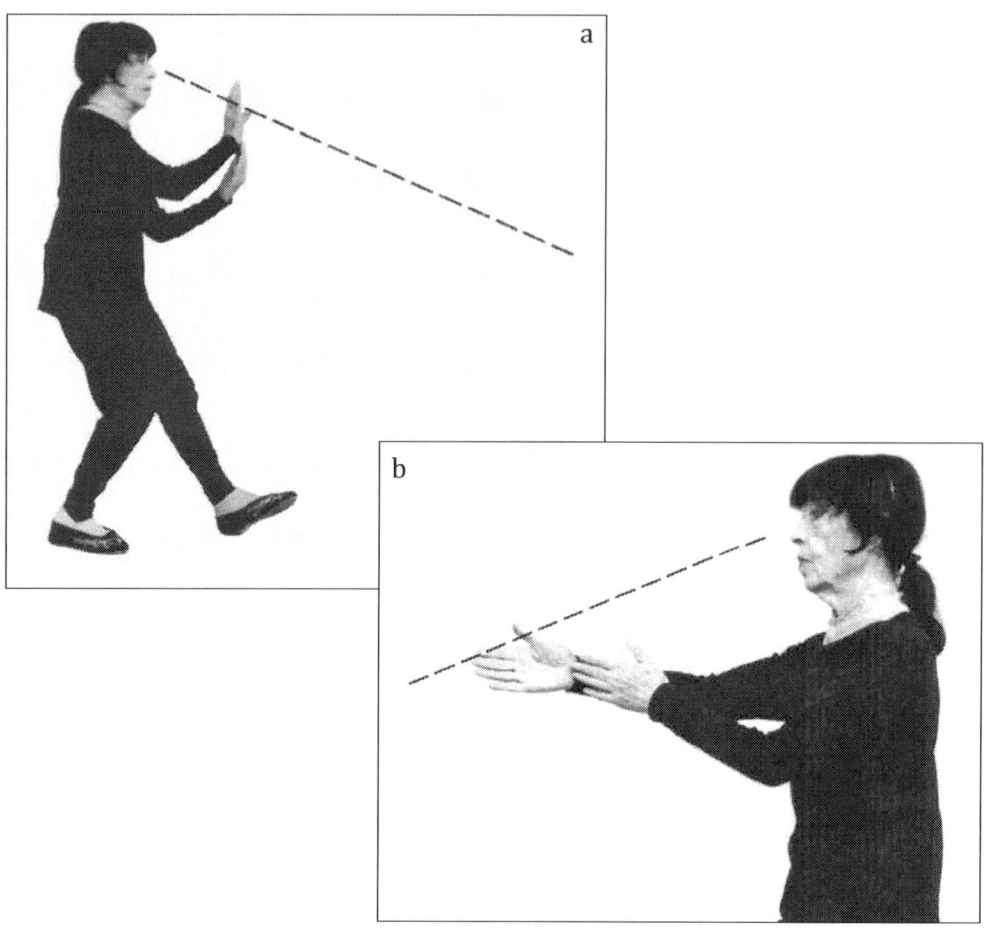

Left: *Hand strums the lute.* The eyes are in the basic 45^0 angle gaze as the right fingertips enter the field of vision causing the eyes to refocus.

Right: *Grasping the bird's tail.* The eyes see out on a long diagonal path. The view is interrupted by the placement of the hands as in hand strums the lute. Therefore, the eyes see the thumb of the right hand.

b) The eye action in the hands strum the lute form occurs frequently with variations, more or less tensed depending on the form. For example, in the Wu Style's third series, when a leg is outstretched and an arm is extended shoulder high with the head turned toward it, the eyes have a "longer look" and are focused on the thumb of that hand; thus, the tension in the eye muscles is lessened. The eye muscles are often stirred by a variety of movements. Eyes are less tense when looking at an object which is far away than when seeing one that is close. The eye muscles are never over-worked in taijiquan since no positions are repeated successively.

c) When the torso sinks or bends forward or sideways and the head and neck remain still, the eyes will, therefore, see the ground closer to the feet, thus activating the eye-muscles, as illustrated above in *a* and *b*. The gaze will remain at a 45-degree angle.

In all the above illustrations, the look has remained unaltered—quiet and calm; the feeling of stillness predominates. All the action, light or strong, is intrinsic, i.e., done according to the physiological laws of nature.

III. The Active (Willed) Eye Movements: the eyes are directed to bestir themselves in coordination with certain movements and forms.

a) For Wu Style cloud-arms form. At certain times the eyes move from a 45-degree gaze to an open-eyed 90-degree gaze in the following way. The eyes look to the right at the palm of the left hand which is placed near the outstretched right arm; the left hand is then moved toward the face, the palm as high as the eyes and about ten to twelve inches away. This eye-level position raises the gaze to a 90-degree angle. Throughout this form, the eye muscles are being activated both to "rest" by returning the eyes to the 45-degree gaze, and to be stirred to a 90-degree gaze and finally to allow the eyes to look far into the distance, thus resting the eyes fully. Such changes, by being consciously directed, extend the range of eye exercise movements.

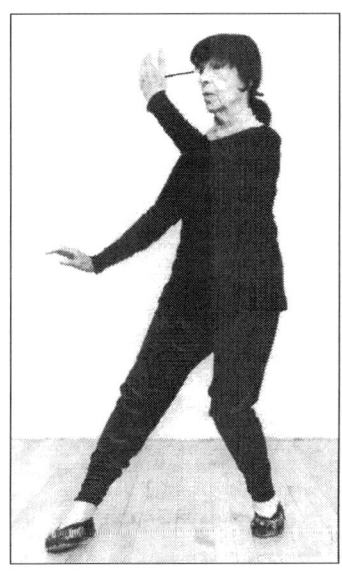

Cloud arms form. The eyes see the palm of the left hand, which is held about twelve inches away from the face. The eyes are opened wide in a 90° gaze.

b) In the flying oblique form, the body position is held unchanged as the right foot, right hand and head are moved. The head is tipped downward slightly toward the right side. The eyes look down obliquely at the upturned right palm which is in front of the right knee. Throughout this complex moving form, the head and eyes hold their position in respect to the right hand, while the torso is regulated to release pressure in the neck. The form ends with the eyes seeing the back of the right hand, the head still slightly tipped. The eyes and head then gently recover the normal position on the next transition movement. There are several transition movements in which the head is tipped to exercise the muscles in a different and more intense way.

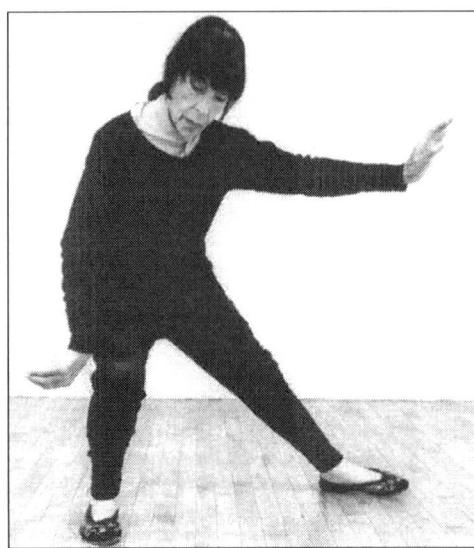 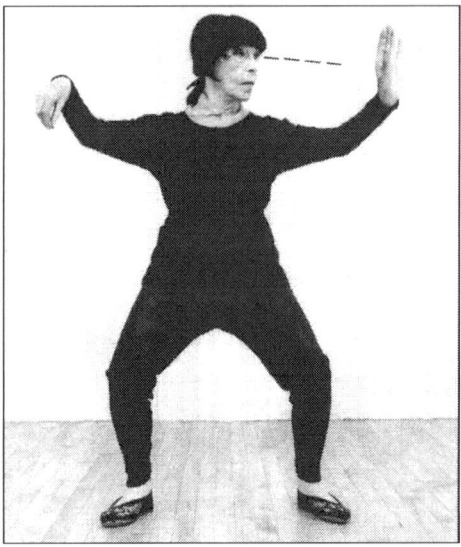

Left: *Transition to flying oblique form.* The head is slightly tucked. The eyes see the right wrist.

Right: *Single whip form.* Occurs nine times in the Wu Style. The eyes experience a variety of dynamic changes during this form.

c) The single whip form appears nine times in the Wu Style. The eyes experience a variety of dynamic changes which are specially designed for this form. The eyes follow the movement of the left hand, which goes at shoulder height from the right side to the left side. The eyes follow the path of the hand as it rises and falls. The eye muscles change in slow succession from a relaxed to a tensed state and back to a relaxed state. In passing from the right to the left side, the hand travels in a parabola. The eyes are then activated more tensely as the palm reaches the center of the curve at chest level because the gaze has moved in a downward and inward path. The gaze then moves upward toward the left, releasing eye pressure as the hand completes the movement at the left side, still at shoulder height. Here the eyes see the back of the hand. The eyes have been slowly activated by a relatively light tension and a strong one, and then "released" to become quietly and evenly relaxed at the end of the arm-hand-head movement. (The head is not tipped downward as it moves from the right side to the left while the eyes follow the hand.)

d) The oblique look: When the eyes are directed to look far right or left, the head must be slightly tipped downward to avoid extreme pressure on the muscles (as in the flying oblique form explained above). In a transition between the single whip and the enfolding form, the head is tipped to the left side and then moves to off-center right to look obliquely at the right upturned palm which is at far right.

This eye position appears only once, perhaps because it is most tense. The eyes recover their neutral position on the next movement and, relatively speaking, have a "rest" in the basic 45-degree gaze.

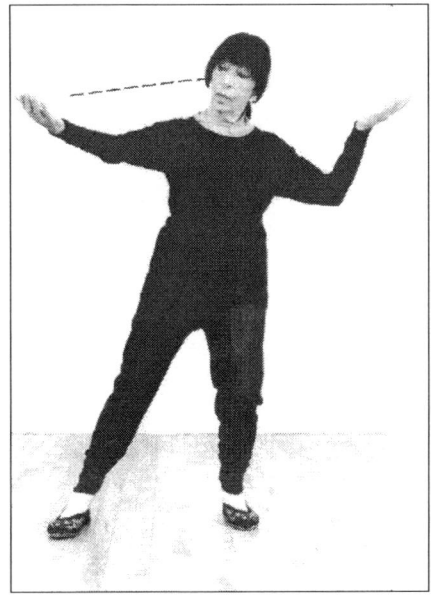

Transition from the
single whip form to the enfolding form.

•••

Suffice it to say that the subtle or obvious eye changes stimulate the agility and the power of the eyes, the movements of which are as necessary to nurture "health and awareness" as are all the other more easily discerned bodily maneuvers.

This analysis encompasses the range of the movements and "stillness" of the eye-action: seeing and looking and not commenting or mentally reacting to what is observed. The eyes function as naturally as does every other part of the body, according to the dictates of the mind and the demands of form, direction, space, time and the dynamic interplay of all these factors.

The eyes become (and remain) intelligent and tranquil and maintain the expressive spirit of the individual personality. They express the essence of taiji-quan: calmness, containment, and the comprehension of some possible potential development of consciousness. The Chinese say the eyes are the "cottage of the spirit," the glow of the spirit of equanimity. S. E. Cirlot, in the *Dictionary of Symbols*, says:

Light is symbolic of

intelligence and of the spirit.

. . . the process of seeing

represents a spiritual act and

symbolizes understanding.

Delza, S. (1992). The life of the hand: Its significance in t'ai-chi ch'uan. *Fighting Arts International*, (71): 31–33.

• 4 •
The Daoist Origins of the Chinese Martial Arts
by Charles Holcombe, Ph.D.

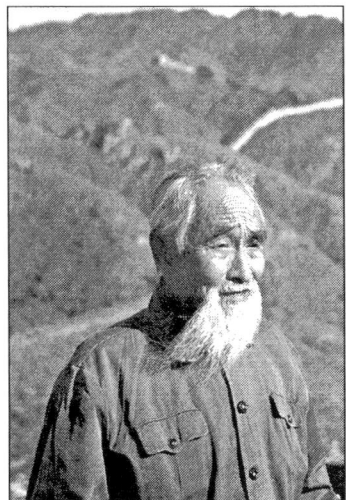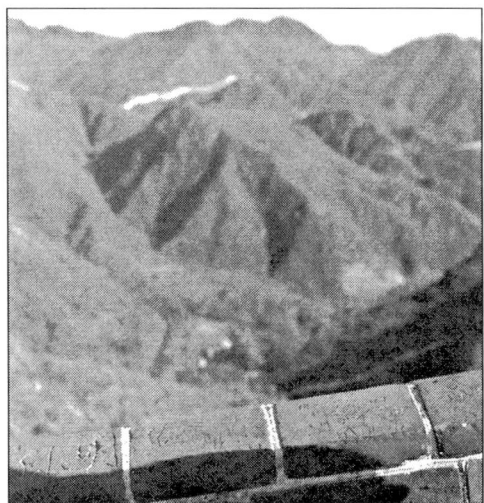

Daoist longevity exercises have greatly influenced China's martial art traditions. Here, an elderly gentleman strolls atop the Badaling section of the Great Wall. Long beards and the long wall are two of the many symbols for long life. Photos by M. DeMarco.

Some three decades ago Joseph Needham offered his opinion that "Chinese boxing . . . probably originated as a department of Taoist [Daoist] physical exercises."[1] This arresting hypothesis manages to strike us as both strange and yet oddly comfortable at the same time. We would expect that religion should have little to do with the deadly business of combat; yet, to anyone even remotely acquainted with the Chinese martial arts, the Daoist imprint is unmistakable. The present chapter is intended to explore the implications of this Daoist paternity. What exactly does it mean to say that the martial arts began with Daoist exercises, and what does that then tell us about the martial arts?

To begin with, it goes without saying that we do not intend to imply that the specific forms of the modern martial arts necessarily derive from older Daoist practices. What we do mean is simply that the basic philosophical underpinnings of the Chinese martial arts are Daoist. Beyond this, I venture to suggest that a technique which is central to the modern martial arts originated in Daoism. This technique is what has relatively recently come to be labeled qigong—*qi*, meaning breath or air, and *gong*, meaning achievement. The art has been defined by a contemporary Chinese scholar as "an active process of physical and mental discipline through the training of the heart/mind, the training of breathing, the training of the body and other means, which takes as its main goal the strengthening of human physical co-ordination."[2] In other words, it is the bending of qi to human intentions or "Daoist breath control."

Qigong has been surprisingly pervasive in Chinese thought. Even staid Confucians advocated its practice. Mencius (c. 372–279 BCE), for example, spoke of "cultivating my overwhelming qi," and in the twelfth century Zhu Xi (1130–1200) advocated the use of qigong breath control in his program of Neo-Confucian self-cultivation.[3] It is with the Daoist school, however, that the manipulation of the inner energies released by breath control is most intimately associated, and it was the Daoists who made the most extravagant claims for that technique. As the distinguished British Sinologist Arthur Waley put it, he who mastered Daoist breath control could "cure every disease, expose himself with immunity to epidemics, charm snakes and tigers, stop wounds from bleeding, stay under the water or walk upon it, stop hunger and thirst, and increase his own life-span."[4]

Such claims are fantastic. That they were, and sometimes still are, taken seriously can only be understood in the light of the Chinese scientific paradigm which took shape in the great eclectic *weltanschauung* of the Han dynasty (202 BCE–220 CE). This Han worldview envisioned the universe to be, in Derk Bodde's words, "a harmoniously functioning organism," the actions of whose component parts were each mutually related.[5] The complex interactions of yin and yang and five basic elements (*wuxing*) produced the manifold phenomena of nature. Elaborate sets of correlations were then devised for each element, and it was assumed that the correlates reacted sympathetically to each other.

This view is nicely illustrated in the following passage from the second century CE Daoist classic *Taiping Jing*:

> The nature of wood [one of the five elements] is humanity. If you contemplate humanity, therefore, you will be transported to the East, since the East is the master of humanity. The five directions [including the center] are all like this. The affairs of the world all follow their own kind. Therefore, if emperors and kings think peacefully, their governments will be peaceful as well, through the appeal of likeness.[6]

Viewed through the lenses of "modern science," it is easy to dismiss the logical process in operation here as "thought magic," in Murakami Yoshimi's words, and rationalize its continued acceptance in otherwise sophisticated Imperial China as an anachronistic relic of more primitive times.[7] In fact, however, this was not "magic" as Sir James Frazer might have defined it, but a mechanical tool for eliciting action at a distance through direct cause and effect, by means of the correlations among the five elements, and physical contact through the universal environment of qi.

Somewhat like the Western concept of the ether, qi was believed to be the substance surrounding and including all things, which brought even distant points into direct physical contact.[8] As the *Liezi* observed perhaps shortly after the fall of Han, "Heaven is merely amassed qi.... When you bend, stretch, or breath, you are always moving inside Heaven."[9]

Since one single substance joined all corners of the cosmos into a single organic unity, it followed that mastery of qi was equivalent to mastery of the material universe. The key was the mind. "What man can imagine, he can always bring about," says the *Taiping Jing*. "The mind and ideas are the pivotal mechanism of heaven and earth and cannot be carelessly moved. If you cause harmonious ch'i [*qi*] to become disordered, calamities will occur daily."[10] It was seriously supposed that the words and actions of a properly cultivated gentleman could affect "places thousands of miles away," and in early Imperial China, at least, such beliefs were not limited to so-called Daoists but were shared by even such stolid Confucians as Fu Xuan (217–278), who pontificated that "the mind... is the controller of all things."[11]

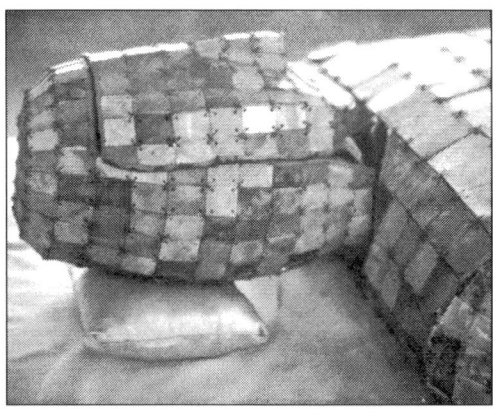

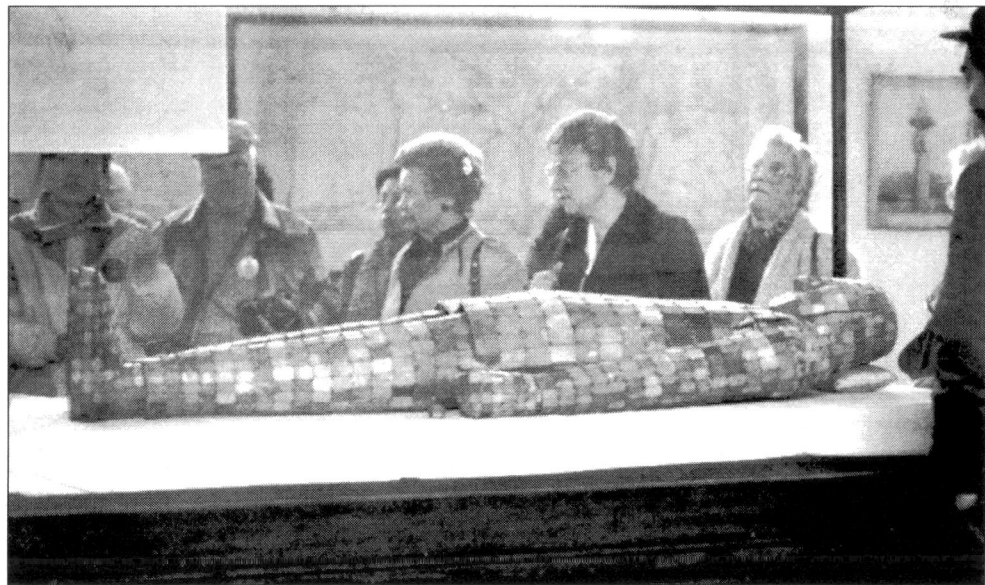

Nanjing Provincial Museum—a 2,000-year-old jade burial suit made of nearly 2,600 squares of green jade. Such "jade cases" were only made for emperors and high-ranking aristocrats. Jade was often utilized in the making of weapons and clothing. Today, it remains a precious stone partly because it is associated with life-prolonging attributes. Top: details of the jade burial suit on display in the Nanjing Provincial Museum. Photos by M. DeMarco.

The Han dynasty theoreticians were principally concerned about the implications of this discovery for government. It was supposed that the true ruler need only approach his task with a cultivated mind and settled heart for all the affairs of his domain to proceed in satisfactory harmony. But the ability of internal cultivation to transform external physical reality also had private significance, which in the long run proved to be of the greatest interest to most people. Specifically, proper circulation of qi could prolong one's life—perhaps indefinitely—and could enable the individual to accomplish otherwise incredible feats.

The technique of manipulating qi for personal satisfaction can be traced back at least as far as the late fifth century BCE, when it was referred to as "moving qi" (*xing qi*) on a jade pendant discovered recently by archaeologists.[12] The practice was evidently quite widespread even before the maturation of its theoretical explanation in the Han dynasty. According to the third century BCE Daoist classic *Zhuangzi*:

> Huffing and puffing, exhaling the old and inhaling the new, the bear pull and the bird stretch, is for long life and only that. This is what the gentlemen of Taoist [Daoist] exercises, men who nourish their bodies, and those who study the long life of P'eng Tsu [the "Chinese Methuselah"].[13]

By the Han dynasty the therapeutic physical exercises—Zhuangzi's "bear pull and bird stretch"—were called *daoyin*. Excellent illustrations of these daoyin exercises dating from the early Han were found in 1973 on silk scrolls unearthed at the tomb complex at Mawangdui.[14] The purpose of these exercises was to loosen up the circulatory system to permit the free passage of qi. As the first century CE skeptic Wang Chong wrote, Daoists "... suppose that if you do not shake, bend, and stretch the arteries in your body they will block up and not circulate, and if they do not circulate the accumulation will cause illness and death."[15]

Daoyin physical exercises were intended to facilitate the circulation of qi and were consequently secondary in importance to the actual manipulation of qi itself, which is often rendered in English as "breath control." This English term encompasses Zhuangzi's "huffing and puffing" without any problem but otherwise does not begin to do justice to the full range of the Chinese concept, since qi is not only breath but the very substance of the universe. Internally, within the human body, qi was envisioned as energy, often in fluid form.[16] When taken literally, as Daoist adepts so often did, this could be understood to mean saliva or the bodily fluids. According to one delightfully mystical text:

> The pure waters of the "jade pond" water the roots of the soul. If you investigate this and are able to cultivate it you can exist eternally. It is called "feeding upon nature." That which is natural is the "glorious pond." The "glorious pond" [refers to] the saliva in one's mouth. If you

breathe in accordance with the rules and swallow it, you will not experience hunger.[17]

Such technologies were understood as ways to physically recycle, conserve, and nourish the bodily qi which the therapeutic daoyin exercises had cleared passages for. A late Han dynasty adept named Wang Chen, for example, "practiced shutting off his qi and swallowing it, calling it embryonic breathing, and swallowing [the fluid] coughed up from the spring beneath his tongue, calling it embryonic feeding."[18]

These early qigong practices may have focused on actual respiration or the circulation of bodily fluids, but mental concentration must have been a necessary concomitant of "breath control" from its inception. With time the role of the mind came to loom even larger. In fully evolved qigong practice the energy of qi is channeled through the body under mental impulse.[19] It was this mental activity, developed into a form of meditation known as "holding on to the one" (*shou-yi*) or "fixed thought" (*cun-si*), which actually unleashed the incredible powers of Daoist "breath control" noted by Arthur Waley.[20] Merely by thinking about it the adept can travel vast distances or cure diseases. As the *Baopuzi* recorded in the fourth century, "if you imagine the ch'i [qi] from your five internal organs emerging from your two eyes to surround your body like mist . . . you can then share a bed with the victim of a plague [without danger]."[21]

The arrival of Indian Buddhism in China shortly after the birth of Christ may have added a new current to the stream of Chinese meditative practice but probably did little more than refine an already existing Daoist tradition.[22] The Parthian monk An Shih-gao, for example, translated a Buddhist sutra on meditation through concentration on breathing (*anapana*) shortly after his arrival at the Han capital in 148 CE, but by that time concentrated thought was also a central fixture of the Daoist tradition as well.[23] The meditative aspect of qigong should, therefore, be considered essentially as part of the main Daoist line of transmission, even while acknowledging the possibility that there were important Buddhist contributions.[24]

The meditative aspect of Daoist qigong in the Han dynasty is nicely illustrated by the following passage from the *Peng Zu ling*:

Whoever moves his qi with the desire of eradicating the "hundred diseases" concentrates on wherever they are located. If his head aches he concentrates on his head, if his foot hurts he concentrates on his foot, combining his qi and sending it to attack it. In the time [the qi] takes to get there [the ache] will have dissipated by itself.[25]

Thus, although the term qigong had not yet been coined, qigong techniques were fully developed by the end of the Han dynasty. At the same time, true Daoist religion also emerged in the last century of the Han, and it soon absorbed and engulfed qigong. The new religion may have had distant precursors in shamanism, but its immediate ancestors are to be found among the *fangshi* ("gentlemen with prescriptions") who began to promote secret arts leading to immortality around the third century BCE.[26] Over the course of the next few centuries these arts evolved and spread until in the second century CE a man named Zhang Daoling (fl. c. 142) instigated a "religious revolution" by organizing a Daoist church dedicated to the pursuit of immortality.[27]

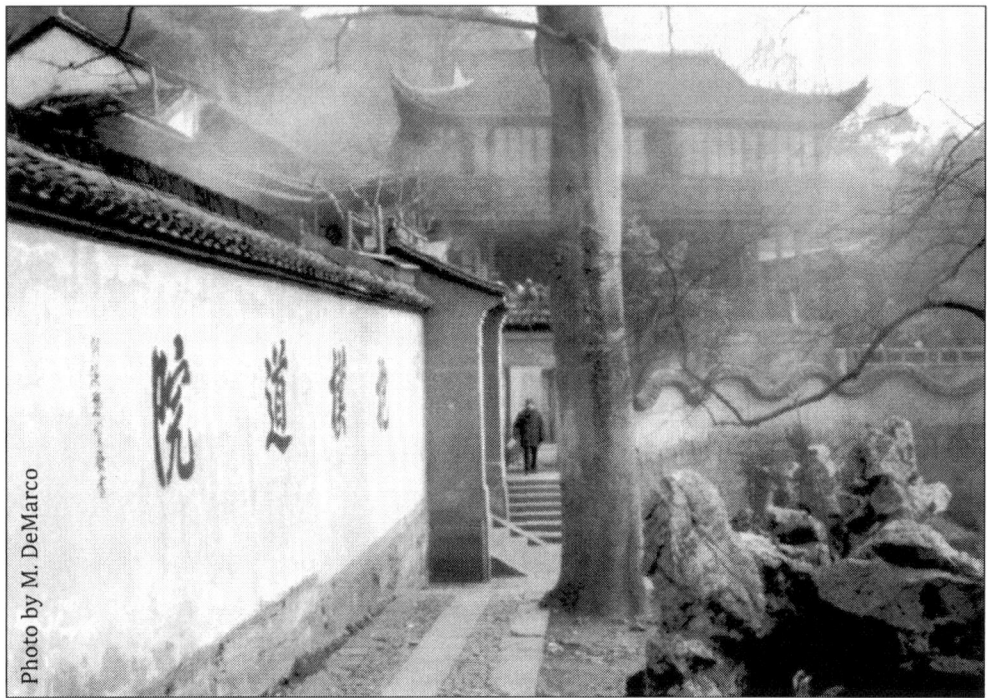

Simplicity Embracing Monastery located on a hill overlooking West Lake in Hangzhou city. It is noted as the place where Daoist Ge Hong alchemically prepared elixirs for attaining immortality.

After a rather conventional beginning studying the classics, the story goes, Zhang had retired to a mountain in modern-day Sichuan to "study the Dao of long life."[28] With divine direction he obtained a sacred text which enabled him to fly and work various other miracles.[29] Because of his new ability to cure disease, "the common people thronged to him and served him as their teacher, the households of his disciples reaching the tens of thousands."[30]

The new faith struck a responsive chord in late Han China, and the quest for immortality soon became all the rage among the elite. In the second century the *Taiping Jing* claimed, perhaps with some hyperbole, that "the perfect gentlemen of the empire eschew office for immortality."[31] After the fall of Han, Chi Yin (313–384)—who strolled about with friends, "settled his heart, stopped eating grain, and cultivated the [Daoist] arts of Huang-Lao [the Yellow Emperor and Laozi]"—was typical of the lofty literati who dominated the era of division that followed.[32] Even Buddhism flourished in the immediate post-Han era largely "as a religion of immortal recipes."[33]

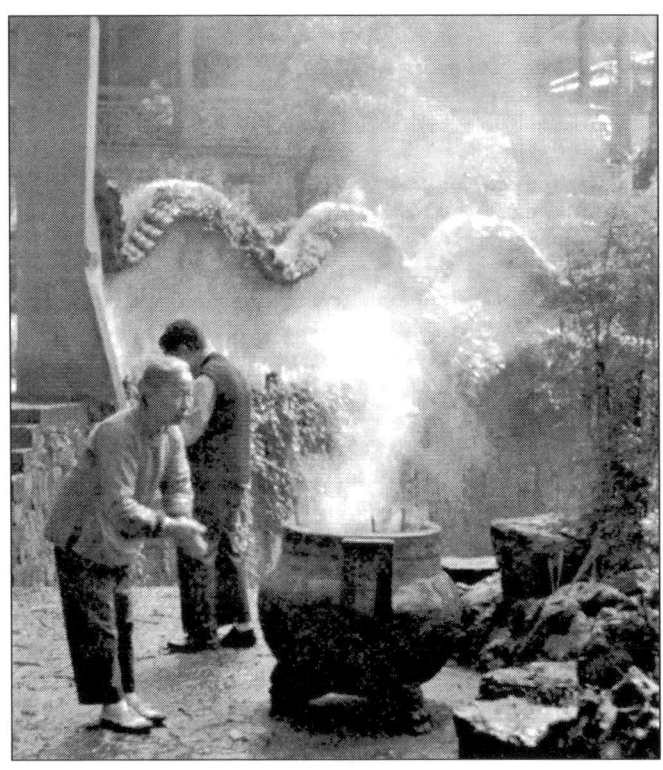

Some believe incense lifts prayers to heaven. In the Daoist tradition, individuals can also be found practicing various exercises for health and spiritual development. Some are obviously martial. Symbolically, incense can represent the movement of qi. Photo by M. DeMarco.

The medievality cult was eclectic and borrowed from every conceivable tradition, including Daoist breath control. Of the adepts (still referred to here as *fangshi*) at the court of the Wei Kingdom early in the third century CE, for example, "[Kan] Shih is able to move his *ch'i* [*qi*] and perform *tao-yin* [*daoyin*] exercises, [Tso] Tz'u is enlightened about the [sexual] arts 'within the chamber,' and [Xi] Chien is good at avoiding [eating] grains. They all claim to be three hundred years old."[34] A text called the *Lai Xiang li*, which may date from the fourth century, listed no fewer than thirty-six different methods for nourishing one's nature and attaining immortality, ranging from "breathing and visualizing the cinnabar field" to "using sacrifices to bring spirits" and eremitism.[35] Qigong mixed freely with cabalistic ideas and talismanic beliefs: the medieval Daoists "also make seals of wood, engraving stars, planets, the sun and moon upon them; and, inhaling ch'i [*qi*] and grasping them, they use them to seal a disease, curing many."[36]

In the Han and pre-Han periods qigong had enjoyed a preeminent position among the arts of longevity. When asked for the secret of his long life by Emperor Wen early in the second century BCE, for example, the 180-year-old Duke Dou supposedly replied: "Your servant [practices] *tao-yin* [*daoyin*]; it is not that I have taken any potions."[37] In the immortality cult that flowered after the fall of the Han, however, it was the elixir of immortality which eclipsed qigong.[38]

Chinese elixirs apparently originated with the shaman's use of intoxicants in antiquity to induce trances. The drugs used for that purpose may have included alcohol, hallucinogenic mushrooms, and other less well-defined "medicines."[39] The *Shan Hai ling*, for example, speaks of a mountain where no fewer than ten shamans "rise and descend, gathering the hundred medicines."[40] This use of drugs was then picked up and elaborated on by the *fangshi* of the early imperial era, and emerged as the path of choice to immortality in the third century CE.

The ingredients of medieval immortality potions included fungi and something known as the "five mineral" powder.[41] Gold was another favorite substance. With typical literal-mindedness some Daoists reasoned that since "it is in the nature of gold that it does not decay.... [so, too,] when the alchemist consumes it, he obtains immortality."[42] However, it was the "refinement of cinnabar" (*liandan*) that was most esteemed by serious adherents of the immortality cult. Cinnabar (HgS, or mercuric sulfide), in fact, came to be a veritable synonym for the elixir itself, and it was in the shadow of that mighty potion that by the sixth century qigong came to be known as *neidan*, or "internal cinnabar," in self-conscious imitation of the more important "external cinnabar" (*waidan*) which was the elixir of immortality itself.[43]

It may strike the reader as odd that intelligent literati were so credulous as to believe in physical immortality. Not all were, but China did have a long tradition of belief in ancestral spirits, ghosts, and other such things. In this the Chinese cannot be said to have been any more credulous than other peoples, but the Chinese were also "rational" enough to question whether it was possible for spirits to exist apart from the material world. Prior to the introduction of the Buddhist belief in reincarnation, therefore, many Chinese suspected that at death "the body and spirit were extinguished together" or at least that their residue was transformed into new material objects.[44] A non-corporeal immortality of the soul in the Christian sense was simply inconceivable, but, this did not mean that spirits did not exist.[45] Like the air itself, which was also composed of physical matter, they were ethereal but physical beings invisible to mortal eyes.[46]

"Immortals" (*xian*), then, were simply deathless spiritual beings who belonged to a more rarefied sphere of matter than mankind.[47] Since all objects in the universe were constructed of a single basic substance, and since all things were in a constant process of transformation, it followed that almost anything could theoretically be transformed into almost anything else if only the necessary preconditions could be met.[48] As Tung Jung-chang (179–219) wrote, "Those who attain the Tao [*Dao*] sprout pinions on their arms, long feathers on their bellies, fly the unscalable blue sky, and pass over the interminable affairs of this world."[49] Medicine seemed a reasonable catalyst for this change, moreover, since the relentless Han expectation of natural symmetry implied that if there were drugs that could kill people, as there certainly were, there should also be corresponding drugs that were antidotes for death.[50]

Unfortunately, the medicines that medieval alchemists brewed often proved harmful or fatal to those who consumed them.[51] It was not unnatural, under the circumstances, for skeptics to point to the absence of evidence for success and wonder, if it were really possible to attain immortality, where all the immortals were.[52]

In his "Essay on Nourishing Life" (*Yang Sheng Lun*), Xi Kang (223–262) began cautiously:

> In this world there are those who say that immortality can be obtained through study, and that through effort one can avoid death. There are others who say that a maximum age of 120 has been the same in antiquity and modern times, and that going beyond this is always a fantastic delusion. Both of these [positions] neglect the facts. [53]

For Xi the records of immortals in the old histories were proof enough that immortals had existed, but he then went on to suggest that they must have been "specially endowed with a different" qi. For modern man to attain immortality, while still theoretically within the realm of possibility, was practically out of reach. Instead, Xi's recipe for nourishing life in the modern world was simply to harmonize with the Dao, consume medicines and drink wine, and nestle into calm inactivity. "Forget enjoyment, and then your pleasure will be sufficient. Neglect life, and then your body will be preserved."[54] In the classic Daoist paradox, since the Dao works through a process of reversal, "those who do not treat life as valuable are the ones who excel at valuing life."[55]

Although Xi Kang did believe in immortals and was actually one of the more prominent third century enthusiasts for collecting medicines and methods of mental and physical self-cultivation, he also clearly possessed a healthy dose of skepticism and had a realistic sense of the possibilities.[56] In the sixth century, Xi's caution was echoed by Yan Chi-dui (531–591), who advised his sons to avoid the futile search for immortality but conceded that nourishing the spirit, breath control, and the proper use of medicine could result in longer life.[57]

The most ardent seekers of immortality were apologetic. In the second century, the *Taiping Jing* warned that [some] "doctors and shamans only want to get people's money."[58] The royal family of third century Wei, who had summoned an assortment of *fangshi* to their court, explained that, of course, "we all consider this to be laughable and do not put any credence in it."[59] And in the most famous of all collections of formulas for immortality, the author of the fourth century *Baopuzi* protested with evident embarrassment that he only wanted "to treat the logic in things exhaustively."[60]

With the waning of the medieval social order after the late Tang dynasty (618–907), the immortality cult gradually diminished in importance. Internal self-cultivation through qigong, often referred to during this period as *neidan*, largely superseded the consumption of elixirs.[61] The mainstream of elite scholar-official interest in the late Imperial period was diverted away from overt religious enthusiasms towards secular Neo-Confucianism, but the religious nimbus surrounding qigong spread now to China's common people through the rise of new forms of popular sectarian Buddho-Daoist religion.

The most famous of these sects was called the White Lotus Society. This sect claimed to have been founded in the era of division after the fall of the Han, but actually seems not to have reached mature form until as late as the sixteenth century.[62] For our purposes the significant thing about White Lotus sectarian religion is that it taught qigong as part of its repertoire of salvationist techniques.[63] It was out of societies like the White Lotus—if not the White Lotus sect itself—that the historical Chinese martial arts first appeared.

No better illustration of the martial arts in practice can be found than the Boxer uprising that erupted at the beginning of the twentieth century. The reason this is such a fascinating example is that the Boxers' so-called "boxing" really consisted of shamanistic dances for inducing spiritual possession and divine invincibility, and not the kind of martial arts combat we would expect.[64] Nor were the Boxers unique in this respect. In many less well-known martial associations as well, such as the early twentieth century Red Spears studied by Elizabeth Perry, ritual magic seems to have been the most prominent feature.[65] The simple explanation for this is that in premodern China "martial arts" were part of a larger matrix of religious belief and practice and inseparable from that religious context.

In the twentieth century, however, "science" and "democracy" became the new watchwords for educated Chinese youth. During the "New Culture" and "May Fourth" movements that began in World War I, the Chinese intelligentsia attempted to remake completely Chinese culture in the Western image. Old religious practices were denounced as "superstition" and rejected as embarrassing reminders of China's backward feudal past.

Qigong was not discarded during this century of modernization, but it was stripped of its burden of religious "superstition." Today qigong is presented as a part of China's lengthy folk medical tradition.[66] It is now considered a "scientific" rather than a religious technique for curing diseases and lengthening life, and, like so much of China's native medical tradition, it is currently attracting worldwide interest. Exciting, if yet unverified, successes have been reported in treating such fashionable diseases as cancer using qigong.[67]

It is certainly not an error to treat qigong as a medical technology in this fashion. In the fourth century BCE *Inner Classic of the Yellow Emperor*, for example, the daoyin and xingqi forms of qigong were already listed as varieties of medical treatment alongside moxibustion, massage, acupuncture, and the consumption of drugs.[68] A Daoist adept in the third century southern state of Wu "fasted to await the patient's cure whenever he moved his ch'i [*xingqi*] to treat someone's illness."[69] A sixth-century bibliographic treatise in the *Sui shu* even mentions a short book in one scroll, "On Methods of Treatment with Qi" (*Lun qi chi liao fang*).[70] In the medieval immortality cult, however, the healing of diseases was but the first step in a continuum that led eventually to immortality. No clear separation was even conceivable between medicine and religion.

It was out of this same religious matrix that the modern martial arts emerged. The fighter and the healer are bound together by their common religious background and by their shared technology of qigong. Many of the popular martial art forms in late Imperial China, such as *taijiquan* (supreme ultimate boxing), *xingiquan* (body and thought boxing), and *baguachang* (eight trigrams hands), show clear evidence of qigong influence.[71] Taiji in particular is interesting. It is the quintessential Chinese martial art, but its practice is marked by breath control, concentration, and graceful dance-like movements. The casual Western observer might never even guess that it was supposed to be a form of combat. And yet the experts all insist it is the deadliest martial art of all.[72] If so, this may be because concentration of the kind developed in qigong really is a way to better health, coordination, and keener combat ability. As the Han dynasty thinkers had realized long ago, the mind really can be the key to many things.

Notes

[1] J. Needham, *Science and Civilization in China, Vol. 2* (Cambridge: Cambridge University Press, 1962), 145–6. See also Wang Hsinwu, *T'ai chi ch'üan-fa ching-i* (The Essential Meaning of the Methods of Taijiquan) (Hong Kong: T'aip'ing shu-chü, 1962), 1.

[2] Li Chih-yung, ed., *Chung-kuo ch'i-kung shih* (A History of Chinese Qigong) (Honan: Honan k'o-hsüeh chi-shu ch'upanshe, 1988), 2.

[3] *Meng Tzu* (Mencius), annotated by Chao Ch'i (Ssu-pu ts'ung-kan edition; Shanghai: Shanghai shang-wu yin-shu-kuan, 1929), 3.6b. For Zhu Xi, see Li Chih-yung, 26.

[4] A. Waley, *The Way and its Power: A Study of the Tao Te Ching and its Place in Chinese Thought* (Guilford: Billing and Sons, Ltd., 1934), 118.

[5] D. Bodde, "The Chinese cosmic magic known as watching for the ethers," *Essays on Chinese Civilization* (Princeton: Princeton University Press, 1981), 351–52.

[6] *T'ai-p'ing ching ho-chiao* (The Collated Classic of Great Peace), ed. by Wang Ming (Peking: Chunghua shuchü, 1960), 27.

[7] Murakami Yoshimi, *Chogoku no sennin–Hobokushi no shiso* (Chinese Immortals – The Thought of the Pao-p'u tzu) (Kyoto: Heirakuji shoten, 1956), 139.

[8] See C. Le Blanc, *Huai Nan Tzu: Philosophical Synthesis in Early Han Thought* (Hong Kong: Hong Kong University Press, 1985), 204; K. DeWoskin, *A Song for One or Two: Music and the Concept of Art in Early China*, Michigan Papers in Chinese Studies, No. 42 (Ann Arbor: University of Michigan Center for Chinese Studies, 1982), 38.

[9] *Lieh tzu*, annotated by Chang Chan (c. 340–400) (reprint; Taipei: Taiwan chunghua shuchü, 1982), 1.14a.

[10] *T'ai-p'ing ching*, 25, 311.

11 For the words of the gentleman, see Wu Luchiang and Tenney Davis, tr., "An Ancient Chinese Treatise on Alchemy Entitled Ts'an T'ung Ch'i," *Isis*, 18.2 (1932), 245. Fu Xuan's text on "Rectifying the Mind" is included in *Ch'üan Chin wen* (Complete Writings of the Qin Dynasty), in *Ch'üan shang-ku san-tai Ch'in Han san-kuo liu-ch'ao wen*, ed. by Yen K'o-chün (1762–1843) (reprint; Kyoto: Chobun shuppansha, 1981), 1733.

12 Li Chih-yung, 9. Murakami Yoshimi defines *xingqi* as "to take in much ch'i [qi] and breathe deeply" (2).

13 *Chuang tzu tsuan-chien* (The Annotated Zhuangzi), ed. by Ch'ien Mu (Hong Kong: Tung-nan yin-wu ch'upanshe, n.d.), 122. *The Inner Classic of the Yellow Emperor* (Huangti neiching) also contains important early references to qigong and may be somewhat older. Francis Ruey-shuang Lee suggests it may date from the fourth century BCE. (*The "Silent Art" of Ancient China: Historical Analysis of the Intellectual and Philosophical Influences in the Earliest Medical Corpus Ling Shu Ching* [Taipei: Linking Publishing Co., 1980], 46).

14 Lin Hou-sheng and Lo P'ei-yü, *Chi-kung san-pai wen* (Three Hundred Questions Concerning Qigong) (Canton: Kuang-tung k'o-chi ch'upanche, 1983), 5.

15 Wang Ch'ung (27–c. 100 CE), *Lun Heng* (An Appraisal of Discussions) (reprint; Taipei: Taiwan chunghua shuchü, 1981), 7.19b.

16 See Ishida Hidemi, "Body and mind: The Chinese perspective," in *Taoist Meditation and Longevity Techniques*, ed. by L. Kohn (Ann Arbor: Center for Chinese Studies, University of Michigan, 1989), 45.

17 *Huang-t'ing ching* (The Classic of the Yellow Court), quoted in T'ao Hung-ching (456–536 CE), *Yang-hsingyen-ming lu* (A record of cultivating nature and prolonging life), in *Tao-tsangyang-sheng shu shih-chung*, ed. by Li Shih-hua and Shen Te-hui (Peking: Chung-i ku-chi ch'upanshe, 1987), 5.

18 *Ts'e-ju yüan-keui* (The Great Tortoise of the Archives) (c. 1013) (reprint; Taipei: Taiwan chunghua shuchü, 1981), 836.9917.

19 The importance of thought in qigong is eloquently stated in Miura Kunio, "The revival of Qi: Qigong in contemporary China," in L. Kohn, ed., *Taoist Meditation*, 337.

20 Murakami Yoshimi, 147. Daoist concentration is described in Li Chihyung, 96 ff.

21 Ko Hung (c. 280–340), *Pao-p'u tzu* (The Master Embracing Simplicity) (reprint; Taipei: Taiwan chung-hua shuchü, 1984), nei-p'ien 15.7a–8a.

22 Chang Chung-yuan ("An introduction to Taoist yoga," *The Review of Religion*, 20.3-4 [1956]) tentatively asserts the relative priority of indigenous Chinese techniques.

23 For An Shih-gao, see Tsukamoto Zenryu, "The early stages in the introduction of Buddhism into China (Up to the fifth century A.D.)," *Cahiers d'histoire mondials*, 5.3 (1960), 557.

24 The modern martial arts are often closely associated with Buddhism especially through the Shaolin school in China and Zen in Japan—but this is a perversion of the important Buddhist belief in pacifism and can be explained in part as a

result of a strong Daoist influence. See P. Demieville, "Le bouddhisme etla guerre, "*Choix d'etudes bouddhiques* (Leiden: E.J. Brill, 1973), 288 and passim.

[25] *P'eng Tsu ching* (The classic of Peng Zi), in *Yang-hsing yen-ming lu*, 14. The text is ascribed to the late Han by C. Despeux, "Gymnastics: The ancient tradition," in L. Kohn, ed., *Taoist Meditation*, 229.

[26] A link between these *fangshi* and the older practices of shamanism has been observed by Li Feng-mao ("Fu-Ch'u-tz'u te k'ao-ch'a chih-i" [Personal Adornment, the Consumption of Medicine, and Shamanistic Tradition: An Investigation of the *Ch'u Tz'u* from the Perspective of Shamanism], *Ku-tienwenhsüeh*, 3 [1981], 89) and others. For shamanism, see E. Harvey, "Shamanism in China," *Studies in the Science of Society*, ed. by G. Murdock (New Haven: Yale University Press, 1937). For the rise of *fangshi*, see Ku Ming-chien (Ku Chieh-kang), *Ch'in Han te fang-hih yü ju-sheng* (Qin and Han fangshi and Confucians) (1933; Taipei: Li-jen shuchü, 1985), 11. Ssuma Ch'ien (145–90 BCE) ascribed the deceits of *fangshi* to a misunderstanding of the scientific principle of the succession of yin and yang. See *Shih-chi* (Records of the Grand Historian) (Peking: Chunghua shuchü, 1959), 1368–69.

[27] M. Strickmann, "On the alchemy of T'ao Hung-ching," in *Facets of Taoism: Essays in Chinese Religion*, ed. by H. Welch and A. Seidel (New Haven: Yale University Press, 1979), 165.

[28] *T'ai-p'ing kuang-chi* (Extensive Records of the Taiping Era), ed. by Li Fang (925–996) (reprint; Peking: Chunghua shuchü, 1981), 55–56.

[29] *Yü-chih-t'ang t'an-hui* (Clustered Conversations of the Jade and Iris Hall), ed. by Hsü Yün-lin (fl. c. 1616) (1875 edition), 17.21a.

[30] *T'ai-p'ing kuang-chi*, 56.

[31] *T'ai-p'ing ching*, 403.

[32] *Yu-chün nien-p'u* (A Chronicle of the General of the Right), ed. by Lu I-t'ung, Mei-shu ts'ung-shu 4.9 (1855; Taipei: I-wen yin-shu-kuan, n.d.), 370.

[33] Tsukamoto Zenryu, *Shina bukkyoshi kenkyo, hoku-gi hen* (Studies in the History of Chinese Buddhism, the Northern Wei Chapters) (Tokyo: Kobunto shobo, 1942), 49.

[34] Ch'en Shou (233–97), *San-kuo shih* (The Annals of the Three Kingdoms) (Peking: Chunghua shuchü, 1959), 29.805.

[35] This text is quoted in *Ch'u-hsüeh chi* (A Record for Initial Study), edited by Hsü Chien (659–729) (reprint; Peking: Chunghua shuchü, 1962), 23.54950. The work is otherwise unknown and undatable, but Lai-hsiang was a place name in the Qin dynasty.

[36] Wei Cheng (580–643), ed., *Sui-shu* (History of the Sui Dynasty) (reprint; Peking: Chunghua shuchü, 1973), 35.1093.

[37] Huan T'an (43 BCE–28CE), *Huan tzu hsin-lun* (New essays of Master Huan) (reprint; Taipei: Taiwan chunghua shuchü, 1976), 11b. Different versions of the story are in circulation.

[38] According to Murakami Yoshimi (143), spiritual immortality could be attained

by union with the Dao through meditation, but immortality of the body required the consumption of medicines, swallowing qi, and so on.

[39] See Chang Kwang-chih, *Art, myth, and ritual: The path to political authority in ancient China* (Cambridge: Harvard University Press, 1983), 55; M. Strickmann, *Notes on mushroom cults in ancient China* (Ghent: Rijksuniversiteit, 1966).

[40] *Shan hai ching chiao-chu* (The collated and annotated Classic of Mountains and Seas) (date uncertain), ed. by Yüan K'o (Shanghai: Shanghai kuchi ch'upanshe, 1980), 16.396.

[41] Chang Hua (232–300), *Po-wu chih* (An account of diverse phenomena) (reprint; Taipei: Taiwan chunghua shuchü, 1983), 7.1b. The so-called "five mineral powder" is discussed in Kuo Lin-ko, "Wei Chin feng-liu" (The fashions of the Wei and Chin), *Chungkuo hsüeh-pao*, 1.6 (1944), 48.

[42] *Ts'an t'ung ch'i k'ao-i* (An examination of variants in the covenant of the union of the three) (c. 142), ed. by Zhu Xi (reprint; Taipei: Taiwan chunghua shuchü, 1983), 12a.

[43] For the appearance of the term *neidan*, see Ko Chao-kuang, *Tao-chiao yü chungkuo wenhua* (Daoism and Chinese culture), Chungkuo wenhua shih ts'ung-shu (Shanghai: Shanghai jenmin ch'upanshe, 1987), 110. Isabelle Robinet ("Original contributions of neidan to Taoism and Chinese thought," in Kohn, ed., *Taoist meditation*, 301) limits the designation *neidan* to only those texts actually using chemical terminology, but clearly the comparison with laboratory alchemy helped shape the identity of qigong practice in general during this period.

[44] Cheng Tao-tzu (5th century), "Shen pu mieh lun" (On the Non-Extinction of the Spirit), contained in *Hungming chi* (The Collection Expanding Illumination), ed. by Seng Yu (435.518) (reprint; Taipei: Taiwan chunghua shuchü, 1983), 5.2a. Cheng, of course, argues for the Buddhist position. For a classic description of the process of death, see *Lieh tzu*, 1.9b.

[45] D. Holzman (*La vie et la pensee de Hi K'ang* [223.262 Ap. J.–C.] [Leiden: E. J. Brill, 1957], 53) observes that for the third century Chinese "une immortalite sans le corps est impensable [immortality with the body is unthinkable]. "

[46] The discussant in Hui-yüan's (334–416) "Sha-men pu ching wang che lun" (Sramana are Not Those Who Honor Kings) (*Hung ming chi*, 5.9a) offers the apparently trite opinion that "although the spirit is a subtle thing, it is certainly still something that is transformed by yin and yang." As much as the coarsest of substances, spirits too were part of the physical world.

[47] See N. Sivin, *Chinese Alchemy: Preliminary Studies* (Cambridge: Harvard University Press, 1968), 41; Yü Ying-shih, "Life and immortality in the mind of Han China," *Harvard Journal of Asiatic Studies*, 25 (1965), 88–89.

[48] See H. Dubs, "The Beginnings of Alchemy, "*Isis*, 38.1-2 (1947), 73, note 76. The third century understanding of fundamental unity amid constant change is noted, for example, in I. Robinet, "Kouo Siang ou le monde comme absolu," *T'oung Pao*, 69.1–3 (1983), 83.

[49] *Ch'üan Hou Han wen* (Complete Writings of the Later Han Dynasty), in *Ch'üan*

shang-ku san-tai Ch'in Han san-kuo liu-ch'ao wen, 89.955.

50 The skeptic Huan Tan was told that since "Heaven produced medicines that kill men, there must be medicines to make men live" (*Huan tzu hsin-lun*, 26a.) Huan's astute reply was that poisons are not actually medicines to kill people, but rather substances which are simply not appropriate to eat.

51 The effects of taking these drugs have been thoroughly studied in Ho Ping-yü and J. Needham, "Elixir poisoning in medieval China," *Janus*, *48* (1959).

52 See Xiang Xiu's third century criticism of Xi Kang, translated in Robert G. Henricks, *Philosophy and Argumentation in Third-Century China: The Essays of Hsi K'ang* (Princeton: Princeton University Press, 1983), 35.

53 *Ch'üan san-kuo wen* (Complete writings of the Three Kingdoms), in *Ch'üan shang-ku san-tai Ch'in Han san-kuo liu-ch'ao wen*, 48.1324.

54 Ibid., 48.1324–25.

55 *Chin-shu* (History of the Qin dynasty), ed. by Fang Hsüan-ling (578. 648) (reprint; Peking: Chunghua shuchü, 1974), 49.1370.

56 Xi's thought is discussed in Horiike Nobuo, "Kei Ko ni okeru shinko to shakai: Sho Shu to no 'yojoron' ronso o chushin to shite" (Faith and Society in Xi Kang–Centering on the Debate with Xiang Xiu over his "Essay on Nourishing Life") *Rekishi ni okeru minshu to bunka: Sakai Tadao sensei koki shukuga kinen ronshu* (Tokyo: Kokusho kankokai, 1982), 109; Holzman, 52.60; and Li Fengmao, "Hsi K'ang yang-sheng ssu-hsiang chih yen-chiu" (Studies of Xi Kang's thought on nourishing life), *Ching-i wen-li hsüeh-yüan hsüeh-pao, 2* (1979).

57 Yen Chih-t'ui [Yan Chi-dui], *Family Instructions for the Yen Clan: Yenshih chia-hsün*, trans., by Teng Ssu-yü (Leiden: E.J. Brill, 1968), 131–133.

58 *T'ai-p'ing ching*, 620.

59 *San-kuo chih*, 29.805.

60 Ko Hung, *Alchemy, Medicine and Religion in the China of A.D. 320: The Nei P'ien of Ko Hung*, trans. by J. Ware (Dover, 1966), 206.

61 See N. Sivin, "Science and medicine in Imperial China—The state of the field," *Journal of Asian Studies*, 47.1 (1988), 55. This movement parallels the simultaneous philosophical shift from Daoist concepts of external transcendence back towards Buddhist and Confucian themes of the immanence of truth within oneself. See Mori Mikisaburo, "Chogoku shiso ni okers choetsu to naizai" (Transcendence and Immanence in Chinese Thought), *Toyo gakujutsu kenkyu*, 23.2 (1984), 124.

62 For an overview of White Lotus sectarianism, see Susan Naquin, "The transmission of White Lotus sectarianism in late imperial China," in *Popular Culture in Later Imperial China*, ed. by D. Johnson, et al. (Berkeley: University of California Press, 1985).

63 The use of qigong in the White Lotus movement is described in D. Overmeyer, *Folk Buddhist Religion: Dissenting Sects in Late Traditional China* (Cambridge: Harvard University Press, 1976), 188, 190–92; Naquin, 275.

64 See Kobayashi Kazumi, "Giwandan no minsho shiso" (The popular thought of the

boxers), in *Koza Chogoku kingendai-shi 2: Giwandan undo* (Tokyo: Tokyo daigaku shuppankai, 1978), 243.

[65] E. Perry, *Rebels and Revolutionaries in North China, 1845–1945* (Stanford: Stanford University Press, 1980), 186–197.

[66] See Linda Chih-ling Koo, *Nourishment of Life: The Culture of Health in Traditional Chinese Society* (Ph.D. dissertation, University of California; Ann Arbor: University Microfilms, 1976), 71–72. Lin Hou-sheng (1), for example, introduces qigong as one of China's folk medical practices.

[67] Cui Lili ("Fitness and health through qigong," *Beijing Review* 32.1 7 [April 24–30, 1989]: 20, 22) reports that qigong has successfully been used to treat "terminal cancer patients" in the People's Republic. It is not clear yet how credible such claims are.

[68] *Ling-shu ching* (The classic of the spiritual axis), in *Huang-ti su-wen ling-shu ching* (The Yellow Emperor's Classics of Common Questions and the Spiritual Axis), annotated by Wang Ping (Ssu-pu ts'ung-k'an edition; Shanghai: Shang-hai shang-wu yin-shu-kuan, 1929), 7.3a.

[69] *Pao-p'u tzu, nei-p'ien* 15.3a.

[70] *Sui-shu*, 34.1046.

[71] See Li Chih-yung, 392. N. Sivin ("Science and Medicine," 68) notes real differences between taijiquan and the ancient daoyin exercises, however.

[72] For the effectiveness of taijiquan in martial arts competition, see "Fang t'ai-chi ta-shih Wang P'ei-sheng), *Jenmin jih-pao* (People's Daily), overseas edition, Aug. 3, 1987, 2.

• 5 •
Taijiquan: Learning How to Learn
by Linda Lehrhaupt, Ph.D.

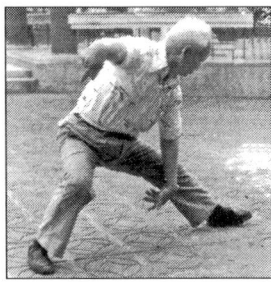 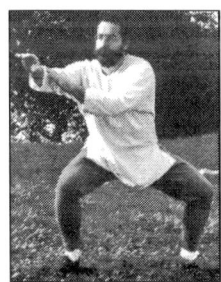 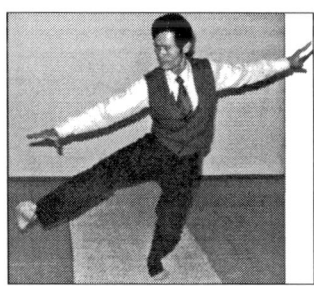

Left to right: Yang Qingyu, Yang Style in Taiwan. Paolo D'Annibala, Yang Style practitioner, Rome. Tu Zongren, Chen Style, Taiwan. Photos courtesy of M. DeMarco, P. D'Annibale, and Z. Tu.

Introduction

When I first began to study taijiquan in 1978, I was attracted to it, like many beginning students, by its description as a form of "meditation in motion." I had visions of flowing in dream-like movements, sensing peace and harmony all around me. I arrived at my first class full of happy expectations, sure that I was about to experience the secret of the Daoist masters. As I watched my teacher move with elegance and gentle power, I became even more excited. That excitement soon turned into frustration and disappointment as I struggled to learn the two short movements she so patiently repeated. At the end of the class, I was sure of only one thing: either my expectations had to go out the door or I did. I chose to stay.

Over and over during the past ten years that I have been teaching, I watch my own students arrive at their first class with the same expectations that I had. They seek to be more peaceful, to find balance, to learn something that will help them cope with stress. Their longing is so great that many hope to reap the benefits of taijiquan from the moment they begin to learn the form. In this mode of wishful thinking and longing for Paradise Now, they often ignore common sense. No one would expect to be a great pianist after one lesson, and yet many beginning taiji students believe that after one short class they will be able to move with the grace and effortlessness of an experienced taiji practitioner.

Most taiji students who stop studying after a short time do so, not because taiji is difficult to learn, but because their expectations are not satisfied quickly enough. The ensuing frustration is so emotionally painful they decide to quit rather than continue to be disappointed.

**When the emphasis is on how and not simply what is learned,
a student embraces everything as part of his taiji practice,
including his feelings and expectations.**

Part of the problem lies in the fact that students approach learning taiji as something to achieve, something to be successful at. But learning taiji, especially in the beginning, is really a process of learning how to learn. Learning how to learn means that what a student discovers about himself is just as important, if not more so, than simply performing a taiji movement correctly. When the emphasis is on how and not simply what is learned, a student embraces everything as part of his taiji practice, including his feelings and expectations. Frustrations, disappointment, or low self-esteem, instead of becoming obstacles to practice, can be transformed into fertile ground for learning about oneself.

In learning how to learn, we discover the essence of taiji as a meditative practice: the study of the self. Here, too, students must often re-examine their expectations of what meditation is. Many think it is the path to an enlightened state of bliss and wisdom, a state in which we are above all problems, free from attachment and desire. But the study of the self is, in fact, the study of the self as it is, not just the narrow view of how we would like ourselves to be. Practicing taiji as meditation invites us to stay open to each moment exactly as it is, to remain present and acknowledge all our experience, not selecting or rejecting anything. By staying open we create space to examine our fears, disappointments, and expectations. Bringing them into awareness allows us to work with them in a healing way. Their power to control us lessens because they no longer remain hidden.

Practicing taiji as meditation, the heart of which is learning how to learn, requires that we cultivate six qualities to support our practice. In the discussion that follows, I would like to examine each of them as they relate to the study of taijiquan.

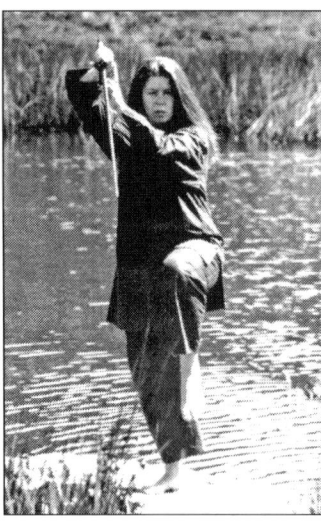 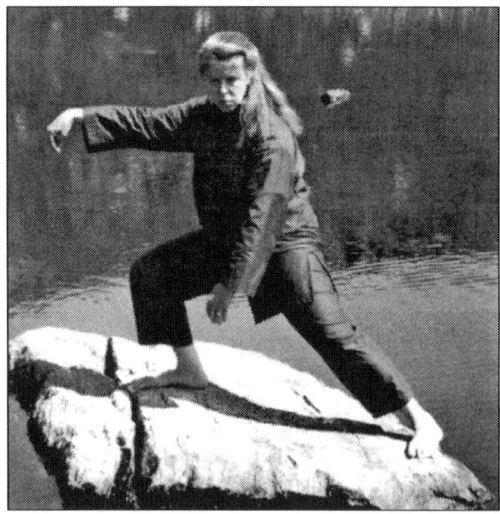

Left: A posture from a taijiquan sword form. Weapons training is a vital aspect of deepening a student's understanding of the taiji principles. Right: The characteristics of water—its flow, softness and ability to accommodate to any shape—are qualities taiji practitioners seek to emulate. Photos courtesy of L. Lehrhaupt.

Effort

Perhaps the most important part of making an effort is taking responsibility for our learning rather than expecting someone else to do our work for us. Though we all would agree that "from nothing comes nothing," we often secretly hope that we can learn something without having to work at it. If we don't learn something, we are quick to blame the teacher or the method rather than examine our own commitment in terms of time and energy.

If there is one hard cold fact about taijiquan, it is that without regular practice we do not progress. We can talk about developing balance or coordination a hundred times, but it will never replace one training session. Developing a consistent practice schedule is not easy; there is so much in our private or work lives that seems to demand our attention. Yet when we don't practice, we set ourselves up for a cycle of disappointment: we don't develop because we don't practice; we don't practice because we don't seem to develop.

When we begin to feel uneasy about how little we practice, we have an excellent opportunity to study ourselves. There can be many different reasons not to practice: we are afraid of not doing it right, we do not feel calm enough, we find it difficult to be alone with ourselves, we feel we are wasting time. Making an effort in this case implies letting these feelings arise and acknowledging them. In doing so, their power to overwhelm or paralyze us lessens, and we can renew our commitment to do it again one more time. We may do this many times, but each time we are getting to know ourselves a bit better. Practicing is something that needs to be practiced. When we give ourselves the chance, the motivation and sense of flow often help us to continue. If we do not choose to continue, then our choice is the result of a conscious decision resulting from the effort to study ourselves.

I have purposely avoided the word *discipline* because I feel we confuse the word *effort* with *discipline*. Discipline often implies forcing ourselves to do something, whatever we feel. Discipline is something we measure in terms of time and amount: the more the better. It often involves ignoring where we are in service to achieving a future goal. Top athletes are said to be disciplined: that many succumb to doping or other unhealthy practices in pushing their bodies beyond human limits is the negative side of this do-or-die attitude to training.

When applied to taijiquan, this kind of discipline hinders rather than furthers practice. We no longer pay attention to our feelings or working with ourselves but emphasize meeting a standard. It is taiji without heart.

Focus

Learning how to learn requires that we develop the capacity to quiet the mind so that we can focus on the work at hand. To quiet the mind does not mean to erase thought, but to dampen and subdue the internal dialogue that occupies so much mental energy. It also does not mean to control thought, but to experience a sense of opening and spaciousness that happens when we are no longer the prisoner of our thoughts and emotions. Mental space is created when we begin to see our thoughts for what they are—just thoughts, and we stop identifying with them as representing who and all we really are.

Simple, clear exercises in which the thinking mind is given a task are the most effective techniques for channeling scattered mental energy into a clear line of focus. Learning a taiji form, which involves repeating each movement over and over, is an excellent practice in this respect. True, not all students experience learning a move as a simple clear task, but when they have the chance to practice over and over, encouraged by a concentrated class environment, their minds have a chance to focus and quiet down. During training they have an opportunity to set aside their mental preoccupation with themselves or with other problems and concentrate on the task at hand. Such concentration, while tiring, can also be rejuvenating and therapeutic.

In taijiquan we have a wonderful opportunity to develop focus—a fine-tuned, laser-sharp concentration that is enhanced by practicing the form and paying attention. Each time we are dreaming, we return to the feeling of muscles and joints moving, the body in motion. It is partly for this reason that learning or teaching a form quickly robs the student of the opportunity to work with precision. Learning a form quickly becomes a rush to get something and display it, rather than experiencing the subtle process of fine-tuning a movement. It leads to a lot of messy, dreamy or even technically competent taiji, but not one that emphasizes the inner development of the practitioner.

Awareness

Joseph Goldstein, a teacher of Vipassana, or insight meditation, describes awareness as "bare attention," which "means observing things as they are, without choosing, without comparing, without evaluating, without laying our projections and expectations onto what is happening, cultivating instead a choiceless and non-interfering awareness" (Goldstein, 1987: 20).

In taiji practice, maintaining bare attention applies to the state of mind in which we learn and teach a movement. For the teacher, it means to emphasize the experience of doing a movement, not demanding millimeter exactness and conformity to some fixed image of the taiji posture. Often the minutely precise corrections that some taiji teachers make are a substitute for good teaching, which involves working with each student personally, where he is at in the moment, rather than simply treating him as clay that can be molded into a dead shape.

Maintaining bare attention for the student means to attempt to be fully present in each moment, to be awake, aware, and able to move and respond to change without resistance. In taiji it means to be here and now when doing the form, not dancing in Dreamland. Moment by moment we experience our body, movement, environment separately and as one. It is the unity and uniqueness of each movement/moment that we experience as the taiji.

Patience

I often tell my beginning students that there is one phrase they are going to hear repeatedly until they think that is all I know how to say. That phrase is, "Once More!" Patience in taiji practice is exercising faith and making a commitment to the learning process of "Once More." What is this process exactly? When we do a movement again and again, our practice is open-ended. Repeating something is not a mechanical re-run of an activity or a determined effort to do something solely to get it right, but a path of discovery. We pay attention to each moment, to experience what we can learn in that moment. It may be something concrete, such as noticing we are not in balance when we take a step, or it may be the joy of experiencing coordinated movement, where effort and flow merge in seamless non-action: doing without doing.

Shunryu Suzuki Roshi, a Zen Master, calls this quality of a discovering mind "beginner's mind." When something is new for us, we are generally open and ready to receive, eager to experience all aspects. When we think we have mastered something, we close down to seeing new perspectives because we've made an investment in knowing. We don't want to risk or challenge this feeling of security. When we lose patience and do not want to try again, we are closing down to life and to learning from our own experience. As Suzuki Roshi writes:

> **In the beginner's mind**
> **there are many possibilities;**
> **in the expert's mind there are few.**
> – Suzuki 1982: 21

Perhaps the most difficult part of repeating something over and over again is learning to work with boredom. In fact, the moment when one is bored is the moment when a deeper level of learning can take place. What we label as boredom is often a simple name that covers much deeper feelings that we do not want to acknowledge: frustration with the difficulty of learning, disappointment at what we label as our own clumsiness, anger at not being quicker to achieve something. Far from being a state of deadness, boredom is a rich field for studying the self and a door to experiencing the preciousness of each moment. It's then that we can go beyond simple mastery or getting a move right and be one with each moment by being awake and aware, with all that is part of it. Being committed to "Once More," to making a gentle resolve to start again in each moment, is the heart of this process.

Gentleness

We often approach learning taiji with a harsh, self-critical attitude that does not allow us to be either patient or gentle with ourselves. We apply the same competitive spirit that is so valued in our world, which leads us to judge ourselves constantly, to set up standards of discipline that are personally difficult to attain, or to emphasize our way as the better one. Perna Chodron, a Tibetan Buddhist nun and student of Chogyam Trungpa, Rinpoche, writes: "Meditation practice isn't about trying to throw ourselves away and become something better. It's about befriending who we already are" (Chodron 1991: 4). If we are to experience taiji practice in the same way—as a continual process of opening to ourselves—then we need to let go of these destructive ideas and practice making friends with ourselves. It is a gentle process of acknowledging our strengths without pride and recognizing our weaknesses without scorn. We try to work with ourselves in the same way we would help a baby stand up after he had fallen. A sense of humor is very helpful in learning to practice gentleness.

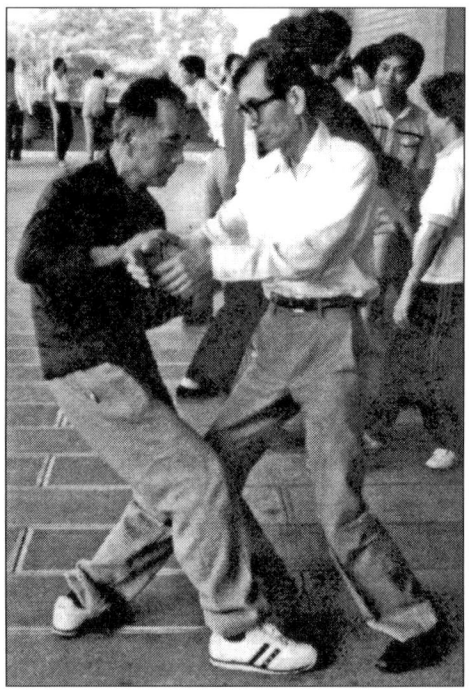

Taijiquan practitioners practicing
push-hands in a park in Taipei, Taiwan.
Photo courtesy of L. Lehrhaupt.

Letting Go

Pema Chodron writes: "The quality of opening or letting go . . . helps us to rediscover this ability that we already must open beyond small-mindedness and to let go of any kind of fixation or limited view. . ... But letting go is not so easy. Rather it's something that happens as a result of working with precision and gentleness. In other words, as you work with being really faithful to the technique in our case, taijiquan, and being as precise as you can and simultaneously as kind as you can, the ability to let go seems to happen to you. The discovery of your ability to let go spontaneously arises; you don't force it" (Chodron 1991: 19).

Letting go of the desire to develop special powers is an important step in taiji practice. There is, unfortunately, a tendency to promote the development of special powers or heightened faculties by teachers and students of taiji and qigong. In one form, it involves repeating stories of famous masters who were said to have such powers as throwing people without touching them or being able to use such powers to bend steel or withstand physical attack without injury. Others talk about mastering qi power and emphasize either its martial arts applications or secret healing techniques. There are investigations of such stories, especially in the sciences of psychology and anthropology, and this is not the place to enter a discussion of whether these reports are true or not. The real problem for students is a spiritual one: seeking extraordinary powers is a misuse of sacred tradition and feeds our ego and need to master others rather than mastering the self.

The most beneficial way to work with the desire to be special is to acknowledge it. Secretly holding onto the wish to be special but denying that we feel this way is a great obstacle to knowing and making friends with ourselves. We all long to be special in some way so that we can feel better about ourselves. When we name it for what it is, we practice being transparent and take the first important step in letting go of the need to be better than others.

In taiji we also experience the difficulty of letting go in learning to relax while doing the form and in practicing push-hands. Letting go in the form means maintaining posture without force, recognizing bad habits, opening to emotional or physical traumas that manifest as unhealthy or stuck body postures—and most of all feeling joy in movement, even if it's clumsy.

Learning to relax in a taiji posture is the most difficult aspect for many taiji students. As a teacher, one often stands before a student whose shoulders are up around his ears as he holds his arms outstretched at chest height, only to be told, "But I am relaxed!" The flood of relief that fills the student's face as he lowers his shoulders when you touch them requires no further comment. What is causing the problem? Poor posture, bad biomechanical habits, inappropriate use of muscular force are all part of the answer, but the source of the problem is that the student is doing the move with his mind, not with his body. When we learn to let go of controlling the movements and let our bodies do the moves, based on correct understanding of how our muscle and skeleton systems work, we discover the great secret of taijiquan as an internal art: effortless power.

Letting go in push-hands includes cultivating a willingness to work with our resistance to close body contact, our fears of getting hurt, our need to win or not lose face. Letting go is supported as we acknowledge our fear, pride, laziness, aggression, lack of self-confidence and any other thing we hide from ourselves, and gently work with them until they no longer control us or remain hidden. Letting go does not mean erasing or blotting out these feelings or pushing ourselves to drop them but making a commitment to face them in gentle awareness.

Wolfe Lowenthal, an American taiji teacher, gives a wonderful description of how we can use push-hands training as a way to study ourselves:

> If in pushing I find my partner straining in resistance, the fault also lies with my use of strength—if I were not being so insistent he could not resist me. Conversely, if I feel my partner's hand force building up on my body, it is because of my resistance—if there were no resistance, he would have nothing to push against.
> – Lowenthal, 1991: 132

When we train in push-hands and let go of the need to win, the person opposite us becomes a partner, not opponent, in our joint effort to explore the true spirit of taiji: what we learn about ourselves through "investment in loss."

When teachers say that taijiquan is a life-long practice, there is often a misunderstanding at to what this means. Often students believe this refers to perfecting the different forms or mastering push-hands to the point where one always wins. But the essence of taiji has nothing to do with perfecting technique or mastering something. It has nothing to do with mastering oneself, if by that we mean controlling our thoughts and feelings or reflecting a perfect image of the Master. It is the practice of learning how to learn or resting in beginner's mind, moment to moment. It is the practice of the student who, frustrated and angry at not getting "it," starts to walk out the door, returns to his training place and makes the gentle vow, "I'll try once more."

References

Chodron, P. (1991). *The wisdom of no escape: And the path of loving kindness.* Boston: Shambhala.

Goldstein, J. (1976). *The experience of insight: A simple and direct guide to Buddhist meditation.* Boston: Shambhala.

Lowenthal, W. *There are no secrets: Professor Cheng Man-ch'ing and his tai chi chuan.* Berkeley: North Atlantic.

Suzuki, S. (1970). *Zen mind, beginner's mind.* New York: Weatherhill.

• 6 •
Thoughts on the Classic of Taijiquan
by Carol M. Derrickson, M.A.

"Using the interchange of yin-yang duality to control one's opponent."

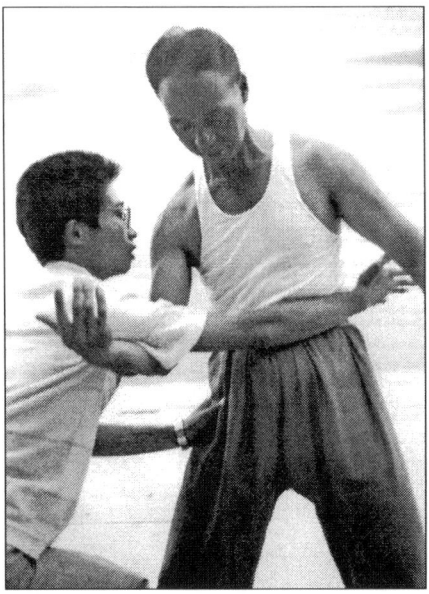

Punch, pull, or push, Mr. Chen Xiqi remains unmovable after many varied attempts were made to topple him. The Chen-taiji stylist lives in Hangzhou, China. Photo by M. DeMarco.

Introduction

Over the years that I have been a student of taijiquan, my teachers have spoken to me of the wisdom of the *Taiji Classics* and I have read a few translations and commentaries of these classics. Somehow, the ideas never quite settled inside me, never quite made sense. Since I know some Chinese, I decided to tackle translating Wang Zongyue's *Classic of Taijiquan* myself. It's written in literary Chinese, a style quite unlike modern spoken Chinese, so the process has been a long and interesting journey toward understanding the wisdom of the classic.

The *Classic of Taijiquan* posits the essentials for completely understanding the workings of the universe as expressed in movement in martial arts. Three aspects dominate the classic as it constructs this framework: 1) defining the meaning and importance of taiji, 2) coordinating all movement in terms of the *shisan shi* or thirteen stances, and 3) using the interchange of yin-yang duality to control one's opponent. Wang argues that these essentials place the practitioner in a superior position which not only allows one to defeat opponents but offers him spiritual growth. Though several significant secondary themes are also woven into the text, these three repeatedly dominate the work.

My Chinese language source was a version edited by Tang Hao of Taiwan. Using the traditional literary Chinese format of adding one's own commentary to an original document, Tang incorporates his editorial comments with the *Classic of Taijiquan* by Wang Zongyue in the volume entitled *Wang Zongyue Taijiquan Ling Yanjiu*. In this study, the classic includes seven parts: 1) *Shisan Shi Lun* or "A Discussion of the Thirteen Stances," 2) *Taijiquan Lun* or "A Discussion of Taijiquan," 3) *Taijiquan Lie* or "An Explanation of Taijiquan," 4) *Shisan Shi Ge* or "Song of the Thirteen Stances," 5) *Dashou Ge* or "Song of Push-hands," 6) *Shisan Shi Xing Gong Xin Lie* or "Expounding on the Central Focus in Performing the Thirteen Stances," and 7) *Shisan Shi Mingmu* or "The Names of the Thirteen Stances."

Tang discusses historical documentation and argues that Wang Zongyue is the author; nonetheless, Wang's authorship is not verified. If Wang were indeed the author, information about him is surprisingly sketchy and inconsistent. Several specialists place him in the Ming dynasty (1368–1644). The piece is written in the literary Chinese of that period, which indicates that an educated person wrote the text. So, if Wang is the author, he would probably have been a member of the educated elite of traditional times. The debate over authenticity and historical documentation continues. Regardless of historical documentation, what is clear is that the ideas of the classic are sufficiently valuable that they have been handed down to succeeding generations. They are the focus of this chapter.

A few quite competent taiji specialists have translated Wang's piece, but the quality of those translations varies considerably. For example, the opening line of Section Two, "A Discussion of Taijiquan" or *Taijiquan Lun*, is translated by Jou Tsung Hwa as follows: "Tai-Chi is born of Wu-Chi. It is the origin of dynamic and static states and the mother of Yin and Yang" (1980: 181). The same line is found in Sophia Delza's *Body and Mind in Harmony* with translation credits given to three other people: "T'ai Chi is infinity, the absolute; it is the mother of Yin and Yang, of everything male and female" (1961: 183). Whereas both translations are basically "correct," Jou's is more readable and direct.

Similar variations can be seen in translations of the next line. T. T. Liang's version in his *T'ai Chi Ch'uan for Health and Self-Defense* reads: "In motion they separate; in tranquility they fuse into one" (1974: 33). In contrast, the same line from Lo's *The Essence of T'ai Chi Ch'uan: The Literary Tradition* reads: "It is not excessive or deficient; accordingly, when it bends, it then straightens" (1979: 31). Liang's translation flows more smoothly and conveys the essence of the idea more clearly.

Part of the problem in understanding the meaning of this classic is in understanding the individual terms with their various spellings, implications, and uses. A background of Chinese philosophy is essential.

The Meaning of Taiji

Clearly identifying and differentiating the two terms *wuji* and *taiji* is the first hurdle. The two major romanization or spelling systems converting Chinese characters into Westernized spellings are Wade-Giles and Pinyin. The Wade-Giles traditional spelling of the two terms are *wu chi* and *t'ai chi*. However, *t'ai chi* is often written incorrectly as *tai chi*. The Pinyin spellings, *wuji* and *taiji*, are closest to their correct pronunciation and will be used here. (When two different spellings for the same word are given hereafter, the first will be Pinyin and the second Wade-Giles, e.g., *qi/ch'i*).

In the term *wuji*, *wu* means "without" or "void"; *ji* is "to the utmost point" or "ultimate." Together they mean "ultimate void" or "ultimate nothingness." In traditional Daoist/Taoist philosophy, wuji is the creative void from which all conscious thought and all ideas spring. *Wuji* gives rise to *yi*, "intention" or "ideas."

So, *yi* means "idea," "intention," or "will," and it is the product of *wuji*. Wang asserts: "Common to everything is *yi* or intention, which does not reside in the outer aspects of movement" (Section One: 2). When the creative forces of *wuji* produce an idea, that intention is put into practice externally as *taiji*, the interplay of yin and yang.

Tai means "very," "much," "excessive," "too." Combined with *ji* as above, taiji means "very ultimate" which doesn't sound quite right in English. So, it may be translated as the "grand ultimate." Daoist philosophy conceives of *taiji* as the workings of yin and yang, the spiraling, ever-changing movement, which is the physical, real-life expression of meaning or thought. From the unity of *wuji* comes the duality of *taiji*.

The duality called *yin* and *yang* is the balance of opposites which characterize the cosmos. The opposites are not in struggle against each other. For one to be healthy, happy, and effective as a martial artist, yin and yang must be in balance in every way. Yang is direct light, the sun. It is hot, aggressive, dominant, the male principle, and it is also expressed in odd numbers, spicy food, cooked food, the governing vessel of the body. In contrast, yin is reflected light, the moon. It is cold, passive, yielding, the female principle, and is also expressed as even numbers, bland food, raw food, the conception vessel of the body. So, taiji is expressed as yin and yang in harmony.

Keeping these concepts clearly in mind, then, I translate the passage referred to above from the original Chinese manuscript as follows:

Taiji zhu	That which is taiji
wuji er sheng	is born from wuji
yin yang zhi mu yeo	and is the mother of yin and yang.
Dong shi ze fen,	When moving it separates,
jing zhi ze he	and when quiet it rejoins
wuguo buji	without excess or deficiency . . . .
	– Section Two: 3

However, more important than individual words and translations are the concepts, the heart of the matter.

This passage means that each person's mind is like *wuji*, the grand void, the ultimate nothingness. It is the creative pool from which ideas, thought, and plans of action spring. It is quiet until the idea is brought into being, until action begins. And it returns to quiet when action is completed.

When movement is initiated and the plan is put into effect, taiji begins. Taiji is movement which expresses the ultimate duality, yin and yang. This interplay of opposites encompasses all movement in taijiquan. For example, in stepping one distinguishes the weighted or yang leg from the less-weighted or yin leg. Ward off is counter-balanced by rollback, and so on.

Simply put, this principle means that in taijiquan one moves when there is a specific reason to do so. The reason may be to respond to an attack or to take advantage of an opponent's vulnerability. Whatever the reason, one moves because an intention or action plan exists which requires movement to execute it successfully.

The *Shisan Shi* or Thirteen Stances

The thirteen stances hold the key to understanding how to move properly and effectively, so Wang devotes much of the classic to discussing the meaning and importance of these movements. Specifically, the content of Sections Two, Six, and Seven focuses on these stances. Wang explains that the thirteen are the combination of movements based on the traditional Five Elements or *wuxing/wu hsing* and the Eight Trigrams or *bagua/pa kua*. The thirteen stances literally form the framework of movement within which taiji is expressed by directing movement to the four major directions, the four oblique corners, and the center. By understanding the subtleties and nuances of the thirteen stances, one learns how to use them to execute any plan of action effectively.

The term translated as "stance" is *shi/shih*. It could also be expressed as "gestures" or "positions of power." *Mathews' Chinese-English Dictionary* also gives the following definitions for *shi*: power, influence, authority, strength, aspect, conditions, and circumstances (1963, #5799: 412). Though the diversity of meanings seems bewildering at first, together they have as a common theme the focus on outer appearance in a position of power or authority. By combining movement based on the Five Elements and the Eight Trigrams, Wang was indicating that such movement was a microcosm, an expression of the entire cosmic order on a small, personal scale. Moreover, the corresponding movement is inherently powerful, and the stances are positions of strength. From this perspective, it is essential to understand the inherent quality of striking energy and the degree of yin-yang quality that exists in each of the stances. Wang, therefore, delineates each in detail in his text. My diagram of "The Thirteen Stances" (see page 71) visually expresses this combination of the Five Elements and the Eight Trigrams and locates the self in the cosmic order.

In traditional Chinese thought, the Five Elements were metal (literally, gold), wood, water, fire, and earth. They correspond with many aspects of health and the body. For example, they are linked with the five internal organs (lungs, liver, kidneys, heart, and spleen), and the five sense organs (nose, eyes, ears, tongue, and lips).

From the point of view of movement, each element also has a corresponding position on the compass, a quality of energy, and type of action. Metal is in the southerly position where the sun is strongest and is, therefore, a strong yang stance. Its energy type is *pi* which means "to split," "chop," "cleave," or "divide." Hence, one can *pi shou* or thrust forth the hand as in a chop. And in overall body movement, metal corresponds to the aggressive, active movement of stepping forward or advancing.

In contrast, the wood element is in the most northerly position which is colder and thoroughly yin in quality. Its energy type is *beng*, which means "to burst," "break open," or "be hit by something." So *beng lie*, for example, would be to break open by a general fist strike or a vibrating palm. In general movement, wood expresses its yin quality by yielding, retreating, or stepping backward. Just as trees or plants are passively yin, so is this type of movement.

The water element is associated with the westerly direction and works with *zuan* energy, which means "to drill," "bore," "get into," "go through," "penetrate," "pierce." For example, *zuan xin tou gu* would be to penetrate the heart and pierce the bone using a strike which shocks one's opponent's entire physical system. Generally, the water element is linked with the act of looking to the left or regarding movement on one's left, since as one faces the north, west is on the left.

In contrast, in the easterly position is the fire element. Its energy type is *pao* which means "to fire" as a cannon; or "to put to fire," as "to fry or roast in a pan." *Pao hong* action is bombardment, pummeling one's opponent. Since east is to the right when facing north, the direction marking the rise of the fiery sun, the fire element corresponds to gazing to the right or regarding movement on the right.

The fifth element is earth which lies at the center. It corresponds to *heng*, a mixture of unrestrained violence with obstructive movement sideways or across a path. *Heng zhu le* is "to block," "to stop," "to parry." The earth element's generalized stance is to be solidly in place in a stable equilibrium. In taijiquan forms this is the stance known as *wuji* or "preparation"; the preparation move sets the stage for the plan of action which is the taijiquan form itself.

Coordinated with the Five Elements are the Eight Trigrams or *bagua/pa kua*. They are best known in the *Yijing/IChing*, which explains their relationship to the cosmos and the meaning of life. Expressed in groups of three lines, the yang lines are solid, and the yin lines have one break in the center. The *bagua* are drawn as yang lines, yin lines, or varying combinations of lines. Identified by their position on the compass, each trigram expresses a type of movement, a characteristic aspect or quality, and an image. Together they guide the practitioner in perceiving the order of the cosmos.

South is expressed by the three solid lines which are completely yang, the source of the sun and heat. Its aspect is creative and dynamic; its image is Heaven or moving upward to the heavens. So, in movement, the southerly trigram is aggressive as *peng* or ward off, a forward and upward movement.

Southwest incorporates yin as its third line; its aspect is gentle or penetrating and its image is the wind. In China, the equatorial winds move from southwest to northeast, so southwest would seem to be the source of the wind. Its movement is *cai*, meaning "to pick" or "to gather," also "to pluck" or "to pull." Wind pulls most strongly over land as a tornado, although it will also often act through simple wind gusts. Though not fully yang, its movement is still powerful. Interestingly, in contemporary Chinese, "to catch a cold" is *shangfeng*, or literally "harmed by the wind." The power attributed to wind has ancient origins.

West is two lines of yin on either side of a yang line; that creates the rudimentary form of the character meaning "water" and water is the image attributed to the west. Its aspect is abysmal. Gradually becoming more yin in quality as one approaches the north, this trigram's movement is *ji* meaning "to push against someone" or "to press." Similarly, as water presses forward it can wear away whatever lies in its path.

The trigram in the northwesterly position is a yang line over two yin lines. Its aspect is that of keeping still or being hard, and its image is that of mountains. Its hardness is yang, but its immobility is yin. The movement for northwest is *kao* or "shoulder stroke," take literally as "leaning against someone." So, in performing the shoulder stroke, one feels solid like the Himalayas, the Kunlun Mountains, or the other mountains which lie to the west-northwest of China.

North's trigram, in counterbalance to the south, is completely yin in nature and is portrayed as three broken lines. Its aspect is receptive, yielding; its image is the earth. Movement is manifested in *lu* which is "to yield" or "to rollback." Just as the earth is receptive and yields to forces acting upon it, in movement one gives way and draws energy toward oneself.

The trigram in the northeast is two yin lines above a yang. Its image is arousing, and its image is thunder. As for movement, *lie* is "to split" or "split energy." With thunderstorms comes lightning, which has an arousing effect on people. Lightning also splits apart trees and other objects. So, in movement one has vibrancy and force to rend asunder.

East's trigram is yang, yin, yang. Its aspect is clinging, and its image is fire. Push or *an* is its movement. The magnificent ball of fire, the sun, seems to push its way up into the heavens from the east, characterizing the nature of this movement.

Southeast is a yin line over two yang lines, creating the aspect of joyousness and having the image of a lake. In movement, it is *chou* or "elbow stroke." In southeast China is a large lake region, including the famous West Lake outside of Hangzhou. One might think of nudging a friend with one's elbow to get his attention to share some happy event or to share the beauty of the lake.

The Thirteen Stances, Five Elements and Eight Trigrams

Trigram's Aspect = shown in ( ). Element's Action = shown in [ ].

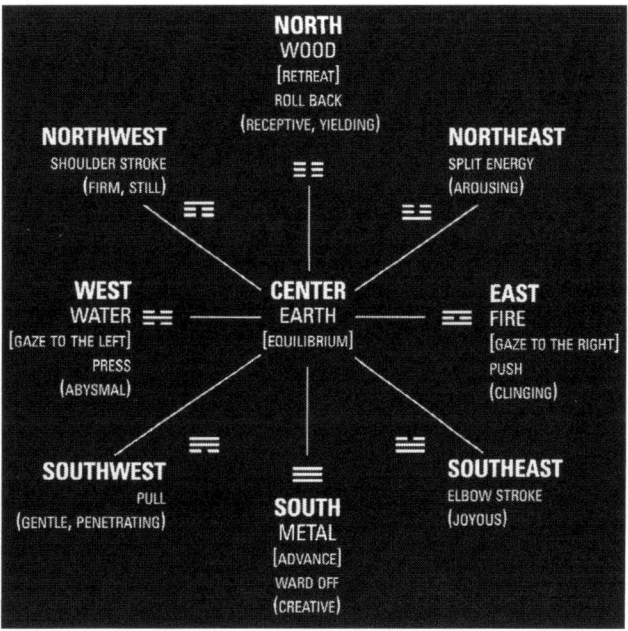

By understanding the subtleties and nuances of these thirteen stances, one can adjust one's own movement to control one's opponent. They are the key to understanding one's own yielding and aggressive energies as a miniature of the cosmic order, a reflection of the yin-yang balance of life itself. Wang remarks in the *Song of the Thirteen Stances*: "The thirteen postures as a whole should not be treated lightly. Their significance springs from the waist. They alter and revolve emptiness and solidity in accordance with the intention one has kept in mind . . ." (Section Four: 8). In movement properly based in the thirteen stances, then, the duality of taiji is clearly expressed. Correctly executing this duality marks the secret of success for taijiquan.

Balancing Yin and Yang Energy

With the thirteen stances, one starts at the center, forming the pivotal focus of one's own microcosm, aware of what is to the left and right and ready to advance or retreat. But as movement is initiated and one plans to move into one of the stances, an interplay of yin and yang also begins.

The classic strongly emphasizes the significance of maintaining a proper balance between the two energies, balancing the dualities in movement:

> Where there is up, there is also down; where there is left, there is also right. If one intends to move upward, then one also entertains a downward intention. If one intends to raise something upward, one must in addition employ the idea of pushing it downward. In this way its roots are naturally severed. This way invites [its] ruin, without a doubt.
> – Section One: 2

Though duality itself is important, how one uses the interchange effectively is what achieves success. In the same section Wang explains:

> [The concept of] emptiness and solidity ought to be clearly distinguished. Anyone place naturally has its own inherent emptiness and solidity, but each place is always in this way also unifying emptiness and solidity. The body is section by section threaded together, so not even an interval the size of a silk fiber or plant thread should be severed.
> – Section One: 2

Defeat is assured if the continuity is severed, and an imbalance is created. Further, success is achieved, and defeat is averted when the ability to yield is the focus of movement:

> By facing forward and yielding backward, one attains a strong position that is like the moving force of the universe. If there are areas which do not have such a strong stance, it is because the body is uncoordinated, and movement is confused. That defect of necessity lies in the failure of the waist and legs. Movements upward, downward, forward, backward, to the left, and to the right are all like this.
> – Section One: 1

And even more specifically:

> If one's left is subjected to weight [from one's opponent], then the left should be emptied. If the right is subjected to weight, the right should be emptied. If [one's opponent) bends downward, then one becomes completely unfathomable. . ... If the other person is moving with haste, then respond hurriedly. If the other person is moving slowly, follow slowly. Although transformed in a myriad of ways, the principle is to be as one string of cash (i.e. to have continuity) . . . The other person won't know me; I alone will know the other person.
> – Section Two: 4

Such movement is also identified by certain terms:

> When the other person is hard and unyielding, and I am gentle and yielding, it is called *zou* or "withdrawing." When I move in accordance with another, it is called *zhan* or "attaching."
> – Section Two: 3

Ultimately, defeating the opponent comes as the result of proper movement incorporating the acts of yielding and attaching.

Spiritual Energy as the Unifying Entity

What has been described so far is like a three-dimensional puzzle or frame. The parts all fit together in a particular way with the self at the center of the microcosm, and movement is in a constantly changing balance of yin and yang based on the thirteen stances. When the opponent challenges that microcosm, yielding and attaching are the primary means for bringing that person under control.

The last dimension to add to the framework is the spiritual or inner aspect. Clearly identifying the terms used in the classic helps. Wang distinguishes between *qi* or "life energy" and *jing*, which is "stimulated qi" or "moving qi." These two terms are primarily dealing with the unseen but physical aspect of life force, as the classic explains:

> As one becomes experienced, one gradually apprehends and understands *jing* or "moving energy." From understanding *jing*, moreover, one by steps reaches spiritual elucidation. In this way one does not use force. Otherwise, how could clear understanding be possible? . . . One must understand yin and yang. Attaching, then, is yielding, and yielding is attaching. Yin is not separated from yang, and yang is not separated from yin. Yin and yang assist each other. In this way one understands how to move energy.
> – Section Two: 4–5

So, on the external side, yielding and not using force are essential. Internally, understanding how to move one's own energy and then moving one's opponent's energy is crucial.

Now this concept of "reaching spiritual elucidation" mentioned above is somewhat vague. The term used here is *shen*, often translated simply as "spirit." I understand the term to incorporate both the physical dimension of what T.T. Liang calls "spirit of vitality" and the internal realm which has to do with the heart and life essence. So, the classic states (Section One: 1): "When the qi is properly excited, spiritual energy [*shen*] is properly practiced within." Jou cites the same idea as the Daoist principle "*lian qi hua shen*," or "transferring physical force into spiritual power" (1980: 213); in other words, through the practice of using the qi, one is transformed spirituality.

One aspect of this process resides in the concept of heart-mind, the term or concept of *xin*. In summary, the classic argues that using *xin* or heart-mind to move the qi makes the qi penetrate the bones. Using qi to move the body, therefore, is deriving benefit from the heart-mind. A light spiritual essence is thus cultivated.

From the martial arts point of view, understanding these concepts and incorporating them into one's fighting technique make one unbeatable. Or as the classic says (Section Two: 4): "A brave hero for whom there is no match is the one who cultivates this in every respect and achieves it." The classic goes even further in its claims that yielding and attaching make one's fighting successful:

> Thus, though there are a wide variety of able martial arts groups, their power and energy differ from that of taijiquan. For the most part, it doesn't go beyond the strong taking advantage of the weak, the slow yielding to the fast, those who are powerful striking the powerless, and the slow of hand yielding to the fast of hand... Note that four ounces can move aside 1000 pounds [by yielding]. It is evident that one is superior by NOT using force. Behold the form by which a seventy or eigthty-year-old person is able to withstand a multitude. How can the fighters who focus on being fast be able to put the principles of yielding and not using force into practice?
> – Section Two: 4–5

This approach is one reason why taijiquan is called the "grand ultimate hand-to-hand combat."

My journey toward understanding the wisdom of the classic, then, goes beyond simply translating terms, creating diagrams, and defining concepts. If these are in fact the fundamental truths of the universe, what is written here goes beyond mere dictums for defeating an opponent. The classic discloses the way that we can be most stable, productive, healthy, and whole in both the physical and spiritual realms.

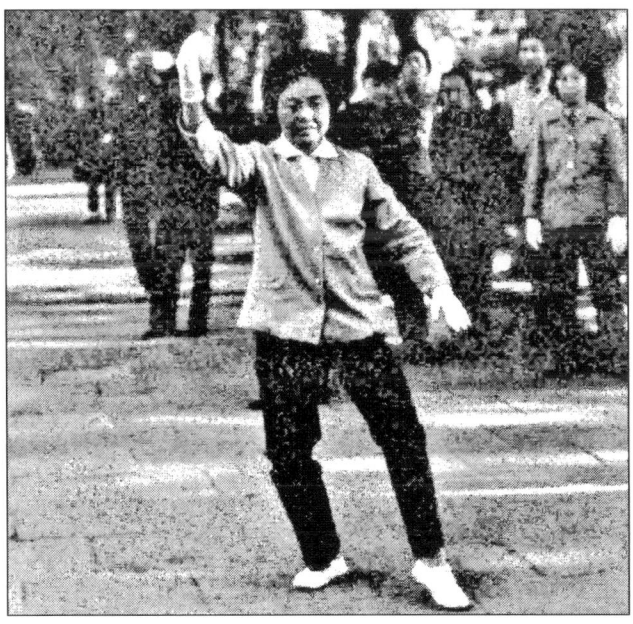

A master exhibiting the harmonizing of yin and yang within the movements of the set. Here, in "white stork spreads wings," one leg is light while the other is weighted; One hand moving high right, while the other is weighted and low left.

The problems of living and moving as a microcosm of life itself are obvious, but not insurmountable. The classic provides many examples, images, and instructions to help its readers understand and execute these important ideas. The following are paramount:

1) Let the creative void of *wuji* give rise to an intention which can be put into practice as taiji;
2) in carrying out the plan, consider the nuances of the thirteen stances and the framework of the Five Elements and the Eight Trigrams in choosing the one(s) which match the problem; and
3) incorporate the harmony of yin and yang as they interplay in yielding and attaching to one's opponent.

These suggestions should not only bring victory but also spiritual understanding, creating a wholeness or melding of the physical, spiritual, and cosmic realms.

References

Cao, Zhiqing. (1988). *Xingyiquan lilun yanjiu*. Beijing: Renmin Tiyu Publications.

Bu, Sophia. (1961). *Body and mind in harmony: T'ai chi ch'uan*. New York: Cornerstone Library.

Jou, Tsung Hwa. (1980). *The tao of tai-chi chuan*. Piscataway, NJ: Tai Chi Foundation.

Liang, T.T. (1974). *T'ai chi ch'uan for health and self-defense*. New York: Random House.

Lo, Benjamin Pang Jeng. (1979). *The essence of t'ai chi chuan: The literary tradition*. Berkeley, CA: North Atlantic Books.

Mark, Bow-Sim. (1979). *Taijiquan genben jiaocai*. Taiwan: Shijian Press.

Mathews, R.H. (1963). *Mathews' Chinese-English dictionary*. Cambridge, MA: Harvard University Press.

Tang, Hao (Ed.). (1971). *Wang Zongyue taijiquan jing yanjiu*. Taiwan: Haulin Publishers.

Wu, Jinrong (Ed.). (1983). *The pinyin Chinese-English dictionary*. Beijing: The Commercial Press.

The Development of Zheng Manqing Taijiquan in Malaysia
by Nigel Sutton, M.A.

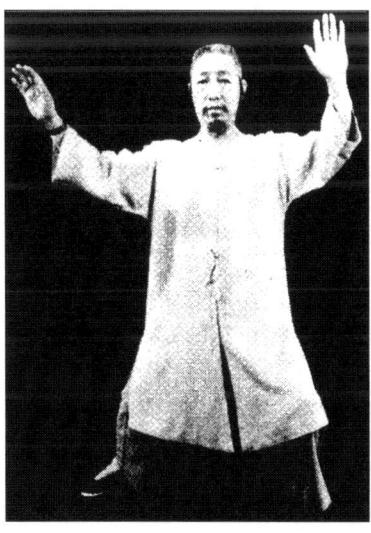

Zheng Manqing moving into embrace-tiger posture.
All illustrations courtesy of Charles E. Tuttle Co.

Most authorities on taijiquan acknowledge the development and existence of five main schools that have come into being as distinct entities during the later part of the twentieth century and the early part of this century. It may be argued, however, that the style most responsible for the enormous growth of awareness and practice of the art on the world stage is that which in Asia is referred to as the Zheng Style, after its founder, Zheng Manqing. While the founder always acknowledged the Yang style origins of his art, his teacher being Yang Chengfu, as time passed and Zheng applied his experience in other related fields to his teaching of taijiquan, it became apparent his art had grown into a distinct style.

To understand the art of Zheng Manqing, it is essential to know something about the man himself. A staunch traditionalist, professor of art, renowned calligrapher, and accomplished doctor of Chinese medicine, Zheng was also an innovator and was thus forced to live on that knife edge, peculiar to Oriental cultures, where demand for the observance of long-established tradition must be weighed against the necessity for innovation and progress. That this state of dynamic tension was of concern to Zheng is illustrated by the reference he made to it in his writings. In essay number 6 of book 3 of his *Manran san lun*, Zheng talks about "understanding change," detailing when change should occur. Although ostensibly writing about painting, everything he writes may be applied to taijiquan. In essay number 8, entitled "Reckoning Mastery," his comments may also be directly applied to his experience of taijiquan (Wile, 1985).

Although in his writings on taijiquan Zheng always named Yang Chengfu as the source of his knowledge, in an article on the development of power in calligraphy he revealed the important role of the Zuo Laipeng system of internal strength training in the growth of his own skill and in his understanding of the art (Wile, 1985: 148). Indeed, it is generally recognized by practitioners of the Zheng Style that it was the injection of the core elements of the Zuo system into his thirty-seven-posture form that made his system unique.

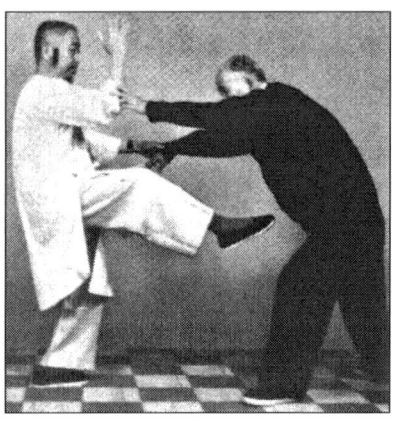

Zheng with T. T. Liang Tongcai.
An application of golden cock stands on one leg.

The thirty-seven postures themselves are based closely, if only superficially, on the Yang Style form, and Zheng gave as his reasons for shortening the traditional form a combination of personal impatience and laziness, as well as the demand for a shorter period of study if the art were to be popularized.

To understand the essence of Zheng's form, we have to look beyond this smoke screen to see that the emphasis is on principle rather than technique, and so contained within the form are all the movement principles that may be found in the traditional form but without so many repetitions of particular movements. So, while it may not contain such moves as fan through back, needle at sea bottom, or part the horse's mane, the principles these postures embody may be found in fair lady plays shuttles, planting punch, and left and right ward off respectively.

What exactly the Zuo system consists of is a source of contention among Zheng's students, and this I will examine later, when discussing the style's practice in Malaysia. Suffice it to say that at this stage it places a greater emphasis on *song* (Wile, 1985: 148), taijiquan's state of alert relaxation, than does the Yang Style.

There is much disagreement, even among Zheng's long-term disciples, as to his personal training history, and probably the closest we come to a definitive version is given in his obituary/biography.[1] It is stated there that in his youth Zheng studied Shaolin boxing but later took up taijiquan for the sake of his health. One cryptic sentence alludes to his studies with Zhang Qingling, from whom he learned the Zuo method. That Zhang was his martial arts elder brother in the Yang family tradition caused some difficulties in that Zheng could not openly refer to him as his teacher.

Song Zijian, one of Zheng's oldest surviving students in Taiwan, asserts that Zheng was sent to Zhang Qingling to learn push-hands, armed with a letter of introduction from his teacher Yang Chengfu. The particular approach to push-hands he was to learn from Zhang Qingling was *song rou* push-hands, which may literally be translated as "relaxed and soft," both of which are hallmarks of the Zuo system and were to become the same for the Zheng system.[2]

While Zheng himself was always passionately interested in the martial aspects of the art, in attempting to popularize it he stressed those aspects he felt legitimized the art, both as the pursuit of a learned gentleman and of a person seeking the widest range of benefits. Because of his medical background and his own experience of being cured of tuberculosis through practice, he stressed the art's strengthening and curative aspects.

As a student of Chinese philosophy, the relationship of the *Yijing* and the *Daodejing* to the philosophical foundation of the art were of great importance to him. Additionally, as a practitioner of the fine arts, both the aesthetic qualities and the striving for perfection of form were of great concern to Zheng's development and approach to taijiquan.

The most obvious changes Zheng made, other than shortening the form, were softening and relaxing the postures, so some exponents of the Yang Style accuse Zheng stylists of doing "old man's taijiquan." It would be a mistake, however, to assume this external appearance of ease means the postures themselves are effortless. Because of the required degree of profound relaxation, a great strain is placed on the supporting leg, so what in Yang Style is often described as being a 70-30 stance becomes a 99.9-0.1 stance, the numbers describing the percentage of weight on each leg. The aim is "to borrow the strength of the earth and the qi of the heavens," which means, in terms of form, the legs do the work while the upper body is kept as empty and relaxed as possible.

In form practice, Zheng emphasized adherence to principle rather than an overemphasis on the techniques represented by individual postures. In Zheng Style the purpose of form is to teach the basic principles such as sinking, relaxation, and the constant interchange of yin and yang, as found in the changes from substantial to insubstantial and then back again.

As well as shortening the form, Zheng only emphasized one of the three traditional taiji weapons, the straight sword, because it most exemplifies and embodies the principles of the art. Zheng also introduced the sword sticking exercises that are another hallmark of his style. In this freestyle exercise, the practitioners keep their sword blades in contact as they maneuver, attempting to attack their opponent without losing the connection. This exercise is a logical extension of push-hands and is particularly effective for training *tingjing*, or sensitivity. In addition, Zheng emphasized a range of auxiliary exercises for the development of *neigong* (internal strength). These exercises are widely regarded as elements of the Zuo Laipeng system.

The exact date when Zheng Manqing first devised the thirty-seven-posture form is unclear, although in his writings he stated that he first taught it in 1937 in Henan Province (Wile, 1985: 192). Song Zijian also remembers it as first being taught then, although he stated that Zheng only had six or seven students at the time.[3] Chia Siewpang, who studied with Zheng in China, relates that he learned the form from him in 1936 (Chia, 1983).

When he went to Taiwan in 1949, Zheng's government connections and, particularly his relationship with Chiang Kai-shek's wife, to whom he was a personal art tutor, ensured that his taijiquan would become popular in certain circles. Indeed, some critics believe Zheng Style is presently in a weak state because his first generation of students in Taiwan was, overall, composed of intellectuals and academics.

Zheng's teaching career in Taiwan spanned a period of twenty-five years, and during this time he taught hundreds, if not thousands, of students. Consequently, students not only reached varying levels of skill but also brought to the art different interests and expectations.

The most obvious differences are in the appearance of the form. Those who learned with him in the earlier years practice a form more closely resembling that of the Yang family, while later students perform in a softer, more rounded fashion. There is much dispute among these students as to whose form is more authentic, although this tends to be debated rather than contested in more physical terms. The one exception to this is the case of the dispute between Wu Guozhong and Chen Zichen (a.k.a. William C.C. Chen). Chen started learning from Zheng while still a young boy, even living at his house for a while. Later he went to America, where he developed a large following.

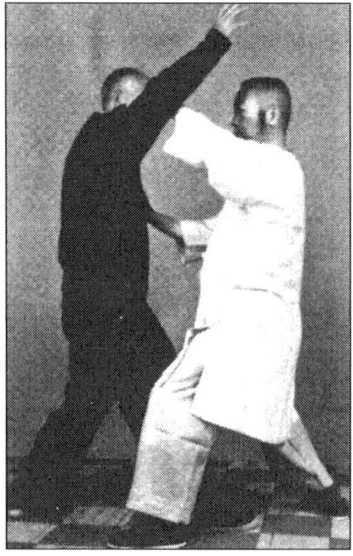

An application of fair lady works at shuttles.

Wu Guozhong, by contrast, only became a disciple fourteen months before Zheng's death, although by his own report he had been training with him for a period of five years or so (Wu: n.d.). Wu claimed, after Zheng's death, to be the only disciple to have learned the "real" taijiquan. Obviously, this claim angered many of his fellow disciples, and this was further compounded by the fact that he was extremely successful, collecting thousands of students throughout Southeast Asia. Finally, in the late eighties, matters came to a head and Chen Zichen took up the gauntlet on behalf of his martial art brothers and sought to arrange a match with Wu. After much dispute over the rules, referees, and formalities, nothing was finally agreed, but the whole incident serves as an illustration of the tensions existing in the Zheng system after his death.

There had, however, been tension prior to Zheng's death, one cause being his decision in the mid-sixties to leave Taiwan for the United States. While the reasons for his move are known among many of his Chinese disciples, they are personal and are not commonly spoken of. Suffice it to say that, to the possible surprise of many of his Western students, it was not for altruistic reasons or to share his art with the world.

Many of his later Chinese students were eager to know just what he taught while in America, and particularly among second- and third-generation students in the East, any information about the nature of his teaching is zealously sought, as are any films featuring him.

No discussion of Zheng's career would be complete without mention of Robert W. Smith, who studied with him in Taiwan and, through his books and articles, made Zheng's taijiquan prowess known through the English-speaking world.

When Zheng's taijiquan was introduced to Malaysia, the pragmatic attitude of the martial arts there necessitated that a visiting teacher be prepared to demonstrate the practical applications of their skills. This was because, for historical and political reasons, the Chinese regard themselves as a threatened minority in Malaysia. They are, it is true, in a minority, and certainly there has been oppression, mostly political and occasionally physical, which has provided some justification for their fears. This oppression has resulted in a wholehearted embracing of traditional Chinese culture, whether remembered and passed down from generation to generation or imported by Chinese experts, initially from Taiwan but more recently from mainland China.

Most Chinese immigrants arrived during the British colonial rule and hailed from the southern provinces of Fujian and Guangdong.[4] Once in Malaysia they settled primarily in dialect groupings, reproducing the settlement patterns of their native land. Thus, one finds Kuala Lumpur and Ipoh predominantly populated by Cantonese speakers, while in Johor Baru the Chinese are mainly speakers of the Fujian dialect.

The immigrants went to Malaysia fleeing injustice and starvation, or sometimes even as indentured slaves. They were primarily from the lower strata of society and generally in China had little or no access to the so-called higher aspects of their culture (Pan, 1991).

Over the years, however, the descendants of those immigrants have prospered and laid the foundations for the emergence of Malaysia's thriving economy. And with their increasing prosperity they have sought to protect and develop their Chinese identity. This has meant the establishment of private schools; the sponsorship of cultural events, such as Chinese opera, art, and calligraphy exhibitions; the establishment and continued support of religious institutions; and the teaching of Chinese martial arts.

In the case of the latter, there was already a strong foundation in place from the early days of the first mass migrations. The clan wars that raged throughout the southern provinces of China during the nineteenth century resulted in mass migration, both voluntary and involuntary, and these disputes, which pitted village against village and dialect group against dialect group, spilled over into the new land so that age-old feuds were continued on foreign soil (Pan, 1991). Many of the masters I have interviewed in the course of my research have recounted tales of "experts" from China being "imported" to solve problems or train students from a particular dialect group so they might defend themselves against other Chinese!

Master Ng Kionghing, a member of the Hakka dialect group who teaches taijiquan in the southern Malaysian town of Batu Pahat, told me his teacher of Li Jia boxing had been invited over from China by fellow Hakka from his region to help protect them.[5] This same master pursued a vendetta against a master of Hong Jia boxing from a neighboring town, ostensibly over lion dance performance rights, but more probably because several generations earlier a master of the Li Style had been beaten by the famed Huang Feihong, the grandmaster of the Hong Jia teacher in the next town.

The settling of disputes through gongfu continues well into the twentieth century, and it was only the increasing prevalence of modern firearms that put traditional fighting skills on the back shelf. The years of fighting and skill testing, however, had established in the Malaysian Chinese martial arts community an attitude of putting one's money where his mouth is and determining the efficacy of technique rather than relying on discussions of philosophy and theory.

While it could be argued that this emphasis on practical application is generally true of Chinese martial arts, the trend, certainly in the latter part of the twentieth century, was to emphasize the healthful and recreational aspects of the arts. Both in Taiwan and China, standardization and an overemphasis on the aesthetics of movement have resulted in a general watering down of the combat elements of the arts.

To a certain extent Zheng himself was involved in this process in Taiwan, but due to his reputation as a person with fighting prowess, a somewhat paradoxical situation arose: while attempting to promote the more cultured aspects of his art, he recruited most of his better students by defeating them in challenges of one form or another. Wu Guozhong, Ong Zichuan, and Yue Shuting all reported it was because of losing to Zheng that they became his disciples.

Probably the first teacher to introduce Zheng's taijiquan to what was then Malaya was Huang Xingxian. A native of Fuzhou Province, he had previously studied Fujian White Crane Boxing and in 1955 was taken by one of Zheng's disciples, Yue Shuting, to become a disciple himself. Then in 1956, he went to Singapore and started teaching. A year later Yue Shuting also went to the Malayan peninsula, visiting Penang, where he decided to settle down and start teaching. Yue was originally from Wenzhou in Zhejiang Province, the same area Zheng came from, and prior to meeting Zheng he had studied Shaolin Boxing. He started studying taijiquan with Zheng in the late 1940s in China.

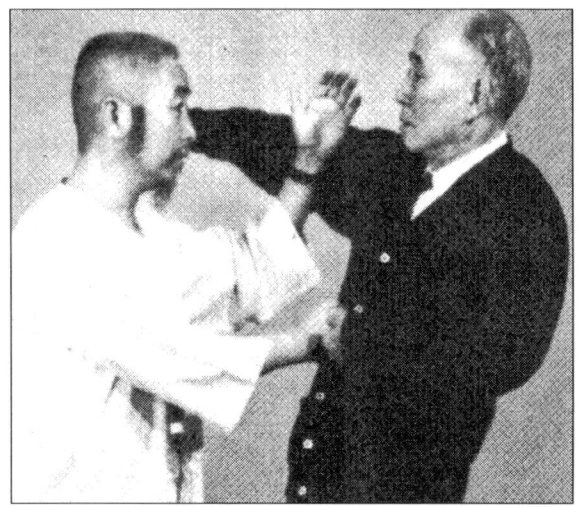

After step forward, deflect downward, Zheng follows with the parry and punch sequence.

Yue Shuting was responsible for starting a taijiquan dynasty that produced probably the strongest fighters in Malaysia and did much to promote the art as a truly effective fighting style. A small man who photographs reveal as thinner and even shorter than Zheng, himself not very tall, Yue soon made a reputation for himself by taking on and beating all comers.

Li Beilei, a teacher renowned throughout Malaysia for his fighting prowess, trained briefly with Yue Shuting before going on to become a disciple of Yue's most famous disciple, Lu Tongbao. Li recalls it was the fact that he was soundly beaten by this little man that made him give up the Shaolin Luohan boxing he had been practicing and take up taijiquan.

When Yue went to Malaysia, he took with him an old friend from China who had trained in Yang Style and who taught the *sanshou* (dispersing hands) two-person form, which Zheng did not teach. Gradually two-person sanshou came to be accepted as a part of Yue's teachings. He also reintroduced some of the moves Zheng himself had omitted, stringing them together into a sequence of eighteen movements he added to the end of the form and simply called the "lower eighteen hands."

These changes reportedly caused Zheng some sadness[6] and he is supposed to have said that some of his students had seen fit to add on extra movements while he, an old man with fifty years of experience, was only really clear about the movements up to the first cross hands (less than a third of the way into the form!). Yue, however, continued to teach his way and, in fact, always referred to what he taught as Yang Style. Indeed, some of his students report that when he first started teaching in Penang, it was the traditional Yang long form he taught.[7]

Yue died on June 16, 1975, only a few months after Zheng Manqing. He was in his mid-sixties and suffering from complications associated with a hole in his heart, which he had from birth. Sadly, he was in Thailand at the time because he had been forced to leave Malaysia due to immigration problems that some aver were deliberately stirred up by jealous rivals.

His most famous student, however, outlived him by another nine years, and was able to pass on Master Yue's unique approach to the art. Lu Tongbao, a heavily built native of Fuqing city, who had previously studied Fujian dog boxing and who owned a tea shop in Penang, trained a whole generation of teachers who are still active throughout Malaysia. Lu died in the early 1980s, but not before he had taught the likes of Li Beilei, Lim Suowei and his brother Lim Souyuan, Chen Huayi, and Lau Kimhong. All of these students suffered and learned at the not-so-gentle hands of Master Lu. Indeed, Lau Kimhong recounts that their sparring mainly consisted of Lu beating them up.[8]

In 1958 Zheng Manqing himself visited Malaysia and Singapore, staying for several months and, according to Song Zijian and Zheng's Malaysian students, teaching a set of neigong exercises that had not previously been taught to his disciples in Taiwan. For some of the time he stayed with Lu Tongbao in Penang, but he also visited Kuala Lumpur, where he gave a demonstration in the Jing Wu stadium, inviting challengers from the audience to come and "try" his gongfu—swiftly and effectively vanquishing all such attempts. After this, Zheng Style taijiquan in Malaysia developed in two main streams: that of Yue Shuting/Lu Tongbao and that of Huang Xingxian.

In the 1980s another teacher appeared on the scene, Wu Guozhong, a former Nationalist soldier who claimed to have learned the "real" Zheng Style taijiquan. His high tuition was based on this claim. Teaching his disciples what he claimed to be the authentic teachings of Zuo Laipeng, he charged anything between $1,000 and $2,000 of the local currency to people wishing to become his disciples, after which they would become eligible to learn the "secrets." The bad blood caused by his claims and by his material success culminated in the previously mentioned challenge match with Chen Zichen. In the meantime, exponents from the Yue/Lu stream had not been idle. Taking exception to his statement in a Malaysian national Chinese-language newspaper that Malaysian taijiquan had gone down a blind alley and was nothing more than dancing, Li Beilei, Zhou Mutu, and Lim Souyuan went to "call" on him during a talk he was giving. They invited Wu to prove his ability with actions instead of words. Unable, for whatever reason, to meet their challenge, in the pragmatic climate of the Malaysian Chinese martial arts world, Wu quietly faded from the scene. Of the several thousands who had flocked to become his disciples, most were disappointed by his failure to prove himself and to reveal any "secrets" of real value, and only two or three hundred are now left.

Each of the three main streams has its unique characteristics. Practitioners from the Yue Shuting tradition tend to emphasize more "muscular" taijiquan and are active on the tournament scene. In the last two international taijiquan championships held in Taiwan, the Malaysian team has been almost exclusively made of exponents of this tradition. Their attitude seems to be very much one of taking what works and applying it, whether it be to push-hands or fighting.

The Huang Xingxian stream in Malaysia, prompted in recent years by Huang's own demonstrations of his seeming ability to send his students flying with just a twitch of his finger, has degenerated into a limp parody of the skill that Huang was reputed to have had in his earlier days. However, in Taiwan, exponents of Huang's approach to taijiquan demonstrate a much more realistic approach to the art with a proven ability in both push-hands and application. The situation that has arisen and perpetuated among Huang's students in Malaysia is due to one of those cases of apparent mass hypnosis that occur periodically in the world of martial arts, whereby a first generation of adoring and overawed students place all their faith in a master figure and attribute their initial lack of expertise and inevitable defeat at the hands of the master to some almost magical power they feel the master will always have over them. This belief then becomes fixed so that, almost despite their best efforts, they feel unable to gain the master's skill. Indeed, the students come to feel this would be impossible because the master has the "power."

This situation then becomes institutionalized, with each successive generation of students "teaching" their successors to respond to the master's touch in the appropriate way. Thus, in many videotapes one can view Huang merely tapping his students, who then engage in gymnastic contortions as they hurl themselves across the room with looks of awe and wonder on their faces. Sadly, in his later years Huang, who died in 1992, seems to have believed in his own ability to perform these amazing feats. When he occasionally encountered those who would not throw themselves at his slightest touch, he either sought to intimidate them by striking them as he pushed with them, or to attribute their failure to "fly" to a high level of gongfu on their part.[9]

Wu Guozhong's students have, however, gone one step further, falling back on a hoary old chestnut: "We cannot practice freestyle push-hands with people outside our school because our qi might damage them." Their reliance on such arguments suggests that the role of hard physical work (*gongfu*) has been all but eliminated from their training program. Inspired perhaps by their master's stories of the secrets of the "real" Zheng Style that he alone learned, at present they rely mainly on long-winded and intellectual expositions of just what exactly their taijiquan is all about, rather than developing the solid skills that would substantiate their claims.

The three main streams of Zheng Style may be further characterized according to the different emphasis of each group. Because of the rough and ready atmosphere that existed at the time Yue Shuting started teaching, a tradition was swiftly established in which exponents proved the validity of their art in a practical and sometimes violent manner. While students of this stream, particularly those who learned from Lu Tongbao, still adhere to this philosophy, there has been a tendency among some students on the periphery of this group to become uneasy about the inability of their teachers to explain the finer points of the theory and philosophy that are the foundation of the art. Thus, these students have often found themselves in a seemingly never-ending search for a teacher who can both explain the principles and apply them. This search has led many to mainland China, yet few have found the satisfaction they seek, as the world of taijiquan is littered with fine "talkers" who prove to be less than adequate "doers."[10]

While Huang started teaching in Malaysia at the same time as Yue, whether by accident or design, he ended up with a different type of student, many of whom seemed to be in search of magic and were not too curious about the exact nature of this magic. Several sources I have interviewed in the course of my research have pointed out that, while the successors of Yue Shuting have gone on to carve out reputations for themselves as master instructors in their own right, none of Huang's students has done the same. Indeed, among his students there is very much a cult of the master.[11]

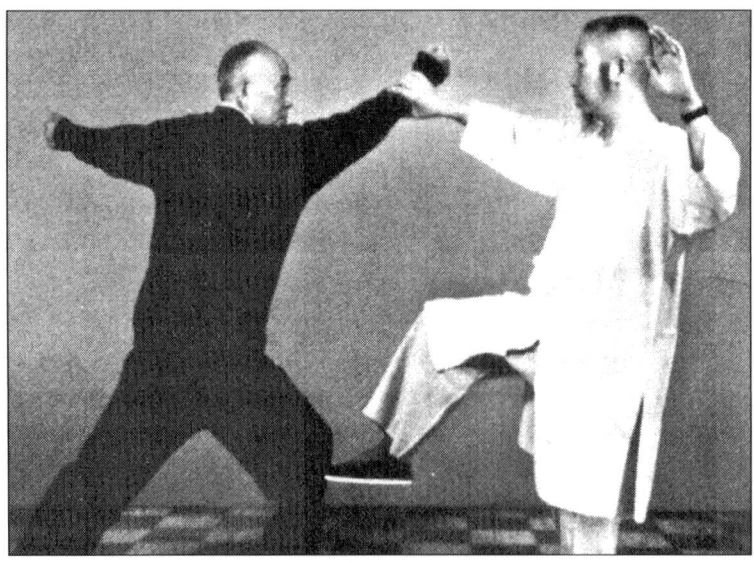

An application of separate right foot.

Wu Guozhong, coming later to the scene with his promise of access to the innermost secrets of Zheng's system, initially attracted students from a wide range of backgrounds, but as his power base in Malaysia became more established, he began to surround himself with intellectuals and high-level businessmen. Cynically, one could observe that these people not only offered the most in terms of material advantage but also posed the least physical threat. Indeed, many of his current students are particularly attracted by the intellectual and highbrow approach he takes in his teaching. Currently one of Wu's leading students, Dr. Wong Bingfeng, teaches a course in taijiquan and related Chinese philosophy at the Malaysian Institute of Arts, a private tertiary education institute in Kuala Lumpur.

In the last two years, Wu's organization has been further weakened by the departure of his chief instructor, Koh Ahtee. Koh might well be typical of the new generation of adherents to the Zheng Style, as his training career has constantly centered on the desire to learn as much as possible about what Zheng actually taught. Koh's defection, taking with him many of Wu's senior students, decimated Wu's Shenlong Association.

Koh Ahtee is interesting to anyone wanting to speculate about the future of Zheng Style in Malaysia, as he has trained extensively in both Wu Guozhong and Lu Tongbao streams. He started studying taijiquan at the age of fourteen, becoming a disciple of Master Lau Kimhong, who was himself a disciple of Lu Tongbao. Lau, intent on proving the efficacy of taijiquan, had early in his career entered a Southeast Asian full-contact fighting championship and taken second in his category, only failing to get first place because of disqualification.

The young Koh impressed Master Lau with his hard-working attitude, and soon he had become one of his best students. Accompanying Lau Kimhong on trips to his various classes around southern Malaysia, Koh had plenty of opportunities to learn from the best of Master Lau's contemporaries. Then, hearing about Wu Guozhong's claims, Koh Ahtee sought him out. At that time, however, Wu was not in Singapore, but Master Tan Chingngee was taking disciples on his behalf. In the Zheng tradition as promulgated by Wu, disciples were often taken into the tradition but not directly by the teacher concerned. Master Tan had visited Taiwan when only eighteen years old in 1974. While there he had trained with Zheng and, according to some, had become his disciple. This claim is open to dispute, but Koh to this day believes it to be true. Wanting to learn more of what Zheng taught, Koh asked Master Tan if he could become his disciple. This was highly irregular, as Koh was already a disciple of Master Lau and, furthermore, Master Lau and Master Tan had been friends for several years.

Out of respect for Master Lau, Koh told him of his intention to become a disciple and Master Lau, furious at his student, punished him by making him kneel in front of a picture of Zhang Sanfeng for several hours. Then, when Wu reappeared on the Malaysian scene after working in America, Koh announced to Master Tan his intention of becoming Wu's disciple. Now it was Master Tan's turn to be furious with his promising student, but all to no avail, for Koh had made up his mind. Showing the same dedication to training that he had with his previous teachers, he swiftly rose to become chief instructor for Wu's Shenlong Association in Kuala Lumpur.

Finally, disillusioned with what he saw as the widening gap between the teachings of Wu and the original doctrine of Zheng Manqing, Koh left to set up as an independent instructor in his own right. Since then, he has sought to adhere strictly to Zheng's teachings and has become a successful professional instructor. Being only in his mid-thirties, he may be able to reach the highest levels of the art. Indeed, Koh might prove to be the helmsman for a new generation, a new breed of Zheng stylist, combining as he does the "show me" attitude of the Yue Shuting stream with the purism and strong theoretical and philosophical base of the Wu Guozhong stream.

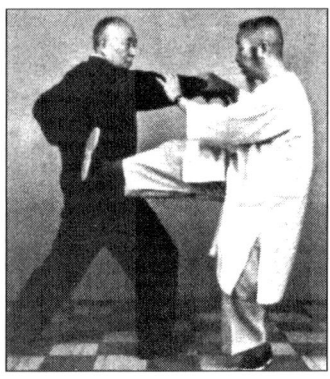

An application of turn body and sweep lotus with leg.

Utterly unintimidated by other martial artists of any discipline, Koh is always willing to demonstrate his skills in whatever fashion is the most appropriate, and in his constant search for more knowledge, he seeks out practitioners of taijiquan with a reputation for having gongfu and seeks to determine whether the reputation is deserved.

Prior to the 1990s, Zheng Style was probably the most popular style of taijiquan in Malaysia, due not only to the efforts of the three streams described above, but also to the relative underexposure to other styles caused by the political situation in Malaysia. In response to the years of the Emergency, when war was waged against the communist guerrillas, the Chinese population came under suspicion and the Chinese government's support of the rebels meant not only did Malaysia have no diplomatic ties with the country, but her Chinese citizens were not allowed to visit the motherland until after retirement. It was only after the final surrender of the remaining communists at the end of the 1980s that this ruling was relaxed and Chinese of all ages could visit China. This political change also opened the doors to a flood of martial arts coaches from the People's Republic of China who previously had only been permitted to teach in Singapore. The new market proved particularly profitable for them, and they now visit in a constant stream, so representatives of all the major styles may now be found running variously thriving associations throughout Malaysia.

Since the mid-1980s there have also been an increasing number of competitions held in Malaysia. These range from competitions only for taijiquan forms and push-hands using Taiwan rules, to the mainland Chinese–inspired wushu competitions, with their standardized forms and emphasis on aesthetics. The presence of these competitions has further divided Zheng stylists with, as might be expected, the Yue Shuting/Lu Tongbao descendants entering and enjoying considerable success, while both Wu's students and Huang's have, overall, been critical and reluctant to participate.

What then are the major differences in training methodology among the groups? As has already been mentioned, practitioners of the Yue stream refer to their art as Yang Style, although most of them have given up teaching the long form. Zhou Mutu reported to me that this is due to the lack of patience of present-day students.[12] They do, however, teach broadsword, which was not a part of Zheng's curriculum. Straight sword is also taught, but not staff or spear. The sanshou solo and two-person forms are taught after the taijiquan solo form and the lower eighteen hands have been learned. Push-hands features prominently with both a series of basic exercises and freestyle being taught. Although the *peng-lu-ji-an* (ward off, rollback, press, push) pattern that was such a vital part of Zheng's curriculum is known, it is not emphasized.

The disciple system is still used widely, although some teachers, such as Li Beilei, have simplified the ceremony while retaining the essence, namely that there is a body of knowledge that is not openly taught. At the heart of this "secret knowledge" is the system of qigong and body conditioning taught by Zheng to Lu Tongbao during his trip to Malaysia in 1958. Many outsiders and even Zheng stylists from Taiwan have denied that such a system existed and say it comes from "external style" martial arts and was probably introduced by Lu himself. Whether this is true or not, all the exponents I have interviewed hold strongly to the view that it came from Zheng. Having talked to people from the different branches of Zheng Style as well as those in Taiwan, I have concluded there are enough similarities in methodology to suggest the system did in fact come from Zheng; such similarities include emphasis on relaxation and gradual progress.

In schools of the Yue/Lu stream, the art is still emphasized as martial in origin and application, and it is not unusual to find sandbags hung in the training hall and on occasion some form of sparring included in the training for senior students. No great emphasis is placed on philosophical explanations or detailed examination of theory; instead, the emphasis is very much on the practical. Perhaps because of this, the students tend to be younger than in other schools, the average age being between twenty-eight and thirty-eight.

In Huang's schools a great deal of time is spent on achieving the elusive state of *song* (relaxation), with a number of auxiliary exercises created by Huang prominent in the curriculum. Practitioners of this stream practice their form at a slower pace than most other exponents, arguing that this better enables them to concentrate on *song*. Huang also devised his own fast form for practicing applications, but how widely this is taught I do not know, only that some exponents refer to it.

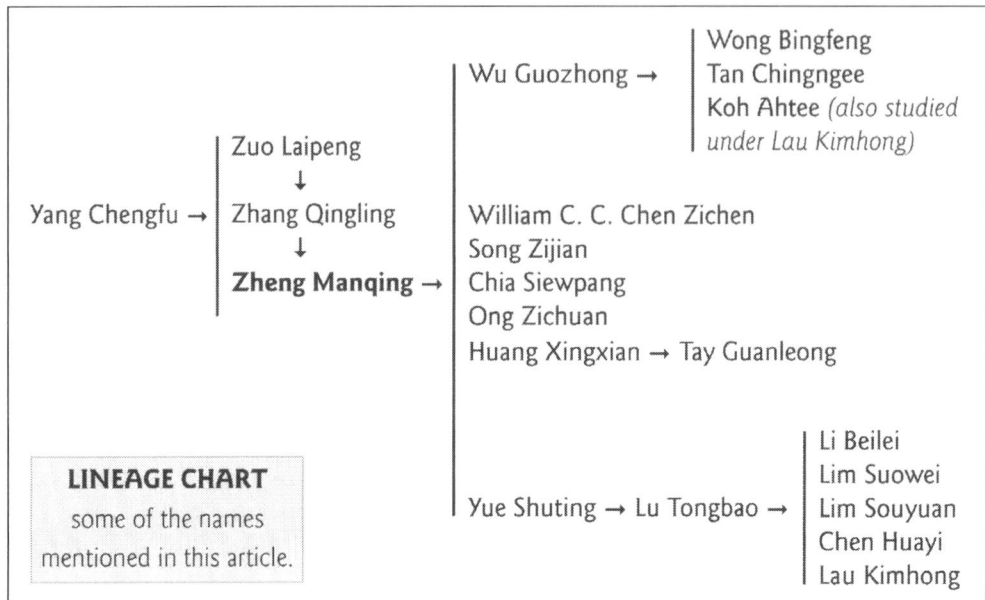

LINEAGE CHART some of the names mentioned in this article.

Huang was reputedly very traditional and secretive, and he certainly took disciples. Indeed, one of his senior students, Master Tay Guanleong, told me when he first approached Huang about becoming a student, after thinking it over, Huang invited him to come and live in his house for three months so he could observe him firsthand and decide whether he were worthy.[13] Other members on the periphery of Huang's organization seem less certain about the value of such secrecy, advocating the open sharing of knowledge and, where their understanding is limited, borrowing from a wide range of sources.[14]

While weapons such as the straight sword are taught, undoubtedly the most important aspects of Huang's approach to Zheng Style are the solo form and auxiliary qigong. Push-hand exercises and freestyle push-hands are both taught, but many of Huang's students, instead of spending their time building a solid foundation, seek to reproduce Huang's magical feats and suffer some discouragement when failing to do so.

The curriculum taught to students in the Wu stream follows what Wu claims to have learned from Zheng, consisting of form, push-hands, and straight sword. A system of qigong is also taught using sandalwood for massage of vital points. As mentioned before, the training emphasizes theory and philosophy, and there is not much room for physical experimentation.

The whole question of application is treated in an abstract manner, an approach that is justified according to Zheng's own writings. In a section on sanshou in the *Thirteen Chapters*, he wrote: "If one is able to interpret energy and master the techniques, one's applications will be successful" (Lo and Inn: 1985). What he does not reveal, however, is exactly how to "interpret energy and master the techniques."

At present, Zheng Style in Malaysia is going through further changes. The death of Huang Xingxian has precipitated a power struggle among his students, despite the fact that, prior to his death, he named his son-in-law as his successor. Wu Guozhong still visits Malaysia from time to time, but his arrival is no longer heralded by large-scale publicity, as it once was. The majority of Lu Tongbao's students who are now teaching are in their fifties and seem to be enjoying some success in training a new generation of students. Their competitive spirit now serves as a major focus for both the development and recognition of skill.

Whatever happens in the future, however, the unique circumstances of the Malaysian Chinese—their desire to explore their Chinese heritage together with their geographical distance from Taiwan, where Zheng Style is arguably stagnant—combine to ensure that Zheng Style will continue to grow, evolve, and flourish.

Notes

1. Published in *Full Circle*, a publication compiled by a group of Zheng's former students in the United States after his death. The biography was translated by Tam Gibbs, and the full text in Chinese may be found on the wall of Zheng's tomb in Taibei, Taiwan.
2. Personal interview conducted by the author, September 1992, in Taibei, Taiwan.
3. Personal interview conducted by the author, September 1992, in Taibei, Taiwan.
4. For more information on Chinese immigration to Malaysia, see Pan, *Sons of the Yellow Emperor*.
5. Personal interview conducted by the author, June 1991, in Malaysia.
6. Personal interview with Koh Ahtee conducted by the author, February 1993, in Malaysia. Koh as a disciple of Wu Guozhong was told this anecdote by Wu.
7. Personal interview with Li Beilai conducted by the author, June 1991, in Malaysia.
8. Personal interview with Lau Kimhong, June 1991, in Malaysia.
9. Personal interview with Koh Ahtee conducted by the author, February 1993, in Malaysia. Koh had such an experience pushing hands with Huang.
10. In March 1993 a guest teacher from China, teaching a variety of forms of taijiquan and qigong and explaining them in relation to the *Yijing*, found his classes undersubscribed, despite initial enthusiasm, after he was bested in push-hands by several local exponents whose skills might best be described, even by themselves, as average.
11. Personal correspondence with a few of his students has confirmed this, as have the squabbles over leadership of his organization that have occurred since his death, as none of the senior students is perceived as having the same high level of skill.
12. Personal interview with Zhou Mutu, June 1991, in Malaysia.
13. Conversation with Tay Guanleong, April 1993.
14. Private correspondence with Huang's students.

Bibliography

Chia, S., and Goh, E. (1983). *Tai Chi: Ten minutes to health*. Singapore: Times Books International.

Lo, P., and Inn, M. (Trans.). (1985). *Cheng Tzu's thirteen treatises on t'ai chi ch'uan*. New York: North Atlantic Books.

Pan, L. (1991). *The sons of the Yellow Emperor: The story of the overseas Chinese*. London: Mandarin.

Wile, D. (Comp. and Trans.). (1985). *Cheng Man-ch'ing's advanced form instructions*. Brooklyn, New York: Sweet Ch'i Press.

Wu, K. (n.d.). *Tao tai chi health*. Self-published.

An Encounter with Chen Xiaowang:
The Continuing Development of Chen Style Taijiquan
by Dietmar Stubenbaum

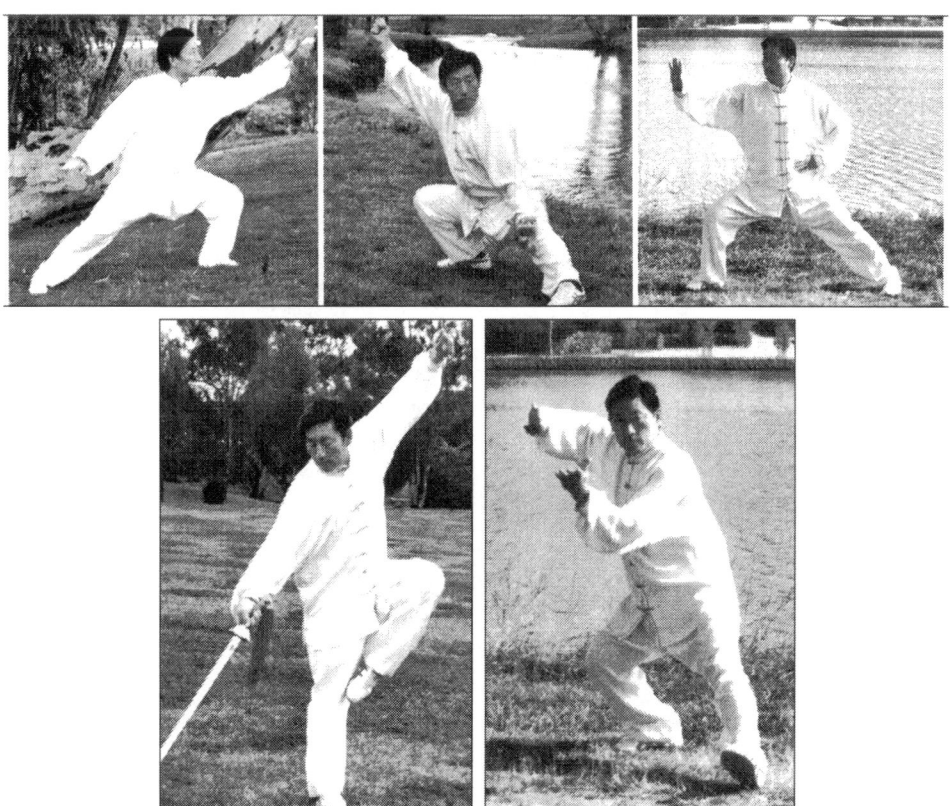

Photographs courtesy of Chen Xiaowang.

Introduction

The following material is provided as a result of a visit made to Chen Xiaowang's house in Australia in November, 1993. I stayed in his home for one week to receive personal instruction in Chen Style taijiquan and to arrange this interview. One of the first things I noticed about Chen Xiaowang is his extremely busy schedule. He is kept busy teaching, giving many private lessons and also instructing various groups. In most of his classes, students are learning the new Chen Style form he created which contains thirty-eight movements. In other classes students are studying the first and second routines of the old family (*laojia*) system, and some advanced students are studying the "sticky spear."

I studied every day with him for about three hours. When could we conduct an interview? It was difficult to find time because he was either busy teaching, interpreters were not available, or there was some such distraction. Luckily, we finally did find time to sit down to talk. Two of Mr. Chen's students, Ms. Pow Yin Chau and Mr. Francis Heng, assisted in interpreting. Without their kind help the interview would have been impossible. But even with their help, it was difficult to conduct an in-depth interview as I would have liked. For example, questions regarding lineage could not be answered satisfactorily since some resource materials which could have provided answers were still in China. Also, there was a collection of photographs in China which could have been used to illustrate the history and evolution of Chen taijiquan. So, in addition to the interview, I present some information regarding the instruction I received personally as well as the general impression I received of this nineteenth-generation Chen Style taijiquan master.

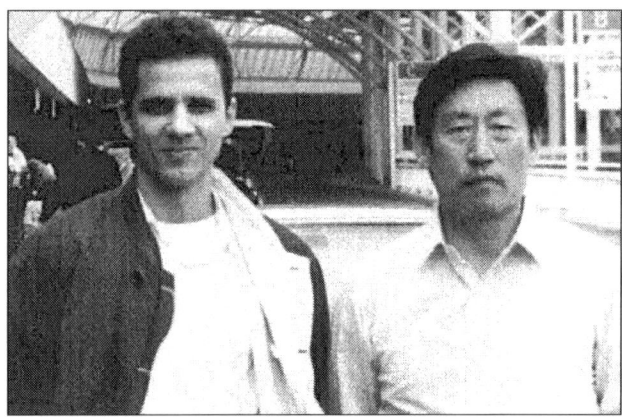

Chen Xiaowang and Dietmar Stubenbaum
at the airport in Australia.

Chen Xiaowang—The Gentleman

As a famous Chinese "cultural treasure," it is surprising to find how friendly Chen Xiaowang can be. Unlike many other martial art masters who choose to remain aloof, Mr. Chen is quite personable. Perhaps it was because his wife and three sons are not yet in Australia that he welcomed my company. Or perhaps part of his openness came from knowing my own interest in Chen Style taijiquan as an adopted "Chen family" member in the lineage of Tu Zongren and Du Yuze, which stemmed from his great grandfather Chen Yanxi. Or perhaps his kindness came simply from his being a gentleman who enjoys being hospitable to guests. When he told me, "Make yourself at home," it was easy to see that he meant it. One of the pleasures this invitation offered was the opportunity to watch hours of his video collection, which proved highly instructional in itself.

Mr. Chen is a quiet person who feels very comfortable here in his peaceful home in Australia. He's a very simple man who likes to relax in between his hectic schedule. When home, he often goes outside to eat fruit, to float in his pool on an inflated raft, or to converse with friends. A big flower garden perfumes the area and draws an array of chirping birds.

Mr. Chen goes to sleep early since he gets up quite early every morning to exercise. Sometimes he goes through the taijiquan forms, but he also spends much time on qigong practice. Nearing fifty years of age, Mr. Chen looks very healthy and much younger than he is. He has a very strong build, especially his legs. Without being muscle-bound, his upper body has very smooth features. He is strong and powerful, continually maintaining a very straight posture in his taijiquan and daily movements.

People from around the world have contacted Mr. Chen for lessons in taijiquan. Many of his students studied from other teachers of various styles. Their past martial art experience helps them to realize how lucky they are now to be studying with Mr. Chen. Much of his personality can be seen in how he teaches. He teaches in his own way. The best way to describe this is to write about my own experience studying with him. Looking back over my years of martial art training in Europe, Japan and Taiwan, this experience proved to be the most insightful.

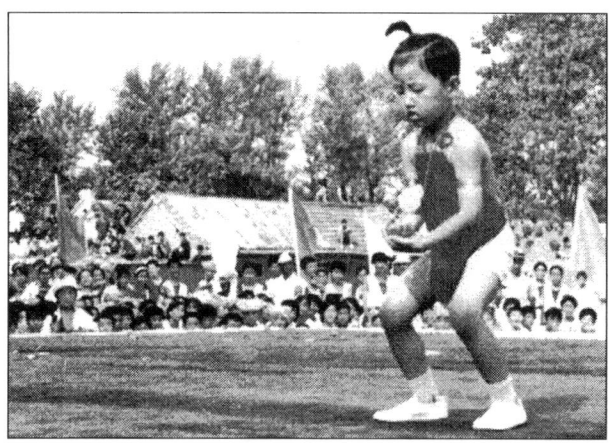

Chen Xiaowang's three-year-old son performing
Buddha's warrior attendant pounds mortar.

Method of Instructing

As mentioned previously, I studied with Chen Xiaowang for three hours per day for one week. Although I already learned the two routines of laojia in Taiwan from Mr. Tu Zongren, Mr. Chen chose to teach me a basic qigong practice to start. This was a standing qigong practice in which one stands erect with both hands extended to the front at chest level, palms facing each other.

Even in this simple posture, Mr. Chen's corrections seemed to offer an endless stream of advice on how to make improvements. The overriding advice was to relax: relax the arms, relax the breathing, relax the legs, feet, little toe. Relax, relax, relax . . .. This basic exercise focuses on letting the qi flow into the hands and to other areas of the body. One ends the exercise by lowering the hands to the dantian, the area a few inches below the navel, and rotating the hands thirty-six times to the left and then to the right.

After I had done this qigong practice for a few days, following all of Mr. Chen's detailed corrections, for the first time ever I felt a very strong feeling of qi moving in my body. Some real changes occurred which I would not have experienced without Mr. Chen's guidance. I felt extremely comfortable even with these basic exercises. I think the primary reason for any progress made was his ability to direct my practice into a deeper state of relaxation than I could have reached before.

Mr. Chen then proceeded to give instruction in individual taijiquan movements, paying attention to movements focusing on single-hand movements, double-hand movements, and the basic steps. Just by visual observation, he can identify any place where one's muscles are tight and where they are relaxed. He points out exactly how the hands and elbows must be, how and why the qi flows or stops. At the same time, he often explains qi movement by referring to acupuncture points. He may show how the qi circulates from the small finger to the shoulder or how it moves from the hands to the back at the same level as the dantian, through reference to the meridians found in acupuncture charts. He teaches these basics in such a detailed fashion that through practice it becomes easier to visualize the internal movement of qi. The results can be felt in better concentration and in the awareness of changes occurring in the body regarding the qi flow.

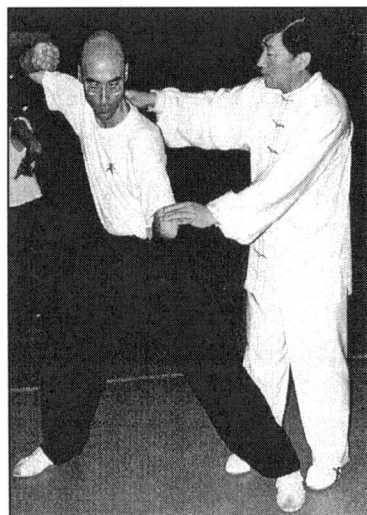 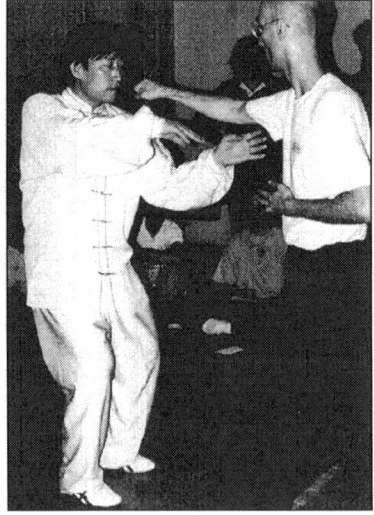

Chen Xiaowang corrects a student's form during a seminar in Italy.
On the right, he is illustrating an application of
Buddha's warrior attendant pounds mortar.

We then incorporated these lessons in correcting my practice of the first of the two routines of the laojia system. The rest of my lessons focused on improving this routine. Even though I had been practicing this set for years, in a short time the set felt much more comfortable under Mr. Chen's guidance. He also showed me some of the standard applications for each technique in the set, including single whip, Buddha's warrior attendant pounds pestle, etc. He used numerous holding techniques (*qinna*) on me. This proved to be an extremely painful experience! Whenever I tried to attack or push him in any way, I quickly found that I just couldn't do anything. At the same time, his techniques flowed easily according to his will. Before this, I thought I had some knowledge about how to push someone. With him, it was just like trying to push a void. I just couldn't move him no matter how I tried. It was impossible. If one were to try to push him, one would be thrown several meters. In fact, I fell quite often following my attempts to topple him. These practical lessons left no doubt about how fully he knows his art.

Mr. Chen is very, very powerful and knows the martial applications to perfection. I have never seen anyone playing taijiquan as well as he, plus his method of instruction is clear and easy to understand. He gives the student all the information he needs to make very fast progress. Of course, Mr. Chen has his price for his instruction, which I found to be worth the investment.

Mr. Chen practices four standard routines of the taijiquan system: *laojia*, first and second routines, and *xinjia*, two routines developed by Chen Fake. In addition, he has developed his own Thirty-Eight Style routine. Two-person practices include push-hands and the sticky-spear routines. He also trains with all weapons, including the single-sword, double-swords, single-dao, double-dao, spear, and halberd. Mr. Chen masterfully performs the competition Yang form and other taijiquan forms. He must know these well since he serves as a judge in many of the taijiquan competitions. His focus, however, remains on the Chen system.

Some Specific Questions Answered by Chen Xiaowang

- *What responsibilities do you have as the nineteenth-generation representative of Chen taijiquan?*
  Simply to pass on taijiquan traditions to the next generation, so all can appreciate it; to preserve the principles of taijiquan; bring taijiquan up to date so people today can accept and appreciate it. Maintain the traditional theories but be able to pass it on; to adapt it to modern situations because people have different requirements today.

- *Regarding your method of instruction, do you consider yourself a traditionalist?*
  I maintain the old traditional methods of teaching, such as the teaching from father-to-son which is a one-to-one concept. I also started teaching in a modern way, adapting to the different cultures, different religions, different people. I can't just show the movements. Taijiquan is not just the feeling of hands; it is the actual feeling of the person. To understand and appreciate the details of taijiquan, I must modify everything to fit different cultural backgrounds, trying to fit my teaching to the psychological makeup of people. In this way I see taijiquan progressing as part of world culture.

It is something I value passing on and will not change it, but I must transfer it through the language and culture of my students so they can fully understand all the aspects of taijiquan.

- *Is there any connections between Chen Style taijiquan and the Shaolin Temple?*
  No influence.

- *Besides the name being derived from Daoism, is there any special religious or philosophical practices which were or still are observed in Chen taijiquan?*
  Daoism, yin-yang, five-element theories ... No doubt about the influence of Daoist principles in the practice of taijiquan. These principles are the very foundation of taijiquan.

- *Are medical aspects part of the study of taijiquan?*
  No matter what walk of life, no matter what race or nationality you are—German, French, Chinese ... differences in height, complexion or whatever—the only thing in common among us is yin-yang and the presence of qi. In this respect, we are all the same. Taijiquan differs from traditional Chinese medicine, but it works on the same principles, e.g., open-close, qi moving up and down. So, the only thing in common among us is the presence of qi. If the qi is balanced, then you are healthy. Therefore, all can study taijiquan. Since Chinese medical practices are based on the yin-yang concept, so taijiquan is part of this system.

- *Have the routines changed much over the years?*
  There have been some minor changes, but the movements are all the same.

- *If you want to learn the whole system, what do you have to practice?*
  Taijiquan is part of our lifestyle and forms a vital part of our daily activity. So, by principle, we traditionally start with the first routine of laojia; afterwards one can proceed to the second level. But this depends on the time we can devote to practice. After one learns the standing qigong, the Thirty-Eight Style, and the first routine and all the basic principles are understood, then it is possible to proceed to the second routine (*paochui*). Xinjia, arranged by Chen Fake, is also included. And now we practice four routines based on the old and new styles.

- *Who are the main teachers in the Chen Village today?*
  There are many very capable teachers. Quite a few.

- *From Chen Style taijiquan came the Yang Style. Has the Yang Style influenced the Chen Style in anyway?*
  No.

- *The teachings in Chen Village were secret. Has this changed?*

There are no secrets anymore.

- *Since there are no secrets, the main obstacle in perfecting one's taijiquan is the limitation of time. How can we make the best of our practice?*
To get the real benefits of Chen taijiquan, even to practice only one form is enough for the health purposes. Studying the Thirty-Eight Style is enough. You can understand how the qi flows and other aspects of the art. But to study the whole Chen system, you need to study seriously for a very long time. I can teach the whole system, but students must study step-by-step; otherwise, they cannot understand the higher levels of practice. One must progress by levels. If you have not mastered the basics, naturally the most advanced levels cannot be taught. If you can appreciate and absorb each level of Chen taijiquan practice and have the time to devote to continue regular practice, then the whole system can be learned.

- *Should one focus on practicing taijiquan movements or on qi flow?*
If your movement is not correct, your qi will not flow.... Every time you move—if you are practicing the routines, push-hands, weapons—every movement, if it is not correct, the movement will be empty. As a result, your form would be purely physical. There will be no qi inside. This is a very important point. It doesn't matter what style you practice. If you practice in the wrong way, you cannot get the full benefit out of martial arts practice. This is why many practice very often but cannot get the full benefit from their work. However, if you are able to master the basics, doing what lets the qi flow, this is the most important point. If you can understand this, then all else is easier to learn.

- *Who were your teachers?*
My father Chen Zhaoxu, my father's cousin Chen Zhaopi and my father's younger brother Chen Zhaokui.

- *We have not read much about your father, Chen Zhaoxu. Can you tell us a little about him and his involvement in taijiquan?*
My father, Chen Zhaoxu, had knowledge in all aspects of taijiquan that went very deep. Even at twenty-two years of age his skills were so high that many boxing masters came to Beijing to see him. This left him satisfied with his youthful talent to the point that he didn't even practice much. But this attitude soon changed. One day a visitor came to see my father. This visitor was also a highly skilled martial artist. In seeking to test the visitor's skill, my father tried to push him from behind. His attempt not only failed to budge the visitor, but my father ended up tossed to the ground. This experience humiliated my father, who returned to his room, closed the doors and didn't talk with anyone. He practiced secluded for three days. My grandfather, Chen Fake, was also very embarrassed by this incident. He tested my father by repeating the same techniques used

when the visitor proved himself superior in the confrontation. My father, with renewed dedication to the art, continued to practice with my grandfather and reached a higher level in taijiquan skills.

Not much later another boxing expert, about the same age as my father, came to visit. The visitor had great boxing skills, but when he tried to attack, my father defended himself quickly and effectively by uprooting the boxer, sending him as high as the house rafters. This was nearly three meters high. My father caught him before he hit the floor so the visitor would not be hurt from the fall.

News of this incident spread quickly. Many heard the rumors of my father's skills, and he continued to have visitors that came to test his skills. His movements became so spontaneous and natural that no one could throw him to the floor again!

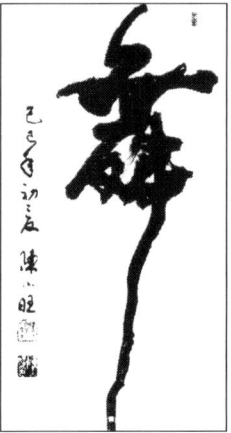

Above: Chen Xiaowang is also well known for his calligraphy.
The character above means "to dance" or "to brandish."
Following: Chen Xiaowang demonstrates some of the taijiquan
movements which were passed down through his family.

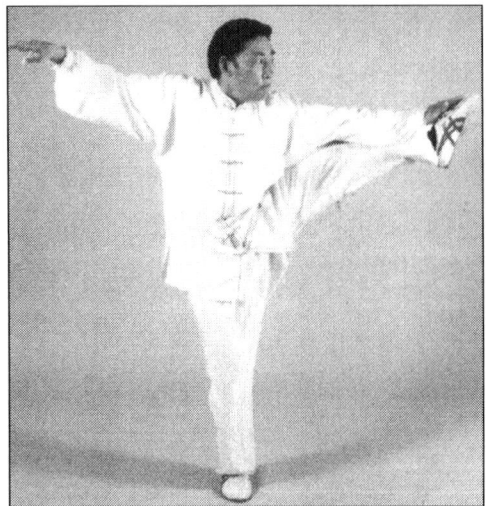
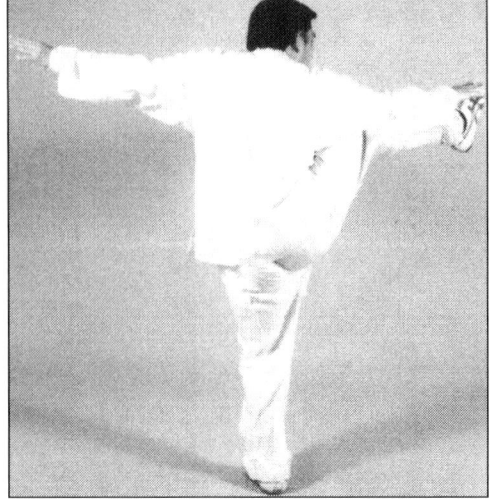

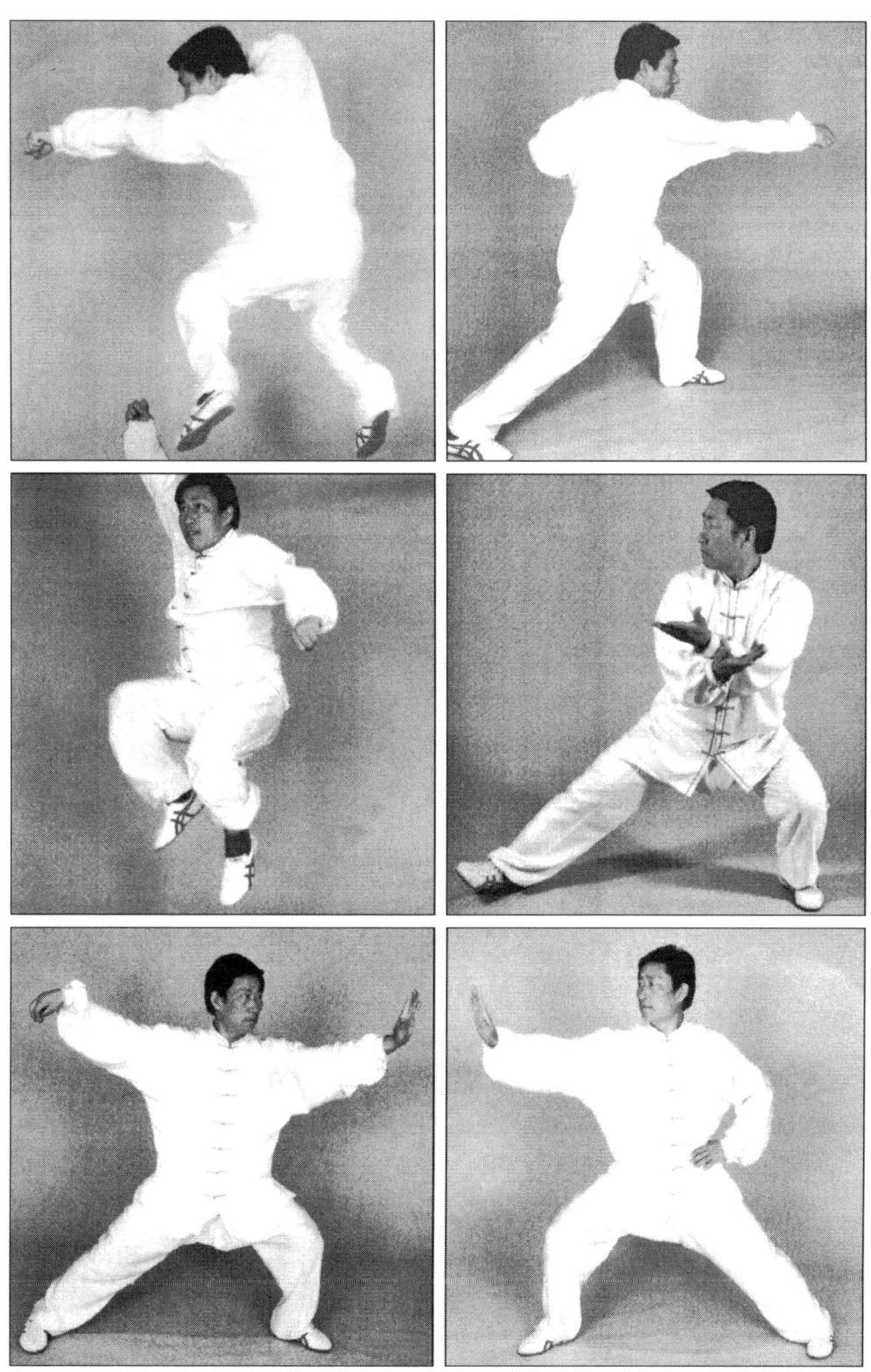

Photos courtesy of Chen Xiaowang.

FACTS ABOUT CHEN XIAOWANG

- Date of birth: October 20, 1946.

- Place of birth: Chen Village, Henan Province, People's Republic of China.

- Awards: Taijiquan gold medalist at three consecutive National Wushu Tournaments in 1980, 1981 and 1982. Taijiquan champion at the first International Wushu Competition held at Xi'an, China in 1985.

- Positions held:
  Taijiquan instructor in China (1980 to 1987).
  Senior Wushu instructor (equivalent to a university associate professor) in China (1988 to present).
  Chairperson of the Henan Province Chen Style Taijiquan Association.
  Technical advisor and official assessor for the standardized competition routine for the Chen, Yang, Wu and Sun taijiquan styles.

- Appointed by the Chinese National Sports Committee in 1985 to draft rules and regulations for taijiquan competitions both domestically and internationally.

- President of the Cultural Exchange Association of Henan Province.

- President of the Society of Chinese Calligraphy and Literature.

- Author: *Chen Style Taijiquan* (1985) and *Chen Style Taijiquan 38 Form* (1984) published by the Sports Publications Centre of the People's Republic of China.

· 9 ·

The Necessity for Softness in Taijiquan
by Michael A. DeMarco, M.A.

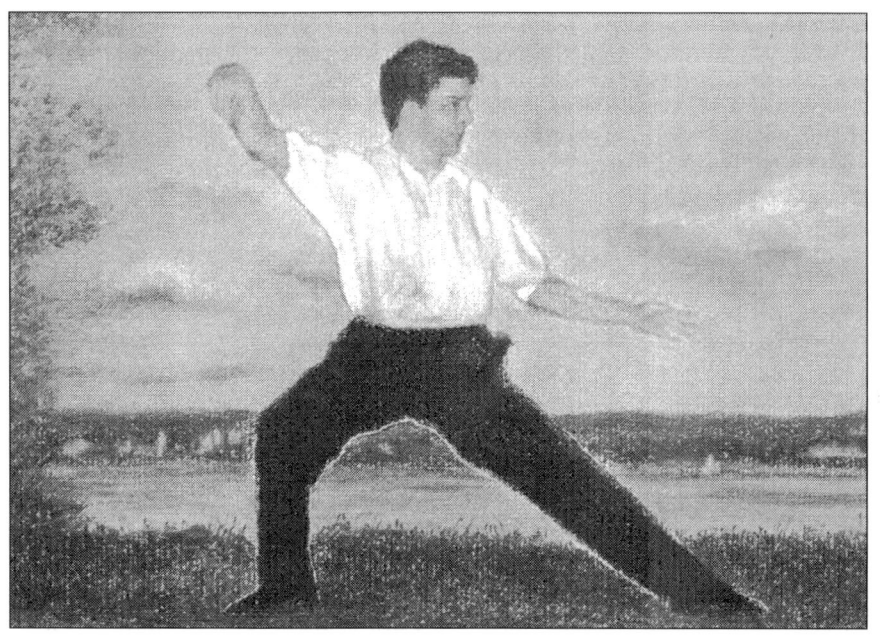

Snake Creeps Downward. Illustration by Mary E. Tanner.

In the whole world, nothing is softer and weaker than water.
And yet for attacking the hard and strong, nothing can beat it
Because there is nothing you can use to replace it.
That water can defeat the unyielding —
That the weak can defeat the strong —
There is no one in the whole world who doesn't know it,
And yet there is no one who can put it into practice.
     *– Ch. 78, Lao-Tzu Te-Tao Ching**

*Henricks, R. (Trans.). (1989). *Lao-tzu te-tao ching*.
New York: Ballantine Books.

For Daoists, water has long been the ultimate symbol for illustrating proper actions. Its unique characteristics offer insights into the Way (*Dao*) of movement which, when applied to the martial arts, gives lessons on how to improve our practice and execution of technique. Through the practice of the various styles of taijiquan that are executed in a relaxed, slow and easy manner, the practitioner can feel the subtleties that allow one's movement to become like water, moving in harmony with the Way.

What is so unique about the nature of water that can be usefully applied in martial arts practice? Water is soft and yielding. However, a river, in travelling thousands of miles from its source to the ocean, must overcome countless rigid obstacles. In the martial arts, someone defending himself must overcome whatever obstacles his opponent may present, be they physical or psychological attacks. Like water with its ability to change form, a person can best defend himself from attack by yielding. Throw a rock into a pond and the water allows the rock to take its course. It yields to the rock while encompassing it. Throw a rock against a tree and see the damage done.

For defense against any aggressive movement, yielding proves to be very effective. A target cannot be hit if it is not present. In the practice of taijiquan, one quickly learns to yield to an incoming attack. In like manner, one learns to flow with the opposite forces which may draw one onward, such as being pulled forwards. When attacks are neutralized in this fashion, it also becomes possible to eliminate any further threat from the attacker by an appropriate technique, i.e., joint lock, throw, or strike. Although relaxed, the response can be executed quite powerfully, much like the concerted force exhibited by a typhoon. Even air, which is often described as "nothing," becomes increasingly dangerous as it transforms from breeze, to wind, to hurricane, to tornado.

In this chapter, we present a few exercises designed to train the martial art practitioner to move more naturally. The following exercises focus on the necessity of softness in order to find the inter-relatedness of unified body movement, the flowing ease of proper technique, and the balance necessary for stability. Above all, these exercises should bring about a "feel" for natural movement that can be applied to the range of self-defense techniques. Some applications from the Yang taijiquan form will then be presented to show how these theories can be applied to any technique.

Exercises: The Way of Taijiquan Body Movement

In addition to softness and yielding, water also illustrates other important characteristics worthy of observation. Because of gravity, water seeks equilibrium as shown in the level surface of a pond. It sinks to the lowest level while remaining even at the surface, much like the well-balanced postures of taijiquan. Water flows and shifts. Since taijiquan is based on the principles of yin and yang, each taiji form flows smoothly one into another. A river moves as one and the techniques strung together to form the taiji set likewise move as one continuous stream. The following exercise will illustrate some of the natural, water-like qualities necessary for doing taijiquan properly.

Exercise One: Taking the First Step

Take a single step. This is something we do every day of our lives, but seldom do we take the time to notice just what the movement entails. Take a single step and ask yourself, "How did I do it?" There are two basic ways to step forward. One is to quickly lift one leg, lean to the front to place the foot down, and fall forward onto the extended foot. The second way follows the taijiquan principles and is shown in the following photos. The complete process for taking a step should be done in a balanced and relaxed manner.

1-A The body is erect and balanced with weight distributed equally on both feet. This position is natural and relaxed.

1-B Slowly shift the body weight totally onto the right leg while keeping the spine straight. This allows the body to remain in balance and frees the left leg for making the step forward. If you did not shift the weight while lifting the foot, you'd fall!

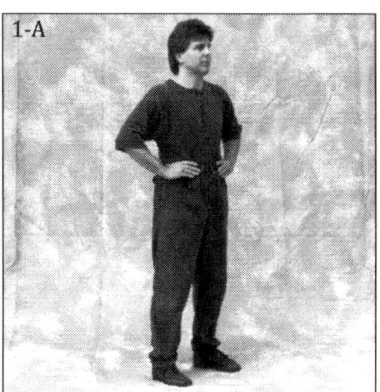
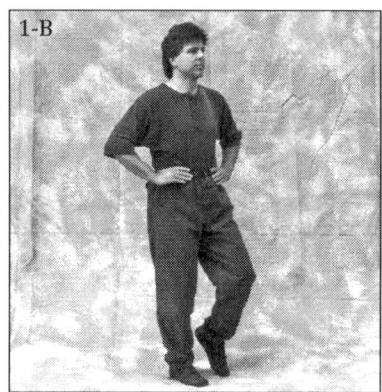

1-C If the right leg remains stiff, the left leg could be placed to the front by the body falling forward. Rather than do this, keep the body erect and sink by bending the right knee.

1-D The sinking movement allows the left heel to be placed forward. The distance of the step depends on how much one sinks. The weight remains on the back leg until the left heel touches the floor.

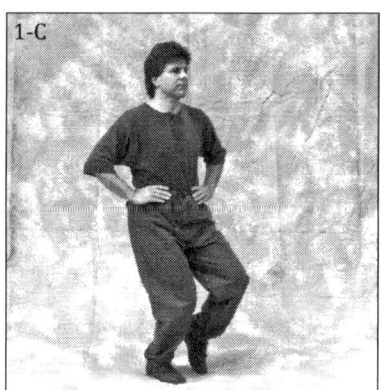
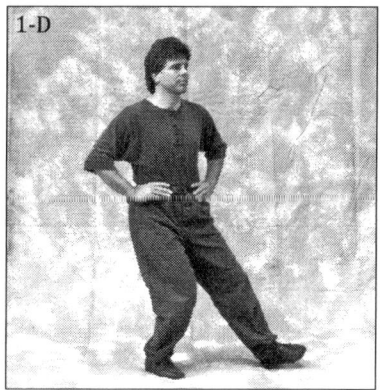

I-E   Slowly shift the weight forward. The toes of the left foot will gradually rest on the floor as the shift occurs. The left knee bends as the back leg straightens. The weight is about 70% on the front foot.

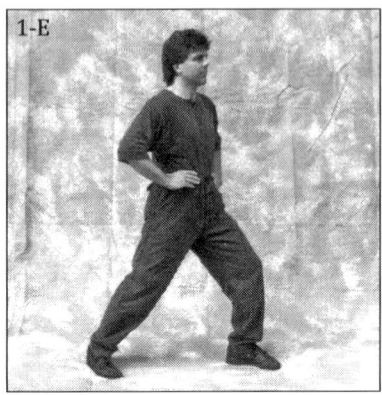

Exercise Two: Letting the Arms Fall Up

Have you seen movies in which a person slips on a banana peel? He loses his footing, as if he had a rug pulled out from under him. As he loses his footing, his hands fly into the air. Some taijiquan movements also illustrate this natural reaction.

2-A, 2-B, and 2-C. Begin as in 1-A, only with the arms hanging freely. Then let your knees buckle and fall freely into a squat. If the arms are relaxed, they will effortlessly move upwards. The movement must be done rather quickly to have this effect on the arms. Just as yin complements yang, the sinking motion is complemented by the rising motion of the arms. If you do this movement in slow motion, it becomes necessary to consciously raise the arms. However, the movement will seem easier and the arms lighter when done after this practice than if one relies solely on muscle power to raise the arms. The movement will seem like the arm movement of a water pump. As one end moves downward (the body), the other moves upward (the arms).

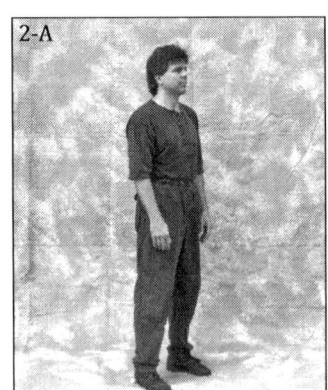 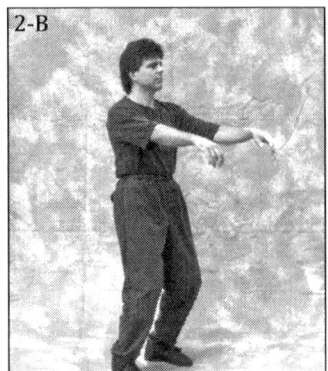 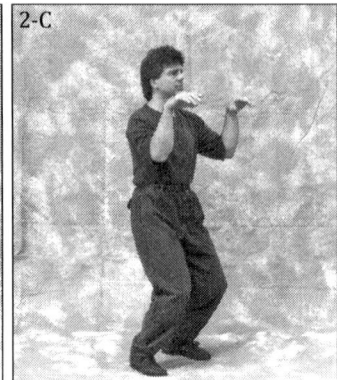

Exercise Three: Interconnected Arm Movement

　　Open a door. It can open only as far as its hinges allow. The following exercise allows one to feel the restrictions a tense body can place on itself. When the whole body moves in a relaxed manner, movements become easier and the body flows freely without straining muscles or joints.

3-A　Stand with the right arm forward.

3-B　While keeping the body rigid, move the right arm as far as possible to the right side. You will feel the right shoulder muscles bunch together and an uncomfortable pulling in the socket. This exercise allows one to feel the effects of doing the movement incorrectly.

3-C thru 3-G. Start again as in 3-A. While keeping the body rigid, let the right arm fall downward by its own weight. Again, you will feel the arm abruptly stop.

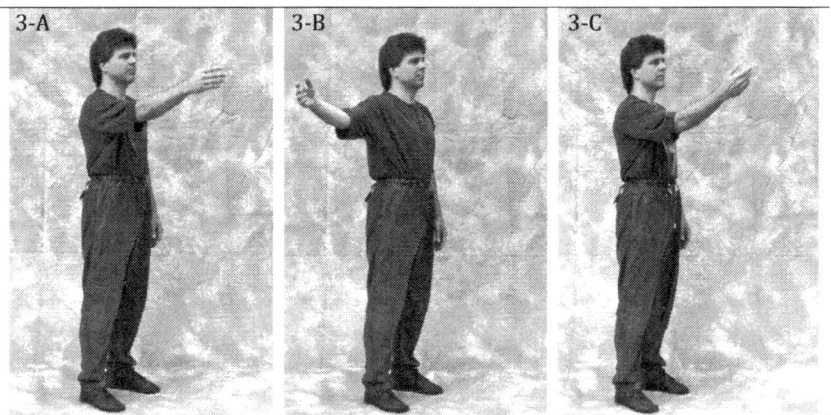

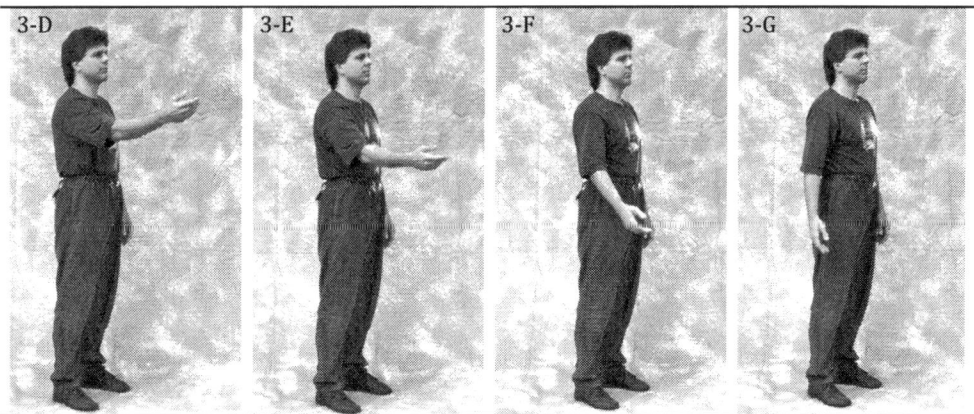

3-H thru 3-K. Try the preceding sequence (3-C thru 3-G) once more, but in a relaxed manner. This will allow your hips and shoulders to rotate with the falling weight of the right arm. The natural arc of the arm falling will be a direct line from front to back and the arm will naturally "fall upwards" due to its own weight and speed during the free-fall. The body will also shift to the right leg and the left heel will rise to follow in the direction of the arm movement. The head will also follow the movement as if you were looking, while pointing with the right hand, at an object behind you.

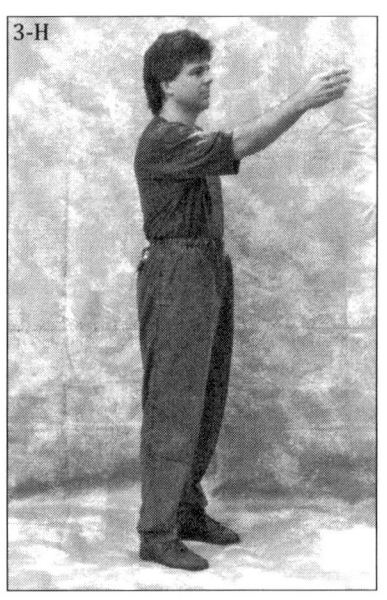
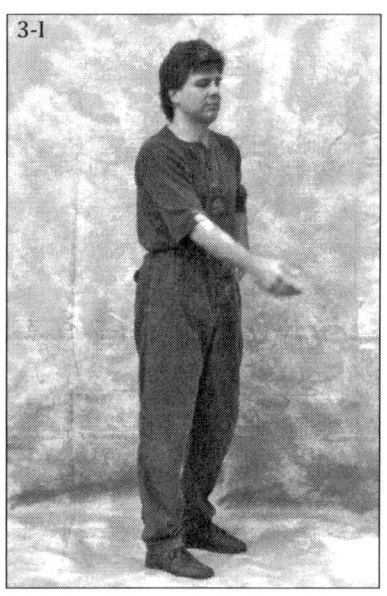
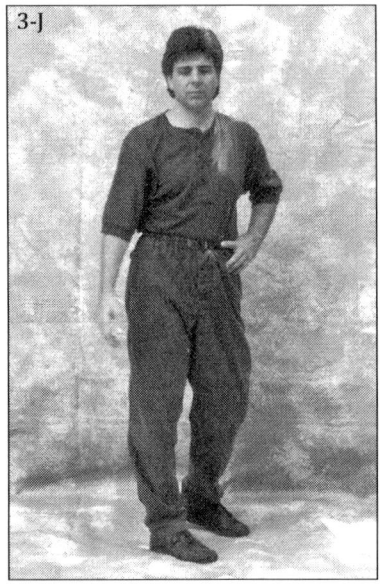
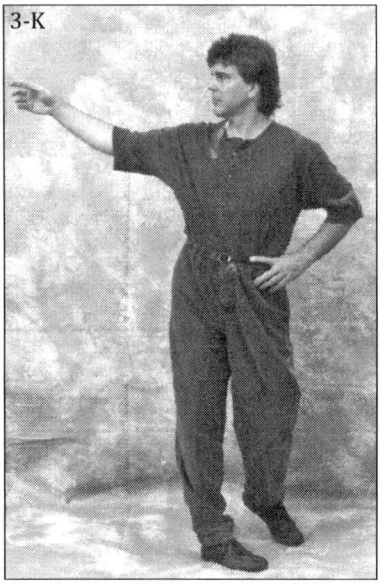

Exercise Four: Interconnected Leg Movement

This exercise has the same purpose as the previous one, except it focuses on the leg and hip movement rather than the arm and shoulder.

4-A Stand with all your weight the left leg (weighted; yang characteristic) and place the right heel out to the right side (empty; yin characteristic). Face in the direction of your right foot.

4-B Turn the head and hips ninety-degrees to the left so that you are looking in the direction of your left foot. You can alternate the movement back and forth from the original position. Did your right foot also turn in the same direction? If not, there may be too much weight on the right leg. Or perhaps the lower body is rigid. Proper shifting of weight, as the alternating between yin and yang, is a prerequisite for smooth, well-balanced movements.

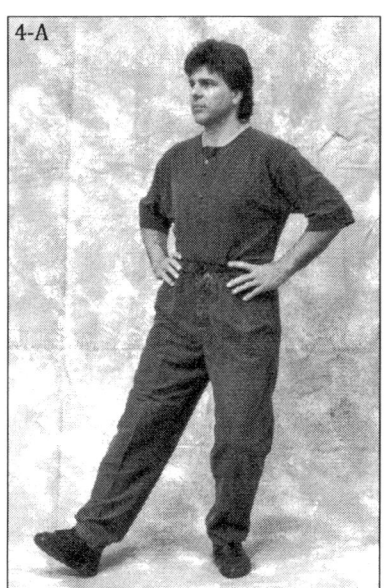

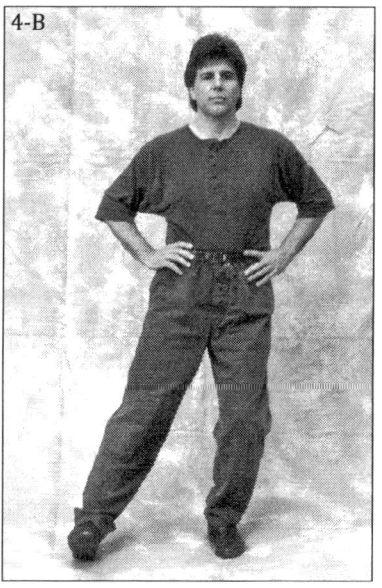

Exercise Five: Rope-like Arms Led by Waist Movement

Taiji Classics state that all movements start in the waist. However, many practitioners execute movements with tensed hands, arms and shoulders. This is true particularly with punches, pushes, and pulls. The body often automatically tenses at the thought of needing additional power. But taiji does not solely rely on arm muscles for power. Power is generated by the integrated body movement. The following exercise can be repeated by alternating the swing to the left and right. In addition to turning the waist on its axis, the player can augment the same movement by shifting his weight by pushing off the back leg, e.g., the left leg when turning right.

5-A thru 5-D. Begin with the stance shown in 5-A and concentrate on letting the arms hang in a relaxed manner as if they were ropes hanging from the shoulders. Turn the waist to the left and feel how the arms swing in the same direction. As the waist turns, the shoulders turn, moving the upper arms and then the forearms naturally follow. This is not a machine-like movement. The parts will follow one another, just as a whip is directed by its handle. But, as the handle is pulled back, the whip's tip is still moving forward until it strikes its target.

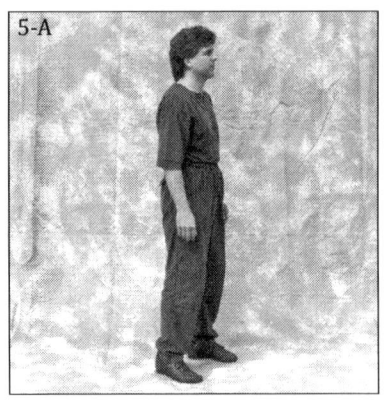
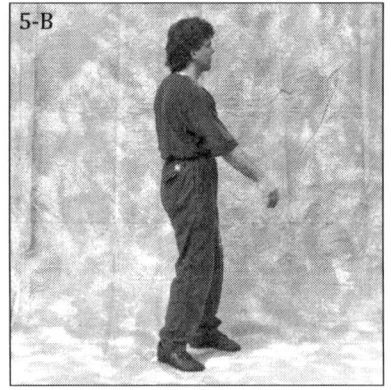
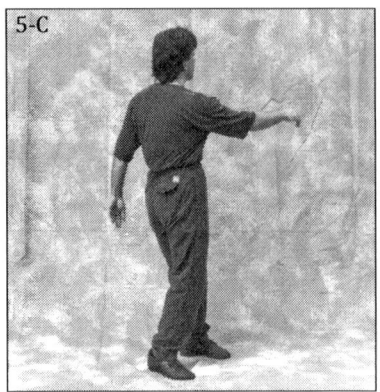
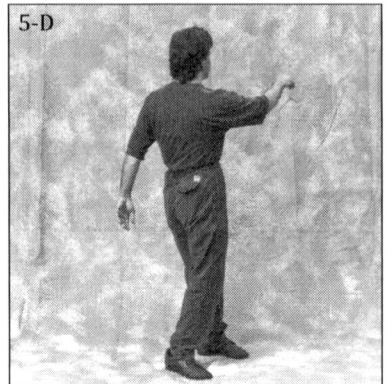

Applications

The following taiji boxing movements illustrate the necessity for softness in executing self-defense techniques. The movements embody the principles upon which taijiquan is based, such as relaxation, balance, fluid change, and integrated body movement. Study the photos and practice the techniques to feel these principles in movement.

While utilizing these principles can greatly improve martial skills, they also are conducive to physical and mental fitness. When smoothness is attained in executing these techniques, the joints and muscles will not be overexerted or overextended, eliminating the threat of injuring ourselves through improper practice. The skeletal system will be in proper alignment with the movements. First practice both the exercises and applications in slow motion. Gradually increase the speed of the techniques but be sure to apply the taiji principles! As a result, the movements should feel powerful, yet relaxed.

Application One: Ward Off

Ward off is a basic but important movement and, therefore, often repeated in the taiji set. The application here shows a technique which can follow a previous block by the right forearm for an incoming right-hand punch. Note that balance is maintained throughout, and the left arm follows the rotation of the waist as the weight is shifted from the right leg to the left. It is not necessary to be tense. Since the attacker's strike was deflected, he chooses to withdraw. The defender simply "goes with the flow" to thwart the attacker from regaining his balance and topples the attacker by accelerating him in the direction of his retreat. Compare this movement to Exercise One.

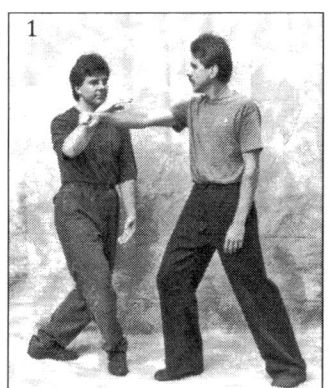
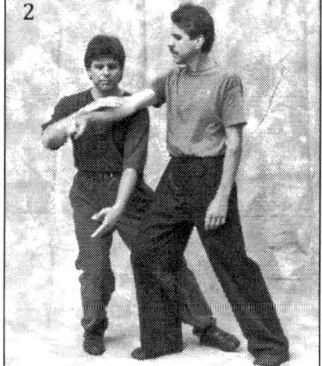
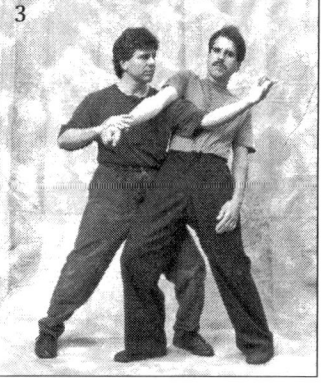

Application Two: Rollback

In rollback, the left hand can be used to intercept a strike and deflect it. While executing the strike with force and momentum, the attacker can easily throw himself off-balance if the strike does not reach its target. The defender, therefore, moves in the same general direction as the incoming force, easily guiding the strike downward and thus drawing the attacker further off-balance to the ground. Note how the defender has shifted his weight from the front to the back foot as in Exercise Three. The hand placed on the attacker's left elbow is an added precaution.

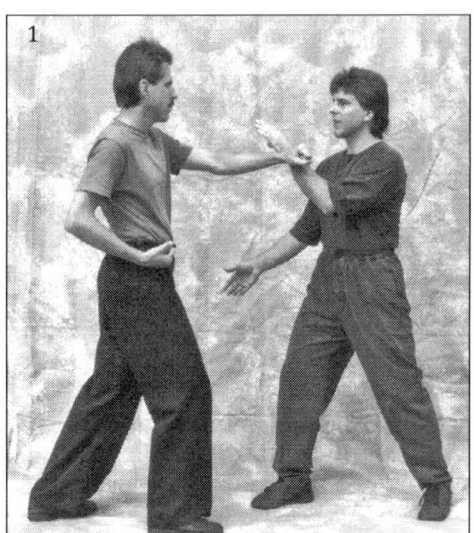
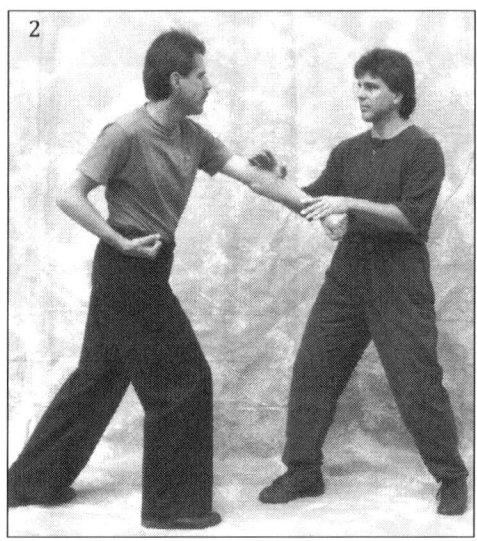
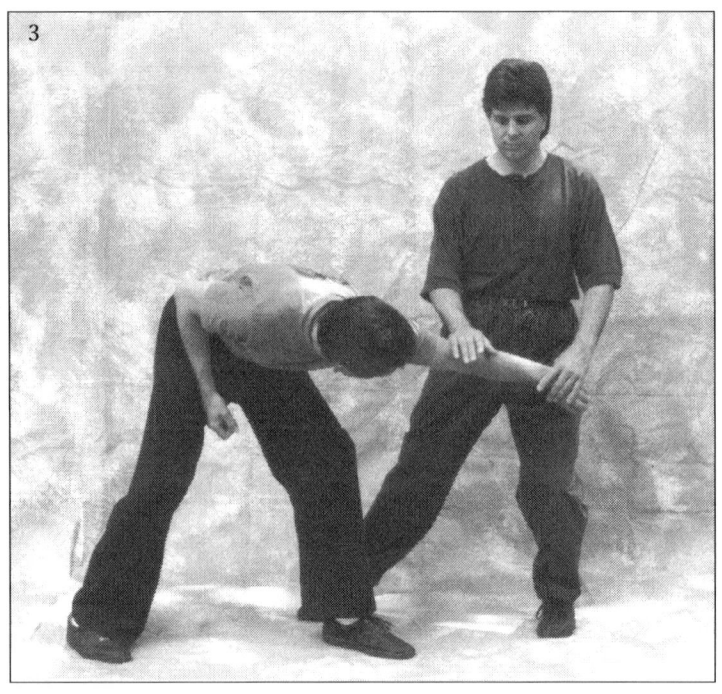

Application Three: Jade Lady Works at Shuttle

One of the applications for jade lady can be seen when an attacker grabs the raised arm of a person with the intent to strike him. Since the arm was raised, he tries to strike at the mid-section. Although grabbed firmly, the defender keeps his right arm relaxed and moves with the slight pull from the attacker. As the attacker steps in to deliver a left punch, the defender turns his waist to the right causing the strike to glance off and be blocked by the left arm. The left arm literally falls into its defensive position by flowing with the body's turn. The attacker, now off-balance, realizes his critical position and starts to retreat. The defender keeps contact by keeping his left arm against the attacker's right arm. Moving with the attacker's retreat, the defender controls the rest of the movement and adds a right-hand push to drive the attacker away. The push could be changed to a strike if so desired. A variety of principles can be found in Jade Lady as shown in the exercises given on the previous pages.

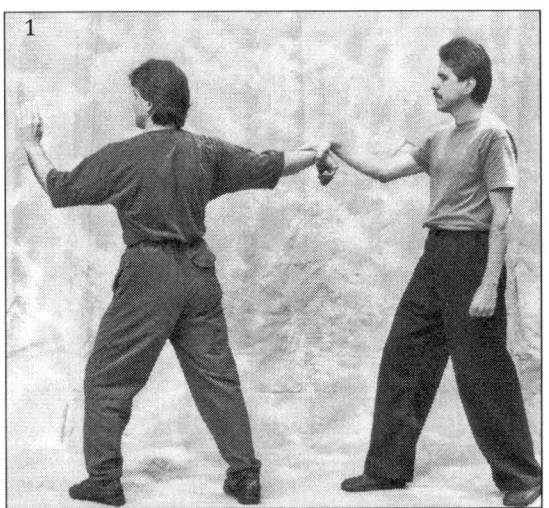
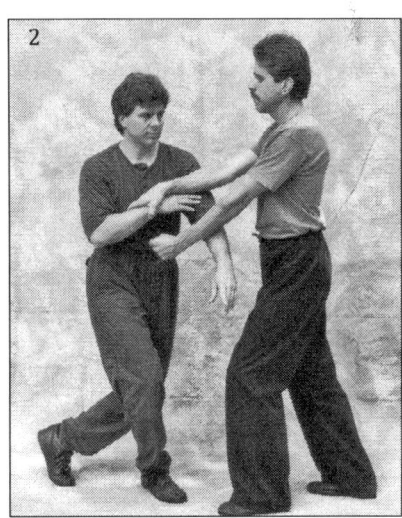
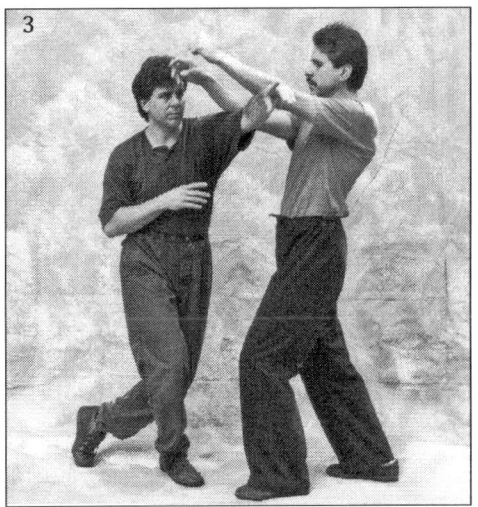
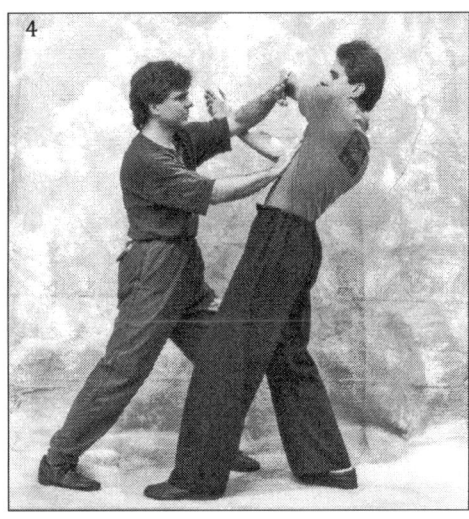

Application Four: Monkey Retreats

By its very name, monkey retreats illustrates a backward movement, which follows the same taiji principles discussed earlier. Some actions in the sequence are the reverse of those executed during a forward movement. For example, rather than step with the heel first, the toe is placed on the ground. The block/deflect is still made in the direction of the attacker's strike and the necessary sinking, shifting and turning remain the same as in forward movements.

The attacker and defender are near each other. As the attacker swings his left fist around at the side of the defender's head, the defender begins his defensive movement. His body shifts and sinks to his left leg, allowing the right leg to be free to step backwards. As this occurs, the right hand "falls upward" due to the momentum and is in position to deflect the attack safely to the side. The defender simultaneously places his left hand on the attacker's chest to check his movement. The left hand could be used to strike the attacker if so desired. Note that the defender's left foot is now empty of weight, and the body's turning pulls the foot into alignment with the hips. If the left leg is tensed or if too much weight remains on it, the toes would remain planted pointing straight forward or even to the left and outside the direction the hips are pointing.

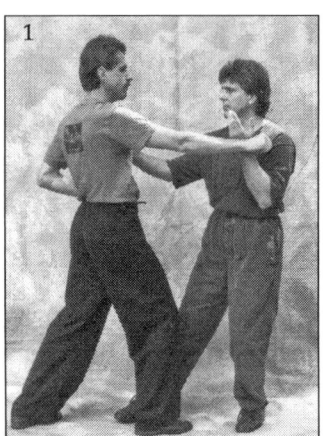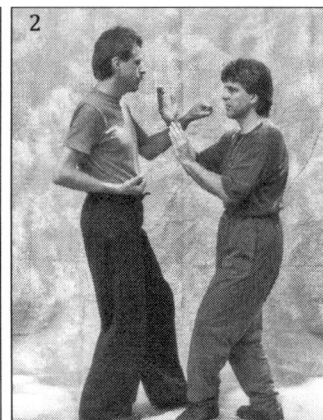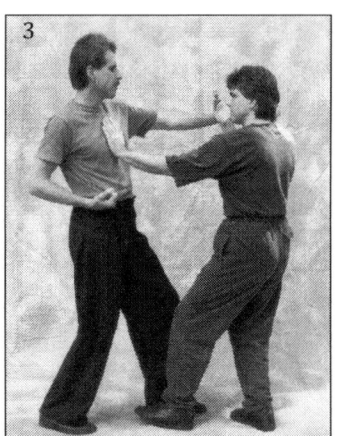

It is hoped that by practicing the exercises and applications presented above, one can come to observe more closely the taiji principles discussed and their importance and usefulness for taijiquan as an art form, a system of self-defense, a moving meditation, and a holistic health system.

All photos by Pete Gool. Special thanks to Peter Danielewicz for his help in demonstrating the techniques with the author.

• 10 •

Zheng Manqing and Taijiquan: A Clarification of Role
by Robert W. Smith, M.A.

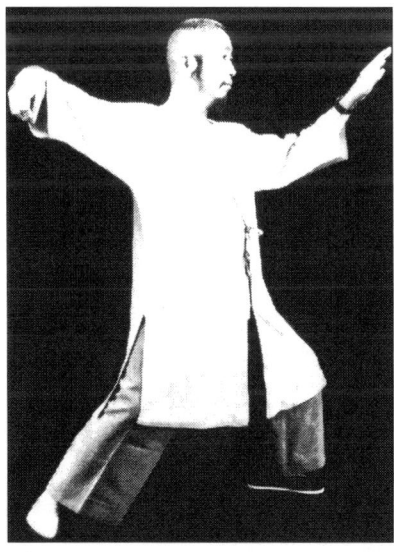

Zheng in single-whip posture, 1965. All illustrations courtesy
of R. Smith, and Charles E. Tuttle Co., except where noted.

In his article on Zheng Manqing's taijiquan (hereafter, simply "taiji") in Malaysia, Nigel Sutton makes some errors of fact and interpretation that I would like to correct (1994: 57–71). A guiding principle to help correct Sutton's commentary is that "the teacher is not the taught." The fact that taiji students do a movement in a certain way does not mean that the teacher did it that way or would even agree to it being done that way. Or, by extension, merely because teachers in Malaysia, Taiwan, or America make comments regarding taiji, what they say does not necessarily reflect what Professor Zheng said or would say on a given aspect of the art.

Sutton goes awry in the first paragraph by stating that Zheng Manqing founded a new system of taiji (1994: 57).[1] This is an error. The long form he learned and taught before World War II was exactly that of Yang Chengfu. There is evidence that Zheng may have been experimenting with a shorter form as early as 1938 when he was director of martial arts in Hunan Province. Given wartime exigencies, he shortened the set by eliminating many repetitions and some postures. But it was somewhat later, in 1947, just before he went to Taiwan, that the shorter form came to fruition.

When I was studying with him in Taiwan (1959–1962), I queried him on the genesis and development of his short form. He was convinced that he'd been right to simplify it. That was said smiling. But then he'd get sterner, saying that it was not a creation of a new system, but rather a rearrangement not affecting basic principles. This form, he said, is the shorter Yang Chengfu system taught by one with half his teacher's skill. Sutton views this as a "new system," but Zheng would not call it so.

Sutton next states that it is generally recognized by students of Zheng Manqing that his incorporation of core elements of the Zuo Laipeng system made his system unique (1994: 58). I know of no one who believes this. We know little of Zuo, but we do know that he did not teach taiji.

To understand Zuo, one must first understand another remarkable person: Zhang Qinlin. The best way to learn about both these men, it seems to me, is through Wang Yannian, a taiji teacher I discussed in *Chinese Boxing: Masters and Methods* (1974). In his book *Taichi* (1988, Taibei), Wang tells how, through a Daoist friend, he met Zhang Qinlin, a taiji teacher over sixty at the time, who had jet-black hair and looked forty. Zhang was born in Hebei in 1887 of a poor family and at fourteen became a yardman at the family home of Yang Jianhou. Over the years, the youngster practiced with Yang Chengfu and other adepts there, becoming quite proficient (Wang, 1988: 1–2, 41–42).

In 1914, Wan Laisheng, a senior student of the famed Du Xinwu, traveled through Hunan and, when he came to Hubei, challenged Yang Chengfu. Zhang took the challenge for Yang and defeated Wan in the first clash—probably injuring Wan's arm.[2] Wan decamped.

Yang Jianhou, who watched the skirmish from inside his house, was taken by Zhang's bravery and skill in beating Wan. Wang Yannian believes that Yang Jianhou's appreciation was also stimulated by the fact that years before Yang himself had a match with Du Xinwu, Wan's teacher, which ended in a stalemate. Lacking corroboration, I tend to doubt that such a match ever occurred.

Be that as it may, Wang writes that Jianhou demonstrated his appreciation by secretly showing Zhang the original Han style of taiji that his father, Yang Luchan, had concealed from the Manchu court when he taught there. Luchan had taught an inferior method, keeping the original Han style for family use only.

Later, Zhang Qinlin met Zuo Laipeng of the Golden Elixir of Life School who taught him *neigong* (internal work) and *tunu daoyin* (breathing methods) esoteric skills.[3] These Zhang blended with his taiji abilities, and his skill became great. In *Chinese Boxing* I tell how Zhang traveled, defeating all boxers until he met Zuo, who tumbled him instantly, commenting, "Your technique, sir, is none too good."[4] Although Wang does not mention the encounter, it is widely believed.

Zhang went to Taiyuan in Shanxi in 1925 to work as a fur merchant and prospered. In the 1929 national martial arts championships held at Nanjing, Zhang, the Shanxi Province champion, became the national champion as well. It is said that he won the honor without breaking a sweat and afterwards berated the principals for not affording him stiffer competition.

Wang Yannian visited me in 1984, and I was able to ask him about Zhang's relationship with Zheng Manqing. After the Nanjing tournament, Wang said,

Professor Zheng approached Zhang Qinlin and asked to study under him. Zhang told Zheng that, since he was already versed in taiji, he would accept him as a student and let him live at his house in Taiyuan but without the customary kowtow.[5]

Wang told me that, physically, Zhang Qinlin was midway between Zheng Manqing and Wang himself but that he had big wide feet, huge hands that seemed to cover one's chest, and was a supple as a snake. His description of Zhang's feet rang a bell: I had heard in Taiwan that he could root so well that his feet sank into the ground. This was the colossus who taught Zheng push-hands and qigong for six months. At the end of the period, Zheng imprudently suggested that they have a real go and was soundly drubbed by Zhang.

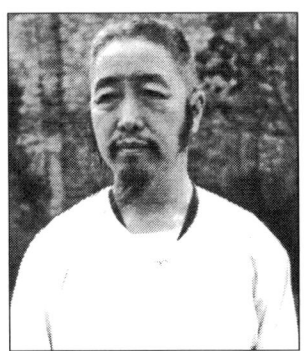 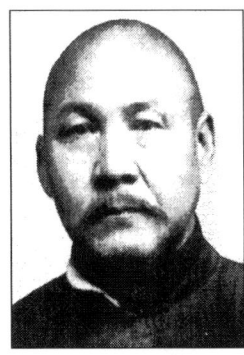 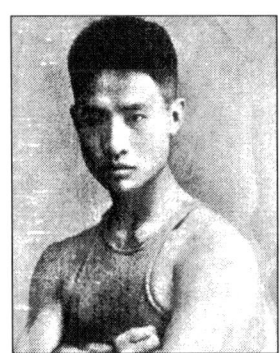

Left: Professor Zheng in 1960. Center: Zhang Qinlin—who taught Zheng neigong (photo courtesy of Wang Yannian). Right: Wan Laisheng.

Some of Zheng's senior students, however, view Zhang Qinlin differently than Wang Yannian did. Liu Xiheng and Ben Lo (Pangjeng) believe that Zheng primarily studied neigong, rather than push-hands, from Zhang and that it was done in Shanghai rather than Shanxi. They reason that, though Zheng practiced push-hands with Zhang as students under Yang Chengfu, his main priority was learning neigong, probably including Zuo Laipeng's teaching, from Zhang.[6] The place may not be important, but it is worth noting that the memorial book of Zheng states that in Taiyuan, Shanxi, he "practiced marvelous techniques of [taiji] energy with [Zhang Qinlin]" (Gibbs, 1985: 18).[7] Mrs. Zheng, however, says that Professor Zheng did not study in Shanxi. Coming from such a strong source, this statement, besides negating Wang Yannian's assertion, adds some weight to the general belief that Zheng never actually met Zuo Laipeng but, instead, derived his neigong from Zhang Qinlin outside of Shanxi, where both Zhang and Zuo lived.

Moreover, Liu Xiheng and Ben Lo say that, when Zhang Qinlin came to Yang Chengfu, he had already learned another taiji form. Yang accepted him and told him that because his form was so good (Professor Zheng told Mr. Liu Xiheng once that it was "very soft, very beautiful") that he needn't study form but only push-hands. Liu further writes, "Some people say this is a secret Yang Family form, but Master Yang's son has denied this and has indicated that it is only Mr. [Zhang's] form." As for Zheng Manqing's challenge to Zhang, as related by Wang Yannian, Liu says, "Perhaps not too much should be made of it, as it would be in the natural order of things in the push-hands class, where these things shift back and forth from day to day."[8]

But what of the mystery man Zuo Laipeng? In his book *Writings on the Way of Taichi*, Wu Guozhong wrote that Zheng Manqing created a new system from a synthesis of Zuo style, Yang style, and his own unique system. This is a major mistake made, one hopes, from carelessness rather than self-serving commercialism. Ben Lo's article in *T'ai Chi* magazine (Lo, 1985) criticizes Wu Guozhong for promoting this error. In his polite but devastating analysis, Lo quotes these words from Professor Zheng's seminal *Thirteen Treatises on Taichi* (Lo, 1985):

> This book is the result of my teacher Professor Yang Chengfu and his taichi book, *T'i Yung Ch'uan Shu*. This book follows my teacher's instructions and is a continuation of his book. Because the traditional form was too long, people lacking patience could not easily finish it and did not continue practicing. Therefore, I simplified the form by deleting the repetitions which were about seventy percent of the form. I called my work *Simplified Taichi*. My classmate, Ch'en Weiming, encouraged my book and urged me to publish it. I believe this work is in harmony with my teacher's idea.

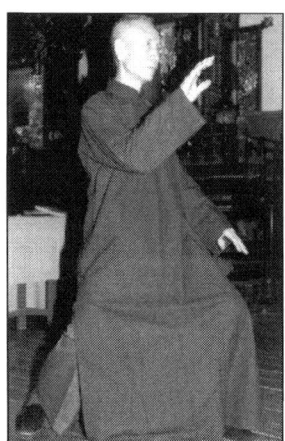
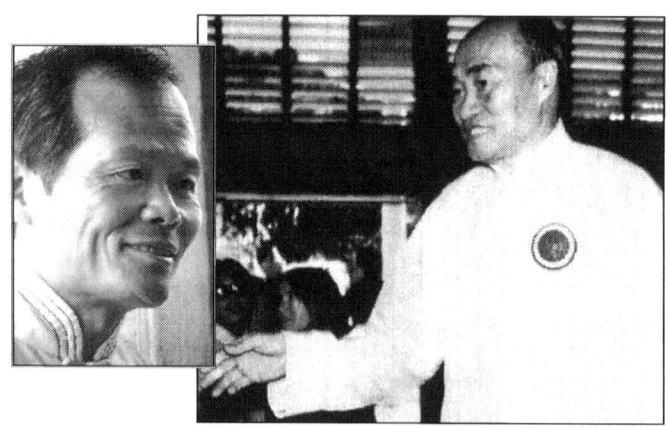

Left: Liu Xiheng—student and confidant of Zheng. Center: Ben Lo.
Right: Huang Xingxian—Zheng's student who spread taiji in Malaysia.

How could Wu, who must have read the *Thirteen Treatises*, miss this passage? Lo then cites Wu Guozhong's book, which quotes a crucial sentence from Zheng Manqing's *Manjan San Lun* written in 1971:

> My fellow student Ch'en Hsiao-lien [Weiming] studied T'ai chi ch'uan for several decades, but when it came to the difference between

strength and energy, he was not able to get to the bottom of it. Not long after that I received the secret teaching of Master [Zuo Laipeng of Shanxi] which stated that the strength issues from the bones, but energy issues from the sinews. In a burst of clarity, I was enlightened. Forty years ago I wrote these words in my Master Cheng's *Thirteen Chapters on Tai-chi ch'üan* ... — Wile, 1985: 148

In fact, Professor Zheng cites the same quote twice in this book (Lo and Inn, 1985: 79, 91). In neither case is it claimed that the words came from Zuo Laipeng. Lo suggests that Professor Zheng may have gotten the words he attributes to Zuo from Zhang Qinlin, student of Zuo's neigong and Yang's push-hands method.

Lo writes that the quote is probably a part of the Yang family tradition rather than the esoteric Daoist one. As proof, he cites Wu Gongzao's *Wu Style Taichi* (1980), which included a photo reproduction of a written manuscript "On Methods of Taichi" passed along by the author's ancestor, Wu Jianquan, who had received it from Yang Banhou. All told, it had been in the Wu family for more than one hundred years (Lo, "Explanation," 1985: 12).[9] The same document was included by Dong Yingjie, a senior student of Yang Chengfu, in his *Taichi Shih-i* [Explanation of tai chi] (1948), thirty-two years earlier.

To Wu Guozhong's contention that he had "learned a final, concentration distillation of fifty years of Professor [Zheng's] experience," Ben Lo answers that there was no difference between the postures of earlier and later periods. "There is only the difference between postures correctly learned and incorrectly learned." Then Lo concludes that Wu "remains inadequate in even the most superficial aspects of the art" (Lo, 1985: 17).

Later, Wu had the temerity to challenge aging Huang Xingxian of Singapore, but this fight was not consummated. (As the challenged given the choice of weapons, Huang should have accepted and specified push-hands in which—even factoring in age—he was clearly superior to Wu.) In due course, Wu's perceived misdeeds brought a challenge from William Chen. After a long play in Chinese newspapers, the pair was unable to agree on modalities and this challenge also fizzled.

The episode hurt everyone and did not help Professor Zheng's reputation. I have always held the view that the Wu-Chen disagreement could likewise have been solved by push-hands (*tuishou*). Since push-hands confirms one's form, a round of it would settle most points in the controversy. A tuishou match is still a possibility. (I suggested this recently to a student of Wu and got this response: "A spot of tuishou? Well, in the last couple months, Wu has published in Chinese in Taiwan a two-hundred-plus-page book on push-hands, which is selling fast. One of the things about this guy is that he doesn't keep secrets." What does a book tell about one's abilities?) If Wu is as bad at taiji as some suggest, then it will be known soon enough. But, if that is true, then Wu already knows and will steer clear of the sportive and opt for what his followers think is his strong suit—the free fight.

According to Sutton, Wu's reputation is that of a Chinese military frogman "who has killed many men" (1994: 64). So why wouldn't he respond to a challenge brought by three of Lu Tongbao's students? The whole affair is full of confusion. I have heard that Wu has recanted the claims attributed to him that stated he was the sole inheritor of Zheng's most important teachings. The evidence adduced against him by Lo and others is far too weighty to perpetuate such claims.[10]

Sutton also writes that Professor Zheng's thirty-seven postures "are based closely, if only superficially, on the Yang style" (1994: 58). This sentence is a paradox and contradicts what Zheng has stated regarding the influence of Yang Chengfu.

Lower on the same page, Sutton claims that the Zuo system places a greater emphasis on *song* (relaxation) than does the Yang style. We know that a Zuo system of taiji does not exist, but we do not know with any clarity what Zuo's neigong method involved. We do know, however, that the Yang system puts a premium on relaxation. The Yang system regarded the *Taichi Classics* as its bible, which contains such statements as Wu Yuxiang's "The softest will then become the strongest" (Lo, et al., 1979: 46). Reflecting Yang Chengfu's direct teaching, Chen Weiming says in *Questions and Answers on Taichi*, "Students who use force can't believe that at the limit of suppleness lies a different quality of strength," and "A poor student is hard and uses force but a good one must be supple without force" (Lo and Smith, 1985: 18). Finally, Professor Zheng says in his *Thirteen Treatises* that Yang Chengfu repeated continually, "Relax! Relax! Relax completely" (Lo and Inn, 1985: 88). I know Sutton joins me in wishing we could relax better. He is right, I think, in believing that Zuo's neigong helped Professor Zheng's taiji. In fact, Zheng acknowledged as much. But we just do not know how or to what degree these practices intertwined. Given its Daoist beginnings, we should not be surprised at change in taiji as it evolves and proliferates. Even in the short form, no two teachers do the form exactly alike. Sutton, like some other recent writers, thinks he sees a difference between earlier and later Zheng style: "Those who learned with him in the earlier years practice a form more closely resembling that of the Yang family while later students perform [sic] in a softer, more rounded fashion" (1994: 22). This, he says, led some exponents of the Yang system to accuse Zheng stylists of, doing "old man's taiji." However, Zheng taught as Yang had taught him. Both had students of varied ages and varied taiji skills.

One must distinguish the teacher from the taught. Sutton thinks Zheng Manqing softened and rounded the Yang postures, but Yang was far softer than Zheng. And the fact that some of Zheng's students do postures one way does not mean Zheng taught them that way. Isn't it just possible that Zheng's teachings involved no changes, but instead simply reflects that he was superb at not changing Yang's system, teaching it as he had learned it? Zheng stressed accuracy first and last. When he learned the rudiments under Yang, he had to master each posture before moving to the next; there was no breezy form class followed by a corrections class. With time, his own form became less energetic and more internalized—compare his 1960 Taiwan film with his 1973 film—but his teaching remained pretty much the same.

I learned and taught taiji across thirty-five years with Professor Zheng and his influence early and late and must correct Sutton on misstatements regarding form. Above all, this must be stressed: the Zheng form is the Yang form shortened, but the postures—the structure and flow—and the principles are all the same.

Without being didactic, let me dilate on the form. Everyone's form will be different—like fingerprints or snowflakes—but the basics will be the same. The structure will be pretty much the same while the flow will come to express some of the personality of the person doing it. Together these two elements comprise the technique of taiji. Professor Zheng would ask taiji practitioners: how much of taiji technique is structure and how much is flow. The answer is that early in one's training, as one learns to apply the basics, structure predominates, but later, flow comes to the fore. Professor Zheng would go on to say that structure and flow together—the technique—make up only 30 percent of taiji. He would then ask, "What is the missing 70 percent?" It is the same as in many arts, in calligraphy— the queen of the Chinese fine arts—for instance. Seventy percent of taiji is naturalness, the intrinsic "you," which can only come from inside you.

That said, it is obvious that there is a complex of factors operating in taiji. Only some of these are visible to the beginning eye. "It is not that fast horses are rare," said Tang scholar Han Yu. "It's just that those who can really spot them are few."

Now, the art would be difficult—Professor Zheng said that taiji was the most difficult of all his "excellences"—even if there were one standard, undeviating model. But there is not. There are two orthodox streams connecting us with founder Yang Luchan, those of sons Jianhou and Banhou. These systems vary somewhat but are still Yang. Zheng Manqing learned from Yang Chengfu, son of Jianhou. Yang Chengfu had a small cadre of top seniors, ranging from Chen Weiming and Dong Yingjie, the most senior, to Zheng Manqing, the youngest. Each had his own style, but each did the Yang system.

Given the history of the Yang family, one should expect some difference in the system as the result of differences in locale, social milieu, teacher, and other variables. With the underdeveloped agrarian economy and poor communications of China, there were few books on taiji that would have helped standardize the system. And then there were the students. To enhance ego, many would stop learning too early before they really understood taiji well enough to teach it; others would learn a different system and then attach the Yang name to it for prestige; and still others would learn the Yang, change it, and then tag their name to the mongrel system. These aberrations tended to dilute the system in many areas. Both Banhou and Jianhou taught a system that could accommodate all physiques and psyches. The system embraced a big method with a high stance, the arms moving in proportionally larger circles; a medium method having a middle stance with greater separation of weight between the feet, the arms moving in smaller circles;

and a small method with the knees deeply bent and the arms moving minimally, most movement being at the waist. Yang Shaohou was proficient in the difficult small method and his trigger-force short energy made him a terror in push-hands. His form was nearly as frightening. A few years ago, a Beijing newspaper interviewed Wu Tunan, a taiji veteran nearing one hundred, who told the interviewer that, when he studied under Yang Shaohou, he was made to do the form under a table for lengthy periods.

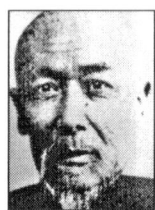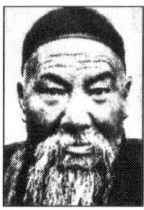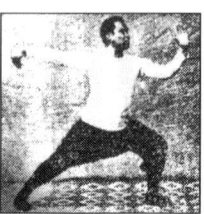

Yang Shaohou, Yang Jianhou (Zheng's grand teacher), and Yang Chengfu, c. 1932.

The key factor distinguishing the low form was simply the height of the form—that is, how much the knees were bent in separating the weight in the stance. I assume, therefore, that the hand position sequence remained essentially the same as in the other forms. I saw a little of this low form in the parks in Taiwan —the hand sequence was the same—but though the players were quite low, the quality of their practice was not too high. Confucius said, germanely, "Some seek Happiness higher than man; others seek it lower. But Happiness is the same height as man."

Continuing our discussion of the form, as time passes, sincere, thinking students will make changes, often contributing beneficially rather than detrimentally to a system's evolution. Something like this occurred in 1938 when Zheng Manqing decided to do as Thoreau advises all of us to, to "simplify, simplify." For largely practical reasons, he reduced the number of postures in a routine from more than a hundred to thirty-seven—still nearly triple the number of postures in the original taiji set (thirteen). And this kind of change is seen in the broad sweep of taiji history.

Chenjiagou, Henan, was the hub of early taiji in China, learning the art from a Shanxi boxer, Wang Zongyue, who visited Henan in the last half of the eighteenth century. Much later, taiji at Chenjiagou split into the so-called old (orthodox) and new (innovative) camps. The split was not decisive in its effect on style, however. The principles and postures of the "new" were not dissimilar from those of the "old." Perhaps a more important change occurred at about the same time. Wu Yuxiang, who had learned the "old" taiji from Yang Luchan and the "new" system from Chen Qingping, synthesized these into his own system. What I want to stress here is the active evolution of the "new" system (see chart on pages 202–203 showing the "new" and "old" lineages in Draeger and Smith, 1980). Wu Yuxiang passed his system to Li Yiyu, who passed it to Hao Weizhen, who passed it to Sun Lutang. Each of these masters modified it and renamed the system after himself. But the "old" system depicted on the right side of the chart shows only Wu Jianquan defecting from the traditional Yang Style. Jianquan was taught by his father, Wu Quanyou, himself taught by Yang Banhou. This Wu system became popular in Hong Kong and southeast Asia.

All of the above lineage details are simply to show the change occurring in taiji over time and in major systems. And there was no end to it on the individual level. Yang Chengfu, in the preface to his *Taichi T'i-yung Ch'uan-shu* [Complete principles and applications of taiji, 1934], wrote that, looking back at photographs made ten years earlier, he saw that his old postures were inferior to those of the new ones (Wile, 1983: 155). In the interim, Yang had grown obese and no longer had the flexibility in left bow-step to turn his waist leftward to the front and to turn his back right foot leftward forty-five degrees from ninety degrees. And yet, looking at the photographs, one readily agrees with Yang: although he had grown fatter, his postures are superior to the old ones.

When the spirit hit him, Professor Zheng would show a few variations for certain postures. In fact, in New York City he taught diagonal flying as a more open posture, with the left arm raised and stretched out leftward like a bird's wing opening, instead of keeping it just outside the left thigh. This and other nuances may have been a factor in some New Yorkers claiming that they had received the "fully evolved form" (an assertion they sometimes used to counter the Taiwan old-timers' contention that Professor Zheng taught them the real form but had diluted it later for "lazy" Americans).

Sutton errs in contrasting the Yang 70/30% front-loaded bow step with the "Zheng" 100/0% (rounded off from his 99.9/0.1%) (1994: 59). Sutton should have asked himself why Professor Zheng would teach the bow step, front-loaded weighting as 70/30% all his life (see the foot-weighting diagrams in all his books) and then a year or so before his death change it to 100/0% for his last student, Wu Guozhong. The short answer is that Professor Zheng did not change the weighting.

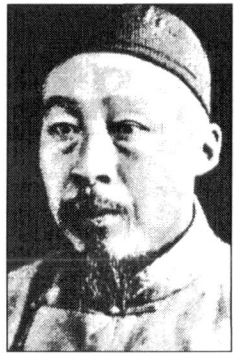 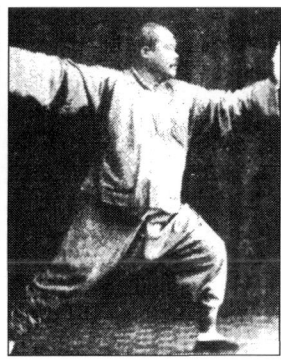 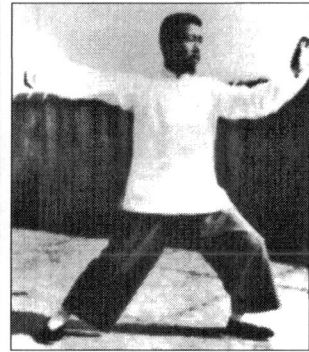

Left: Chen Weiming. Single-whip postures of Yang Chengfu (center),
ca. 1933 and Zheng Manqing, ca. 1948.

In our collaboration, *T'ai-Chi*, I asked Professor Zheng whether auxiliary exercises to enhance correct breathing, the postures, and overall agility were beneficial. He responded that the postures themselves are so fully founded, variable, and beneficial that additional exercises would only detract from a student's progress. Sutton's assertion that Professor Zheng taught a range of auxiliary exercises for the development of neigong, exercises regarded as coming from the Zuo Laipeng system, is, therefore, inaccurate (1994: 59). Zheng was a quick study and if he concentrated on a thing he would have it. He was an encyclopedia of the esoteric, the ultimate dilettante in the best sense. He tried a myriad of neigong methods and, if he added the variable of time to concentration, he got a thing good. No one around today knows what he learned from Zuo Laipeng, but Zheng was impressed with Zuo's wisdom as imparted by Zhang Qinlin, from whom he probably received Zuo's teachings as well.

But in his preface to Zheng Manqing's *Thirteen Treatises*, Chen Weiming writes that, after Zheng arrived in Sichuan (1939), "[H]e met an extraordinary man, studied with him, and made great progress" (Wile, 1985: 1). Chen was close to Zheng and knew that he had an uncanny ability to attract great men wherever he went. Thus, this may mean that—even for Zheng—the Sichuan man was exceptional. Professor Zheng never noted the man by name, unusual perhaps for someone who had helped him progress. Could it have been Zhang Qinlin or even Zuo Laipeng relocating, as Zheng had, westward away from the invading Japanese? Ben Lo believes that Zheng stayed in Shanxi during World War II, but we do not know for sure. It remains a puzzlement.

Professor Zheng was often jocular and during such moods would often show snatches of neigong, but he believed that students are easily diverted into laziness and wanted to have them use their time in taiji itself. Late in life he did develop "eight methods," a splendid set for older people. He did not teach it in a regular class, but I learned half of it from Tam Gibbs before his death and of this I retain the slenderest memory. In New York City, he taught several massage methods and ways of nurturing qi, and these can be learned from Wolfe Lowenthal's insightful first book on Professor Zheng, *There Are No Secrets* (1991: 112–122).

I never met Yue Shuting, Lu Tongbao, and Li Beilei, leaders of the second of three streams of Professor Zheng's teaching in Malaysia, nor did Zheng ever mention them to me (he did speak favorably of Huang Xingxian). I have heard from a reliable source that Yue's lungs were affected by wounds he received from the Japanese in World War II. If what Sutton writes of Yue's group is true, however, I shake my head sadly. He writes that they had a more muscular taiji than Huang Xingxian, that they prevailed in tournaments, and that Mr. Lu was known for sparring with and beating up his students (1994: 63–64).

Let us take these in order. Muscular taiji, like free love, is a contradiction in terms. Zheng Manqing taught that there was no hard in taiji—only different degrees of soft. Echoing Yang Chengfu, Chen Weiming wrote, "Those people who say you must use force usually have excess strength or practice with a hard style and won't give it up, thus never obtain the essence of taiji" (Lo and Smith, 1985: 18), and again, "People using force cannot benefit from taichi . . . they have failed to internalize the art" (Lo and Smith, 1994: 42). Professor Zheng wrote that we must "completely spurn muscular force" and that we should "relax completely and not exert muscular force" (Cheng, 1962: 13). It seems unlikely that anyone who would stress a more muscular taiji is practicing the taiji of Professor Zheng.

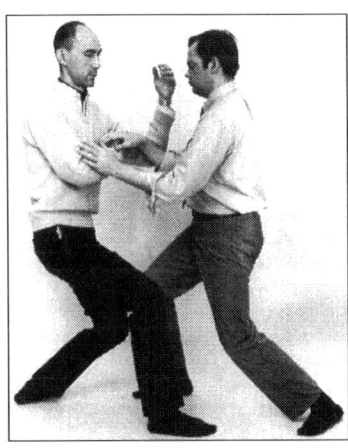

Tam Gibbs (right) doing push-hands
with Ed Young in New York City.

The fact that the Yue stream won more tournaments suggests a correlation between muscle and tournaments that should make Sutton pause. Tournaments are anathema to taiji. I have seen several. I cannot remember ever seeing relaxation there—only tension and force.

Taiji, to the extent that it becomes commercial and overly competitive, is no longer the real taiji that Chen Weiming loved so well. After all, taiji comes from Daoism which opposes all competition. Moreover, push-hands is meant to be a quiet means of testing and confirming one's form with another person while adhering to the basic principle established centuries ago of "no resistance and no letting go." Push-hands is not for commerce and ego. This principle was violated by Mr. Lu's sparring with and beating up students. I don't know what Sutton means by this, but it smacks of something other than taiji.

Some critics, Sutton writes, believe that taiji is presently weak because Professor Zheng's first generation of students in Taiwan were mainly intellectuals and academics (1994: 59). Who asserts this and what is the evidence? Sutton should give such critics a wide berth.

In fact, contemporary taiji is vibrant and hardy. Thousands of people everywhere have better health and a richer life thanks to Professor Zheng's taiji. Today, it is strong—and getting stronger—in substance and spirit. True, many gentries were drawn to him by his Olympian accomplishments. But he accepted people from every station of life (in New York City, he had problems with local Chinese because he flung open his door and heart to the hippies of that time). Even if the contention that he taught the elite were true, there is no correlation between gentry and weak taiji. I think Sutton is talking of "tournament taiji" and muscular push-hands, which are not taiji at all. He must read again the *Classics* and Zheng's *Thirteen Treatises*, both of which condemn muscularity. For myself, I think the ideal student for push-hands is a person with little or no athletic background whatsoever.

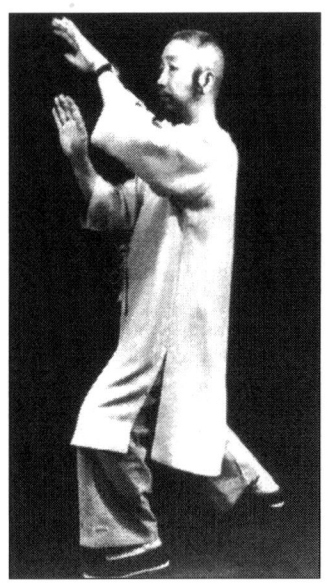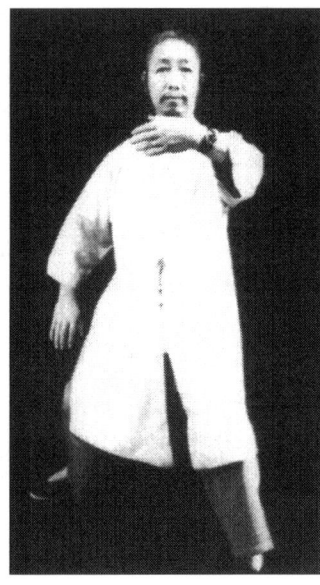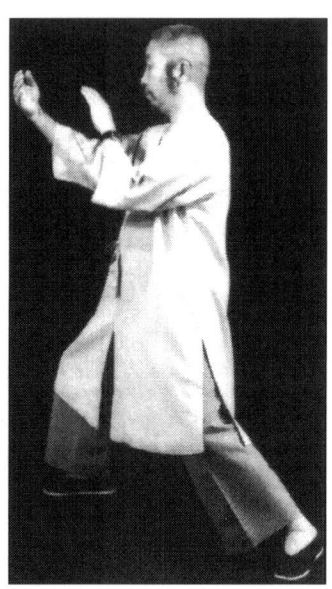

Zheng Manqing in lady works at shuttles, ward off, and rollback.

When Sutton writes that Zheng Manqing, while trying to promote the cultural aspects of his art, "recruited" most of his top students by beating them in challenges of one form or another, he is being too sanguinary (1994: 62). The verb "recruited" should be deleted—Zheng did not have to recruit anyone—and "challenges" ought to be softened. Probably most challenges were simply push-hands tests in which the outsider found no place for push or pull and, at once enthralled by Zheng's body brilliance and frustrated by his own ineptitude against it, just gave up.

I say this with some understanding. When Professor Zheng came to New York City in the 1960s, I visited his studio frequently. On my first visit, during of a lecture, he called me to the front and introduced me to the class as a boxer who had travelled around southeast Asia challenging all and sundry. This was not quite so. I did seek out taiji teachers for push-hands and got on famously with them, for courtesy and friendship prevailed. This does not mean that Zheng could not or would not wreak exquisite havoc if someone strayed outside the structured confines of push-hands (this too, I know from personal experience).

The point I am making is that Zheng was no gentle ruffian or thug. Sutton's bias toward muscular taiji would have bored Zheng. Whenever I or anyone else dwelled too long on combative matters, he invariably would start yawning, softly take the arm of the miscreant—often me—and blast him off the wall. True, he loved to talk with me about the Yangs, Du Xinwu, and other greats, but this was more in the historical rather than combative context.

Sutton's chief undoing, I think, is that he believes too much of the gossip, forever rife, in boxing circles. For example, he states that Professor Zheng's decision to leave Taiwan for the US in the midsixties was not made for altruistic reasons or to share his art with the world (1994: 60). But then he does not drop the other shoe; he neglects to tell us why Zheng went. I had spoken with Professor Zheng about a trip to the West shortly before I returned to the US from Taiwan in 1962, during the Cuban missile crisis. He went in January, 1964, to show his art at the Cernuschi Museum in Paris; he was the first artist ever to give a one-man show in the fifty-year history of that institution. This show was followed the same year by a one-man show at the World's Fair in New York, in 1968 at the FAR Gallery in New York, and in 1973 at the Hudson River Museum. All these shows met with lavish critical praise. Professor Zheng was honored but had to take out a bank loan to cover expenses for the first show. I only learned of the loan recently. It says something for his altruism that he never asked his students to support the trip financially, which all of us would have done without a second thought. On the way home from Paris in 1964, Zheng visited old friends and made new friends in New York City—artists, literati, and taiji aficionados—many of whom urged him to relocate here and promised him support. In due course he accepted. In any case, it strikes me as journalistically unethical on Sutton's part to claim to "know" something bad about a person and indict him with a hint and wink, but never name the fault.

Sutton ends his article by criticizing Zheng Manqing for being abstract on function, quoting from *Thirteen Treatises*: "If one is able to interpret energy and master the techniques, one's applications will be successful" (1994: 70),[11] then complains that Zheng does not reveal exactly how to interpret energy and master the techniques. But he does. He tells us continually in his writing and teaching to persevere in the postures and push-hands and to follow the basic principles of the Classics faithfully with belief, to become familiar with correct touch, to learn listening energy (*tingjin*), and to gradually comprehend interpreting energy (*dongjin*). Some of these lessons are provided in the very chapter from which Sutton quotes (Lo and Inn, 1985: 204).

No other person in taiji history has shed so much light on the more esoteric aspects of the art as has Zheng Manqing. When he first published *Thirteen Treatises* in 1950, he even wrote a series of articles in the major newspaper in Taibei telling his all-Chinese audience how to understand the more arcane subject matter in the book.

Zheng said he could not give us a pill (they don't make pills like that). Taiji is a microcosm of life. One must work at it and work hard, through its agonies and exultations, and only then will it yield its favors. Why else did Zheng say that, of all his excellences, taiji was the most difficult? So, though his words can guide us and help us, they cannot do our job for us nor even fully help us understand it. Confucius said, "When I have presented one corner of a subject to anyone and he cannot from it learn the other three, I do not repeat the lesson" (Legge, n.d.: 203).

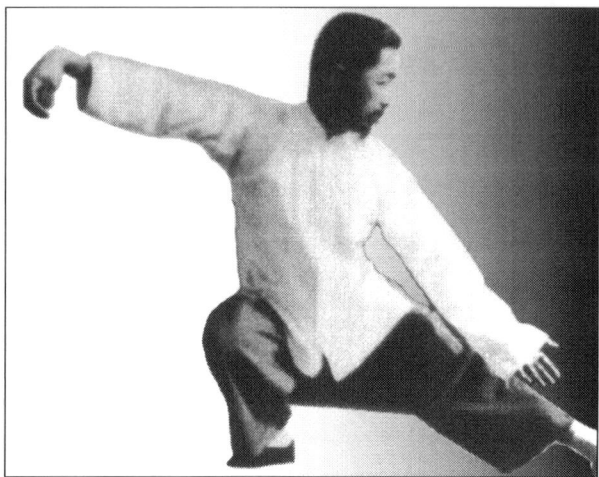

Squatting single whip, ca. 1948.

Professor Zheng, while alive, was often the target of gossip by inferior boxers, largely in Asia. Envy is a great stimulus. The villains, "boxers of the mouth corners," had only to approach him to be educated, but they avoided the opportunity like Dracula did garlic. Now that he is dead, it is worse—Zheng's own students sometimes behave poorly out of egotism. This is a shame. Add to which he is accused of keeping secrets by a writer who will not read or consult,[12] apparently cannot understand, and whose attitude cries out for infinitely more practice in "quiet minding." Put simply, Professor Zheng stood for good. I hope Mr. Sutton can come to see this.[13] In writing to protect Professor Zheng's estimable name, I am no sycophant, but just a person who wants to right a wrong. Here I have tried to "use all gently" (as the Bard says). But if Mr. Sutton finds my words harsh or in need of corrigenda, he should let me know so that I can correct them.

Notes

[1] See page 57. In the first paragraph, the writer also suggests that the growth of taiji on the world stage is largely because of Zheng Manqing's style. This assertion can only be correct if one leaves out the influence of China itself with its millions of practitioners, relatively few of whom do the so-called Zheng Style or even know of Zheng.

[2] Wang Yannian recently wrote me correcting the year of the match from 1914 to 1924 (Julia Fairchild letter to R. Smith, October 16, 1994). Additionally, Liu Xiheng writes that a Mr. Hong, a student of Yang Chengfu who later lived in Hong

Transliteration of Chinese

Wade-Giles	Pinyin	Wade-Giles	Pinyin
PEOPLE		Wu Yu-hsiang	Wu Yuxiang
Chang Ch'in-lin	Zhang Qinlin	Yang Pan-hou	Yang Banhou
Ch'en Ch'ing-ping	Chen Qingping	Yang Ch'eng-fu	Yang Chengfu
Ch'en Wei-ming	Chen Weiming	Yang Chien-hou	Yang Jianhou
Cheng Man-ch'ing	Zheng Manqing	Yang Lu-ch'an	Yang Luchan
Han Yu	Han Yu	Yang Shao-hou	Yang Shaohou
Hao Wei-chen	Hao Weichen		
Huang Hsing-hsien	Huang Xingxian	**PLACES**	
Li I-yü	Li Yiyu	Pei ching	Beijing
Liu Hsi-heng	Liu Xiheng	Ch'en-chia-kou	Chenjiagou
Lu Tung-pao	Lu Dongbao	Nan ching	Nanjing
Sun Lu-t'ang	Sun Lutang	Shanshi	Shanxi
Tso Lai-p'eng	Zuo Laipeng	Szechwan	Sichuan
Tu Hsin-wu	Du Xinwu	T'aiyüan	Taiyuan
Tung Ying-chih	Dong Yingjie		
Wan Lai-sheng	Wan Laisheng	**PRACTICES**	
Wang Tsung-yueh	Wang Zongyue	nei-kung	neigong
Wang Yan-mian	Wang Yennien	t'ai chi ch'üan	taijiquan
Wu Chien-ch'uan	Wu Jianquan	t'ai chi shih-i	taiji shi yi
Wu Ch'uan-yu	Wu Quanyu	t'ing chin	ting jin
Wu Kuo-chung	Wu Guozhong	tung chin	dong jin
Wu Kung-tsao	Wu Gongzao		
Wu T'u-nan	Wu Tunan		

Kong, saw the Zhang–Wan challenge match (letters to R. Smith, May 7 and 9, 1991). So, the match occurred. But in *Chinese Boxing* (p. 38), I write that when Wan and Zhang squared off "the fight went nowhere: both injured their hands at the outset, and it was postponed." The source for this was Zheng Manqing himself given orally to me. At the same time, he told me that earlier Wan had tested Yang Chengfu and was easily dispatched, saying as he left "two years" (meaning he would train for that period and return). When Wan challenged Yang again, Zhang intercepted. I tend to accept this version: Zheng knew both Yang and Zhang well and there was no need to slant the story. And it does not diminish Zhang—his glory days were ahead of him.

[3] Wang Yannian inexplicably renders Zuo's given name as "Yifeng."

[4] See page 38 of *Chinese Boxing*. The next sentence reads: "[Zheng] stayed with this man a while and derived a new method of doing the postures." I can't remember the source or even having written the sentence. The source certainly was not Zheng Manqing. I hope these words were not an ingredient in Wu Guozhong's claims. Lacking any corroboration for these words, since they were written over twenty years ago, I now disavow them.

⁵ Conversation with Wang Yannian in Bethesda, Maryland, September 24, 1984.
⁶ Letters from Liu Xiheng, May 7 and 9, 1991; Phone conversation with Ben Lo, August 1994.
⁷ See Tam Gibbs (1985). This article is dated November 2, 1978, and is an expansion of the memorial tablet largely written, according to Ben Lo, by Yao Menggu, an artist colleague of Professor Zheng. Gibbs fleshed out the text of the memorial for this article and his translation was done in the presence of Mrs. Zheng as she transliterated the classical language (*wen yen*) of the original into vernacular Chinese (*pai hua*) so that Gibbs could understand it and translate it into English.
⁸ Letters from Liu Xiheng, May 7 and 9, 1991.
⁹ Wu Jianquan's father, Wu Quanyou, was a top student of Yang Banhou.
¹⁰ I never met Wu Guozhong. A decade or so ago, he wrote me urging me to let him put my name with his on a book he had written (presumably, the old Cheng-Smith nexus would then become Wu-Smith). The proposal struck me as strange, and I declined his offer.
¹¹ The writer incorrectly attributes this to Ben Lo and Martin Inn's translation of *Thirteen Treatises*, but the words are from D. Wile's *Advanced T'ai-chi Form Instructions*, p. 112. There is no substantive difference, however, in the two translations.
¹² Sutton should have consulted with me. If he had, many of these errors could have been avoided. He had erroneously stated that I made Professor Zheng's prowess known through the English-speaking world (p. 61). In this article and elsewhere, Sutton attributes Zheng's fame to my writing, confusing the message with the messenger. Let me be plain: Professor Zheng's reputation is the result of his extraordinary ability in taiji. His towering taiji earned him a deserved recognition. Sutton's error is the ultimate example, it seems to me, of confusing the teacher and the taught.
¹³ Since Sutton is one of the few writers in the martial arts genre combining writing craft and style—and we must encourage such talent—it has been hard for me to criticize him. But the issues demanded it. Germanely, in passing, permit me to bow to karateka Graham Noble of England, who can bridge Eastern and Western martial arts in his facile writing; to Dave Lowry; to Canadian judoka Paul Nurse; to Hunter Armstrong, keeper of Donn Draeger's flame—who has that rare quality in the fighting genre—common sense. Last, but probably at the top of this short list, I would place the taiji teacher from Australia, Paul Lynch, whose writing stands and moves and is always lubricated by intelligence and wit. With the advent of the *Journal of Asian Martial Arts*, I am sure this short list will become longer.

Bibliography

Cheng, M. (1962). *Taichi chuan: A calisthenics for health and self defense*. Taibei: Shih Chung Tai-chi Chuan Center.

Draeger, D., and Smith, R. (1980). *Comprehensive Asian fighting arts*. Tokyo: Kodansha.

Gibbs, T. (1985). Cheng Tzu: Master of Five Excellences. *Full circle, 1* (2): 13–21.

Legge, J. (Trans.). (n.d.). The Confucian analects. In *The four books.* Also in *The Chinese classics*, vol. 1. Oxford: Clarendon Press (1893).

Lo, P., and Inn, M. (Trans.). (1985). *Cheng Tzu's thirteen treatises on t'ai chi ch'uan*. Richmond, California: North Atlantic Books.

Lo, P. (1985, August). Explanation of Tso-style t'ai chi ch'uan. T'ai chi ch'uan. Taibei: Taiwan.

Lo, P., Inn, M., Amacker, R., and Foe, S. (Trans.). (1979). *The essence of t'ai chi ch'uan: The literary tradition*. Richmond, California: North Atlantic Books.

Lo, P., and Smith, R. (Trans). (1985). *Ch'en Wei-ming, T'ai chi ch'uan ta wen* [Questions and answers on taijiquan]. Richmond, California: North Atlantic Books.

Lowenthal, W. (1991). *There are no secrets: Professor Cheng Man-ch'ing and his tai chi chuan*. Berkeley, California: North Atlantic Books.

Sutton, N. (1994). The development of Zheng Manqing taijiquan in Malaysia. *Journal of Asian martial arts, 3*(1): 56–71.

Wang Y. (1988). *Taijiquan*. Taibei, Taiwan: self-published.

Wile, D. (Comp. and Trans.). (1985). *Cheng Man-ch'ing advanced form instructions*. Brooklyn, New York: Sweet Ch'i Press.

Wile, D. (1983). (Trans.). *Master Cheng's thirteen chapters on t'ai-chi ch'uan*. Brooklyn, New York: Sweet Ch'i Press.

Wile, D. (1983). *T'ai chi touchstones: Yang family secret transmissions*. Brooklyn, New York: Sweet Ch'i Press.

Yang, C. (1975). *T'ai-chi ch'uan t'i-yung ch'uan shu*. [Complete principles and practice of t'ai-chi ch'uan]. Taibei: Chunghua wushu chupanshe.

Principles and Practices in Taijiquan
by Peter Lim Tian Tek

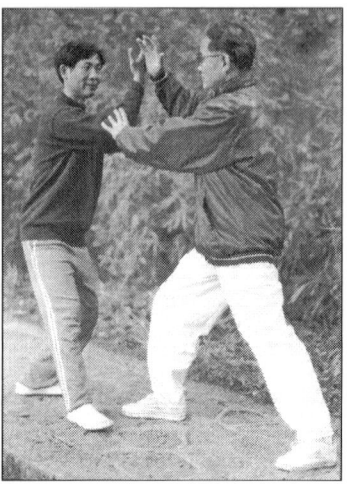

Mr. Xia Tao (L.), President of the Hangzhou Wushu Association, practicing tuishou with Mr. Jiang Jialun. Photograph courtesy of Don Mainfort.

Taijiquan is both a martial art and a health art and its correct practice brings benefits in both areas. To practice correctly, a proper understanding of the theories behind the practice is required. The following is a short discussion of some of the more important theories pertaining to both health and combat.

BASIC PRINCIPLES

Loose with No Tension (*song*)

Relax and loosen all the joints so that they are flexible, connected and able to integrate properly. Proper posture is held with the minimum of muscular exertion. Gravity provides the downward stacking mechanics that establishes a power source from the feet being rooted to the ground. Proper relaxation provides more efficient use of muscles resulting in a pliable strength rather than tensed strength.

I prefer to translate *song* as "no tension" rather than "relaxation," which too often implies limpness. Why is there a need for *song*? Very simply because if you are not *song* the muscles are not able to work efficiently. Muscles tense when the antagonistic muscle groups have in some way impeded the motion of each other, as such tension is the retained energy of the movement. This results in reduced mobility, promotes fatigue and reduces power. *Jing* travels through a strike much like a wave or pulse with relaxed musculature conducting it with no retained tension. This is like a whip which has no tension but is able to deliver a telling strike.

Stability by Sinking (*wen, chen*)

Stability is a result of coordinating our body structure with the downward pull of gravity creating a net force against the earth from both body weight and the downward projection of mass through a single point identified as the "root." Lowering the center of gravity is essential to stability. Therefore, we should become aware of our center and thus feel the resulting stability in our movements.

Agility (*ling*)

Agility is a result of not being double-weighted or having a "dead rooting." By maintaining only one point of substantial contact with the ground you can gain the ability to move quickly, much like a ball which moves easily across the ground because it only has one point of contact with it.

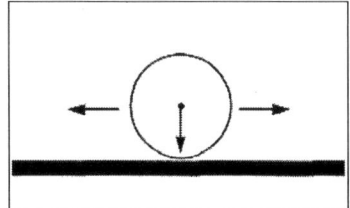

A ball has only one contact point with the ground and so can move freely in any direction.

The key is the word "center." We should avoid dead rooting. The idea is to lower your center of gravity to your proper focus at the dantian. There it should have a net downward force but be hung from the torso in the correct location. This would give you a centered but light feeling. If you are trying to get your center to the root of your feet, that is not centeredness. Ask yourself where the center of your body is and there is where the mass of the center should be. Some methodologies involving external and internal practices were adopted to train for this centering. The external way of training is to force the center down as far as it can go by sinking. This causes the musculature supporting the downward force to return a force from the feet back up toward the center. The internal method would first locate the center of gravity and then develop proper body posture to support it. When that is done, one should slowly lower the stance over time without sacrificing proper balance and body alignment.

Sensitivity (*ming gan*)

One of the keys in taijiquan combat is to train by focusing the mind (*yi*) on each motion. Focus the conscious mind, but also allow the subconscious to respond and become more aware. We need sensitivity to detect where our center is and where there are flaws in posture that can be exploited by an attacker. This sensitivity likewise allows us to detect an opponent's energy and movement.

Roundness (*yuan*)

The roundness of physical movement denotes a smooth connection and efficient transfer of force and energy. Hence, in the taiji postures, seek roundness. Roundness also helps in the dissipation of incoming energy.

Not Losing Contact, Not Resisting

Budiu buding means literally "not losing contact, not resisting" and is perhaps one of the most descriptive terms of taiji combat. *Peng* and its characteristics are what enables this to occur. *Peng* is expansive in nature; it has the qualities of sticking and buoyancy and stability. If your opponent retreats, it follows, if he advances, it sticks and redirects.

In cultivating this principle, we need to understand that sticking is necessary to "listen" to your opponent's strength and understand it so you can counter it by turning it against himself. Proper "listening" makes it possible for you to detect gaps and flaws in his posture and turn them to your advantage. At the same time, the buoyant quality makes it hard for your opponent to detect your center.

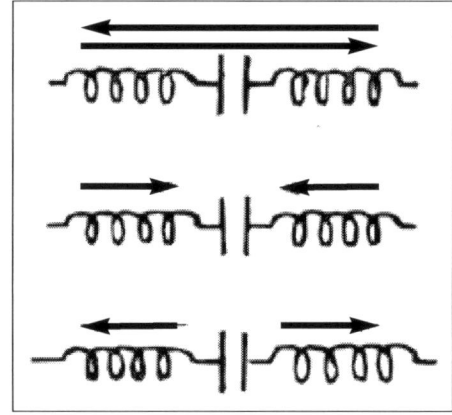

Top: Not letting go; Not resisting.
Middle: Resisting.
Bottom: Letting go.
Drawings of springs help illustrate the above concepts.

Breathing

Breathing initially should be natural and abdominal. As you learn how to "swim in air," the air assumes a heavy quality not unlike water. You will find that it takes relaxed effort to generate the movement. As a result of this, the breathing pattern will naturally change to your abdomen, expanding when you push out, the way it does when you are pushing a car. This is the point where reverse breathing becomes natural. It should be a natural transition and should not be forced. Practicing reverse breathing by itself to isolate the dantian and its movements in qigong should also not be forced. Reverse breathing occurs when the abdomen is pulled inward on inhaling and extend it on exhaling.

PRACTICES
Three Heights and Four Frames

The three heights are high, middle and low; the four frames are slow, fast, large, small. These denote the different ways of doing the taijiquan routine, each for a specific purpose.

The Three Heights

- *Middle:* This is the normal way we practice with the knees slightly bent and the body lowered. Here is where we learn the movements, their coordination, transition and focus.
- *Low:* At this level, our thighs should be at least parallel to the ground. One gets to this level progressively from the middle frame. It adds to the difficulty of the form and aids in further development in regard to endurance, body connection and coordination, stability and strength.
- *High:* At this level, we refine the body connection and coordination so that the techniques can be effected with minimal movement.

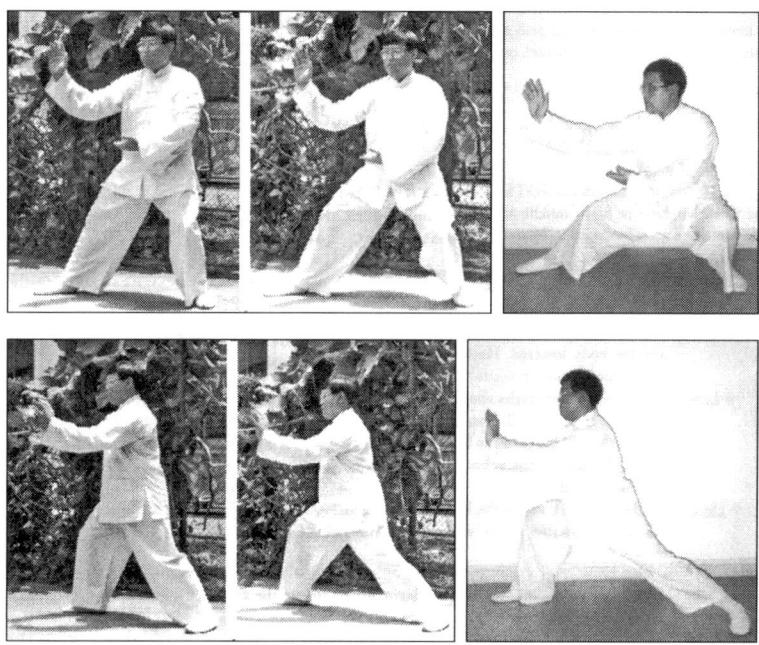

The author demonstrating the rollback (top) and push postures in three heights: high, medium, and low. Photographs courtesy of Peter Lim Tian Tek.

The Four Frames

- *Slow:* By practicing in this manner, we learn to coordinate the taiji movements and transitions and establish the foundation that make good taiji boxing skills.
- *Large:* Practicing movements in an extra-large fashion facilitates stretching and develops resiliency, good circulation and proper

muscular development. It also allows the movement comprising each technique to be savored and fully understood. It is usually done slowly as well.

• **Fast:** The techniques can also be executed quickly but without losing the qualities obtained by training slowly and with large movements.

• **Small:** This practice refines taiji techniques to their essentials so that they can be effected with minimum effort and movement. Normally in training, after learning the middle-height set and slow frame, one may commence to a fast set at a slightly lower height. However, one must retain the same qualities as before, being relaxed, sunk, and connected. Then a practitioner may move on to an even lower height at a slower speed with large movements. Lastly, one finally practices at a high height with small movements. This was the way Yang Banhou trained his students.

Form and Training

The form teaches us the content of the art, allowing us to know ourselves and how we function. Tuishou and other two-person exercises expand on this knowledge and teach us also how to know others. In knowing ourselves and knowing others we can "conquer them a hundred times out of a hundred." The form teaches us how our body can function efficiently and how it moves, what makes it live and what makes it effective. We learn here how to experience and control what we loosely refer to as "energy," "vitality principle," "vector energy," "*jing*" or "*qi*." The form is a means to experience, cultivate and learn how to effectively use this energy.

This energy is manifested through what is called "opening and closing" and has its origins in breath. This energy movement denotes the internal form (*nei xing*) and the physical movement denotes the external form (*wai xing*). In the beginning, the internal form comes from and is molded by the external form, but later the external form follows the dictates of the internal form. In the beginning, the mind directs the movements and is distinct from it. Later, the mind and the movement are one. The mind and body, internally and externally, fuse to become one entity, one reality. This is necessary for quick reactions and for the body and mind to act together to make the most of the situation.

This mind-body coordination and synthesis should become instinctive. As one becomes more dependent on the internal form and the flow of internal energy, the focus on the external form diminishes. The internal energy will be manifested through the external form. The mind and energy become the primary considerations at this level of practice. This is where the energy acts as the mind dictates; the body acts as the energy dictates. Ego and thought have no place as one moves according to the principles of the energy, to blend and balance with and to nullify the incoming flow of energy from an opponent's attack. The physical weapon is activated by the force within it although this force is an energy that is distinct from the weapon. This is internal boxing and its internal strategies for combat.

Push-hands (*tuishou*) and Sparring Hands (*sanshou*)
In taijiquan, tuishou is a practice to achieve several major goals:

1) To develop sensitivity to your opponent's motion and its origin.
2) To develop the ability to effortlessly redirect your opponent's motion by detecting and utilizing the weak vector of his motion.
3) To apply and practice a flexible rooting with fixed and moving steps while responding to your opponent's strength and motion.

Tuishou was also called *roushou* (soft hands) to emphasize non-resistance. It is not a combat practice. *Sanshou*, which is the application of the sensitivity and effortlessness developed through tuishou in a combat situation (blows, kicks, locks, grabs, etc), is the actual combative training in taijiquan. Free fighting is free form *sanshou* and is as close as you can get to combat without actually having someone out to hurt you. The Yang school has an eighty-eight posture (forty-four per person), fixed-form *sanshou*, which is akin to fixed-form sparring. The set was designed to slowly prepare the practitioner for free-form fighting or sparring. *Tingjing* (listening to *jing*) is paramount in taijiquan, since it is only by being sensitive enough to detect your opponent's motion, its qualities and its origin (this is the most important) that you can control him.

The two-person taijiquan set has specific training methodologies and goals. Fixed steps train one's sensitivity, stability and power within a limited range of motion. Moving steps expand this training to a simple back-and-forth motion by moving with self-controlled balance while avoiding being controlled by your opponent. *Dalu* (great rollback) adds the corner movements so that the repertoire is not limited to back-and-forth. Besides including the remaining four fundamental techniques, *dalu* teaches that retreat is also a form of attack. Free-form push-hands combines all the elements but still limits practice to the basic push-hands parameters. The following are goals for free-form push-hands:

1) To achieve sensitivity through contact.
2) To use that sensitivity to find the flaws in the attacker's defense. This is done by neither resisting nor letting go of an opponent's attack. The movements should be proactive in that you do not resist his motion but redirect it using its inherent flaws. In this way, the defensive movement need not only neutralize the attacking motion but may be turned into a counterattack as well.
3) To apply the principles cultivated in the form (correct posture, rooting, sensing energy, knowledge of your own center, etc.) in a reactive situation with a partner.
4) To learn the basics of attack and defense using effortless power born of proper rooting, posture and motion.

"Attracting to emptiness" simply means presenting the opponent a target which is actually a trap to lead him into emptiness (neutralizing and causing his force and momentum to act against himself). When this is done properly, your opponent's "thousand-pound force" can be deflected and used against him by the simple application of "four ounces" on the weakest vector of the incoming force to alter its trajectory back to the origin. One of the keys of taijiquan is never to use more than four ounces and never to receive more than four ounces (not exactly four ounces, mind you, the term simply indicates a light force). Accurate distancing and timing are necessary to accomplish such advanced techniques.

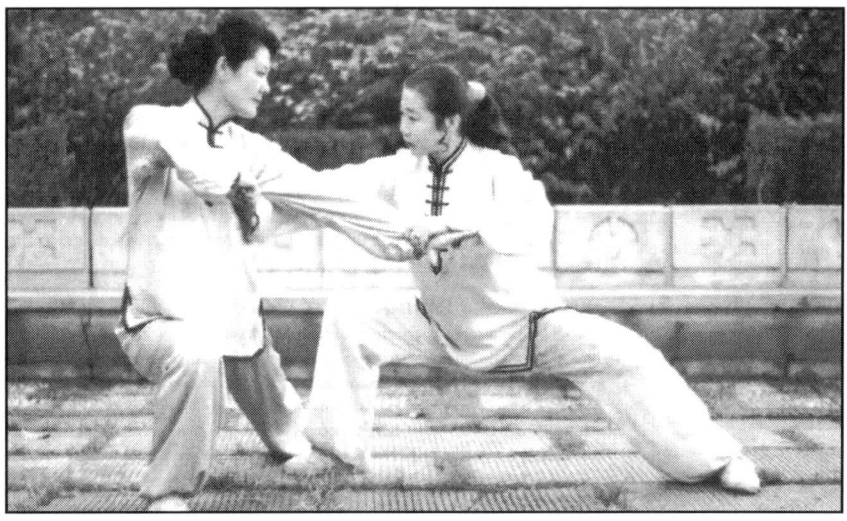

In Hangzhou city, Jin Huiying (right) practices taiji applications with her student Wu Hangxin. Two-person practices help develop sensitivity necessary to improve one's form and technique. Photograph courtesy of Don Mainfort.

Is push-hands a win or lose competition? No, it isn't. It is a form of training in which both parties benefit. Oftentimes good teachers will let one party do the pushing and the other do the countering. This teaches one to detect the center and the other to avoid detection and to counter. Winning or losing should not be important at this level of training as the goal is for the partners to train each other in knowing themselves and each other.

Beating Big with Small, Fast with Slow

"Beating big with small" usually means overcoming a big force with a lesser one. This is attained by not directly opposing the big force but redirecting it to our advantage by adding a smaller force to change the trajectory of the larger force. "Beating fast with slow" means beating a faster moving opponent with a slower technique. How is this achieved? No matter how fast an attacking limb is, it is always slower than the body behind it or the last joint between it and the body. By affecting the body directly via the center, by avoiding the fast-moving end and attacking the middle or last joint of the limb, we need not move as fast as we would normally need to meet the fast end of the limb and stop it. It is also easier to change its ultimate trajectory by affecting it closer to the trajectory's origin. Ultimately, by focusing on the origins of the attacker's strength—at his center and root—we need not move as fast as his attacking limb since that is not the object of our focus.

Training the Mind's Eye

The "mind's eye" is the way we perceive the outside world in relation to ourselves. In taijiquan we alter the normal perception via the way we practice. In doing the set slowly and with full intent, we become aware of the transition of the movement through time and create our own internal division of time according to the flow of taiji movement. Although the movements may be done quickly, this internal division of time still applies because it was previously set at a slower pace. Movements made quickly still appear to have a slow-motion quality when seen through the internal "mind's eye," allowing one to function at high speed without losing perception due to it.

Much of how we perceive time, space and movement is determined by how fast that information reaches the seat of our consciousness. If our attention is divided, external stimuli, even if slow moving, will appear quick and catch us by surprise. Fear and discomfort are two major causes of such internal noise that clouds our ability to perceive real time. Hence, there is the requirement for martial arts practitioners to develop a clear mind. By calming ourselves, sinking and relaxing to reduce tension and discomfort, losing our ego to put aside the fear of loss, we can see what is coming much more clearly. The quick is no longer that quick because one knows where it's coming from and going to and when it will arrive.

Point Focus in *Jing* Generation

Taijiquan techniques are manifested by having the qi in the body's meridians power the muscles. According to Chinese medical theories, qi is what gives the muscles the tenacity or tonus to manifest the techniques using the bones as a base. Qi originates at *yong quan* (called "bubbling well," the place where qi is stored; point K-1) and travels through the meridians causing the muscles to be qi-filled. Qi is directed by a mental focus, which is why there is the saying that the "mind leads the qi." The resulting muscular tenacity is what gives the "five bows" of the body (i.e. the back, which is the main bow, and the four limbs which are the secondary bows) the stored potential energy which can be released or shot into an opponent.

The back needs to be loose but straight to allow the unrestricted use of the muscles connected to it. Proper posture allows mental signals to pass from the nerves emanating from the spinal cord to instantaneously reach the muscles. The connecting path and the manifesting energy are referred to as *jing*. Hence, taijiquan movements are often described as "propelled." Qi is present in the body all the time, but it is its specific gathering, focus and transmission that makes it relevant in terms of martial arts.

Afterword

The above are some of the principles and practices of taijiquan. Practice according to the principles will not only bring good health but also the necessary fundamentals for application in combat. The best references for the art are still the *Taiji Classics*. Read them often and apply the principles therein to your practice. You will find as you progress that a new understanding of what they mean will become apparent. Most of all, enjoy your art and make it your very own by living and practicing it.

ENGLISH	PINYIN	CHINESE
press	an⁴	按
not losing contact, not resisting	bu⁴ diu¹ bu⁴ ding³	不丢不頂
sink	chen²	沉
vigor, power, strength, energy	jing⁴	勁
light sensitivity	ming² gan³	明感
internal form	nei⁴ xing²	內形
gas, air, vital energy	qi⁴	氣
soft hand	rou² shou³	柔手
scattering hands	san³ shou³	散手
relax, loosen	song¹	忪
listening energy	ting¹ jing⁴	听勁
push-hands	tui¹ shou³	推手
external form	wai⁴ xing²	外形
stable, steady, firm	wen³	穩
round, circular	yuan²	園
mind, idea, meaning	yi⁴	意
gushing spring	yong³ quan²	涌泉

References

Chen, W.M. (1925). *Taijiquan shu*. [The art of taijiquan]. Hong Kong: Wushu chubanshe (reprint, n.d.).

Chen, W.M. (1927). *Taijiquan dawen*. [Questions and answers on taijiquan] Taipei: Hualian chubanshe (1969 reprint).

Chen, Y.K. (1947). *Tai-chi chuan: Its effects and practical applications*. (Zhang Guoshui, Trans.). Shanghai: Kelly and Walsh, Ltd.

Chen, Y.L. (1943). *Taijiquan dao jian gan sanshou hebian*. [Taijiquan, broadsword, two-edged sword, staff, and sparring]. Shanghai: Shanghai dichan yanjiusuo.

Hsu, Y.S. (1921). *Taijiquan shi tujie*. [Illustrated manual of the postures of taijiquan]. Taipei: Hualian chubanshe (1982 reprint).

Hsu, Z.Y. (1927). *Taijiquan qianshuo*. [Introduction to taijiquan]. Shanghai: Taijiquan yanjiushe.

Lee, Y.A. (1968). *Lee's modified tai chi chuan for health*. Hong Kong: Unicorn Press.

Liang, T.T. (1977). *T'ai chi chuan for health and self-defense*. New York: Vintage Books.

Sieh, R. (1992). *T'ai chi chuan: The internal tradition*. Berkeley: North Atlantic Books.

Wang, Y.Q. (1990). *Yangshi taijiquan shuzhen*. [Authentic Yang style taijiquan]. Beijing: Renmin tiyu chubanshe.

Xu, Z.J. (1991). *Yangshi taijiquan*. [Yang style taijiquan]. Beijing: Beijing tiyu yuan chubanshe.

Yang, C.F. (1931). *Taijiquan shiyong fa*. [Self-defense applications of taijiquan]. Taipei: Zhonghua wushu chubanshe (1974 reprint).

Yang, C.F. (1934). Taijiquan tiyong quanshu. [Complete principles and practices of taijiquan]. Taipei: Zhonghua wushu chubanshe (1975 reprint).

Yue, T. (1961). *Taijiquan yao suo*. Shanghai: private publication.

Zhang, Y.J. (1986). *Taijiquan li chuanjen*. [The true principles of taijiquan]. Dazhong Shuju.

Zhang, Z.X. (1993). *Taijiquan duanlian yaoling*. [Principles of taijiquan training]. Guizhou: Guizhou kexue jishu chubanshe.

Zheng, J. (1933). *Yang Chengfu shi taijiquan*. [Yang Chengfu style taijiquan]. Guangxi renmin chubanshe (1993 reprint).

Zheng, M.C. (1946). *Zhengzi taijiquan shisan pian*. [Master Zheng's thirteen chapters on taijiquan]. Taipei: Lanxi tushu chubanshe.

Zheng, X.F. (1991). *Taijiquan pu*. Beijing: Renmin tiyu chubanshe.

• 12 •

Inner Circle Taiji Training Exercises
by Stuart Kohler, M.A.

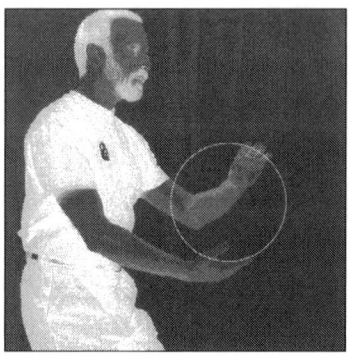

Photographs courtesy of Jim Eaton.

The taiji classics offer insights into the art for taiji players of all levels: and can also help resolve common frustrations for the practitioner. Students, particularly new students in the West, often feel they must invest years of training time and effort before they will master a form which yields the return they seek. One response is for teachers to offer a "short" form, while another is to offer training in which feeling is emphasized over precision of form. Some traditional training styles focus more on exactness of individual postures, which will later be linked into a single, flowing whole.

A study of the taiji classics suggests a method by which accuracy of postures need not be sacrificed for feeling in order to attain experiential understanding of continuous energy flow. This insight is derived from the delight of the "effortless effort" to be found in the practice of taijiquan, which cultivates the circulation of energy which, in turn, promotes health and, for the martial artist, power. I call this approach "Inner Circle Training."

The following quote from Song Chijian's "Twelve Guiding Principles," based on his *T'ai Chi Ch'uan Hsueh* [Taijiquan Xue], points to an essential circularity in the movements comprising the routine:

> The movements of [taijiquan] all advance in a circular line. When the forward and backward movements of [taijiquan] are connected, large or small circles are formed. If one's movements can be rounded out, then they will be lively and agile. If the body moves like a cartwheel and the hands follow the body movements, then the movements will naturally be circular. In this way the forms turning left and right, rounded and lively, will be like shooting stars.
>
> – Gallagher, 1989: 29

Simply stated, the premise of "Inner Circle Taiji Training" is that all postures are circular in nature, even those which may first appear to be strictly linear. By encouraging "play" to find the circles and deliberately exaggerating those circles, students are often able to experience a flow of energy much earlier in their taiji careers than would otherwise be possible.

One additional comment about inner circles also applies to all of the external or observable circles throughout the form. While circles are composed of inward and outward energy, a true circle is not composed of two pieces which are joined together (no matter how smoothly). Inbound energy is often gathering or coiling energy, as in press or push, in other words, a loading of the spring which will be released as part of the same single, fluid motion on the outbound phase. (The reverse may also be true, as in a posture such as needle at sea bottom [*nai di zen*]. The extension may be seen as the "loading" energy, while compression is the releasing energy. The intention here is to stress continuous fluid movement over linear sequences, no matter how seamlessly connected.)

Before examining postures taken from the taiji routine, we must first consider the gesture of a simple circle made by the hand. Notice that a fluid circle made by the hand is actually articulated by the wrist and elbow, and, to a lesser extent, the shoulder and waist (the involvement of the lower joints will be noted later). As the circle is made smaller and more subtle, it may be observed that the smallest and most subtle hand-circle is principally formed by the wrist. As one continues to refine the size and subtlety, external (observable) movement ceases, but there remains the sensation or intent of circular movement. This is the experience of the "inner circle."

As a first example from the routine, consider the postures ward off and rollback and, in particular, the transition between them (this and all following examples are taken from Yang Style taiji). From the rounded peng energy of ward off, the right hand extends out, fingers rotate up and the hand spirals inward as rollback is formed. There are actually several places in this sequence where continuous energy flow may be interrupted. Any interruption establishes a "dead spot" in which energy has been exhausted and has not yet been renewed. Yang Chengfu in his *Ten Essential Points of Taijiquan* states:

> When the old strength has been exhausted and the new is not yet developed, one can very easily be controlled by an opponent.... From beginning to end it [mind-intent rather than muscular force] continues fluidly without interruption; completing a cycle and beginning again, it flows in an endless circle and is never exhausted.
> – Gallagher, 1989: 22

Such an interruption may occur if the right hand extends outward, stops at its fullest extension, then reverses direction to form the upright arm of rollback (Figures 1a–1c). To form what Yang Chengfu calls an "endless circle," it is helpful to imagine the lead hand as making a "flicking" movement, rolling the focus of energy from the center of the hand at ward off out to the fingers and fingertips at the fullest extension and then allowing the energy focus to return to the palm as rollback is formed (Figures 2a–2e). Another inner circle is found in the forward hand of rollback as it circles in and up into the forward hand of press. This circle keeps the forward hand from waiting (exhausted energy) while the rear hand circles up to join and form Press.

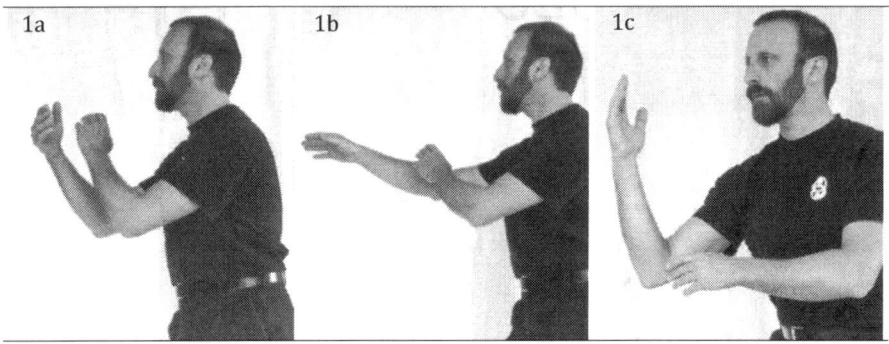

1a–c: Incorrect rollback sequence.
2a–e: Correct rollback sequence.

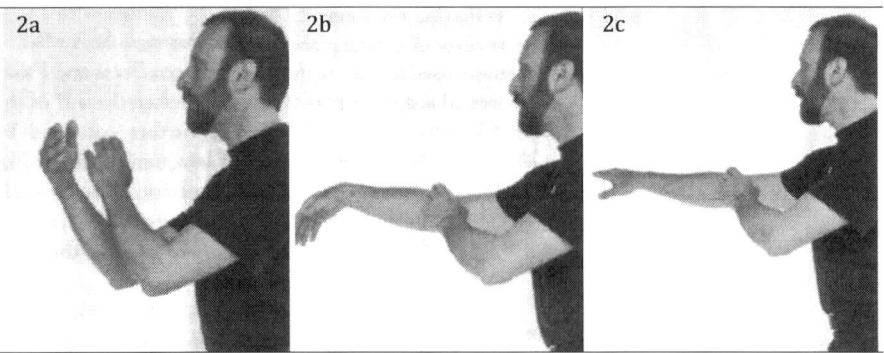

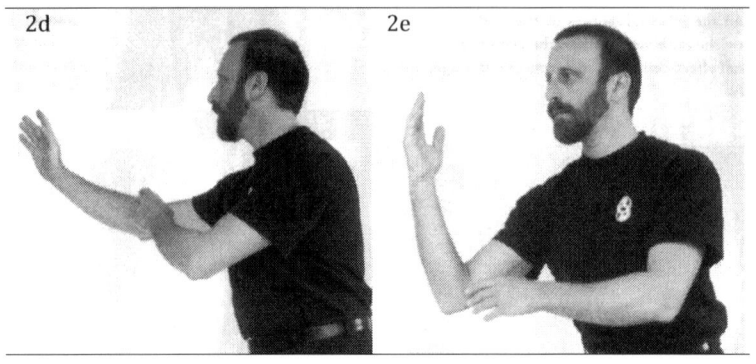

Following the formation of press is the transition to push. The analogy of catching and immediately passing a basketball is sometimes used to convey the transition between press and push. This mental image suggests fluidity, the "unbroken thread" of the taiji classics. This visualization may be further enhanced by adding a circular image. Thus, instead of imagining a piston-like in-and-out motion, which is linear (and, therefore, has a "dead" moment of transition between in and out, Figures 3a–3c), thinking of this motion in terms of a subtle circle can improve the energy flow in this transition (Figures 4a–4f).

Incorrect press-push sequence.

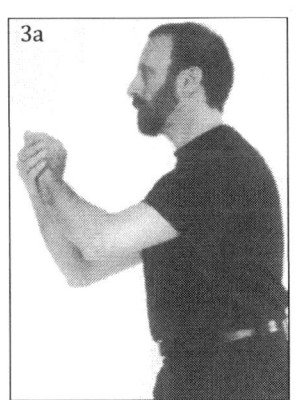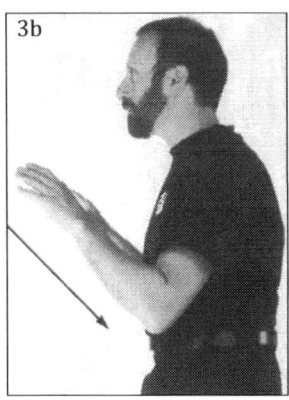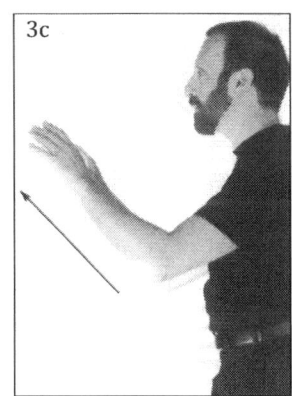

Correct press-push sequence.

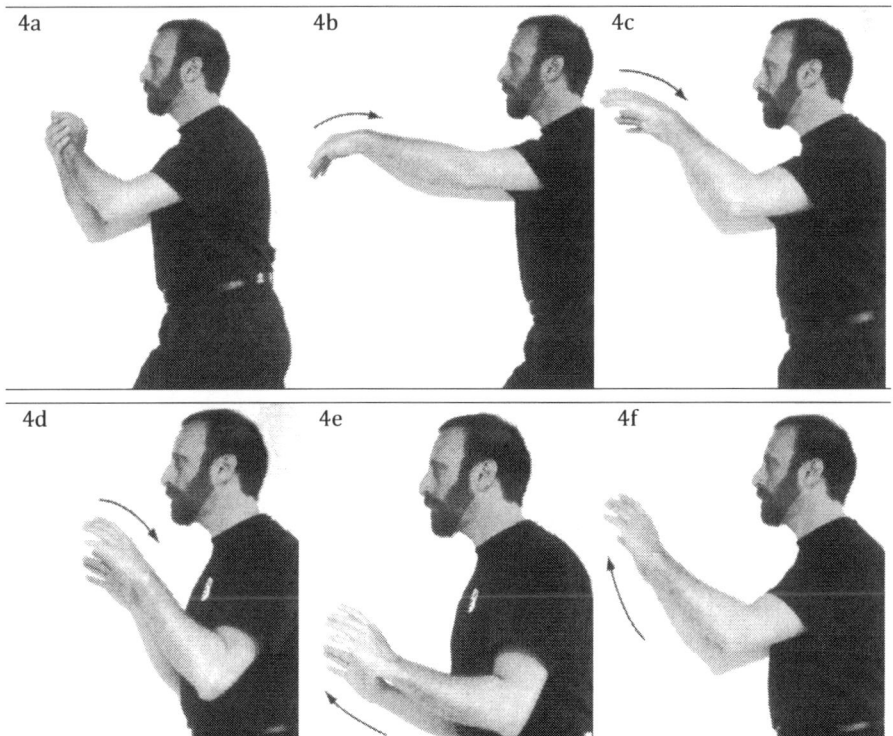

In playing with the inner circle concept here as well as in all postures, one would be well advised to follow Wang Zongyue's advice in his *Mental Elucidation*: "At first let your movements be open and expanded; later make them small and compact" (Gallagher, 1989: 49). In training, gestures can be deliberately exaggerated to show the circle, later to refine and reduce the size of the gesture while still retaining the feeling found in the larger gesture. Thus, on the inbound motion of push, the arms lift as well as retreat; on the outbound motion, the arms depress as they extend, the overall effect being a subtle vertical circle executed in front of the body.

Thrusting hand/palm (*chuan zhang*), found in the third section of the traditional Yang Style long form, offers an inner circle in a posture usually considered inherently linear. From the completion of high pat horse (*gao tan ma*), the left hand must drop, however slightly, to clear the right arm. The common error here is to move the left arm as a piston which established a "dead spot" at the transition between the inbound and outbound motion (Figures 5a–5c). A circular gesture made by the left hand and arm creates an uninterrupted flow of energy which also incorporates the adjustment of height necessary to clear the right arm (Figures 6a–6f).

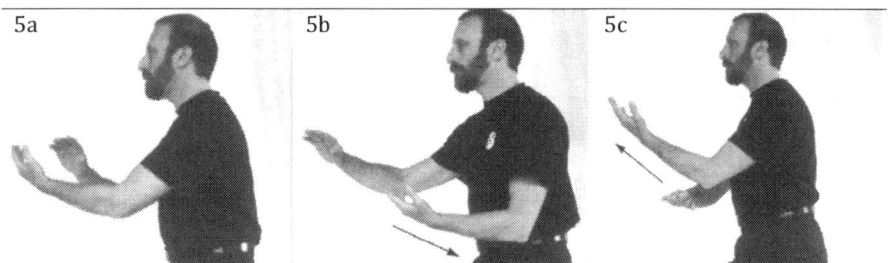

5 - Incorrect thrusting hand sequence.

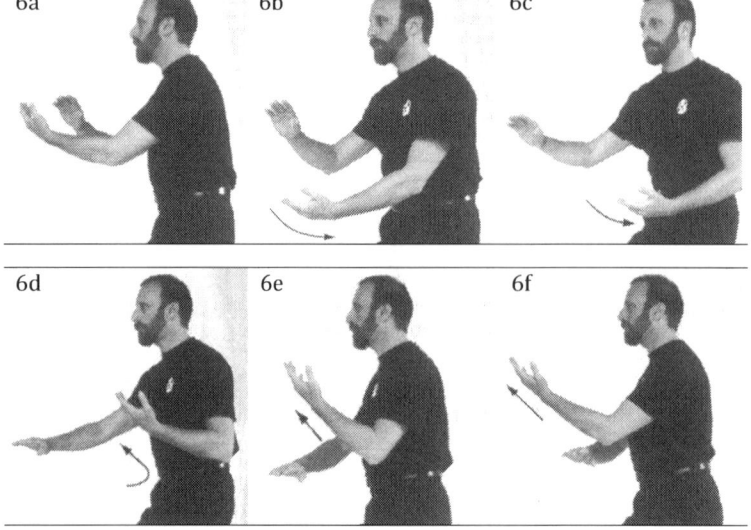

6 - Correct thrusting hand sequence.

As a third example, let us examine the beginning posture (*qi shi*). Traditionally, students are instructed to allow the arms to rise, wrists leading (as if balloons were tied by strings to their wrists) until the forearms are shoulder height or roughly parallel to the floor. Next the fingertips extend, making a single line from the shoulder. The common linear flaw here is that these gestures are treated as two separate movements, thereby occasioning the possibility of a "dead spot" between the point at which the arms have finished rising and before the fingertips begin their extension. To help prevent this, create the mental image of a single rounded movement, beginning with the rising arms, which is extended by moving energy out to the fingertips, again in almost a "flicking" gesture from the wrist.

Continuing with the beginning, the elbows become heavy as the hands draw in towards the body. At the completion of this gesture, the fingertips rotate up and then the hands arc down from the elbows to complete beginning. An inner circle may be found as the hands draw inward rather than coming to a stop at the closest point and then allowing the fingers to rotate up. The inner circle here connects the motion of the hands as they draw inward, arc back, up and around, and "flick" forward from the wrist to form a circle to the front. This is followed by the hands moving in a rounded arc downward, which traditionally completes beginning. No matter how smoothly these movements are connected, unless the player internalizes the associated inner circles, beginning may only aspire to be a series of smoothly connected linear pieces.

A reference to the continuous flow of inner circles may be found in the first line of the *Zhang Sanfeng Classic*: "In every movement the entire body must be light and spirited and all its parts connected like a string of pearls" (Gallagher, 1989: 47). Imagine the flow and arc of a string of pearls (even better if imagined underwater or moving in slow motion) in this same movement. In most of the examples cited in this chapter, the focus has been on the arms, hands and fingers as forming the "string of pearls." It is important to remember, however, that our brief discussion gives us only a partial view and is, therefore, only partially accurate. As found later in the *Zhang Sanfeng Classic*:

> The energy is rooted in the feet, rises through the legs, is controlled by the waist, and is formed in the fingers. From the feet to the legs to the waist, all must act as an integrated whole, so that in advancing and retreating, one can attain the proper preconditions and the position of strength.
> – Gallagher, 1989: 47

An example of a full-body generation of energy would be the waist circling of rollback. Energy from the rooted feet and legs sets the waist circling in motion, which in turn generates the circular movement of the arms. Specifically, from the extension of the leading arm, it is the turning of the waist which pulls that arm into its circle (Figures 7a–7b). The importance of this insight can be seen in the difference between pulling a rope with just the arms and shoulders and pulling that same rope with energy generated from the rooted feet, legs and waist-in effect, a classic form of "wind-up."

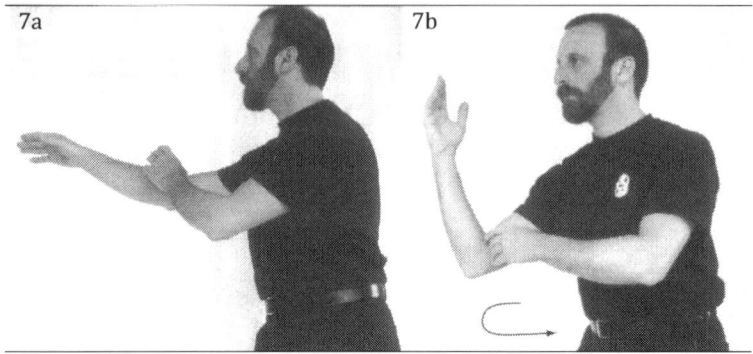

The waist in rollback sequence

Revisiting thrusting hand/palm, notice that again it is the waist circling to the left which generates the inbound circling of the thrusting hand (Figures 8a–8b). If the waist remains stationary, the thrusting hand has only isolated arm and shoulder energy and power. Similarly, the outbound part of the thrusting hand circle is generated by the waist circle to the right.

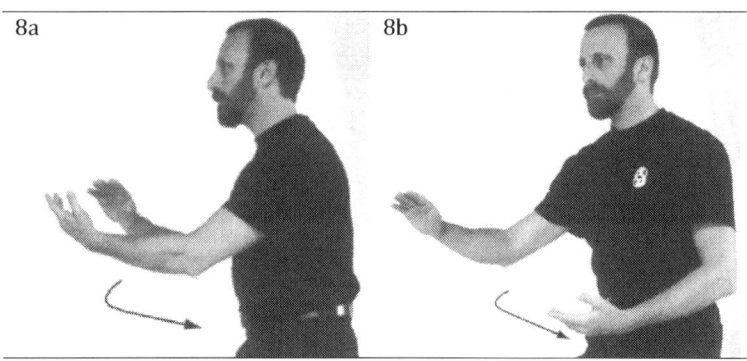

The waist in thrusting hand sequence

Again, it should be stated here that the exaggerated, "overt" circles are training exercises only; they are not meant to be taken as instruction in the correct execution of any given posture. Rather, it is a training technique intended to assist in achieving an experiential understanding of energy flow continuity in the form and the real, if subtle, sources of power in the postures. As a training technique, one should work to develop fluidity by exaggerating the circles, refining them later by reducing the external size while retaining the inner circular intent. This style of training in no way condones a form which lacks precision by encouraging one posture to be mindlessly merged into the next. In fact, when undertaken with sincerity, inner circle training will lead to a much higher level of mastery in doing the forms precisely.

Practice with the mind-intent of seeing circles in every gesture, especially those which appear to be inherently linear. The true goal of inner circle training is to internalize the circles so that they indeed become unobservable to others. All that should remain observable of inner circle training is greater smoothness, the absence of jerky start/stop linear gestures and the experience of the entire body as "light and spirited and all its parts connected like a string of pearls."

	Wade-Giles	**Pinyin**	**Chinese**
People	Chang^1 San^1-feng^1	Zhang^{1}San^{1}feng^1	張三丰
	Yang^2 Cheng-fu^3	Yang^2 Cheng^{2}fu^3	楊澄甫
	Wang^2 Tsung^1-yueh^4	Wang^2 Zong^1 yue^4	王宗岳
Classic	T'ai^4 Chi^2 Ch'uan^2 Hsueh^2	tai^4 ji^2 quan^2 xue^2	太極拳學
Movements			
Beginning posture	ch'i^3 shih^4	qi^3 shi^4	起勢
Sea Bottom Needle	hai^3 ti^3 chen^1	hai^3 di^3 zhen^1	海底針
Push	chi^3	ji^3	擠
Press	an^4	an^4	按
Thrusting Hand/Palm	ch'uan^1 chang^3	chuan^1 zhang^3	穿掌
High Pat Horse	kao^1 tan^1 ma^3	gao^1 tan^1 ma^3	高探馬

Reference

Gallagher, P. (1989). *Drawing silk: A manual for t'ai chi*. Guilford, VT: Deer Mountain Taoist Academy.

• 13 •

Remembering Zheng Manqing: Some Sketches from His Life
by Robert W. Smith, M.A.

"Draw your chair up close to the edge of the precipice and I'll tell you a story."
—F. Scott Fitzgerald

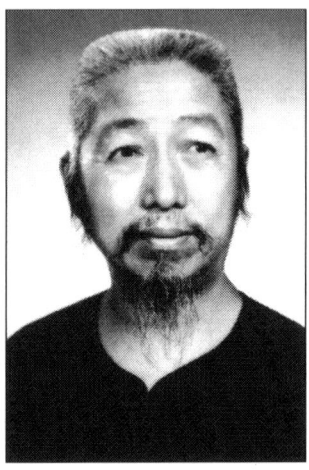

"I never wanted to become a Buddha;
I wanted to become a man." — Zheng Manqing

Photos courtesy of R. W. Smith except where noted.

Sometime after Professor Zheng died in 1975, Tam Gibbs, one of his senior taiji students, called me from New York City saying he had had an exhilarating talk with Mrs. Zheng. He said in this discussion she described some events that occurred during the early years of her marriage to Zheng. A young, cultured woman—her father was a top figure in the Chinese Air Force—she was awed by the brilliance and energy of the forty-year-old Zheng. And often she didn't quite know what to make of his friends. She cited two boxers, man and wife, who would come to the Zheng home and never bother to knock at or open the outer gate—they simply jumped over it and strode in. Another boxer one night rose from his chair in the living room and bade her turn off the lights. She did. He then did a form in total darkness and all she could see were sparks and lights from his qi. When she turned the lights on and examined him for electrical sources, she found none.

Tam Gibbs urged me to interview Mrs. Zheng, saying I knew the history and liked a good story. I wrote her and suggested it. She politely declined, saying she was young then and her recall of names was so faulty that it would, she felt, negate the value of the story. She also owned that recalling the old days just then would trouble her emotionally. So I backed away.

Another of the stories she had told Tam that day concerned a young Western-style boxer, Guo Qinfang, the lightweight champion of China, who knew Professor Zheng well in the early 1940s. One day in Chongqing the Professor took Guo with him to see a "strange" boxer named Wang Xiuai.[1] When they got to the boxer's modest house, an emaciated man who looked like a coolie opened the door and politely invited them in. They sat down in chairs while the "coolie" huddled against the wall. After a little while, young, impatient Guo inquired of Zheng where the master was. Zheng pointed to the "coolie" and said, "That's him." Zheng spoke to the man and he answered. Zheng then told Guo to go stand before him, which Guo did. The boxer gently took Guo's hand, smiled, and without force—at least Guo felt no force, only an exquisite energy—put him facedown onto the floor. Guo got up and squared off with the man. No blows were struck, but the boxer suddenly appeared behind the stupefied Guo. The three then drank tea, talked awhile, and the visitors left, Zheng laughing, Guo enthralled but puzzled.

In 1992 I wrote Danny Emerick, studying under Liu Xiheng in Taiwan, and urged him to interview Mr. Guo. Sometime later, Danny sent me the manuscript of an interview in which he and translator Michael Schnapp, another longtime student of Liu, asked the questions to which Guo and, at one point, his boxing brother, Xu Yizhong, responded.

Guo Qinfang Meets Professor Zheng

"I [Guo Qinfang] first met Professor Zheng Manqing in 1930 at a Shanghai university. He was dean of the Chinese Arts Department, and I was attending one of his classes.

"Ten years later, during the war against Japan, I participated in a boxing match for the war effort against a 160-pound boxer named [Song] at Chongqing.[2] At the time I weighed 130 pounds. Since the bout was billed as an exhibition, I queried Song beforehand on how we should fight.

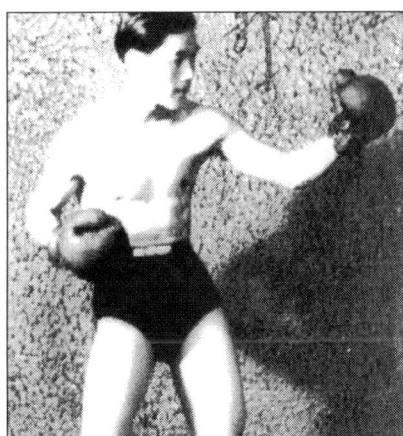

Guo Qinfang: Lightweight champion of China in the late 1930s.
Photo courtesy of Guo Qinfang.

"'You'll see when we get into the ring,' he said curtly, letting me know that he was serious and not in an exhibition mood.

"In the first three-minute round we felt each other out and went to our corners to the sound of general hissing; clearly the audience wanted more action. Song responded by coming out for the second round with a barrage of blows. But I was ready and avoided his volley easily. In the third round, when he failed to react to a few of my jabs, I moved in with heavier punches to his head and soon he was hurt and hanging on. When he clinched, I concentrated my attack on his midsection.

"In the fourth round, because he hadn't connected once to my head, he went to my lower body. When this had no effect on me, he tried to hit me below the belt, bringing an avalanche of boos from the crowd and a stoppage of the fight by the referee. He left the ring forfeiting, and many in the crowd who had paid for six rounds demanded refunds. Trying to save the situation and his 'face,' I, the winner, told the crowd that Mr. Song had not violated the rules intentionally and that the money spent for tickets went to a good cause.

"Of course, I knew the low blows had been intentional. Later on, I learned that Mr. Song had moved to America and was famous for being 'the boxing champion of China.'

"It so happened that Professor Zheng was there watching the fight. He saw that Song had broken the rules and was concerned that I had been injured. He didn't know that I had been one of his many art students a decade before, but he thought my skill had been outstanding and sent Zhang Zigang, one of his senior students, around to talk with me. Zhang approached me, saying that his teacher really admired my gongfu and asked whether I had been hurt. I told him no, that I had dodged Song's punches and he had only hit my gloves. He said that his teacher would treat me if I liked. When I asked his teacher's name, he told me Zheng Manqing. I asked him what his teacher was and he said a doctor. I told him: 'Your teacher is my teacher and my teacher is a painter!'

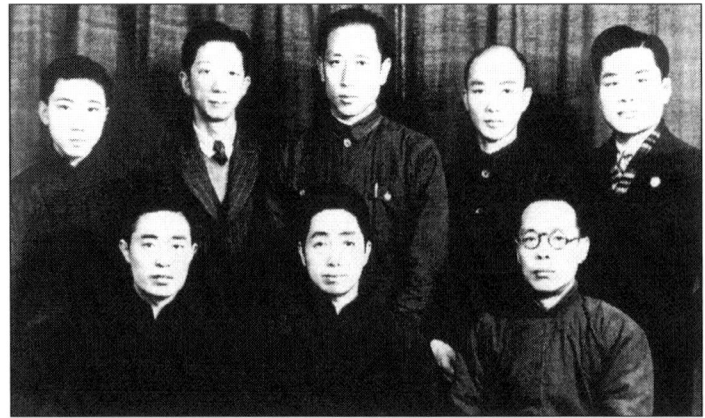

Photo of Zheng Manqing (center front), Guo Qinfang (rear row, far right with scarf), and Zhang Zigang (behind Zheng) in 1943. Others are unidentified. Zheng Manqing said Zhang probably was the most skilled taiji master on the mainland at that time.

"Later I studied taiji from Professor Zheng, but my main emphasis was still on boxing and how taiji could be applied to boxing, not quite the same as those who focused their energies solely on taiji. But with time, I was able to get a thorough understanding of Professor Zheng's teaching. When I box, I substitute for force his idea of overcoming the hard with the soft. I slip and duck my opponent's blows so that he can't land a single punch round after round. Of course, I'm speaking of head blows. I don't worry about body shots; special training has made me immune to these. But I never permit a head punch and so have never been injured there—unlike my teacher, Chinese Australian Chen Hanqiang ["Tacky"], an outstanding area pro of the 1920s and 1930s, whose ears were shifted out of place from head shots.

"When I teach a novice boxing, I first teach him to avoid and dodge so that he never takes a punch before I teach him to attack. If at first you teach him to attack rather than defend, he will be hit and will often become afraid. So, I teach him not to let himself get hit. This approach, of course, takes time and patience in the basics, such as jumping rope, hitting a ball or bag, and abdominal training so that you can take punches there. On the latter, you work until you can take just about any blow there. The abdomen can be trained in this way, but the head cannot. You can train only to avoid being hit but not to take punches to the head. If you take too many head blows, your brain will be damaged.

"Beyond this Western boxing training, I also was able to study some qigong. My teacher Huang in Chongqing was so versed in this mysterious art that [with permission] one could hit him in the head with a brick and it would have no effect. [In general practice] Huang would let anyone hit him anywhere except in the head—presumably, because of the eyes—without discomfort. One of his students, and a brother-student of mine, had practiced the art to such an extent that he would let a car run over his abdomen without injury.

"These abilities had more to do with qi than with muscular development. But there is another way: I trained, as I said before, with abdominal exercises. And this can be expanded to other parts of the body using a punching board. For instance, the lower arms can be trained by first hitting a wooden pole, starting lightly. Train until your arms become red, then purple, then black, and finally recover their original color. And then you are done—you then can take blows to the arms. In the end, you strike a steel pole. My students hit my arms, which are so hard that it hurts them. This is hard training and has nothing to do with technique. At first, you strike the pole twenty times progressing over time up to a hundred repetitions. Then you can work in pairs, striking each other's arms like this [demonstrating].

"One of Professor Zheng's students, the late Shi Shufang, has a special method of taking punches [Mr. Shi shows this ability in the 1960 film on Professor Zheng made in Taiwan], and he once challenged me to an arm-striking contest. I told him I hadn't practiced this for a long time. He replied that he had challenged people all over the island and that there was no one who could beat him but that I shouldn't be afraid; after all, I was a famed boxer. I accepted and we went at it. After twenty or thirty of my strikes, he gave up.

"But he still would not accept defeat. He suggested slapping with the hands. When I was young, however, I had practiced 'steel-sand hand,' and so it took only ten or twelve of these exchanges before he surrendered. Steel-sand hand is so devastating that, once learned, it can never be used because the opponent's nose and head will bleed. I was supposed to train three years, but by the time I reached the halfway point I could not chance hitting anyone. In my painting practice, the brush in my hand began to feel like a nail, with no feel at all. So, I thought to myself: 'This is wrong. My hands are numb—what good is it? Even as a fighting tool, it is too terrible, impossible to use without inflicting serious injury.' So, I told my students not to train this way.

"In steel-sand practice, you really use steel sand, but you start with green peas and add the steel sand later. I was able to use this open-hand tactic against an opponent's arm in boxing as a block, but, of course, it was illegal against the head.

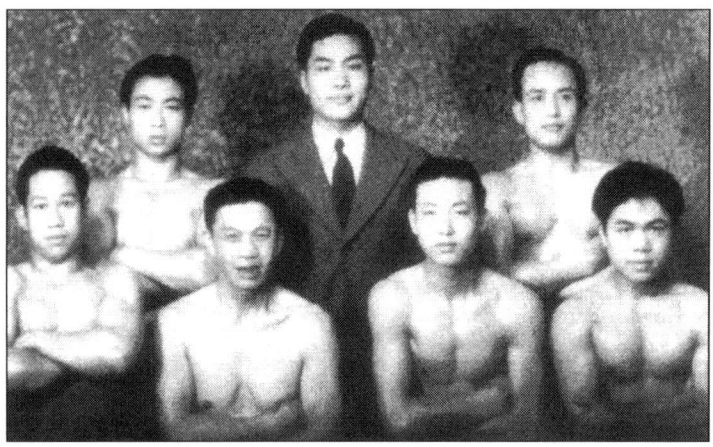

Guo Qinfang with the Jing Wu Boxing Team on occasion of his win over Topolesky, the Russian lightweight champion, at the 1937 International Boxing Tournament in Shanghai. Guo is suited and standing in the middle of the group. Seated in the first row, second from left, is Cheng Hanqiang (Tacky Chen). Seated fourth from left is Guo Huitang. Standing on the left of Guo is Pan Guohu. The identities of the others in the group are unknown. Photo courtesy of Guo Qinfang.

"Coming back to Professor Zheng, he was always studying many things. While we called him our teacher, he had people whom he called teacher. One, especially gifted, was the man who led warlord Feng Yuxiang's broadsword troop. Once, when I went to the Professor's house, he was upstairs practicing a method of this man's. When he came down, I asked what he'd been doing and he responded, 'Practicing *dianxue* [the art of attacking vital points].' This art was closely held and few would be taught its secrets. Zheng Manqing's maternal aunt, Hong Lei, said that the adept who headed the famed broadsword troop—I've forgotten his name—used to be rather short but suddenly grew taller when he got married. I asked how this could be and she replied that he used to be very heavy and liked to practice *qing gong* [light gongfu]. He became superb at jumping skills, leaping over walls and onto roofs. He would sleep hanging vertically on a wall in a hammock. So his heaviness and spurt in height might have been a result of this. One time, three men simultaneously attacked him. Two immediately fell and one ran away. Oh, his gongfu was exceptional! At the time, the Professor's aunt introduced them and he began to teach the Professor. This adept was about fifty.

"Occasionally, Laoshi [Since he taught at a university and was a taiji instructor, the titles of "Laoshi" (teacher) and "Professor" are often used when talking about Zheng Manqing] would call me over and say, 'Young Guo, let's play a bit.' But I knew all he had to do was to get me once on a vital point and it would be over. And, at this time, he'd only learned to attack points, not how to cure the results of an attack. So, I would tell Laoshi that, if we put on boxing gloves, I would be willing to 'play.' But I wasn't willing to play empty handed. Therefore he would often test my gongfu wearing boxing gloves, and every time there was a boxing exhibition at the British Embassy he would take me along.

"One couldn't tell many of the great boxers of the past simply by their appearance. I often admonished my students at Shi Da [Shi Fan University] that they should not take what I taught them to the streets and get into fights. You can never tell who has gongfu. You may think that an old guy on the street may be easy to bully, but the moment you act, you find yourself on the ground injured. Even now, if someone starts to attack me, as soon as he makes a move, I sense it and my strike hits him before he hits me.

"The famous Du Xinwu mastered *qing* [light], *ying* [heavy], and Dao [Daoist] gongfu. Once in Chongqing, a friend he was visiting wanted to spar with him, but Du, then past eighty, declined, suggesting instead that each of them demonstrate some aspect of gongfu. For his part, Du showed qing by jumping onto the back of a chair and taking three steps with it. Then he sat down and rocked like this [demonstrating], but it was so difficult that his friend could not do it—only Du's bones could stand it.

"Later, he went into seclusion in a Daoist temple in Hunan Province to practice the Dao. Zhang Shijun, a renowned doctor in Chongqing, was a student of Du and once went to visit the octogenarian former transport guard at the Hunan temple. When Dr. Zhang first arrived there, he couldn't see Du but, after a search, found him meditating in a corner. One of the students with Dr. Zhang put his hand under Du's nose and, horrified, found that Du was not breathing. He was dead. The other students with Dr. Zhang began crying, lamenting Du's passing. The lamentations stopped in about a half hour, when Du awoke to announce that he had been on a 'little trip.' In fact, he had been gone for eight to ten days and only came back then because of the commotion. As he came to and his paleness turned to pink and light returned to his eyes, his students asked him how he could still live without breathing for so long. He told them that he had not been breathing through his nose but rather through his abdomen. He seemed like a god able to go out on such trips. Of all the great ones I've seen or heard of, he was the most advanced."

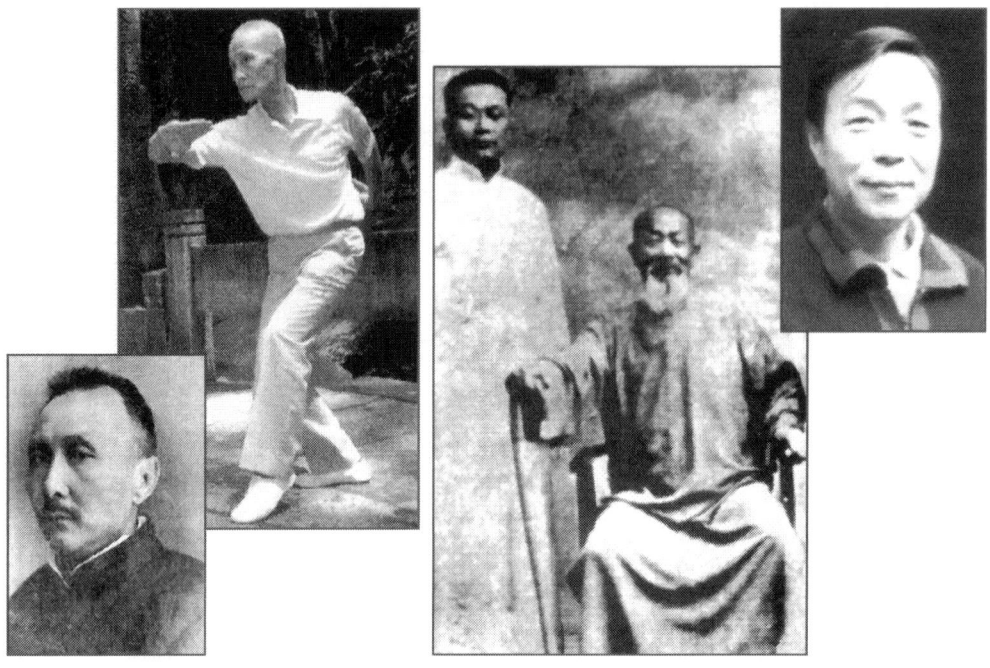

Left to right: Boxing legend Du Xinwu; Wan Laisheng, protégé of Du Xinwu, whose match with Zheng Manqing never occurred; Wu Mengxia, who beat Wan but not Zheng to the punch, with his bagua teacher Gao Yisheng; Xu Yizhong, a senior student of Zheng Manqing.

Xu Yizhong Interpolates

"I've heard that once Du Xinwu sought out the young and talented Zheng Manqing. When Du asked Zheng to show his form, the brave Zheng demurred; he wanted to get right to the boxing. So they began. When Du attacked Zheng Laoshi, Zheng sat back into his rear leg, eliminating Du's energy. Feeling this, Du broke off, saying, 'Anyone who can fight on just one leg is really good!'"

[See Smith, 1974: 39, for comments on this match. Mr. Xu's account seems to give Professor Zheng the best of it. As I recall his words, however, Zheng told me that, when the elderly Du visited him, they ate, talked awhile, and then went to bed. In the middle of the night, Zheng was awakened by Du, who said, "Let's play awhile." Zheng got up and they went at it. Zheng said it was like an avalanche of softness: everywhere he turned, however he changed his posture, Du's foot was in his face. Obviously this was a friendly match, the strikes divorced from power. Zheng recalled that Du praised him for his ability to get into one leg, but, mainly, Zheng was saying he felt helpless in that blizzard of feet.]³

Guo Qinfang Continues

"Another famous taiji teacher was Li Huangze, so skilled in gongfu that he could drop a person from a distance without touching him. In push-hands, if you touched his arm, out you went. He had studied in Germany and was a college professor. I wanted to learn from him, but the war and my job situation prevented it.

Once he pushed hands with a Mr. Yao, a corpulent xingyi adept. In the midst of the proceedings, that worthy launched a fist at Li. At this, Li took a couple of steps back as though he had been thrown away by the impact. When they stopped, Mr. Yao found some black spots on his body and realized he had been injured. These could have been caused by Li's use of mind [*yi*] rather than qi. Li, who not only had this 'touching' ability, but could also cure it, offered to do so. Instead, Mr. Yao went for treatment to Li's teacher, a woman, who had studied Buddhism in Tibet and combined that esoteric teaching with taiji. There are many mysterious things in China—things that can't be explained scientifically. These people worked diligently from their early years to master these methods. And they did not divulge their secrets easily. Even if offered large amounts of money by someone seeking to become a disciple, they would not accept the person unless he or she had an unblemished character."

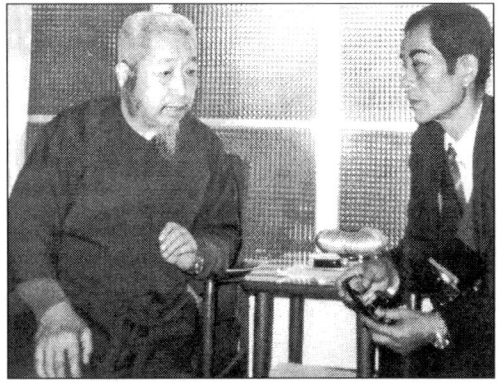

Two old friends talking. Zheng and Guo Qinfang at Zheng's residence in Yungho, Taibei, 1968. Photo courtesy of Guo Qinfang.

[See Smith, 1974: 35. "I was there the day that the daughter of a former Chinese ambassador to the United States, a visiting taiji student, told Zheng Laoshi of Li Huangze, her taiji master in Shanghai. Zheng nodded that he knew the man. The woman then said that he had special powers. Zheng asked her to explain. She told how she had tired of push-hands and asked Li what he would do against a real attack. He urged her to attack. She attacked, but as she neared him a force propelled her back and she began bouncing up and down. When her feet began to hurt, she implored him to let her stop. With a pass of his hand, he permitted her to stop bouncing. She also said that, when he touched a student, his hands generated sparks. Zheng laughed at all this. 'I knew Li,' he said. 'His taiji was not too good. He could do the thing you mention, but only because you are a student. The trick will not work against an equal or a superior.' Zheng later told me that Li had learned taiji from Dong Yingjie (another senior student of Yang Chengfu) and subsequently had gained a special skill of 'knocking down without touching.' The skill depended on student awe, however, and would not work against a good boxer." I include this excerpt because of the interesting contrasting views on the same man by Zheng

Laoshi and Mr. Guo. Essentially it was a matter of angle of slant: Zheng was looking down, Guo, up.][4]

Mr. Xu Comments

"Doctor Hong Shihao was important in Zheng Laoshi's life. Hong is a ninety-two-year-old legal consultant—a Ph.D. from Harvard—who lives in Hong Kong and knows a lot about Zheng Laoshi's early years. I've seen him recently and he is quite healthy. When Laoshi left Beijing to teach at the university in Shanghai, Dr. Hong befriended him and took him to Yang Chengfu for taiji. When he first relocated south to Shanghai from Beijing, Yang had few students and it was Dr. Hong who brought him judges, lawyers, and other powerful people to learn taiji. Here Laoshi met Zhang Qinlin and others. Zhang himself had studied taiji elsewhere and his push-hands was excellent.

"Dr. Hong sponsored young Zheng. And when Dr. Hong came to class, Yang Chengfu would single out and teach Zheng more. But Hong was extremely busy with many foreign clients and, so, wasn't able to go to class all that often. Usually, Master Yang himself would not teach much; he stayed upstairs and let his son do the teaching. But when Dr. Hong came, Mrs. Yang would tell her husband he had arrived and Yang would go downstairs to teach. His students would then seize the opportunity to ask Master Yang about various aspects of taiji. Because Yang didn't teach much, his students behind his back would make remarks about him, such as saying that he was going to take his art into the coffin with him. But Zhang Qinlin had studied taiji and *neigong* [internal work] before he came to Master Yang, so often they would practice in the back. Zhang's gongfu was quite high and it was Professor Zheng's way to learn from anyone who was better than he was. Even though that person might be a brother of his, he would still call him 'laoshi.' So, Professor called Zhang 'Laoshi.'

"Wang Yannian, who lives here [Taiwan], studied under Zhang Qinlin on the mainland for a short time. So, when Wang first came to Taiwan, he visited Professor Zheng and told him he had also studied under Zhang; hence they were 'brothers.' That was really forcing it, but because Laoshi kindly called Wang 'classmate,' we then called him 'Uncle.'

"Now, another reason Master Yang gave Zheng Manqing special training was that Laoshi treated and cured Yang's wife of a debilitating illness. Thereafter, it was not only the influence of Mr. Hong, but that of the ever-present Mrs. Yang that ensured Zheng priority instruction. It helped also that he himself attacked the problems of taiji energetically and sopped up Yang's instruction like a sponge.

"Relaxation will bring good gongfu and also good health. In taiji we talk of 'body' and 'function.' The 'body' emphasizes health, and, of course, the 'function' stresses the martial side. Practice over time will enliven the body and reveal and refine fighting use. In taiji there is an advanced level in which I know that my opponent is going to use energy before he actually does, so I don't attack him. Only if he attacks will I respond and my counter will arrive first. Zheng Laoshi was outstanding in this kind of gongfu. [There is an apposite phrase in the *Classics*: "If my opponent does not move, I don't move either, but when he does I have already started moving and will arrive before he does."] Taiji also insists that it is the waist, not the hands, that moves. When you begin to understand what it means not to move your hands, then you have entered the door of the art."

Guo Qingfang Resumes

"Laoshi was really a good person, one always willing to learn from anyone more skilled than he and willing to teach anyone inferior in skill. Once, when I went to his house, I found him practicing a kind of gongfu that involved striking layers of tofu with a slender strip of bamboo held between his thumb and finger. He mobilized his qi and tapped lightly against the top layer of tofu. After a while, when we looked at the tofu, it was unscathed, but when the top layer was removed, we saw that the bottom layer had turned to mush. Incredible! I don't know how he did it, but I'm sure it was genuine and not trickery. He put effort and energy into everything he did. When he set his mind on something, he wanted to become the best. And he was the best at many different things. If he could not be best at something, he would not even claim to be good at it. He was second best at a lot of things.[5] For instance, he was brilliant at Chinese-style chess. One time he played against the Chinese national grand champion and won two and lost three of the five games, but refused to be second best and so didn't pursue competitive chess any further.[6]

"Laoshi truly was an Olympian. Perhaps a superman. We've already told how intelligent he was, how quickly he could absorb something. This was his strong side. Everyone was in awe of his taiji. It made him famous. But he wouldn't teach just anyone. Based on a person's sincerity, he would decide whether or not to accept him as a student. With me, he sought me out because of my boxing skill. Now, I am his student. Good teachers are this way. They see natural ability in a person and they go out of their way to teach him or her without any condition. I'm that way with my students. It is sincerity, not money, that determines whether or what I teach.

"Once, Zheng Laoshi saw a classified ad in a newspaper about a man who claimed to have excellent gongfu—there was no match for him anywhere on earth. Zheng sought him out and announced that he had seen the ad and he would like to try him out. They squared off and one blow from Laoshi left the man with blood all over his face. This man had a reputation as a street fighter who liked to challenge gongfu types. Now, this local hoodlum had been beaten at his own game.

"I remember, too, a time in Chongqing when Laoshi was giving a demonstration for the American advisor group. He asked me to accompany him. To get from my office to his, I had to take a bus. While waiting in line, a fellow tried to cut in front of me. I told him that he had to get in line at the end. Suddenly he—pah!—threw a punch. I dodged slightly to the side while punching him at the same time. He fell to his knees. I told him that, since he broke the line, which was against the rules, I wasn't worried about him reporting the incident to the police. It turned out he was a plainclothes policeman, and, when we went to his unit, his superior said that I had hurt him. I replied that, if he were injured, I would be responsible for healing him. So, I went to Laoshi and told him about it, and he wrote a note telling the policeman that he was a doctor and would treat him for free.

"The next day, Zheng Laoshi was surprised when he examined the chap and found his jaw swollen on the side opposite to the one receiving the blow. The shock of the punch doubtless caused this. Laoshi asked him if he knew the man he had fought with and, when the man shook his head, Zheng told him that it was the boxing champion of China! Laoshi further told him that I had only used 50 percent; had I punched full force, his face would have been shattered. Notwithstanding this, the policeman still filed charges against me, but Zheng Laoshi quashed the charge. I felt sorry about the incident, of course, but when he threw that punch, I countered instinctively. It couldn't be helped."

Son Patrick Remembers His Father

In December 1989 I met with Professor Zheng's son, Patrick, a restaurateur and taiji teacher in Asheville, North Carolina, close to my home. After a tasty repast at his restaurant, he recalled some incidents that involved his father.

Recalling his childhood, Patrick said he and his brother Wayne often got into scrapes. Although his mother usually had the task of punishing the errant boys, occasionally his father would do it. But when he did, he invariably used a small stick and was careful never to use his hand when paddling his sons. Patrick learned later the reason that his father never used his hands to paddle them. It was simply too dangerous for Professor Zheng to use hands trained in *dianxue* (the art of attacking vital points) to punish his young sons.

Patrick's mother told him in 1992 that, when his father first joined the Yang Chengfu circle, the top student, Chen Weiming, was away for a time. When he returned, Master Yang introduced him to the newcomer and suggested they do some *tuishou* (push-hands). They did and, though Chen tried to push him, he couldn't find him. Young Zheng merely neutralized his every endeavor. Chen Weiming was greatly impressed and the two became close friends.

In Taibei one day, the pedicab in which his father and mother were riding was hit by an errant bicyclist. Professor Zheng reached up and flipped the bicycle and rider over so they couldn't hit Mrs. Zheng, who emerged unscathed. He, however, did suffer a small abrasion on one leg.

When Patrick was seven or eight, the Professor took him to an ancient master in southern Taiwan. The old man lived in a barnlike structure, and what really caught Patrick's attention on entering was a sword hanging from the ceiling, perhaps fifteen feet above them. This puzzled Patrick and he politely asked the oldster if the sword were his. When the master nodded, the young boy asked what it was doing in a place where no one could get it. The old man smiled and said, "Oh, I can get it," whereupon he rose into the air, hovered, got the sword, and brought it down so the boy could see it! As Richard Burton would say, "There ensued incredulity." Patrick acknowledges that if someone told him such a tale, he wouldn't believe it, but he has to—he saw it.[7]

A famed taiji teacher was coming down a gangplank from a boat when he was accosted by four bandits. Instantly he sent them sprawling. A renowned doctor and man of good will, he addressed the downed brigands individually: A, you see me in seven days; B, in fourteen; C, in a month; and D, in six months. They each became sick and came for treatment at the times he had specified. A taiji senior told me he knew this story and the teacher probably was Zhang Xiulin (died c. 1930), a master of taiji, bagua, and dongpi, a man about whom little is known. Zheng Laoshi mentioned him once to me, eyes bright, and said that he had not met him, but solid sources pronounced him "truly marvelous." So, this tale only concerns Zheng tangentially, as the teller.

When Patrick was managing a restaurant in New York City, he came down with a bad wisdom tooth. The dentist gave him five shots and had to break the tooth into four parts to get it out. His jaw was swollen and the pain so intense he couldn't sleep at night. Soon, he was a shambling wreck and went to his father for help. Laoshi began by telling him he had done right by letting the dentist do what he could and he, Laoshi, was interposing merely to manage the trauma. He told Patrick to sit in a chair and went behind him. Telling him to relax completely, he put his hand on Patrick's head and, in the time it took him to sense his father's hand, he was out. He woke the next morning miraculously refreshed and ready to take the medicine Laoshi had sent out for. The pain was gone. Patrick asked him, "Father, how did you do that?" to which Laoshi made a face as if to say, "It's much too deep to tell you."

I end with an occurrence relayed by Patrick to me from Mrs. Zheng in June 1993. This story still leaves me wondering. Mrs. Zheng told of attending an automatic-writing session with a woman friend and Tam Gibbs in Taibei after Laoshi's death in 1975. They entered a place where there was a sandy pit with a man seated at each corner. A seven-year-old girl held one end of a six-foot pole, and a male doctor in his thirties held the other end, effectively bisecting the square. A slender piece of wood was attached to the middle of the pole and hung down into the sand below. As questions were asked in Mandarin Chinese, the mediums—the girl and the man—held the pole lightly, and it responded by moving and, with its central wooden "arm," writing answers in Chinese characters in the sand. The four men at the corners—one of whom had lived in the US and was skeptical about the proceedings—transcribed the answers. After some general dialogue, Mrs. Zheng thought to test the mediums by switching to a Zhejiang dialect unknown to those there. The answers came back written in Zheng's unique "grass" writing, which she could read but the four transcribers could not. This shocked her greatly, as did what happened when she put a glass of his favorite cognac in the center of the sand. Without spilling a drop, the arm moved the cognac through the sand out of the way; it apparently was interfering with the writing! One of her questions, incidentally, was how Laoshi liked his favorite cognac. His answer: "Very much!" Other questions were on past events known only to the two of them.

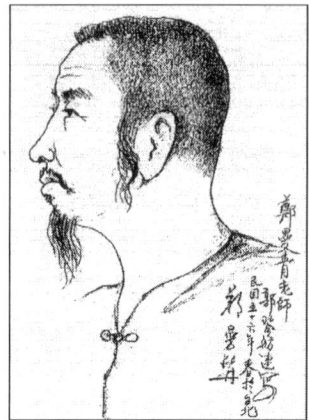

Teacher Zheng Manqing. Sketch by Guo Qinfang, spring 1967. The Professor was so delighted at how Mr. Guo had caught his spirit that he signed the sketch himself. Courtesy of Guo Qinfang.

I proffer no opinion on the authenticity of the proceedings, but would give a pretty penny to have been present. There was a popular craze (notice how those two words go together?) in automatic writing in England and America at the turn of the century, but much of it was fakery with questions limited to simple yes or no answers. This episode in Taibei, however, was not of that kind. It was, in fact, a full-fledged intimate conversation between a bereaved widow and her departed loved one. Readers must do their own mulling on this one. But enough! Though Mae West once quipped that "Too much of a good thing is wonderful," Confucius cautioned that we shouldn't talk too much, too loudly, or too often. There are other stories of this gifted, giving man, but they must await another time.[8]

Notes

[1] Conversation with Ben (Pangjeng) Lo, April 4, 1975. Tam Gibbs's version of this story was identical to Ben Lo's, but Mr. Lo was able to supply the name of this mystery man. Alone with Professor Zheng and Mrs. Zheng in New York City in the 1960s, Zheng told me about the great *dianxue* (vital points) teacher of this name he had trained under, but did not give the locale, and I assumed wrongly that this was one of two dianxue teachers he had studied with in Nanjing.

[2] Mr. Guo states that, in 1992 in a US martial arts magazine, the boxer he fought claimed to have TKO'd him. Despite this severely skewed account of the bout, since the boxer did not identify Guo by name, Mr. Guo believes he should accord him the same courtesy. So I call him "Song"—not his real name. Germanely, the *New Shu* (*Shu* is short for Sichuan Province) *Newspaper* of January 10, 1943, re-

Transliteration of Chinese			
Wade-Giles	Pinyin	Wade-Giles	Pinyin
PEOPLE		Tung Ying-chih	Dong Yingjie
Chang Ch'in-lin	Zhang Qinlin	Wan Lai-sheng	Wan Laisheng
Chang Hsiu-lin	Zhang Xiulin	Wang Hsiu-ai	Wang Xiuai
Chang Shih-chun	Zhang Shijun	Wang Yen-nien	Wang Yannian
Chang Tze-kang	Zhang Zigang	Wu Meng-hsia	Wu Mengxia
Ch'en Han-ch'ing	Chen Hanqiang	Yang Ch'eng-fu	Yang Chengfu
Ch'en Wei-ming	Chen Weiming		
Cheng Man-ch'ing	Zheng Manqing	**PLACES**	
Feng Yu-hsiang	Feng Yuxiang	Chekiang	Zhejiang
Hsu I-chung	Xu Yizhong	Ching Wu	Qing Wu
Hung Lei	Hong Lei	Chungking	Chongqing
Hung Shih-hao	Hong Shihao	Hunan	Hunan
Kao I-sheng	Gao Yisheng	Pei Ching	Beijing
Kuo Ch'in-fang	Guo Qinfang	Szechwan	Sichuan
Kuo Hui-t'ang	Guo Huitang		
Li Huang-tse	Li Huangze	**PRACTICES**	
Liu Hsi-heng	Liu Xiheng	pakua	bagua
P'an Kuo-hua	Pan Guohua	hsing-i	xingyi
Shih Shu-fang	Shi Shufang	tien-hsueh	dianxue
Tu Hsin-wu	Du Xinwu	tung-pi	dongpi

porting on the boxing card of the day before, said, in part, "The highlight of the entire event was the match between Guo Qinfang and [Song], which was especially exciting. After four rounds, despite his smaller stature, Guo beat [Song] by virtue of his quick and agile movements" (translation by Michael Schnapp).

[3] Wan Laisheng, a student of Du Xinwu, and Zheng Laoshi had an open challenge going through World War II, but they never clashed. I learned from Zheng himself that, at a party in Chongqing during the war, the host, famed Wu Mengxia, brought Wan Laisheng over to introduce him to Zheng and, while Zheng was warily watching Wan, host Wu lashed out at Zheng, who among the dropping teacups countered to Wu's eyes, momentarily blinding him. The defeated Wu specified "three years," meaning he would return in three years, but never did (see Smith, 1974: 37).

[4] Professor Zheng told me in 1964 that Li Huangze, who had heard of Yang Chengfu from one of his math students, came to Yang and kowtowed seeking instruction. Yang said no, that he must kowtow to Dong Yingjie, who would be his student. Li did and later learned the special method.

[5] Reminding one of Irish poet James Stephen's line describing Stephen Mackenna, that translator of Plotinus and greatest talker in Ireland: "He was wildly in love

with everything he couldn't do." I was forever finding new arrows in Zheng's quiver. I visited the New York studio once to learn that someone had put a staff in his hands one day and he had taken the thing and trounced everyone there, repeating the course for some New York University fencers brought in a day or two later. There was simply no end to the man. This doesn't mean he was an overly competitive lout, but rather underscores his abiding interest in life and people.

[6] Some experts informed me that Zheng was only second in certain arts—in calligraphy and as an authority on Laozi or Confucius, for instance. Other experts would dispute these assertions, putting him first, but even if true, a small catalog of seconds isn't bad. One thing was not in dispute. No one ever called him second in taiji.

[7] Recalling Groucho Marx's classic quip, "Who do you believe—me or your eyes?" It is said that V. Nijinski, the greatest dancer the world has seen, did not levitate as some suggested. No, he leaped and what gave the appearance of levitation was that at the apex of the leap he hovered. This old man seeking his sword from on high had gravity against him and a boy's eyes and imagination for him. Obviously skilled in *qing gong* (light gongfu) he leaped high and got his sword, but he didn't hover. The boy's mind did that. But I could be wrong about this.

[8] I can't resist a last story from Patrick Zheng deserving the rubric "strange" that concerns Professor Zheng's clothes. Laoshi designed his own clothes (he wouldn't wear a collar, the symbol of a slave in old China) and had them tailored by an old friend who didn't believe in machines and did all the work by hand. After Laoshi's death, his shade appeared to a senior student and asked why he hadn't been buried with an undershirt. When the student asked why he didn't ask his widow, the shade said he didn't want to frighten her. So, the student sought an answer from Mrs. Zheng who, not knowing, asked the long-retired tailor who had made and fit all of Laoshi's coffin clothes. Puzzled, the tailor asked her, "How do you know about the undershirt? Only I know [that fact]." Then he explained that when he tried to put the undershirt on Laoshi, his body was so stiff it was too difficult to fit it on him. The tailor said he left it off, knowing no one would be aware of it anyhow. Someone apparently was.

Reference

Smith, R. (1974). *Chinese boxing: Masters and methods*. Tokyo: Kodansha International.

Acknowledgments

Thanks go to Guo Qinfang for wonderful help with the text and, especially, with the graphics. Michael Schnapp, Danny Emerick, Russ Mason, and Dan Johnston also had oars in the water. Messrs. Liu Xiheng and Xu Yizhong kept me from making too many errors. Lastly, I bow to Juliana Cheng and Patrick Cheng and also to Ben Lo, superb teacher and researcher on taiji, for his help in preparing this article.

• 14 •

In Search of a Unified Dao:
Zheng Manqing's Life and Contribution to Taijiquan
by Barbara Davis, M.A.

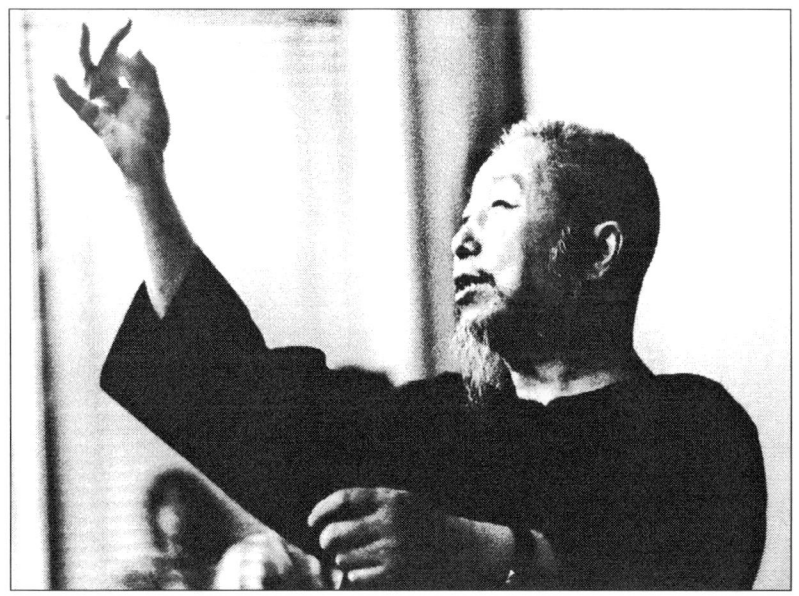

Zheng Manqing lecturing at the Shizhong (a.k.a. Shr Jung) school in New York City, where he delivered a number of talks on taijiquan, philosophy, and health. All photos courtesy of Ken van Sickle, except where noted.

In little over 150 years, taijiquan has grown from being a family-held tradition in a small village in northern China to become an international phenomenon. Of the many people who have been involved with its growth in the twentieth century and in its movement to the West, one of the most influential figures was Zheng Manqing.

Like his predecessors in the Yang family lineage, Zheng was instrumental in helping taijiquan reach new audiences. His erudition, skill, personality, and his social connections all helped in this. Zheng brought to his teachings a thorough knowledge of several disciplines, and to his writing a depth of classical learning that the taijiquan world had until then not seen.

As a result, Zheng Manqing indisputably has had a great impact on how many of us now think about and practice taijiquan. Now, decades after Zheng Manqing's death, it is helpful for us to examine the details of his life and the cultural and historical environment that nurtured his ideas, so we may better understand his unique contributions to the world of taijiquan. As many readers may not be familiar with the full scope of his writings, an extensive bibliography has been appended that lists Zheng's many works, and those written about him.

The World of Traditional China

To talk about Zheng Manqing, or any Chinese traditionalist for that matter, we must start with Confucius. Over 2,400 years ago, the great sage said to his disciples, "My Dao is that of an all-pervading unity." These deceptively simple words (yet so difficult to implement) became a motto for his followers throughout the centuries, including the young Zheng Manqing.

Confucius's ideas are rooted in humanism, and are expressed in proper behavior and relationships. After his time, his ideas became codified in traditions, curricula, and laws. He is revered in China as "the First Teacher." He promoted respect for the ancients, broad learning, and careful reflection. Confucius and his teachings became the very symbol of traditional China, and had a profound impact on all aspects of Chinese society and that of much of East Asia.

A twentieth-century paragon of Confucius's teachings, Zheng also became a teacher, one who welcomed all who were serious about study, regardless of nationality. He emphasized in all of his work an unrelenting quest for the ideals of Confucius and his early interpreter, Mencius.

However, by the time Zheng was born, at the beginning of the twentieth century, the traditional society that Confucian ideas had so influenced was crumbling away, torn from inside and outside by the forces of change and modernization. Yet throughout his life, Zheng remained drawn to the world of the traditional scholar, or literati, a world steeped in poetry, art, philosophy, and history.

Zheng and his peers struggled to understand their circumstance at the turbulent nexus of tradition and modernity. Many chose to cast away the old ways and pursue Western-influenced sciences and social structures in hopes of building a new society that would be unfettered by the weight of history and tradition. On the other extreme, for many traditionally minded people, the task was one of accepting the dominant trends toward modernization, but maintaining and utilizing the strengths of the past. Zheng argued for this latter ideal his whole life.

Zheng wove together his many talents and interests with seeming ease, untiringly guiding others. He followed the Dao, or Way, of Confucianism, which emphasized above all else human relations. Zheng coupled this with an unswerving loyalty to family, friends, students, and country.

Accomplished at painting, poetry, calligraphy, taijiquan, and medicine, Zheng was known in his later years by the sobriquet Master of Five Excellences. Today his followers still respectfully refer to him as "the Professor," and he is recognized around the world for his contributions to taijiquan. In Taiwan in particular, his paintings and calligraphy are prized possessions. Among his students, friends, and patients, his medical skills were considered superb and subtle. Beyond these accomplishments, he is remembered by many as an eloquent and gifted teacher and writer. His wide-ranging interests and multiple talents provided him with a rich ground for cross-fertilization of ideas. These talents, together with the circumstances of his life, presented him with opportunities to make unique and influential contributions.

Even now, decades after his death in 1975, Zheng Manqing has continued to accumulate taijiquan followers through his books and through the continued efforts of his direct and indirect students. But what made Zheng so influential? What was unique about his work? To answer these questions, we will first look at the life and surroundings of this multidimensional man.

Zheng Manqing's Life

Zheng was born in the waning years of the Qing dynasty, on July 29, 1902.[2] His given name was Yue. He later took the name Manqing (Man-ch'ing), and used *Manran* (Manjan, "Beautiful Whiskers") in his fifties.[3] He often used pen names in concert with these names, including Hermit of the Jade Well, Host of the Tower of Long Evening, and Old One Who Never Tires of Learning.[4]

Zheng was a native of the Yongia district in the fertile province of Zhejiang (Chekiang), on the southeast coast of China. This small port town and surrounding district, all now known as Wenzhou, is on the mouth of the Ou River, a short distance from the coast of the East China Sea.[5]

Zheng was the youngest of six children.[6] His father died when he was very young, and the family was poor.[7] Zheng's mother's surname was Zhang.[8] During his childhood, she taught him herbal medicine, calligraphy, and poetry. He tells that when he was a child, he would tug at her sleeve and plead with her to recite Tang dynasty poetry to him.[9] When he was six, she began to teach him calligraphy. Her sister, Zhang Guang, also known as Old Lady Redfern, was a painter of some renown who later helped him develop his skills at the "outline" style of painting.[10]

Zheng was precocious and had a photographic memory, but his childhood was also marked by illnesses and a major accident. When he was nine, he was hit in the head with a brick from a crumbling wall and fell into a coma for several days. When he came to, he had lost his memory. To help him recuperate, the family used herbal remedies, and then apprenticed him to a local painter, Wang Xiangchan, in hope that simple work like grinding the painter's ink would be therapeutic.[11] As he recuperated, the many hours in the studio made a lasting impression on the young boy, and he began to practice painting, at first on leftover paper wrappers from his grandmother's medicines.

By the age of fourteen, Zheng had mastered painting well enough that his teacher sent him out on his own. In the traditional manner, Wang gave him a studio name (Wisteria Flower) and set prices for his paintings, thereby initiating him into a professional life that would span decades and continents. Zheng spent the next several years in nearby Hangzhou, a renowned center of the arts, where he studied painting, poetry, and calligraphy. He was soon able to support his family by means of his artwork. Even in these early years, his painting favored the expressive xieyi style of brushwork; as for subjects, he concentrated primarily on flowers and plants.[12]

When he was seventeen, Zheng went to Beijing. It was 1919, just as the May

Fourth reform movement was reaching its height. This movement was made up of students and intellectuals who questioned the old structures of governance, education, and society. They sought to open up China to new ideas from Japan, Europe, and the United States, in an effort to shed what they thought of as a stagnant past. They also promoted the use of vernacular Chinese in writing, rather than the classical Chinese that had been the mainstay of the written word since long before Confucius.

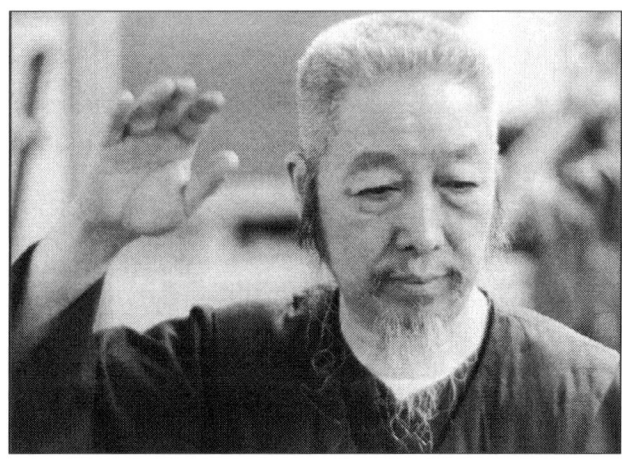

Zheng Manqing moving through the taiji forms.

In Beijing, Zheng became a member of several circles of poets and painters, who were for the most part older gentlemen of a traditionalist bent. These connections eventually led to an invitation to teach poetry at Yuwen University in 1924. That same year, Cai Yuanpei, chancellor of Beijing University and a fellow native of Zhejiang Province, recommended him for a teaching position at National Zhinan University in Shanghai.[13] In Shanghai, Zheng was invited to be director of the painting department at the Shanghai School of Fine Arts and was later involved with the start up of the College of Culture and Art. In 1925 he had a solo art show at the Shuixie Pavilion in Beijing's Central Park, and was sent by the Ministry of Education to Japan to do research on the arts. The next year, he assembled his first collection of paintings.[14]

Zheng began to study medicine more rigorously in his midtwenties. Building on the base that he had gained from his mother, he began to study around 1926 with Dr. Song You'an of Anhui Province, whom he had met in Shanghai. His medical training encompassed both practice and theory, and became a major part of his livelihood, as well as an important aspect of his understanding of taijiquan.

Zheng had a weakened body since childhood. He contracted tuberculosis while in Beijing, and still was suffering from it when he went to live in Shanghai. When a friend suggested he take up taijiquan to regain his health, Zheng assented. Earlier in his life he had studied some taijiquan as well as exercises such as *baduanjin* and *yijinjing* in efforts to strengthen himself.[15]

In the mid-1920s, Yang Chengfu (1883–1936), one of the well-known members of the Yang family lineage of taijiquan, began teaching in Shanghai with his senior disciple Chen Weiming (1881–1958). They founded the *Zhi Rou* [Attaining Softness] Taijiquan Society.[16] In 1932 Zheng Manqing was introduced by an acquaintance to Yang Chengfu and commenced close to six years of study with Yang.[17] Zheng won Master Yang's favor after healing Yang's wife from a serious illness. At her urging, Yang taught Zheng without holding anything back. Zheng was a quick learner, and after only a year made great progress. Zheng also briefly studied with Zhang Qinlin, who was from Taiyuan, Shanxi Province.[18]

By 1930 Professor Zheng had retired from college teaching, and spent time in neighboring Jiangsu Province, where he studied essay and poem writing with Qian Mingshan.[19] He was soon able to put his improved writing skills to good use, as Yang Chengfu called upon him to write a preface for, and, as many assert, to ghostwrite Yang's 1934 book *Taijiquan tiyong quan shu*.[20] Zheng's preface draws in ideas from the *Yijing*, the *Book of Songs*, and the *Daodejing* among others, demonstrating his early efforts to synthesize classical learning with taijiquan. In his hands, taijiquan was not merely exercise or boxing. It was part of the Confucian Dao he so admired.

The War Years

In 1895 the Japanese took control of southern Manchuria and Taiwan, and forced many humiliating concessions from the Chinese. The encroachments continued until 1937, when the Japanese launched a brutal war against the Chinese. This lasted until the Japanese surrender at the end of World War II. The two main players in China, the Communists and the Nationalists (the Kuomintang or Guomindang), were able to put aside their differences for a time to unite against their common enemy. But as soon as peace was declared on the international front, full-scale civil war broke out at home. At the time the Sino-Japanese War began, Zheng Manqing was practicing medicine full time. He had previously taught taijiquan at the Central Military Academy (formerly named Huangpu or Whampoa) in 1933. He now assisted the military in the war efforts by teaching taijiquan in Hunan (for the provincial government) and Sichuan (for the Central Military Training Group), and by writing medical prescriptions useful to the military.

The Nationalist government relocated westward to Chongqing in 1939, in Sichuan Province. Zheng moved along with it. Now thirty-seven, he continued to practice traditional medicine and teach taijiquan. With his colleagues he formed and then served as president of the National Chinese Medical Association. This group's purpose was to help promote traditional medicine, which was under attack by modernizers enamored of Western science and medicine. Zheng served as a member of the National Assembly for the Construction of the Constitution in 1946, and as a representative for the Community of Doctors of Traditional Medicine to the National Assembly in 1947. He married Ding Yidu when he was forty. She was the daughter of an Air Force official and had studied medicine at Beijing University.

Together they had five children: three girls and two boys.

It was during this period that Zheng worked on condensing the hundred-some moves of the Yang family taijiquan form he had learned from Yang Chengfu down to thirty-seven moves. In 1946, while still in Nanjing, he completed work on his first taijiquan book, *Zhengzi taijiquan shisan pian* [Master Zheng's Thirteen Treatises on Taijiquan]. This book was aimed at the serious practitioner and in its first part delved into the deeper philosophy and medical substantiations for taijiquan practice. The second part was a thorough examination of the martial application of the moves, along with photographs. The war interfered, however, and the manuscript was not published until 1950, when Zheng and his family were safely in Taiwan. The book received support from high places. Among its calligraphed dedications are ones by President Chiang Kai-shek, Control Yuan President Yu Youren, and elder classmate Chen Weiming. Chen's support was particularly important, due to his high status among Yang Chengfu's senior students and as a well-educated early taijiquan writer himself.[21]

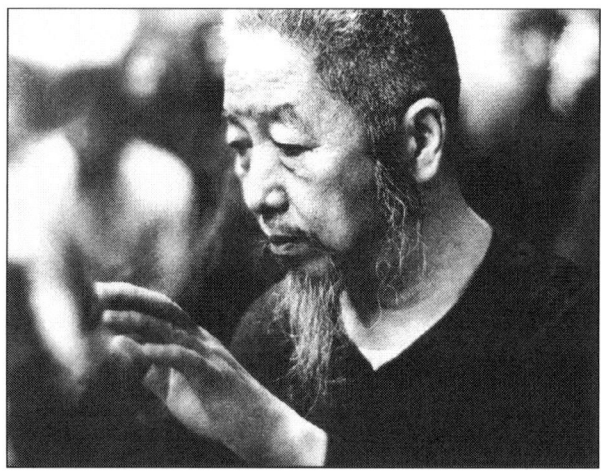

Zheng Manqing moving through the taiji forms.

In Taiwan

The Nationalist government was to relocate yet one more time. When the mainland fell to the Communists, millions of people who had been connected to the Nationalist effort took refuge on the island province of Taiwan, a hundred miles off the southeast coast of China. The nationalist governmental seat was now activated in Taibei. Under the guidance of Chiang Kai-shek and the Guomindang, a governing body for all of China—in absentia—was put in place. The civil war ostensibly over, a cold war ensued, with martial law kept in place on the island until 1987.

The mainland refugees considered Taiwan to be a temporary haven until the mainland was retaken. From behind the cold war barricade, the Nationalist refugees turned toward developing Taiwan economically, creating a free China that would prove their politics correct. The Nationalist government presented itself in international politics as the "true China," holding the much-coveted United Nations seat until 1971. They continued to seek and receive United States aid, and served as an important outpost and staging ground for it in the Korean and Vietnam conflicts.

In this atmosphere of resettlement, Zheng Manqing quickly reestablished a sense of normalcy. He started new poetry and calligraphy circles, and became involved with the national arts scene by helping to start and run the Republic of China Fine Arts Society. One of his more influential painting students was Madame Chiang Kai-shek. He was invited to teach poetry, painting, and calligraphy at the graduate school of the College of Chinese Culture in Taibei.

Zheng taught taijiquan publicly for several years at the request of the Taibei mayor. Usually, however, students came to him via personal introductions. If they did not yet know the taijiquan form, a more senior student would be assigned to teach it to them. Students would gather informally on the weekends to work out in the courtyard of his home in Yonghe (a Taibei suburb). Zheng titled his group the Shizhong [Correct Timing] Taijiquan Center, which continues to operate to this day under the guidance of his direct students.

In 1961, at the age of sixty, Zheng published his second collection of paintings, *Manran xieyi*, as well as a short work on gynecology and his first volume of poetry. In 1962, perhaps sensing the future of taijiquan's growth, he published an English instructional book, *Taijiquan for Health and Self-Defense*, through the Shizhong Center. This book, aimed at the beginner, illustrated his simplified form and articulated his philosophy of taijiquan. In 1965 a Chinese book, *Zhengzi taijiquan zixiu xinfa* [Master Zheng's New Method of Taijiquan Self-Cultivation] came out. This book described the moves in detail, with photographs and foot charts, and also contained a reprint of the thirteen chapters previously published in *Zheng Zi taijiquan shisan pian* [Master Zheng's Thirteen Treatises on Taijiquan]. In 1967 he published a second English-language text, *T'ai Chi*, in collaboration with his student Robert W. Smith, an American martial arts historian.

Like many of his contemporaries in Taiwan, Zheng felt the pain of separation from his family. Torn from each other by years of war and exile, his writing showed little of his feelings. It is only in his poetry that the depth of this hurt and the conflicts it raised are revealed, as is shown in "Receiving a Letter from Home":

> After New Year's a letter from home arrives
> My soul is cut off from a dream, it is difficult to return.
> My younger brother has died from who knows what illness,
> Mother is aging, with no one to lean on,
> In her desolate hut, tries to make a living from a tiny piece of land,
> Passing the days, suffering unending hunger.
> In the waning night, in tears longing for her son,
> Sobbing, not daring to wipe away the tears.[23]

A low-grade state of war was still in effect between the mainland People's Republic of China and the Taiwan-based Republic of China. There was no way for him or others to communicate directly with their families left behind on the mainland. This sense of isolation and loss, combined with the terrible weight of not being able to fulfill their filial duties toward their parents, was a burden never resolved for many of his generation who found themselves in exile.

The American Years

In 1964 Zheng travelled to Europe and the United States to mount exhibits of his artwork. He had a one-man show in Paris at the Cernuschi Museum of Chinese Art, and then exhibited at the Republic of China pavilion at the New York World's Fair. While in the United States he gave a demonstration of taijiquan at the United Nations, and met up with many old friends from the Chinese mainland. One of these friends encouraged him to stay in New York City so as to be able to write and teach.24 Zheng decided to settle in Manhattan with his family and yet again he set about establishing venues for his practice of medicine, painting, and taijiquan. Within a short time of his arrival in New York City, he had established the Shizhong Center for Culture and the Arts in Chinatown with the help of local sponsors. This center soon became the locus of many of his activities. It was here that he taught taijiquan, saw patients, and gave lectures.

Zheng was one of taijiquan's earliest and foremost proponents overseas. He said, "I not only desire my country to be strong, I would also like to share the benefits of taijiquan with all mankind."[25] He willingly taught non-Chinese as well as his fellow countrymen, men and women equally, and made full use of his books, lectures, articles, and even movies to disseminate his ideas.

The Shizhong Center, initially on Canal Street in Chinatown, quickly began to attract an interesting mix of students.[26] Word had passed quickly around in both Chinese and martial arts circles that a taijiquan master had come to town. Among his early students were overseas Chinese, who ranged from businessmen to restaurant workers. There were many Americans, including serious martial artists, as well as a large number of hippies.

Zheng seemed to care deeply for his students, regardless of their nationality, and treated their foibles with a sense of amusement. He seized the chance to influence them, both in the Chinese tradition of teacher as surrogate parent, and as a representative of Chinese culture.

Now in his sixties, Zheng had come to the United States at a time when many American youth were rebelling against their parents and teachers, and against the draft and the war in Vietnam. Demonstrations and fierce political debates were commonplace, as were "free love" and the use of drugs. Anyone in a position of authority—or anyone over thirty—was automatically suspect.

Into this social turmoil walked Zheng, who, as a "master from the Far East," could neatly sidestep this politicized atmosphere. His physical appearance—a slight sixty-five-year-old man in Chinese scholar's robes with a graying crew cut and sparse, long whiskers—did not fit the young Americans' image of one of their own authoritarian elders. Besides, he was different: he was an artist, poet, and herbalist.

Ironically, the traditions these American students were so eager to absorb from Zheng were at the same time being violently rejected by their counterparts in China. Mao Zedong's Cultural Revolution in the People's Republic of China was underway, and its destructiveness was not known yet in the West. Zheng also avoided the controversy over American involvement in Vietnam. Though many of his American students were involved in leftist antiwar protests, and he himself was an ardent anticommunist, Zheng steered clear of public debate.

Toward his Chinese students and friends, Zheng's mission was slightly different. He viewed it as his responsibility to help keep traditional culture alive for them, and to keep them engaged with it. He frequently wrote of the importance of keeping Chinese youth linked to their moral and ethical roots.[27]

In Zheng's hands, taijiquan and the Shizhong Center became vehicles for the promotion of Chinese culture.[28] With the help of translators, he taught taijiquan and delivered lectures on Confucius's *Doctrine of the Mean*, Laozi's *Daodejing*, and health. Beyond taijiquan study, philosophy, art, and culture, students also unconsciously absorbed Chinese attitudes about the teacher-student and student-student hierarchy. These relationships to some extent replicate Chinese family structure, with the teacher as parent. For example, when teaching in New York City, Zheng did not hesitate to comment on the length of the male American students' hair, and when one of the more serious students cut his hair, Zheng observed that he had become more human.[29]

Many of Zheng's students revered him. Zheng advised them on their marriages, jobs, and health. They would come, as did many nonstudents, to consult with him on health matters. He would sit at his desk at the studio, read their pulses, and then write out a prescription for them to have filled at the nearby Chinese herbal pharmacies.

Zheng knew of the temptations of the free love and drugs with which the students were surrounded. He knew how poor the American diet and lifestyle was, and taught them about the need for balance of food and rest. He recognized their search for answers to the upheaval in society and their own lives. He talked to them about the Dao, giving them answers to questions that at the time they themselves didn't even realize they were asking.

Zheng painted at his study in his home, which was high up in an apartment building on Riverside Drive in the Upper West Side. He named his study Tower of the Long Twilight for its view of the sunset over the Hudson River. The curator of his Parisian exhibit praised his work, saying Zheng Manqing, "more than any of his contemporaries, pushed to its extreme limits the role played by the discipline of the mind. His entire work is suffused by the unmistakable strength of his brush."[30] In 1967 Zheng wrote on one of his paintings of bamboo with what had by then become his characteristic blunt-tipped calligraphic style:

> Painting is like catching a fleeting glimpse of a galloping
> white horse through a crack. In communicating one's spirit,
> the brush must move as if chasing the wind.[31]

Zheng Manqing held to traditional culture through all of his years away from China. Even after close to ten years of living in New York City, he still maintained his traditional scholar's appearance. He had a sense of the importance of tradition and held to Confucius's admiration of the past, as shown in this poem from 1973:

> Whose brush can excel both old and new?
> With every rub of my eyes I recognize the distant hills anew.
> Last night a clear dream inspired a poetic thought.
> The single stroke of the green mountain
> Contains all my heart's yearning for antiquity.[32]

At the same time, Zheng noted in his painting essays that there were those artists who felt that an overadmiration of the ancients (in this case, painters) stifled innovation and ignored today's masters. To admire past masters did not mean to be "mired in traditionalism." Rather, one should build on a solid foundation of understanding the past, and that ultimately, it was most important to follow Nature.[33]

Zheng received the title of director of fine arts, the Republic of China Cultural Renaissance Movement, American Branch. The Renaissance Movement, initiated by Chiang Kai-shek, aimed to reinforce traditional culture and all its values, as a response to the destructive forces of Mao Zedong's Cultural Revolution. The Nationalists felt themselves to be protectors and guardians of traditional Chinese culture and its treasures, and later felt a sense of vindication when the true devastation of the Cultural Revolution became known.[34]

Even under criticism from some of his friends, Zheng continued to write in classical Chinese his whole life.[35] Language had been a part of the cultural battleground in China from the early 1900s. Educational and governmental reforms brought to an end the monopoly that classical Chinese had over the written language, and ushered in a flowering of vernacular writing. But for some traditionalists such as Zheng, the written language was sacrosanct, and to become cut off linguistically from the wellsprings of the past was a grave mistake.

Zheng wrote copiously while in New York City. It was a time for reflection and distillation of his ideas, resulting in commentaries on the *Daodejing*; the Confucian classics of the *Analects*, *Great Learning*, and *Doctrine of the Mean*; and the *Yijing*. A collection of his original essays on the arts, *Manran san lun* [Manran's three treatises], was published in 1974 in Taibei.[36] As one of his last books, *Manran san lun* brought together under one cover essays on three of his "excellences": painting, calligraphy, and poetry. Perhaps nowhere else is his ability to weave together his interests as visible as in this book. In his preface he remarks:

Calligraphy and painting are rooted in the same source. [As is said of the early poet and painter] Wang Wei, "In his poems are paintings, and in his paintings are poems." Guang Wen's *Three Excellences* [painting, poetry, and calligraphy] came forth from the same hand, and met together on the same page, united by sentiment.[37]

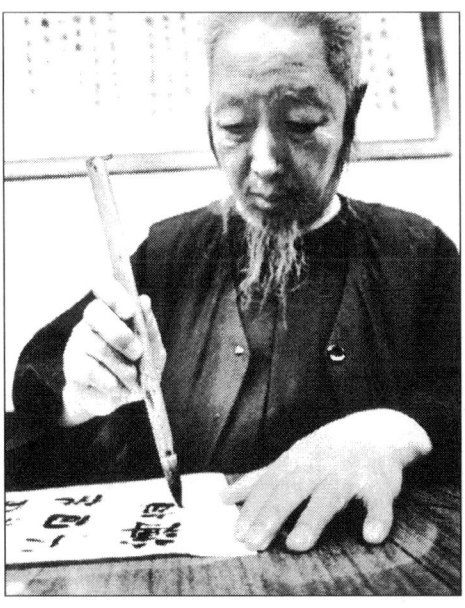

Zheng completing a poem. In China, well-developed calligraphic skills are highly respected. Calligraphy requires great inner concentration and control.

In the same preface, he links painting to the medical concepts so familiar to him as an herbal doctor:

> As for brush and ink, it is just like harmonizing the qi and blood. If the brush has too little ink, then it will be dry; if the ink has no brush [i.e., the ink is not used] it will congeal. In the same way that the qi is able to command the blood to move, we can see that the brush leads the ink's movement.[38]

In a similar fashion, Zheng's essays on calligraphy are permeated with taijiquan-like metaphors. In "Establishing the Foundation," he describes the formation of qi and strength using language that just as easily could be describing taijiquan:

> How does the calligrapher lay a foundation? Sink the qi to the dantian. The sole of the foot is planted in the ground, that's all. He moves his qi to his shoulder, elbow, wrist, the fingers, and then reaches the tip of the brush.[39]

Zheng himself never stopped studying. In fact, late in life he took the nickname the Old Man Who Never Tires of Learning. In his introduction to his *Yijing* commentary, Zheng said that in his search for the book's core ideas, he found the most primary one was *ren* or "human conduct." Zheng went on to lament that "to not see Confucius's Dao is like the sun and moon not shining, which is a misfortune for all of humankind."

Professor Zheng went back to Taiwan several times during his sojourn in the United States. On each trip he saw to the publication of his books, exhibited his artwork, and lectured on taijiquan, philosophy, and medicine. In 1974 Zheng planned to go for a third visit to Taiwan. He designated six senior students to run the New York Shizhong school in his absence.[41] Zheng left for Taiwan with his assistant Tam Gibbs to oversee publication of his commentary on the *Yijing* that had been the focus of his scholarly work for a number of years. After reading the proofs he paraphrased Confucius, that now, having finished the *Yijing*, he could die without regret.[42] Just ten days before his old acquaintance Chiang Kai-shek passed away, Zheng himself died of a cerebral hemorrhage, March 26, 1975.

Zheng Manqing's Legacy

Zheng was mourned by his family and many friends and students. At the funeral in Taibei, hundreds of mourners came and kowtowed at the memorial service. His family and representatives of the diverse groups of people with whom he had associated were all present: the highest circles of government and military, medical doctors, artists, and taijiquan colleagues and students. Floral wreaths and calligraphic banners mournfully sang praises of his "five excellences."[43] Students and friends also held memorial services in Singapore and New York.

In 1982 the National Palace Museum arranged with Zheng's widow for a retrospective exhibit, for which twenty-five of his paintings and works of calligraphy were selected. This was a great tribute to him, as the Palace Museum did not routinely exhibit modern artists. A catalogue of this exhibit was published for the occasion that included a reprint of a preface written by Madame Chiang Kai-shek to an earlier collection of his paintings.[44]

Since Zheng Manqing's death, his seminal works on taijiquan have been translated into other languages, and his students have carried on his mission of spreading taijiquan through their own work. Though it has been decades since Zheng passed away, his influence has continued to spread. Already there are thousands of third- and fourth-generation students practicing within his lineage, as well as thousands of adepts from other schools who rely on his writings for guidance in their taijiquan study. Zheng, along with other Nationalist colleagues, has also been "rehabilitated" in mainland China, so that one can now find him and his writings listed in martial arts materials.[45]

Zheng Manqing's Innovations in Taijiquan

The original role of martial arts study had been grueling professional training for men who would work as guards, bodyguards, or boxers. However, as the use of modern firearms grew, some martial arts began to shift from a primary focus on fighting application toward use for health and self-cultivation.

New methods of training evolved that did not require as high a level of time commitment, physical ability, or exertion. This was particularly true in the case of taijiquan, as its focus on softness and relaxation made it more appealing to a broader segment of the population, such as members of the educated elite and women. With this growth of interest, the martial arts became known as cultural treasures and as a means of defending national interests:

> Just as a segment of late Ming literati abandoned their traditional disdain for martial pursuits in the face of Manchu aggression, so a number of early twentieth century intellectuals embraced *guoshu* (Chinese martial arts) as part of a program of self-strengthening to counter Japanese imperialism and Western models of modernization.[46]

Taijiquan changed to fit into the social climate of the late Qing and early Republic, even in the manner in which it was taught. Typically martial arts had been taught in a master-disciple manner, and were usually transmitted within family lines, often from father to son. Yang Luchan (1799–1872, Zheng's great grand-teacher) and his offspring marked the beginning of public teaching of taiji. Yang had been allowed to study within Chen family circles (where taijiquan was said to have originated), but soon began to see the merit of teaching publicly. As Yang was purported to have said in the late 1800s, taiji was not

> to challenge others but for self-defense, not to bully the world but to save the nation.... We are poor because we are weak; truly weakness is the cause of poverty.... the best method of saving the nation is to make saving the weak our highest priority. To ignore this is to be doomed to failure.[46]

By the early 1900s Yang's sons were participating in the newly formed "ecumenical" martial arts organizations in Beijing, and took the lead in offering taijiquan to the public.[47]

A natural evolution of styles of taijiquan took place. The influence of each practitioner's physique and abilities, as well as interests and goals, all left a mark on the actual taijiquan forms. By the 1900s, this resulted in at least a dozen substyles of taijiquan within both Chen and Yang family circles.[48] But more significantly, forms were modified to appeal to a wider audience. Yang's grandson, Yang Chengfu, modified their family form, taking out the more strenuous and martial moves specifically to reach a wider public.

Zheng Manqing and others of his generation, such as Chen Weiming, Dong Yingjie, and Xu Yusheng, continued the work of spreading and refining taijiquan study and teaching in public forums. They chose to place the "needs of the nation" above the "filial" demands of private lineages. Zheng himself felt that the keeping of secrets would ultimately diminish the art.

As Zheng matured in his own practice, he began to see the wisdom of his Yang predecessors in their promotion of taijiquan as a health exercise for the general populace. He knew from his own personal experience its profound health benefits and saw it as a means of improving his countrymen's health. As he later wrote:

Without sound health, as without education, what good can one do to one's nation or social order, kith and kin, or neighbors? None at all![49]

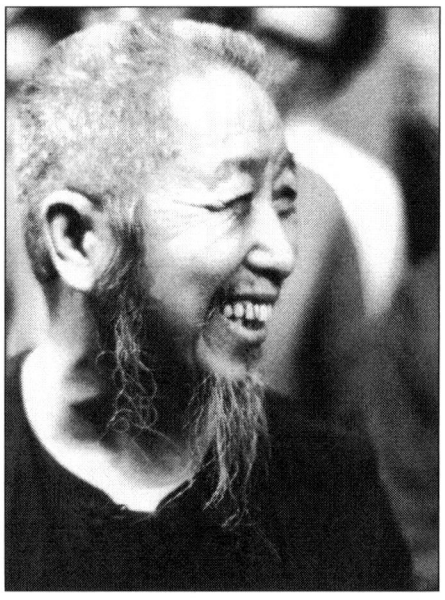

Zheng drew many followers, not only because of his knowledge, but also because of his warm personality.

Zheng saw how the Chinese people were suffering from sickness and poor self-esteem. Zheng felt that improved health and mind-set would help to "clear from us Chinese the undignified appellation of the 'infirm people of the Far East.'"[50] Thus, when Zheng writes that to withhold this gem was to ruin the country, or that on behalf of one's kin and country, one should study taijiquan, it should not be dismissed as a mere slogan.

Zheng's first dozen years of teaching took place during the upheaval of the Sino-Japanese War. It was clear to him that there were several problems inherent in the teaching and practice patterns of the past: the length of study needed to master taijiquan, the amount of time necessary for practice each day, and perseverance in study and practice.

As a result, over the next decade, Zheng Manqing decided to rework the Yang family taijiquan form because, citing national interests, he said, "I had to simplify the form in order to spread it, and I had to spread it so that it could make the people and the country strong."[51] By eliminating repeated moves he was able to condense the 128-move "long form" into a thirty-seven-move "short form." He felt this condensed form did not sacrifice the variety of moves nor adversely affect the potential quality of practice. This reduced the amount of time needed for a practice session from over a half hour to under ten minutes. He ultimately asserted, "I believe this book is in harmony with my teacher's [Yang Chengfu's] ideas,"[52] and received the support of his elder classmate Chen Weiming.

In his effort to popularize taijiquan practice, Zheng recommended ten minutes, morning and evening, of practice, rather than the hours of practice each day that were demanded in a traditional school. Zheng also cited other more practical reasons for doing taijiquan as opposed to other kinds of exercise: convenience, time, and low or no cost. It was safer than swimming and was not overly strenuous.[53]

Zheng also describes his internal struggle over what should or should not be shared openly. Could he follow the traditions of holding secrets back, potentially risking diminishing the art as well as the health of the country? No, he said. "If I also keep one secret or if I keep all of them, I would then be guilty of saving a pearl while my country went to ruin."[54] Yet he was nervous that he might be passing these secrets on to the wrong person. In the end, his desire to share the great benefits of taijiquan with the world won out.

It was in part because of potential health benefits that he felt taijiquan was particularly well suited for women. As a doctor of Chinese medicine, he applauded the emancipation of women from centuries of social and physical "restraints" (i.e., foot and breast binding and seclusion), and admonished that

> The health of a nation depends on the health of its women.
> Healthy mothers usually give birth to healthy babies while
> unhealthy mothers to unhealthy ones. Like sowing seeds,
> fertilized soil yields rich crops while barren soil poor ones.
> Since taking exercises is so important to women's health,
> it is most advisable for them to adopt taijiquan.[55]

He feared though that too much stimulation and activity would interfere with women's metabolism. He cited the traditional medical concept of women's health being based on "blood"[56] and that "blood being normally tranquil, so to speak, too strenuous activity for a woman will adversely affect her circulation."[57]

Beyond taijiquan's use as a health exercise, Zheng found in it one more vehicle for the teaching of the Confucian Dao. He was in a unique position to both add taijiquan to the repertoire of the gentleman-scholar, as well as to expand the reach of taijiquan ideas with an infusion of Chinese philosophy. Confucian, Daoist, and Neo-Confucian philosophy were important elements of his teachings of taijiquan. During a time when much of the writing on taijiquan focused on the physical aspects of practice, Zheng brought to his works fresh ideas from *Mencius*, the *Analects*, the *Yijing*, *The Art of War*, and the *Daodejing*, along with later philosophers such as Wang Yangming.

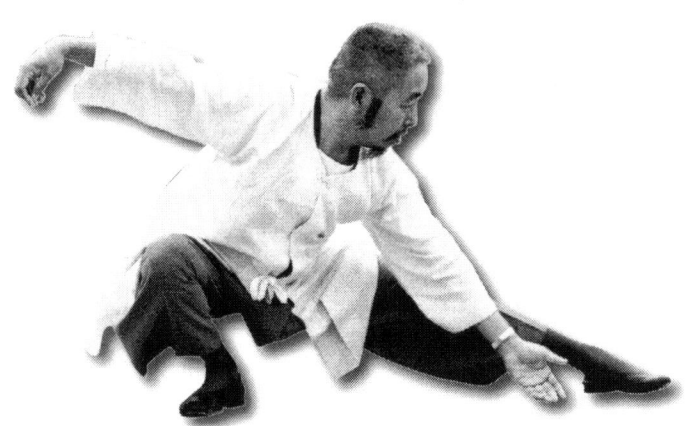

Photo courtesy of Robert W. Smith.

Conclusion

Zheng Manqing was a true Renaissance man who stepped beyond the bounds of traditional scholarship into the arena of martial arts. He brought with him the fruits of his previous studies, and in doing so, helped enrich taijiquan for people of all ages and nationalities. He incorporated into all of his work the ethics and philosophies of traditional China. Above all, Zheng Manqing, a man who indeed-never tired of learning, was able to put into practice Confucius's words: "My Dao is that of an all-pervading unity."

<u>Pinyin</u>	<u>Wade-Giles</u>	<u>Pinyin</u>	<u>Wade-Giles</u>
Chen Weiming	Ch'en Wei-ming	Yang Luchan	Yang Lu-ch'an
Cai Yuanpei	Ts'ai Yuan-p'ei	Yongjia	Yung-chia
Ding Yidu	Ting I-tu	Zhang	Chang
Dong Yingjie	Tung Ying-chieh	Zhang Guang	Chang Kuang
Guang Wen	Kuang Wen	Zhejiang	Chekiang
Qian Mingshan	Ch'ien Ming-shan	Zheng Manqing	Cheng Man-ch'ing
Shizhong	Shih Chung, Shr Jung	Zheng Manran	Cheng Man-jan
Song You'an	Sung You-an	Zheng Qian	Cheng Ch'ien
Wenzhou	Wen-chou, Wen-chow	Zhi Rou	Chih Jou
Yang Chengfu	Yang Ch'eng-fu		

Notes

Many people have freely given ideas, information, and editorial assistance over the many years and versions of this article. I am deeply indebted to the many students of Zheng's with whom I have been able to associate through my years of taijiquan study and research work, as well as to classmates of mine who have shared an interest in exploring Zheng's life and works in depth. I would like specifically to thank Robert W. Smith for assistance on many details of Zheng's life; and from the University of Minnesota: Richard Mather (professor emeritus of Chinese) for help with Zheng's poetry, Romeyn Taylor (professor emeritus of Chinese history) for cogent criticism and encouragement, and Dr. Yuan Zhou and Yuh-shiow Wang (East Asian Library). Previous drafts have benefited from the feedback of historians Cynthia Brokaw, Jon Saari, and Ann Waltner, and anthropologist Margery Wolf. The late historian Angus MacDonald challenged me with some overarching questions at the beginning of this project, but passed away before seeing the fruits of his suggestions.

Biographical information for this article was drawn in the main from *Zheng Manqing's Memorial Book* [Zhengzi ai si lu], and an amplified English version of the same ("Cheng Tzu: Master of the Five Excellences" in *Full Circle*, 1: 2, 13–21). Other sources are indicated in the notes, which include autobiographical information from Zheng's numerous articles and books.

Western dates are used in this article. Every effort has been made to corroborate dates as accurately as possible; however, there are occasions where information available does not yield a clear timeline (also see note number 2). For consistency's sake, Pinyin romanization is used for transliteration of Chinese, including quoted material, except for names more familiar in other forms and published works that use other systems. Translations are my own unless otherwise indicated.

This article was presented in slightly different forms for the Midwest Council for Asian Affairs (1991) for a master's degree paper in the Department of East Asian Studies, University of Minnesota.

Abbreviations

Simplified Methods *T'ai Chi Ch'uan: A Simplified Method for Health and Self-Defense.*
Thirteen Treatises *Cheng Tzu's Thirteen Treatises on T'ai Chi Ch'uan.*
Chinese Painting *Traditional Chinese Paintings of the Southern School: Works by Man-jan Cheng.*
ZGJXD *Zhongguo jinxiandai renwu minghao da cidian.*

[1] *Analects of Confucius*, book 4, chapter 15.
[2] Zheng's Chinese birth date is Guangxu 28th year, 25th day of the 6th moon. I have arrived at the Western date by consulting the standard reference, *Liangqian nianlai zhongxi li duizhao biao* [Comparative Table of Chinese-Western Calendars for Two Thousand Years, Beijing: Sanlian Publishing, 1956]. There are a

fair number of discrepancies between dates or ages in various material on Zheng. This may be attributed to confusion between different methods of calculating ages (one is considered to be one year old at birth, and another year is added at New Year's) and translation between the traditional and Western dating systems. Thus all ages given for Zheng (within this article as well as other people's material) should be taken as accurate within two years.

[3] One's given name would have been used within the family, or by teachers, and a *zi*, or style name, was taken at twenty. It was common, particularly among the educated and artistic, to use alternate names, such as pen names, nicknames, and studio names. For well-known people such as Zheng and many of his associates, these names can be found in special indexes (e.g., ZGJXD).

[4] These names will be found on his paintings, calligraphy works, and books, in signature and chop. Hermit of the Jade Well was one of his most commonly used appellations, which he used from at least the late 1940s on.

[5] Throughout China's thousands of years of organized governance, placenames have changed, often back and forth between two names, as in the case of Yongia (Yung-chia) and Wenzhou (Wen-chou or Wenchow). Geographical dictionaries, gazetteers, and historical maps can be consulted for these changes.

[6] *Manran san lun*, p. 9.

[7] According to one source, Zheng's family had been wealthy in previous generations, but a fire had destroyed their property (Su Shaoqing "Wujue laoren," p. 6).

[8] It is customary for a woman to maintain her own family name even after marriage. Her offspring would bear her husband's surname.

[9] *Manran san lun*, p. 9. The Tang dynasty (618–905) was one of the richest periods in Chinese poetry, producing such famous poets as Du Fu, Li Bai, and Wang Wei. Their poems are memorized in school and are used as models for writing.

[10] In her later years, Zhang Guang (c. 1878–1970) used the style name Old Lady Redfern (Hongwei Laoren) and, in her earlier years, Virtue Harmony (*De Yi*). Zhang specialized in the "birds and flowers" genre of painting. She worked at a number of jobs, including as principal of a teachers' training school and as a professor of art in Shanghai, Beijing, Hangzhou, and Guangdong (ZGJXD entry no. 4702). The "outline style" of painting, also called "detailed brush" (*gongbi*), uses carefully executed fine outlines that are then filled with color.

[11] Wang's given name was Ruyüan. He lived from 1867 to 1923 and was from Longxiang, Zhejiang Province. His style name was Xiangchan (also written as Xiangquan). His studio was named Fragrant Leaf (*Xiangye Lou*). He was an expert at flower and plant paintings and landscapes and had many disciples, the young Zheng among them (ZGJXD entry no. 4303).

[12] *Xieyi* literally means "writing the thoughts." It is a very fluid, expressive style that demands great mastery of the brush, ink, and paper.

[13] Cai Yuanpei (Ts'ai Yuan-p'ei, 1868–1940) was one of the most influential educators of early Republican China. He was educated within the traditional system and passed the highest exam (*jinshi*, received scholar) at the very young age of

twenty-two. Cai served as minister of education, chancellor of Beijing University, and was founder and president of the Academia Sinica, the national research institute. In his work he sought a synthesis of Chinese and Western intellectual processes. Cai supported the practice of taijiquan and wrote prefaces for a number of taijiquan books, including those by Yang Chengfu (1933) and Xu Longhou (1921).

[14] This early album appears to be the same as one entitled *Zheng Manqing xiesheng jiapin* [Zheng Manqing's paintings from life], dated 1924, which is reproduced in *Zheng Manqing huaji*, plates 31–34. Among the well-known people who wrote calligraphic inscriptions for it (dated 1926) was Cai Yuanpei.

[15] Ben Lo, one of Zheng's senior students, reports that Zheng did not study Shaolin boxing, but rather "internal exercises" for qi cultivation such as *baduanjin*. Shaolin gongfu refers to a wide range of popular exercises that were associated with Shaolin Temple traditions (Ben Lo interview, September 1995). In a similar fashion nowadays, these kinds of exercises are often associated with qigong practices.

[16] Chen established the society in 1925, after eight years of study with Yang. It is not clear from material consulted whether Yang moved to Shanghai or was visiting and teaching on a regular basis (see Chen, *Taijiquan dawen*).

[17] There is some confusion about the precise dates of Zheng's study with Yang Chengfu. Some sources (e.g., *Zheng Manqing xiansheng aisi lu*, p. 4) state that Zheng began with Yang at twenty-seven *sui* (approximately twenty-five to twenty-six years of age in the Western dating method), which would be around 1927. However, Zheng himself wrote in his preface to Yang's 1934 book, *Taijiquan tiyong quan shu*, that he was introduced to Yang in *Renshan zhengyue* (February 1932) by a Mr. Po Qiucheng. That would place Zheng's period of study with Yang from 1932 until 1936, when Yang passed away. Chen Weiming's calligraphed preface (dated 1947) to Zheng's *Thirteen Treatises*, p. 1, states that Zheng studied with Yang for six years.

[18] See R. Smith, (1995). "Zheng Manqing and Taijiquan: A Clarification of Role." *Journal of Asian Martial Arts*, 4(1), 52–53.

[19] Zheng was studying both with Qian and Yang during the same period. Qian Mingshan (c.1875–c.1944) had the given name of Qian Zhenhuang. He was from Yanghu (today's Changzhou), Jiangsu Province. He passed the jinshi examination in 1904 and, after leaving work in the government, became known as a scholar and calligrapher (ZGJXD no. 7642).

[20] It is generally considered that Yang was not literate, or not literate enough to write the books that appeared under his name. His first book, *Taijiquan shi yongfa*, is said to have been ghostwritten by another senior student, Dong Yingie, in 1931. Additionally, Chen Weiming wrote three books under his own name (*Taijiquan shu*, *Taijiquan hen*, and *Taiji jian*), though in each of these books he mentions that he was recording Yang Chengfu's words (See Wile, *T'ai-chi Touchstones*, p. iii–iv.)

[21] This book is translated in full in Lo and Inn's *Cheng-tzu's Thirteen Treatises*. It was completed in 1947 and published in 1950 after Zheng moved to Taiwan. Yu's inscription is dated November 1948. Chen's preface is dated April 1947.

[22] When Zheng departed for the United States, the association was left in the hands of his senior student, Liu Xihong. It is currently headed by Xu Yizhong. Shizhong is a philosophical term meaning "at the right time." (The Taiwan group romanized the term as *Shih Chung*, the American group as *Shr Jung*.) Information on the Taiwan Shizhong group is culled from Smith, *Chinese Boxing*; Smalheiser, "Push Hands . . ." (interview with Abraham Liu); *Taijiquan zazhi*; and Ben Lo (interviews, August and September 1995).

[23] "De jia shu," from *Yujing caotang shi xuji*, vol. 2, p. 4. In *Manran san lun*, Zheng indicates that he was the youngest of six children (p. 3). This reference to a younger brother may be poetic license, or may refer to the youngest of his elder brothers. Zheng may also have been simplifying the reference so as to fit the poetic meter.

[24] It was arranged for Zheng to use the Columbia University Library. For a writer or researcher, the open stacks at the library would have been a great temptation, especially as compared with the closed-stack system common to Chinese libraries (Ben Lo, interview, August 1995). In appreciation, Zheng donated copies of some of his works to a number of university libraries across the United States.

[25] *Thirteen Treatises*, p. 108–109.

[26] Information on the New York Shizhong school is culled from discussions with Zheng's students between 1979 and 1994, including Ed Young, Maggie Newman, Lori Reinstein, Ken Van Sickle, Jane Faigao, Bataan Faigao, Carol Yamasaki, and Wolfe Lowenthal, and from numerous articles in *Full Circle* and *T'ai Chi Player*.

[27] This is an overarching theme in his book *Renwen qianshuo*.

[28] Zheng Manqing was not the first Chinese person to be interested in promoting Chinese ideals to foreigners and overseas Chinese. In 1895 reformer and Confucian follower Kang Youwei (1858–1927) had suggested in a memorial to the Qing emperor that not only should Confucianism continue to be spread among the Chinese, but that Confucian academies should even be set up overseas. See Spence, *Gates of Heavenly Peace*, p. 42.

[29] Ed Young, "Character Study," p. 3.

[30] *Chinese Paintings*, p. 2.

[31] *Chinese Paintings*, p. 20.

[32] From the painting Green Mountain, in *Chinese Paintings*, plate 6, dated 1973, with my editing.

[33] *Manran san lun*, p. 72–73.

[34] See Zheng's *Renwen qianshuo*, author's introduction, ch. 39, "The Cultural Renaissance"; as well as Anon., "Principles for the Promotion of the Chinese Cultural Renaissance Movement"; and Uhalley, "Taiwan's Response to the Cultural Revolution."

[35] See *Renwen qianshuo*, author's introduction.

36 Among Zheng's publishers were such well-respected presses as the Commercial Press, Zhonghua Shuju, and the National Palace Museum. He also self-published a number of books, a common custom among Chinese scholars.

37 *Manran san lun*, p. 2. Both Wang Wei (699–759) and Guang Wen (fl. 742–755) flourished during the culturally rich Tian Bao reign period (742–755) of the Emperor Xuanzong in the early Tang dynasty. Wang Wei is credited with having founded a style of painting called *pomo* (broken ink) that spawned the more expressive ink painting styles popular in scholarly and amateur circles. Guang Wen, whose actual name was Zheng Qian, served in the Tang court as assistant chief musician and later as head of the *Guanwen guan*, the Office of Director of Studies. Zheng presented one of his paintings to Emperor Xuanzong, who was a great patron of the arts. The emperor inscribed the painting with "Three Excellences Zheng Qian," referring to Zheng's skill at painting, poetry, and calligraphy. After a while, Zheng became known in learned circles as Zheng Guang Wen, which literally means "Broadly Learned Zheng" (see *Xin tang shu juan* 202, p. 5766–5767, by Ouyang Xiu, Beijing: Zhonghua shuju, 1975). Zheng Manqing admired Zheng Qian's breadth of learning and carved a seal in admiration that he used occasionally on his artwork. The seal bore the inscription "Born 1,200 Years after Guang Wen" (see e.g., *Zheng Manqing xian-sheng shuhua tezhan mulu*, pl. 15).

38 *Manran san lun*, p. 2.

39 *Manran san lun*, p. 44. The dantian, or "field of cinnabar," is an important energy point in the body, located a couple of inches below and internal to the navel.

40 *Yiquan*, author's introduction, p. 3.

41 The six senior students were Tam Gibbs, Ed Young, Maggie Newman, Lou Kleinsmith, Mort Raphael, and Stanley Israel.

42 "In the morning hearing the Dao, in the evening die without regret" (in James Legge, *Confucian Analects*, bk. 4, ch. 8). Confucius also said, "If some years were added to my life, I would give fifty to the study of the *Yi[jing]*, and then I might come to be without great faults" (*Analects*, bk. 7, ch. 16, Legge).

43 These are among the material in *Zhengzi ai si lu*.

44 *Zheng Manqing xiansheng shuhua tezhan mulu* [Catalogue of Mr. Zheng Manqing's special exhibit of calligraphy and painting] p. 1–3.

45 Zheng is now listed, for example, in mainland-published martial arts biographies and bibliographies such as the *Zhongguo wushu da cidian* [Dictionary of Chinese martial arts, p. 489, p. 504], in Yang lineage charts found in martial arts books, as well as the ZGJXD.

46 Wile, *T'ai-chi Touchstones*, p. x. This is not to suggest that the educated men who took up taijiquan were not able to fight. Zheng himself took on many challengers. See Smith, *Chinese Boxing*, p. 25–46.

47 Wile, *T'ai-chi Touchstones*, p. 153. These are supposed to be Yang's words as spoken to Yang Chengfu. As Yang Luchan was already dead before Yang Chengfu was born, we could speculate that these words may actually reflect Yang Chengfu's attitudes, and were being purposely antedated (as is common practice

in China) to make a point with more authority.

[48] For more on the history of taijiquan, see Draeger and Smith, *Asian Fighting Arts*, p. 35–39, and DeMarco, "The Origin and Evolution of Taijiquan."

[49] *Simplified Method*, pp. 26–27.

[50] *Simplified Method*, p. 57.

[51] *Thirteen Treatises*, p. 104.

[52] *Thirteen Treatises*, p. 108.

[53] *Simplified Method*, p. 52.

[54] *Thirteen Treatises*, p. 87.

[55] *Simplified Method*, p. 54.

[56] In traditional Chinese medicine, "blood" (*xue*) incorporates more than the Western physical blood. It provides nourishment, maintenance, and moisture through the body, moving through the blood vessels and meridians. It is moved by the qi of the heart and chest. See Kaptchuk, *The Web That Has No Weaver*, p. 201.

[57] *Simplified Method*, p. 53.

Bibliography
Works by Zheng Manqing (Zheng Manran, Cheng Man-ching, Cheng Man-jan)

Books

Note: Zheng's taijiquan writings can be divided into five "books," which have been published in varying combinations in both Chinese and English editions, noted as follows:
- *Zhengzi taijiquan shisan pian* [Thirteen treatises] Section 1
- *Zhengzi taijiquan shisan pian* [Thirteen treatises] Section 2
- *Zhengzi taijiquan zixiu xinfa* [New method]
- *T'ai Chi Ch'uan: A Simplified Method* (in English)
- *T'ai Chi* (in English)

Cheng, M., and Smith, R. (1967). *T'ai chi*. Rutland, VT: Charles E. Tuttle Co. Gibbs, T. (Trans.).

____. (1981). *Lao-tzu: My words are very easy to understand*. Berkeley: North Atlantic Books. [Translation of Laozi yizhi jie.]

Lo, B., and Inn, M. (Trans.). (1985). *Cheng Tzu's thirteen chapters on t'ai chi ch'uan*. Berkeley: North Atlantic Books. [Authorized translation of *Zhengzi taijiquan shisan pian*, sections 1 and 2.]

Tseng, B. (Trans.). (1981). *T'ai chi ch'uan: A simplified method of calisthenics for health and self-defense*. Berkeley: North Atlantic Books.

Wile, D. (Trans.). (1983). *Master Cheng's thirteen chapters on t'ai chi ch'uan*. Brooklyn: Sweet Ch'i Press. [Translation of *Zhengzi taijiquan shisan pian*, section 1.]

Wile, D. (Trans.). (1985). *Cheng Man-ch'ing's advanced t'ai chi form instructions*. Brooklyn: Sweet Ch'i Press. [Translation of *Zhengzi taijiquan shisan pian*, section 2 and additional material.]

Zheng, M. (n.d.). *Guke jingwei* [Subtleties of orthopedics]. Text not extant. Zheng, M. (n.d.). *Tang shi zhen du* [Probing and measuring Tang poetry]. Taiwan: n.p.

Zheng, M. (n.d.). *Manqing zixuan* [Manqing freestyle poetry]. Text not extant. Zheng, M. (n.d.). *Yujing caotang shiji* [Jade well grass hall poetry collection]. Vol. 1. Taibei: self-published. [c. 1961].

Zheng, M. (1950). *Zhengzi taijiquan shisan pian* [Master Zheng's thirteen treatises on taijiquan] Sections 1 and 2. Taibei: n.p.

Zheng, M. (1961). *Nuke xinfa* [Essence of gynecology]. Taibei: National Traditional Chinese Medical Research Institute.

Zheng, M. (1962). *T'ai chi ch'uan: A simplified method of calisthenics for health and self-defense*. Taibei: Shih Chung T'ai-chi Chuan Center.

Zheng, M. (1965). *Zhengzi taijiquan zixiu xinfa* [Master Zheng's new method of taijiquan self-cultivation]. Taibei: Shizhong quanshe. [Includes *Zhengzi taijiquan shisan pian*, section 1]. Reprinted 1977.

Zheng, M. (1966). *Tan ai ba yao* [Eight important points on cancer]. Taibei: Guoli zhongguo yi yao yanjiu suo. Pamphlet.

Zheng, M. (1971). *Laozi yizhi jie* [Lao-Tzu: My words are very easy to understand]. Taibei: Zhonghua shuju.

Zheng, M. (1971). *Lunyu shizhi* [Explanation of the meaning of the Analects]. Taibei: Zhonghua shuju.

Zheng, M. (1971). *Xueyong xinjie* [New commentary on Great learning and Doctrine of the mean]. Taibei: Commercial Press.

Zheng, M. (1971). *Yujing caotang shiji* [Jade well grass hall poetry collection], Vol. 2. Taibei: self-published.

Zheng, M. (1973). *Renwen qianshuo* [A simplified explanation of man and his culture]. Taiwan: self-published.

Zheng, M. (1974). *Manran san lun* [Three treatises of Manran]. Taibei: Zhonghua shuju.

Zheng, M. (1974). *Yiquan* [The complete Book of changes]. Taibei: Meiya Publishing.

Articles

Gibbs, T., and Young, E. (Trans.). (Fall 1983). The Professor lectures. *T'ai chi player*, 1, 1–2. [First introductory lecture on zhongyong.]

Gibbs, T. (Trans.). (Dec. 1986). Professor Cheng on self defense. *T'ai chi player*, 4.

Hennessy, M. (Trans.). (1971). The story of strong man (Qiangren zhuan). Manuscript. [Autobiographical essay.]

Hennessy, M. (Trans.). (1988). Principles for living. Manuscript, 3pp.

Hennessy, M. (Trans.). (1989). Cheng Man-ch'ing's last statement concerning t'ai chi ch'uan. Manuscript, 2pp. [Signed "Man-jan, Spring Day, 1975."]

Hennessy, M. (1995). *Cheng Man-ch'ing: Master of Five Excellences*. Berkeley: Frog.

Zheng, M. (n.d.). *Xingben lun* [Discussion of man's original nature]. [Appendix to Xueyong xinjie.]

Zheng, M. (June 10, 1968). Meditation corresponds perfectly with medical principles; It is the bridge to better health and the path to longer life. Zhongyang ribao. [In *Cheng Man-ch'ing's advanced form instructions*, 121–125.]

Zheng, M. (July 20, 1970). *Principles of wisdom in taijiquan*. Taijiquan yanjiusuo.

Zheng, M. (July 20, 1971). A glimpse at the fifth anniversary of the Taijiquan Research Association. Taijiquan yanjiu suo.

Zheng, M. (Dec. 16, 1974). *Man tan wuchin xi zhi xiong jing* [An explanation of the constant bear movement from the five animals]. Changliu. Taibei: Taiwan Railway Bureau. Revised ed. Taijiquan zazhi, April 1983.

Zheng, M. (July 1984). Professor Cheng on the chung-yung. *T'ai chi player*, 1–3.

Zheng, M. (April 1984). Taijiquan yu tiyu [Taijiquan and physical education]. *Taijiquan zazhi*, 10–14.

Zheng, M. (July 1985). Professor Cheng on the chung-yung. *T'ai chi player*, 1–2.

Lectures

Gibbs, T., and Young, E. (Trans.). (Jan. 1974). Professor Cheng's health lecture. Manuscript, 11 pp. [New York City.]

Zheng, M. *Zhongyong* (Doctrine of the Mean). Lecture series for Shizhong Center, New York City. See under "articles" and "secondary sources".

Zheng, M. (June 20, 1971). *Kongzi yu Laozi zhi yitong* [Similarities and differences between Confucius and Laozi]. Taibei: Ministry of Education, Department of Culture. [Pamphlet.]

Zheng, M. (April 1984). Tan taijiquan [Speaking about taijiquan]. *Taijiquan zazhi*, 32, 6–7. [Feb. 26, 1975, at Miaoli Detective Bureau Hall.]

Painting Collections and Calligraphy

(1926). *Zheng Manqing xiesheng jiapin* [High quality paintings from life by Zheng Manqing], or *Zheng Manqing huace* [Painting album by Zheng Manqing]. [Reproduced in *Zheng Manran shuhua ji*, 31–34.]

(1961). *The art of Cheng Man-ch'ing* [Manran xieyi]. Taibei: Heritage Press.

(1971). *Zheng Manran shuhua ji* [Collection of Zheng Manran's calligraphy and painting]. Taibei: Zhonghua shuju. [Catalogue of exhibit at Taibei Provincial Museum.]

(1973). *Traditional Chinese paintings of the southern school: Works by Manjan Cheng*. Yonkers: Hudson River Museum.

(1982). *Zheng Manqing xiansheng shuhua tezhan mulu* [Special exhibition of painting and calligraphic works by Mr. Zheng Manqing]. Taibei: National Palace Museum. [Reprinted from *The Art of Cheng Man-ch'ing*.]

Movies

Yang style t'ai chi ch'uan. Produced by Shr Jung Cultural Center. Color. Narrative, form, push-hands, sword, approx. 20 min.

Untitled. Taijiquan form and pushing hands. New York City. B&W, approx. 10 min.

Untitled. Taijiquan demonstration. Taiwan. B&W, approx. 10 min.

Secondary Sources

Anon. (Oct. 29, 1973). Hold it! *New Yorker*, 35–36

Anon. (Dec. 10, 1974). The brush. *New Yorker*, 41.

Anon. (1975). *Zheng Manqing xiansheng ai si lu* [Mr. Zheng Manqing's funeral and memorial book]. Taibei: n.p.

Anon. (April 25, 1975). Cheng Man-ching is dead at 73; Calligrapher, painter and poet. *New York Times*, 32.

Chen, W. (n.d.). *Taijiquan shu* [The art of taijiquan]. Hong Kong: Wushu chubanshe.

Chen, W. (1929). *Taijiquan hen* [Questions and answers on taijiquan]. Shanghai: n.p. [Reprint, Taibei: Zhongguo taijiquan xue shu yanjiuhui, 1967.]

DeMarco, M. (1992). The origin and evolution of taijiquan. *Journal of Asian Martial Arts, 1*(1), 8–25.

Dong, Y. (1975). *Taijiquan shiyi* [Principles of taijiquan]. Hong Kong: Zhonghua shuju.

Draeger, D., and Smith, R. (1974). *Asian fighting arts*. NY: Berkeley Medallion.

Faigo, B. (1984). Here it is: A conversational portrait. *Full circle*, 1:1, 2–12.

Gibbs, T. (1984). Tam Gibbs' notes from Prof. Cheng's class. *T'ai chi Player*, 2, 5.

Gibbs, T. (Trans.). (1985). Cheng Tzu: Master of the five excellences. *Full circle*, 1:2, 13–20. [English rendition with Madame Zheng.]

Hennessy, M. (n.d.). Translation and commentary on Cheng Man-ch'ing's "principles for living." Manuscript. 3pp.

Lad, J. (1983). What does it mean to say that t'ai-chi ch'uan is scientific? *T'ai chi player*, 1, 6–8.

Lad, J. (1984). On mobilization of ch'i: Activating a mechanism or giving a signal? *T'ai ch'i Player*, 2, 6–8.

Lerhman, F. (1975). Untitled. *Shr Jung Newsletter*, 1:1, 7. [In memory of Professor Cheng.]

Lo, B., and Smith, R. (Trans.). (1985). *T'ai chi ch'uan ta-wen* [Questions and answers on taijiquan]. Berkeley: North Atlantic Books.

Lo, P. (1985). *Zuojia taijiquan shiyi* [Settling the uncertainties about Zuo family taijiquan]. Taijiquan zazhi, 40, 8–14.

Lo, P., et al. (1979). *The essence of t'ai chi ch'uan*. Berkeley: North Atlantic Books.

Lowenthal, W. (1983). The wonder of t'ai-chi ch'uan. *T'ai chi Player*, 1, 2–3.

Lowenthal, W. (1984). The virtue of t'ai-chi ch'uan. *T'ai chi Player,* 2, 5–6.

Lowenthal, W. (1985). The negative aspect of t'ai-chi ch'uan. *T'ai chi Player*, 3, 10–11.

Lowenthal, W. (1991). *There are no secrets: Professor Cheng Man-ch'ing's t'ai chi ch'uan*. Berkeley: North Atlantic Books.

Lowenthal, W. (1994). *Gateway to the miraculous: Further explorations in the Tao of Cheng Man-ch'ing*. Berkeley: Frog.

Mu, B. (n.d.). Wujuede shuhuajia Zheng Manqing [Painter-calligrapher of five excellences Zheng Manqing]. *Taijiquan zazh*i, 25, 6.

Smalheiser, M. (1990). Push hands is a game of skill. *T'ai Chi*, 145. [Interview with

Abraham Liu.]
Smith, R. (1974). *Chinese boxing: Masters and methods*. Tokyo: Kodansha.
Smith, R. (1975). A Master Passes. *Shr Jung Newsletter*, 1:1, 2–7.
Smith, R. (1984). A defense of Cheng Man-ch'ing. *Inside Kung-fu*, 11:2, 6. [Letter to the editor.]
Smith, R. (1995). Zheng Manqing and taijiquan: A clarification of role. *Journal of Asian Martial Arts, 4*(1), 50–65.
Su, S. (April 1983). Wujue laoren: Zheng Manqing gong xiao zhuan [Old man of five excellences: A short biography of Zheng Manqing]. *Taijiquan zazhi*, 6–7.
Wile, D. (1983). *T'ai chi touchstones: Yang family secret transmissions*. Brooklyn: Sweet Ch'i Press.
Xu, L. (Xu Yusheng). (1982). *Taijiquan shi tujie* [Illustrated explanation of taijiquan]. Taibei: Hualian chubanshe.
Xu, Y. (April 1983). Dao'en shi, zhi yishi [Mourning our beloved teacher, some anecdotes]. *Taijiquan zazhi*, 8.
Yamasaki, C. (1986). Notes from Professor Cheng's class. *T'ai chi Player*, 3, 4–5.
Yang C. (1983). *Taijiquan tiyong quan shu* [Complete book of substance and application of taijiquan]. Taibei: Laogu wenhua shiye.
Yang C., et al. (1984). Taijiquan xuanbian. Beijing: Beijingshi Zhongguo shudian.
Young, E. (July 1985). Some notes on translation. *T'ai chi Player*, 3.
Xinhua Press. (1992). *Zhongguo jinxiandai renwu minghao dacidian* [Dictionary of alternate names of modern Chinese personages]. Zhejiang: Xinhua Press.

Background Material

Chang, E., and Etzold, T. (Eds.). (1976). *China in the 1920s: Nationalism and revolution*. New York: New Viewpoints.
Dennerline, J. (1988). *Qian Mu and the world of seven mansions*. New Haven: Yale University Press.
Furth, C. (1976). *The limits of change*. Cambridge: Harvard University Press.
Kaptchuk, T. (1983). *The web that has no weaver*. New York: Congdon and Weed.
Legge, J. (Trans.). (1971). *The Analects, Confucius*. New York: Dover.
Liu, F. (1956). *A military history of modern China 1924–1945*. Princeton: Princeton University Press.
Lowe, H. (1983). *The adventures of Wu*. Princeton: Princeton University Press.
Rankin, M. (1986). *Elite activism and political transformation in China: Zhejiang province, 1865–1911*. Stanford: Stanford University Press.
Saari, J. (1990). *Legacies of childhood: Growing up Chinese in a time of crisis, 890–1920*. Cambridge: Council on East Asian Studies, Harvard University.
Shieh, M. (1970). *The Kuomintang: Selected historical documents, 1894–1969*. New York: St. John's University Press.
Smith, R. (1983). *China's cultural heritage: The Ch'ing dynasty, 1644–1912*. Boulder: Westview Press.
Spence, J. (1982). *Gates of heavenly peace*. New York: Penguin Books.

Spence, J. (1990). *In search of modern China*. New York: Norton.
Schwarcz, V. (1986). *The Chinese enlightenment*. Berkeley: University of California.
Taylor, R. (1990). *Religious dimensions of Confucianism*. Albany: State University of New York Press.
Uhalley, S. (1967). Taiwan's response to the Cultural Revolution. *Asia Survey*, VII, 824–829.
Wolf, M. (1991). *Thrice-told tale: Feminism, postmodernism, and ethnographic responsibility*. Stanford: Stanford University Press.

• 8 •

The Luoshu as Taiji Boxing's
Secret Inner-Sanctum Training Method

by Bradford Tyrey and Marcus Brinkman

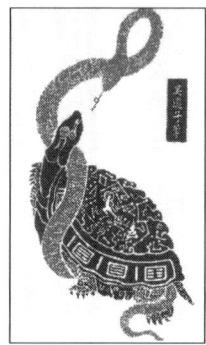
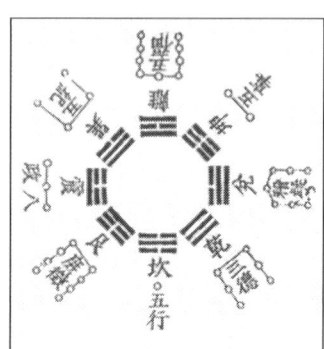

Ink rubbing of a snake and tortoise originally painted by Wu Daozi, a famed painter who lived during the Tang dynasty (618–907). From the collection of M. DeMarco.

Within the old practices of taiji, there exists a training method that is obscure and nearly lost. This method, passed from Chen Zhangxing to his student Yang Luchan, was born out of the Luoshu, colloquially referred to as the "Magic Square."

Ancient Daoist writings reveal that there was a need to understand how and why certain celestial principles interacted to bring about change and transformation in the heavens. From out of the Great Void, an answer mysteriously appeared for all to behold. According to Chinese mythology, Yu the Great discovered a celestial and cryptic chart, the Luoshu, on the shell of a great tortoise which was emerging from the sacred waters of the Luo River.

The tortoise, appearing majestic and heavenly, embodied and represented both heaven and earth. Its back, being convex, symbolized the canopy of heaven, and the tortoise's belly, being flat, symbolized the earth. The four feet, each with four toes, symbolized the four seasons. As the seasons changed, so did the colors of the feet and toes. The colors and their corresponding seasons were said to be dark green (spring), yellow (summer), white (fall), and black (winter). Upon the turtle's body there also appeared twenty-eight constellation formations and their locations in the heavens.

The Luoshu in its most general interpretation, represents the post-heaven diagram of change. Emperor Wen was said to have found profound inspiration from the arrangement on the tortoise's shell in formulating the foundation of the *Yijing* (Book of Changes). In its very essence, the Luoshu is a diagram of change which evokes the positioning of the eight *gua* (trigrams in the *Yijing*).

Using a heavenly numerological arrangement, the Luoshu forms a Daoist ritual dance pattern which is drawn or envisioned upon a floor. In old taiji boxing practice, this diagram was taught as the essential element to enhance and transform the post-birth qi and spirit into a mysterious union within the practitioner. Special patterns, fistic sets, and methods of bodily motion were derived from Luoshu's pattern. While one moves within this pattern, he should regulate his breath and properly swallow the jade-dew (saliva) in order to arouse the qi and thus nourish the primogenial breath of the Inner Palace. By this means, the Luoshu is a guide to taiji boxing practice, which leads to the threshold of immortality.

The Luoshu is a divine and magical square in which the number fifteen (15) can always be reached by adding three numbers in a straight line. The arrangement is as shown below:

$$
\begin{array}{ccc}
4 & 9 & 2 \\
3 & 5 & 7 \\
8 & 1 & 6
\end{array}
$$

4 + 9 + 2 = 15	4 + 3 + 8 = 15	8 + 5 + 2 = 15
3 + 5 + 7 = 15	9 + 5 + 1 = 15	6 + 5 + 4 = 15
8 + 1 + 6 = 15	2 + 7 + 6 = 15	

In 1937, Chen Weiming gave an account of how his teacher, Yang Chengfu, learned a treasured lance-training process passed down to him from Yang Luchan, who had been taught this secret method by his teacher, Chen Changxing, in the Chen Village during the 1800's. Chen Weiming had also shown to many of his original students an old handwritten manuscript on taiji lance training that was compiled by him and another student of Yang Chengfu. The manuscript, complete with drawings of lance exercises, specific notes on where to move and hold qi within one's body, and how to express qi outwardly through the lance, also provided insights into why lance training, when combined with the Luoshu, is one method by which man can attain the highest excellence in corporeal form and spiritual decorum.

A manuscript of similar content was also held by Sun Lutang, according to one of his "inner sanctum" students, Jiu Hao. Jiu, a prolific researcher and writer of taiji practice, wrote that Sun's manuscript was a repository of information encompassing taiji boxing and the Luoshu, which he had compiled based on the teachings of his masters, his talks with Yang Chengfu and Yang Shaohou, his visits to the Chen Village, and personal insights into the *Yijing*. Jiu, in his teachings, explained the importance of Luoshu training in taiji, xingyi, and bagua, by giving an excerpt from one of Sun's lectures to his students:

> Through the practice of taijiquan, the yang essence is nourished and brought forth. Through the practice of taiji lance, the yin essence is aroused and enfolds. Through the union of the yang with yin, the five forces of water, wood,

earth, fire, and gold come into being and merge within and throughout the body and lance. Through the Luoshu, one embarks to be inscribed upon the Register of the Immortals.

In his writings, Jiu Hao explained that Sun devoted his earliest morning hours to special forms of meditation, followed by a period of studying and interpreting the *Yijing* and its spiritual meanings and interrelations with the Luoshu. Sun then applied his interpretations to his practice of xingyi and bagua, both refining the stealth of his physical applications and cultivating himself spiritually. Jiu wrote that "Sun, over the years, changed his postures and manner of practice to be more attuned to his knowledge about qi development and his perception of the *Yijing* and Luoshu." Because these changes became so prevalent in Sun's later years, Sun remarked to his students that he practiced *bian quan* (changing fist). Some of his students misinterpreted this comment as a new fistic art that Sun had created. In actuality, Sun was referring to the significant number of changes he was making concerning postures, applications, and ways to practice. Sun wrote a book on these changes though it was said to have been stolen by a student or guest who had visited his home.

He had apparently decided not to rewrite this book. Jiu Hao, having read the book, later wrote down what he could remember, a document amounting to more than sixty pages. Jiu further annotated these pages with additional information that Sun taught. This newly compiled book on Changing Fist was later passed on to one of Jiu's inner-sanctum students.

Sun, who was well-known for his amazing feats with a lance, also wrote a text on lance practice and application that both Chen Weiming and Jiu Hao had read. This book cited numerous methods of using the Magic Square for stepping methods, lance attacks and counters, xingyi five-element lance, solo and partner training, and standing qi circulation exercises. There was also a section on lance studies applied to the Magic Square. This book, not surprisingly, was also stolen before it could be published, as was Sun's personal diary that he had written in for over forty years. Jiu Hao, once again, wrote extensive notes on Sun's lance book and accounts from the diary.

Chen Weiming wrote and published a short manuscript in Shanghai in the latter 1930's in which he explained what Yang Chengfu had been taught during one of his three-month stays in the Chen Village. The following is a partial translation:

> The Luoshu, according to many Chen family elders, is composed of both an inner and outer form, both halves embracing a myriad of meanings. The inner, in relation to the human physique, refers to the inner movement and location of qi as actuated by the five influences [elements] and the mind's will to govern the qi in movement. The outer, refers to a number of specific areas, some of which are: standing practice—in

preparation for movement; combat—areas to strike and guard; and weapons—areas to focus one's attack for maiming and overcoming the opponent using lance, sword, knife, and so forth.

Chen went on to explain, based on his contact while training with certain teachers, that some schools emphasized discipline and instruction derived from their understandings of the Magic Square:

These methods are especially taught by some of the elder teachers of the Chen taiji boxing style, Yang Luchan's original version of the Yang family art, and the Sun Lutang school. My master, Yang Chengfu, said that Yang Luchan learned both the inner and outer Luoshu applications and thus was able to attain supreme boxing skills. He passed on this knowledge to his sons, but it was Yang Jianhou who most ardently practiced his boxing according to his ever deepening understanding of the Luoshu though it was Yang Banhou, in his later years, who began teaching these guarded methods outside the Yang family circle.

The Magic Square, as applied to the exterior of the human body, is adjusted according to one's posture and purpose of practice. In taiji, bagua, and xingyi boxing arts, Magic Square principles remain identical. Briefly presented here are the five major variations of this method as outlined by lecture notes from classes taught separately by Sun Lutang and Yang Chengfu. For easy reference, Yang Style drawings are used as examples.

Solo Boxing Practice

The practice of each posture must be in accord with the Luoshu. To attain such accord, one must first study the respective positions related to both the inner and outer parts of the human body and then accommodate these positions to seasonal, daily, earthly and heavenly interactions. As one comprehends both the meanings and correlations of the magic numbers, one then shall uncover the secrets of movement according to the Luoshu. One mysterious factor is the sum of fifteen.

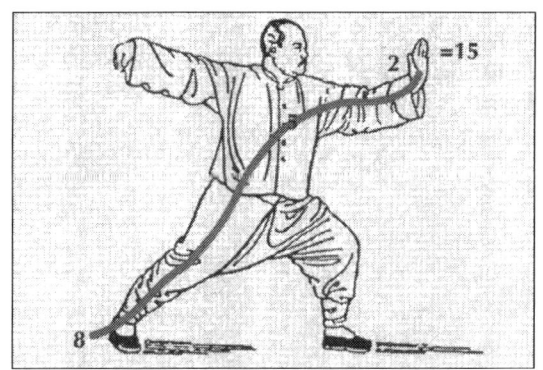

Lance Practice

The Luoshu, in regard to lance practice, is divided into four parts. Respectively, they are the Luoshu of one's stationary body (posture), that of the body moving with the lance, that of spearing outward towards configurations of the Luoshu, and that of paired-lance practice.

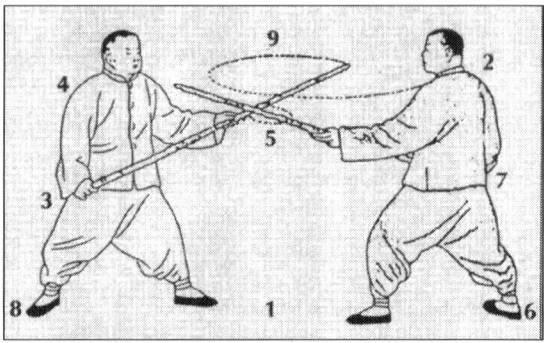

Saber and Sword

In both saber and sword, the blade's angle of attack dictates the arrangement of the Luoshu. An outward thrust expands the numerical positioning, while an inward (yielding) action contracts the numerical positioning to its origin.

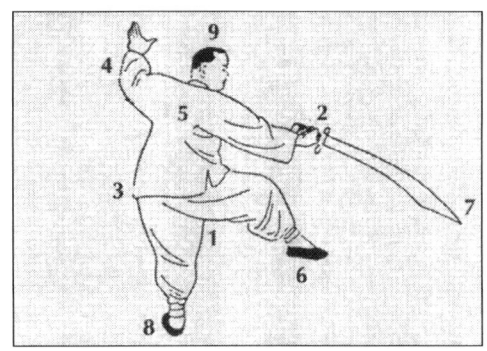

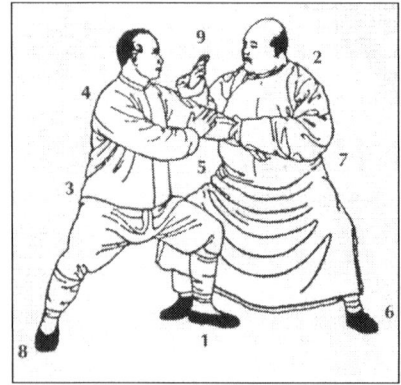

Two-Person Practice

As in paired-weapons practice, each person contains his own inner and outer Luoshu. When two people touch in practice, the Luoshu are said to unite between the practitioners. Changes in the positioning of the Luoshu depend upon posture, yielding, and the issuance of force at a specific point. One's success hinges upon attaining the sum of fifteen, whether yielding or overcoming.

Conclusion

The Luoshu, as one of the inner-sanctum secrets, touches upon every aspect of taiji training. Jiu Hao, in one of his visits to the Chen Village, recorded what he was taught concerning the two drawings. His recordings differ from what has been published in an old book on the Chen Style which contains these same drawings. Jiu explains in his writings that "being in the presence of teachers, one is given information and insight that will not be written. The Chen family, in particular those with long beards, hold to this way steadfastly."

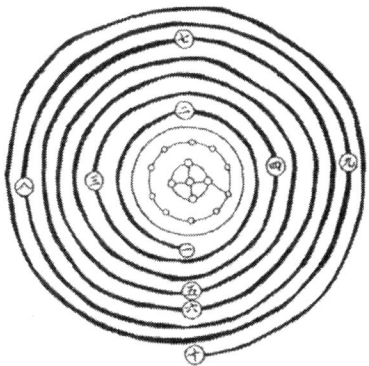 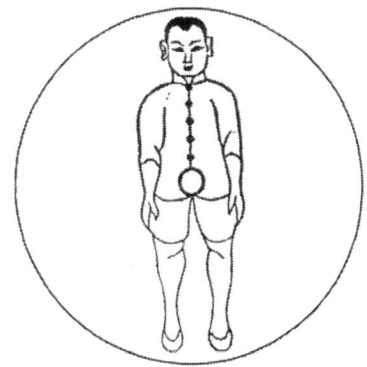

The following is an excerpt from Jiu's manuscript:

Taiji boxing's inner *jing* [force] spreads throughout the body, initiating from a single-most point. It is in a constant state of expansion and contraction. Though one is tranquil, jing coils as a dragon in the heavens.

Even within a single action, the jing is continuous from one action into another. As a spider's web, once you touch it [one's web of jing], you cannot escape. As in a whirlpool of water, the force swirls, and if touched, though it cannot be seen, its vortex pulls you in and no escape is possible. The jing has many perpetuating circular forces and though, if skillful enough, you may escape from an outer web of jing, you cannot escape from the center of the vortex which is limitless in its progressive strength.

Man, though in a posture inducing tranquility or in a posture of movement, has the jing web within and without concurrently, both reinforcing the other, as do the yin and yang. The inner jing and outer jing are likened to yin and yang. The Luoshu, having its arrangement within man's jing web, interior and exterior, is the heavenly thread by which all is united within the body. In this manner, the heart, the spirit, the breath, and the Luoshu may find harmonious abode in the cavity of the body, dwelling permanently within.

• 9 •
The Combative Elements of Yang Taijiquan
by Peter Lim Tian Tek

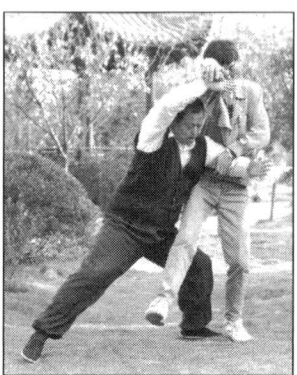

Wang Xianggen, who teaches in Hangzhou, China, topples a student.
Photo courtesy of Don Mainfort.

Other than the fact that its name can be translated as "The Supreme Ultimate Fist," taijiquan (or simply taiji for short) has always been noted as a highly effective combat art. It first became widely noted as a combat art when Yang Luchan brought it to Beijing where he taught at the imperial court. Yang was challenged many times, but no one ever came close to defeating him. So great was his skill that the martial artists bestowed on him the title "Yang the Invincible."

More recently, Yang Luchan's grandson, Yang Chengfu, promoted the art until it spread far and wide. Yang Chengfu taught his art as a combat art which can be used to strengthen the body. His three books attest to this fact. There is no substance to the widespread assumption that Yang Taiji is solely health oriented and not combat effective. By practicing taiji as a martial art, one can also gain the health benefits. Yang Chengfu, in his book *The Practical Application of Taijiquan*, wrote:

> In taijiquan, the ability to cultivate oneself physically and spiritually, but not to defend oneself, is civil accomplishment. The ability to defend oneself, but not to cultivate oneself, is martial accomplishment. The soft taiji method is the true taiji method. The ability to teach the art of self-cultivation and self-defense, both cultivation and application, is complete civil and martial taiji.
>
> – adapted from Douglas Wile's translation.

In these modern times, with the advent of modern weapons of both individual and mass destruction, the civil or health-giving aspects have been emphasized over the martial. The full art, however, as the above words explain, consists of both civil and martial aspects. One without the other is incomplete. The civil aspects of taiji have been much written about but the martial or combative principles, applications, etc. are little known and in danger of being lost.

As a martial art, taiji is very different from the hard-hitting, external martial forms. What is combat taiji then? It is certainly not about great power even though taiji is capable of generating great power. The classics state clearly that the art is not based on great power. Once, when Yang Banhou had bested an opponent and was proud of himself because of it, Yang Luchan, his illustrious father, pointed to Banhou's torn sleeve and said that he was happy that Banhou had won but did he use taiji to win? The implication is, of course, that a torn sleeve is a sign of inappropriately used power. Yang Luchan's own boxing was so soft that it was nicknamed "cotton fist" or "neutralizing fist." It was once berated as not being combat effective because of its softness, a point which Yang refuted by promptly defeating the antagonizer.

The following are some of the key elements used by taiji exponents in combat. The author and his student, WSU Taiji Club President, Desmond Tan, demonstrate some simple applications to illustrate the points discussed in this chapter.

COMBAT PRINCIPLES

A Word About Anatomical Weapons

The anatomical weapons in taiji are not rigorously hardened as in external styles of martial arts. This is because it is not hardness of the weapon but the energy within it that is the effecting component. If the correct structure of the anatomical weapon is maintained, then structurally it will be substantial and able to deliver telling blows with much power without recourse to hardening. The appropriate and efficient use of strength usually does not require great excess to obtain the desired effect. The principles behind the adage of "deflecting a thousand pounds with four ounces" hold true in taiji.

■ "Not Letting Go; not resisting"

The combat principle of "not letting go, not resisting" is first cultivated in push-hands (*tuishou*) practice and later refined in sparring hands (*sanshou*) practice. The key element in this principle is sticking (*nian*) and it operates through sticking energy (*zhan*). This is because without sticking, one cannot "hear" the opponent's energy and its qualities and so be able to control them effectively. And, if we resist, then we give the attacker a base for which to effect his attack. That is why instead of deflecting, resisting and absorbing an opponent's attacking force, taiji exponents evade, redirect and blend with it. "Evade" means simply to move out of his way. In any attack, there are only limited points to attack, so simply removing yourself out of his attacking focus by a change of position negates it. Contact should not be a hard block, but a blending with the attacking part by yielding, sticking and following the opponent's momentum, joining his energy and redirecting it to your advantage.

Through sticking energy we can then develop listening energy (*tingjing*), which is the sensitivity to detect the opponent's strength, its origin, trajectory, magnitude and component vectors. Once we are able to detect his energy movement and center of mass, we can effectively know his intent and control it by affecting the energy flow and center of mass efficiently.

APPLICATION: Not Letting Go, Not Resisting
(A-1) Mr. Tan attacks with a left punch. (A-2) Mr. Lim, "not resisting," neutralizes the punch by leading it into emptiness. (A-3) Tan realizes he is over-extended and so withdraws. (A-4) Lim, by "not letting go," sticks to Tan, following him while adding on to his momentum and utilizes the opportunity for a push. Sequence photos courtesy of Lim Tian Tek.

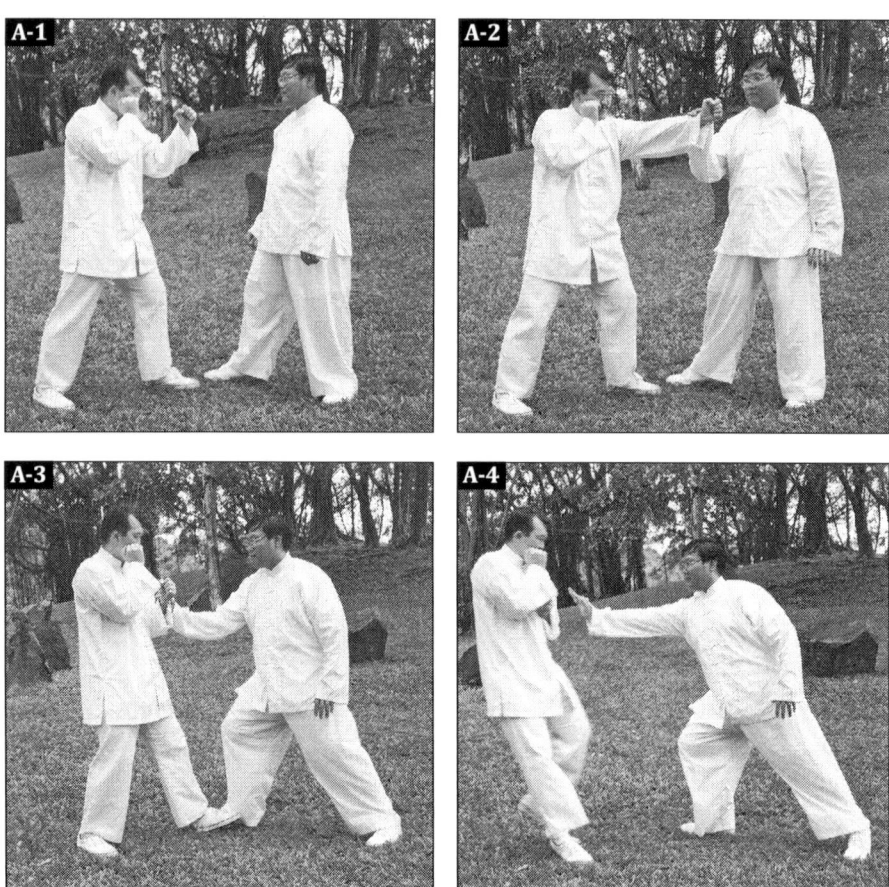

■ "Following His Posture; Borrowing His Strength"
Sui ren zhi shi, jie ren zhi li simply means to follow your opponent's structure and adapt to it so that it is ineffective. This is practical application of the principle of *bu diu bu ding* by yielding and following him. Rather than a rigid application of learned postures, the applications should occur spontaneously in response to the opponent's movement.

"Borrowing his strength" is essentially utilizing the opponent's own strength against him, either by causing it to overextend or to channel it through your own body structure back to him. He is literally then hitting himself and there is little expenditure by way of energy for the taiji practitioner.

This following of the opponent's structure is first learned from push-hands, which is why it is important that push-hands not degrade into a choreographed exercise. Sensing the opponent's movements and responding to them is correct rather than just going through the motions and not sensing them. If he does not move, you should not move. Even in a static position, there will be structural flaws that can be detected by the touch, and one can attack them by moving first. But be always aware of a possible trap, even during an attack. Sensing plays a very important role in avoiding traps by responding in midattack and countering the trap.

APPLICATION: Following His Posture, Borrowing His Strength
(B-1) Mr. Tan punches, but the strike is neutralized by Lim's ward off block (B-2). (B-3) Tan follows with a roundhouse kick, but Lim sticks to Tan and follows his movement by rotating and stepping forward. Lim thus redirects the power from the kick with his left arm, transfers the power into his right arm, and utilizes it to pin Tan's right arm. (B-4) Since Tan is now defenseless, Lim easily follows with a palm strike to an accupoint near the shoulder (known as *lu* 1).

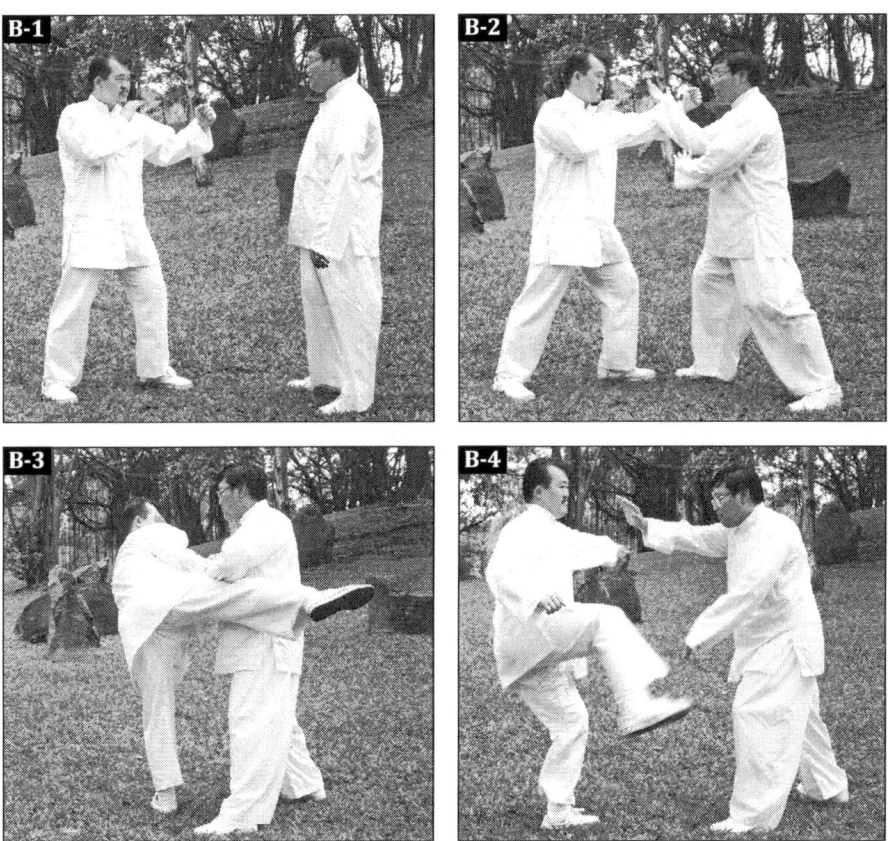

■ "Attract Into Emptiness"

Yin jin ru kong, "attract into emptiness," is one of the most common tactics used in taiji. It is exemplified by the posture "rollback" which implements the opponent's entry into emptiness. The tactic essentially is presenting a false target for the opponent to attack, and when he does, you spring the trap of letting his own momentum and mass be his own undoing by overextending it. Finding no target, he is naturally unbalanced and is easy to counter.

■ "Emitting Energy"

Used when the taiji practitioner attacks, *fajing* refers to the emission and transmission of energy out of the practitioner's body and into the enemy or target. The whole process is of an explosive nature, but at no point in it is the body or limbs rigid. Taiji practitioners are noted for their great power when it comes to uprooting or bouncing an opponent out. This power, however, is applied appropriately and efficiently. Having a lot of power but not knowing where to use it is quite useless; hence, the importance of sensitivity. Sensitivity allows you to know not only the opponent and avoid his power, but also to know where to apply your power to greatest effect.

So, is the appropriate use of great power then the key to self-defense? No, it isn't. Power in excess of what is required to achieve neutralization and control is inherently unstable. One must refine the process till it becomes so efficient that minimum power can produce maximum effect. Then, even an old man can best a young and strong one, not with more power but with the intelligent and efficient application of the body.

That is why masters like Zheng Manqing can send a 200-pound man flying across the room but finds a bowling ball too heavy to carry on with the sport (Lowenthal, 1991). This is no paradox once the underlying principles are understood.

■ "Long Energy"

Zhang jing (long energy) is the most common type of energy emission used in taiji. It develops from the feet, and because the energy path is long—through all the joints and ending at the fingers—it is called "long energy." It is commonly seen when taiji practitioners "bounce out" their push-hands partners. The whole body of the opponent is physically pushed away by moving his center of mass. If it is done correctly, both his feet should leave the ground when he is propelled away. This is why the technique is called "uprooting."

The energy can be developed from the rear foot, the front foot or from one to the other. All the joints in the body work coordinately and smoothly, without tension, to transfer, amplify, and focus the generated energy to the point of attack. This type of energy is usually the first to be manifested by the practitioner and, though it can be spectacular, it does not cause very serious injury.

APPLICATION: Long Energy

Long Energy (*zhang jing*) is the most common method of energy emission seen in taijiquan. It can be spectacular but seldom causes serious injury. It is often used in push-hands practice to uproot the opponent. Sequence photos courtesy of Lim Tian Tek.

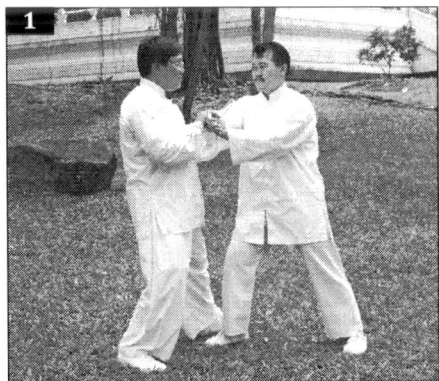
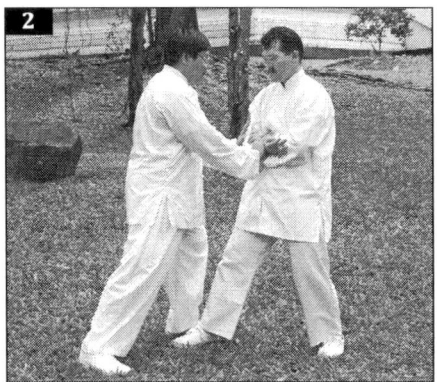
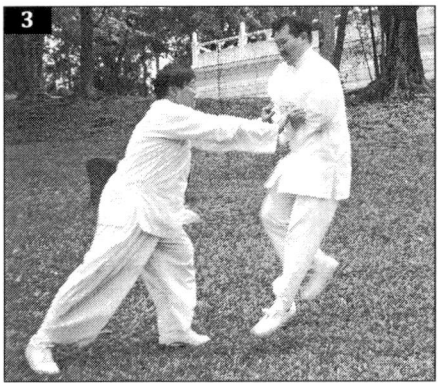

■ "Short Energy"

Short energy emission (*duan jing*) is less common and is considered a rather advanced method. The energy transmission path is shorter than that of Long Energy and originates at the center of mass which is supported by the rooting leg. The energy emission begins at the center of mass and propagates outwards, down the root and out through the limbs. It is aimed at and acts directly upon the opponent's center of mass, using it as a base for a crushing attack that ruptures organs, rends musculature and breaks bones. The fastest application of such energy is called cold energy (*leng jing*) because the emission is so sudden that it catches the opponent by great surprise, so great that it frightens him and causes him to break out in cold sweat.

APPLICATION: Short Energy

Short Energy (*duan jing*) is directed at the center of the opponent's mass in an explosive manner. The opponent is not bounced out as with a Long Energy application, but is usually dropped on the spot.

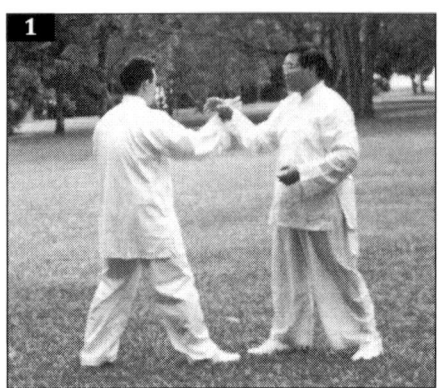
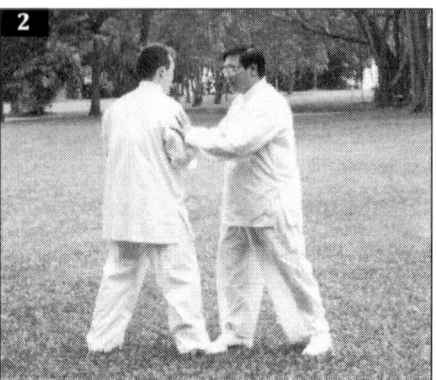
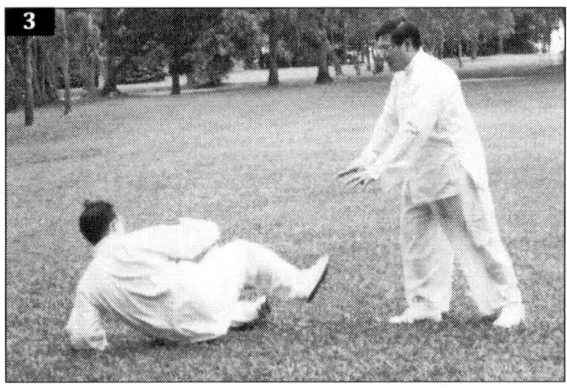

- "Intercepting Energy" or "Receiving Energy"

Jie jing skill has always been associated with the great masters and we know that Yang Luchan, Yang Chengfu, and Zheng Manqing possessed this skill. It has been said to border on the mysterious and it is hard to attain such skill. It can only be attained after one is learned in the "tenths, hundredth and thousandths" parts in taiji. At lower levels of attainment, jie jing is expressed mainly through the hands. At higher levels, where the entire body is responsive, it can be expressed from almost any part of the body.

With jie jing skill, one meets an incoming object by sticking, yielding and attaining almost the same speed as the object. This means that since the acceleration of the object and the contact point is nearly the same, their relative speed to each other is small. By "listening" to the object's center and vectors, one can apply an appropriate minimum vector to change the object's trajectory. If it is a balanced object, it can be easily pushed; if it is not, it can be easily redirected. This is what Zheng Manqing meant when he said that in jie jing one must first attract the object, then throw it away.

APPLICATION: Intercepting/Receiving Energy

Jie Jing can be translated both as "intercepting energy" or "receiving energy." The point of contact is the point of neutralization and also the point of counter-attack. Normally the opponent's energy has not fully reached the defender when the counter occurs. Sequence photos courtesy of Lim Tian Tek.

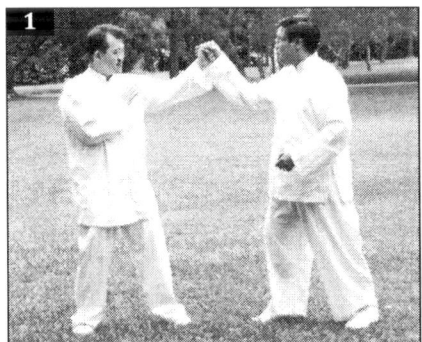
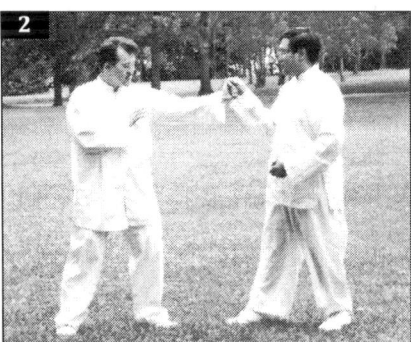
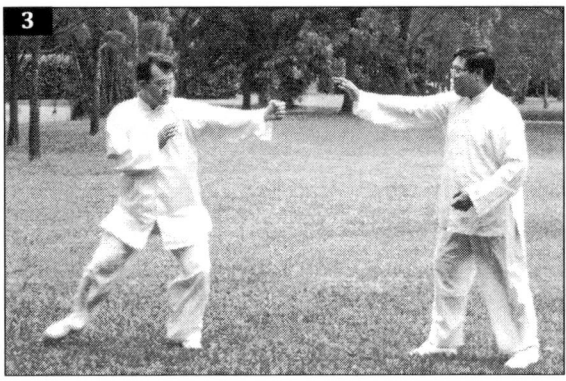

- "Tenths, Hundredths, and Thousandths Parts"

It is possible to divide each taiji movement into ever finer gradations of movement, technique and jing flow. Each part is then meaningful and has an application in a combative context. The refinement of movements to efficiency is but the beginning. Later, each part of the movement has meaning, as does each part of every part, and so on.

This practice also ensures that the mind is conscious of every part of the movement and every tiny movement of the body. Sensitivity is thus trained to a very fine degree as is the response to minute stimuli. The classics state the goal quite clearly: to be so light and sensitive that "a feather cannot be added nor a fly alight."

The Four Advanced Yang Taijiquan Combat Skills

There are situations in which the skills and principles discussed above require some augmentation to make them even more effective. This situation usually occurs when the opponent's skill level is so high that an effective counter is not possible using less injurious means. In such situations, stronger discouragement is required, and to anticipate such eventualities, Yang Taijiquan has four advanced combat skills. These four skills can only be learned and applied effectively after one is able to understand each individual portion of any technique. In other words, one must be able to comprehend and put into practice the "tenths, hundredths, and thousandths parts" in taijiquan.

These four skills are recorded in the handwritten manual handed down from Yang Luchan. It must be noted that the four skills are not used entirely on their own but are integrated to form a comprehensive system of attack and defense built upon the basics of stability, sensitivity, agility and efficient use of the body and energy.

■ "Sealing Accupoints"

Bi xue, known as "hitting accupoints," is more commonly known among Chinese martial artists as *dian xue* (dotting accupoints) because the majority of these kinds of attack make use of the fingertips. Attacking accupoints is by no means unique to taiji, but the way it is done is certainly quite unique. While other martial arts often make use of serious conditioning of the anatomical weapons and vigorous body conditioning to develop the strength and resistance required to hit accupoints, taiji uses positional and structural advantage to let the opponent provide the power to hit himself with his own power and mass.

Accupoints are divided into fatal and non-fatal accupoints. Fatal accupoints are only used in a life-and-death situation as they can cause death very quickly and should not be used indiscriminately. Non-fatal accupoints are used to simply disable or incapacitate the opponent without causing too much harm. There are also accupoints that are more effective at different times of the day depending on the qi flow in the body. These timed strikes are of a more insidious nature as they are used for delayed killing or assassinations.

A sample of some of the accupoints used in taiji is provided. However, readers are advised against using them unless absolutely necessary and to refrain from experimentation as the recovery techniques should be properly understood before one practices with accupoints. Even then, it is advisable not to practice them with any sort of impact since any accupoint strike on the body is a severe disruption of the body's systems and will have both long term and short term effects on the health of the body. In most cases, even after remedial massage and accupoint treatment is carried out, herbs are taken to strengthen and stabilize the body in order to eliminate any aftereffects.

GRASP SPARROW'S TAIL
- **Ward off (*peng*):** wrist and forearm points
  (LI 4/5/7/10/11, SI 6/7, Lu 5/6/7/8, H 2/3/6, P6, TW 5)
- **Rollback (*lu*):** wrist and upper arm points
  (TW 11/12, LI 13, P 2)

- **Press (*ji*):** center of chest
  (Ren 15/17, K 23, and flank, Liv 13/14, Sp 21, GB 24)
- **Push (*an*):** ribs (K 23, ST 19) and floating ribs (LI 13/14)

■ "Grasping Muscles"

Grasping musculature in taiji is akin to the specialization of *qinna* (grasping and holding), which is an advanced skill in many forms of Chinese martial arts. The difference is that in taiji, the use of positional advantage, momentum and structural advantage is of more importance than super-strong fingers. The sensitivity of combat taiji permits one to use the opponent's structure, position, mass and momentum against himself causing him to literally lock and tie himself up with his structure with the taiji practitioner simply "helping" him do it. The result of this is that the opponent becomes unstable and, therefore, vulnerable to serious injury should the taiji practitioner choose to press his advantage. The locks and holds also cause sprains, tears of the musculature and dislocations of bones at the joints, which further disable the opponent.

■ "Sectioning Fascia"

Sectioning fascia (*jie mo*) is directed at restricting blood flow so as to render the body ineffectual in the execution of attacks. This is done primarily by structural control so that the position and state of the musculature and soft tissues of the opponent are such that the blood flow to certain parts of the body is restricted. Blood-flow pressure points, or "gate points" as they are referred to in Chinese, are also used to effect this. This technique can cause the limb to "go to sleep" or cause a knock-out. Also part of this skill is the restriction of air flow by attacking the respiratory system and the musculature that powers it. Strikes are sometimes used to effect this.

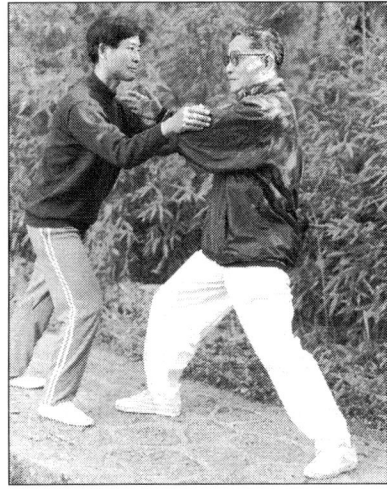

Xia Tao (left), President of the Hangzhou Wushu
Association, practicing push-hands with Jiang Jialun.
Photo courtesy of Don Mainfort.

Positional and structural advantage and use are essential to restrict and control the opponent's body. This is possible to a high degree through the tactile sensitivity attained through diligent practice in push-hands and sparring hands.

■ "Holding Vessels"

Holding vessels (*na mai*) refers to the grasping, holding and pushing of the qi meridians and accupoints with the purpose of disrupting and controlling the qi flow in the body. This technique impairs the body's function and movement, thus rendering the opponent vulnerable. Whereas grasping muscle attacks the physical structure of the body and sectioning fascia attacks the circulatory system, holding vessel attacks the internal vital-energy flow, which is distinct from the accupoints and the striking of them.

Good knowledge of the body's qi meridians is necessary as is the results of their disruption and blockage. As with the above skills, the opponent's own body and energy are used against himself through superior information via tactile sensitivity and appropriate and efficient application to obtain the desired result.

Healing and Harming

The knowledge and skill to cause destruction and death of the body can also be used to restore health and prolong life. The four advanced skills mentioned briefly above all require a thorough and intimate knowledge of the body and its functions. This knowledge can be used to heal injuries and cure illnesses by opening blockages to qi and blood circulation, restoring proper musculature position and function.

Often, this healing function is learned first before the harming function is taught. This ensures a proper disposition and respect for the skill as well as firm grounding in the theoretical base and its practical application. It is because these skills are so destructive that they are seldom taught and many practitioners of the art are not aware of their existence. They are passed on only to the most trusted of disciples who will not abuse them but use them for the benefit of all mankind.

The Taijiquan Martial Artist

Above all, taiji exponents are encouraged to be moral people. A sense of righteousness, chivalry, kindness, compassion, nobility and being a benefit to society should always be the code of conduct for the taiji practitioner. A practitioner should embody the principles of his art and apply its stratagems and philosophies in his dealings with all things.

The aim of taiji as a martial art is to stop violence conclusively without recourse to more violence. Most of the time, violence is redirected against itself or rendered ineffectual. Hence, taiji practitioners usually overpower their opponents by just turning their own violence against themselves, educating them rather than hurting them. Violence begets violence. In taiji practice, violence is shown to act against itself. By employing taiji theory in self-defense, the destructive cycle is broken and a more rational, less confrontational solution is found to be the most effective.

Can taiji be used as an attacking art? Yes, but violence should only be the last recourse, never the first. Ego has no place in taiji as it gets in the way of efficient practice and usage of the art. Taiji itself is an art to prolong life, in peace and in combat. In practicing taiji as a combat art, peace is learned and cherished. We learn the art that we may never have to use it. With the knowledge of violence and its consequences, we choose to avoid the destructive path.

▼●▼

English	Pinyin	Chinese
not letting go, not resisting	bu^4 diu^1 bu^4 ding^3	不丟不頂
following his posture	sui^2 ren^2 zhi^1 shi^4	隨人之勢
borrowing his strength	jie^4 ren^2 zhi^1 li^4	借人之力
attract to emptiness	yin^3 jin^4 ru^4 kong^1	引進入空
emitting energy	fa^1 jing^4	發勁
long energy	chang^2 jing^4	長勁
short energy	duan^3 jing^4	短勁
intercepting/receiving energy	jie^1 jing^4	接勁
sealing accupoints	bi^4 xue^2	閉穴
grasping muscles	zhua^4 jin^1	抓筋
sectioning fascia	jie^4 mo^2	節膜
holding vessels	na^2 mai^4	拿脈

References

Lowenthal, W. (1991). *There are no secrets: Professor Cheng Man-ch'ing's t'ai chi ch'uan*. Berkeley: North Atlantic Books.

Wile, D. (Trans.). (1983). *T'ai-chi touchstones: Yang family secret transmissions*. Brooklyn, NY: Sweet Ch'i Press.

• 10 •

Breathing in Taiji and Other Fighting Arts
by Robert W. Smith

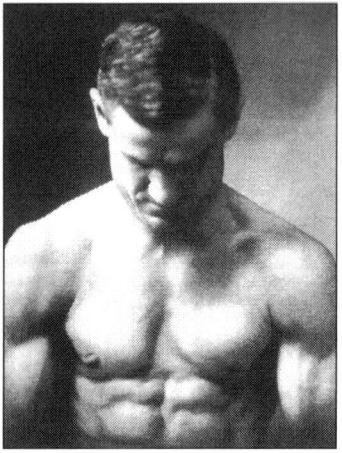

E. J. Harrison
Courtesy of The Overlook Press.

**"You cannot do it," explained the Master,
"because you do not breathe right."**

– E. Herrigel, Zen in the Art of Archery

Early on, I found breath a curious and fascinating thing. We use the same breath to cool coffee and to warm our hands. The nose, the agency of breath, is likewise strange. Why is it that we can smell another's halitosis, but not our own? As a youngster, I experimented with a number of breathing methods and early came to question the chest or intercostal breathing in vogue in the West since before the turn of the century.[1] I liked the Indian yoga breathing, which favored deep, abdominal breathing over shallow, chest breathing, but I was bothered by its holding of air and its extraordinary "cleansing" methods (swallowing cotton into the stomach, and so on) and so left off.

Judo in the 1940's—especially E. J. Harrison's seminal *The Fighting Spirit of Japan*—really focused me on abdominal breathing. Chinese boxing in the 1950's kept me there while introducing me to natural and reverse breathing. It is a huge subject seemingly with as many variations as shown in the Kama Sutra. This confusion of voices gave me, as the French say, furiously to think and resulted in this chapter. When the librarian asks the small boy how he liked the book on walruses he was returning, he answers, "It was all right, but I didn't want to know that much about walruses." I risk the same reaction from readers before they finish this screed, asking only that they look at it as a small trip down that road called

Dao. Because of its subject, this piece must be considered provisional until better minds address the subject. If I have abused the facts, I trust *Journal of Asian Martial Arts* readers will bring their corrigenda down my corridor.

Subject and Focus

How should one breathe in practicing taiji? One should breathe naturally. Watch how a baby breathes, easily without thought or effort, its tiny belly expanding with each inhalation and falling with each exhalation. On inhale, the dome-shaped diaphragm—the muscle separating the thoracic from the abdominal cavity—contracts and flattens downward; and on exhale, relaxes upward, expelling the air. Inhalation is the work phase; exhalation, the passive phase.

The skeletal muscles of the rib cage and the diaphragm are the effectors of breathing that can be controlled voluntarily to some extent though most breathing is done automatically from a control center in the brain stem (Sebel, 1985: 39). In seeking the natural, one should watch or become like a child—ancient wisdom urged by the Daoists and Jesus alike. Or if this isn't proof enough, glance at the religious statuary throughout Asia. Even when the subject is male, invariably the abdomen is swelling, indicating that deep belly breathing is present (Durckheim, 1962: 81, 144–145). This is compelling evidence given the religious and meditative mix permeating the Asian martial arts from early times.

My focus here is on the breathing mechanics of taiji, especially the taiji of Zheng Manqing. I follow the spoor through other methods, old and new, internal and external boxing alike. There is a considerable literature on the *qi* (intrinsic energy) refined from gross air by the mind in the *dantian* (psychic center just below the navel) during respiration. But my survey tries to stress the physical over the psychophysiological; and the actual breathing, over how one sits or stands while practicing it.

Zheng Manqing's Natural Breathing

Professor Zheng once wrote, "When you practice the form, once you move, you should follow the [*Taiji*] *Classics*. If the movement follows the *Classics*, it is correct" (Lo, et al., 1979:15). And in the same way, if you want to understand breath, you should heed the *Classics*. And we do. "Let the *qi* (breath) sink to the *dantian*" first and foremost. "Being able to breathe [properly] leads to agility. The softest will then become the strongest" (Lo, et al., 1979: 46).[2] Then come Li Yiyu's cogent words:[3]

> Let . . . the inhalation and exhalation be smooth and unimpeded throughout the entire body. The inhalation closes and gathers, the exhalation opens and discharges. Because the inhalation can naturally raise and also uproot the opponent, the exhalation can naturally sink down and also discharge (*fa fang*) him . . .
> – Lo, et al., 1979: 75

These words enabled Professor Zheng to teach how the breathing coordinated with the movements in the form, namely that, when the body expands (into a posture), the qi gathers in the dantian by inhaling, and when the body contracts (into a transition), the qi "opens" or empties from the dantian by exhaling.

In his early works, Professor Zheng said little on the subject of breathing, even writing, "Initially, it is best not to be concerned about breathing: first learn the techniques of the postures and then incorporate the breathing" (Cheng and Smith, 1967: 11). In his towering *Cheng's Thirteen Treatises on T'ai-Chi Ch'uan* (Lo and Inn, 1985), he writes that when the qi sinks to the dantian the internal organs can relax and move, and open and close with each breath. Further, he says, "The breathing should be long, fine, quiet, and slow," but doesn't return to the subject again (Lo and Inn, 1985: 62, 114).[4] He believed that if one really understands these characteristics, it would keep the student breathing properly. His first text in English, printed in Taiwan in 1962, had nothing on breathing mechanics. Five years later, our collaboration was nearly as stingy, advising that breathing was unimportant initially, that one inhales through the nose as the arms are extended outward and upward and exhales through the nose as the arms are retracted or lowered (Cheng and Smith, 1967: 11).

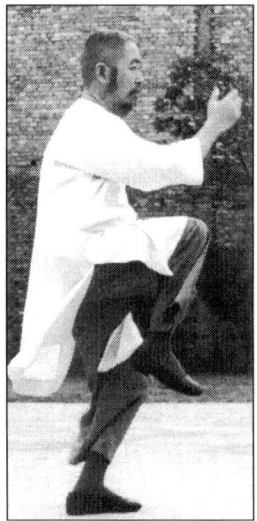

Zheng Manqing: In his movements, such as "golden rooster stands on one leg," Zheng followed nature. Photo courtesy of R. W. Smith.

In 1968, the year after our book appeared, Zheng overcame his seeming reticence and published a lengthy delineation of breathing in a Taipei newspaper (Wile, 1985: 114–115). There, he begins by portraying we humans as so surrounded by troubles that there is no solace, no rest for the mind, even in sleep. The one avenue to peace, he says, is meditation. It had cured or alleviated the tuberculosis and other maladies afflicting him earlier. The basis of meditation, he writes, is deep breathing that enhances blood circulation, speeds the absorption of nutrients, and eases the metabolic process. Nutrients carried by the bloodstream must be combined by the oxygen from breathing for oxidation to occur, and the carbon dioxide resulting from oxidation must be eliminated to keep the proper metabolic balance. Thus, breath is even more important than food. He goes on to explain the physiology of air and blood. After condemning shallow chest breathing, he describes his method:

> [We use] ... abdominal breathing. As we inhale air, the lungs expand and fill to capacity, allowing it to deeply permeate the air sacs, thus maximizing its distribution. Simultaneously, the diaphragm is pushed downward, causing the belly to protrude. When we exhale, the belly contracts, pushing upward and completely expelling the stale air in the lungs. In this way, the exchange of gases in the lungs realizes its greatest efficiency through this kind of exercise for the internal organs.

Zheng continues his discussion with this verse:

> Lightly close the mouth; the eyelids hang like curtains.
> Using abdominal breathing, rid all random thoughts.
> – Wile, 1985: 114–115

And he continues with more instruction (Wile, 1985: 114–115):

> Inhale the air deeply to fill the lungs but do not expand the chest. The pressure of the diaphragm downward expands the lung capacity and causes the belly to protrude slightly. When one exhales, the belly empties as the diaphragm is pressed upwards, completely forcing the stale air out. The breathing should be deep, long, fine, even, light, slow, and quiet.

In his last book, *New Method of Self-Study for T'ai-Chi Ch'uan* (Wile, 1985: 13–14), Professor Zheng differentiates the taiji process of qi since Laozi ("Concentrate your qi and develop softness ... can you become like a child?" [Ch. 10]) from the hard qi system of the Buddhist Damo (Bodhidharma) in his Sinew-Changing and Marrow-Washing Classics. The path of taiji qi, writes Zheng, rises up the *du* meridian in the back of the body to the crown of the head (*ni huan*) transforming sexual essence (*jing*) to qi and qi to spirit (*shen*). Taiji's qi comes from the bones but Damo's qi moves with the breath up the front, rising along the ren meridian to the face and head. This is external because it circulates only in the sinews and can't be changed to spirit. Zheng then writes that sinking the qi to the dantian takes a long time and to expedite it gives his four-word formula for breathing: fine, long, calm, and slow.

This is the extent of Professor Zheng's writing on breathing, but we also have data from his teacher, Yang Chengfu; his colleague, Chen Weiming; his seniors; and other internal teachers to buttress and confirm his written word. But first, let me dilate on an experience we shared once.

A visit to Professor Zheng in New York City in 1964, still green in memory, gave me a hands-on demonstration of his breathing. Zheng, his wife, and I were together for several hours at their apartment on Riverside Drive, muddling along in a linguistic wilderness: between Mrs. Zheng's spare English and my tortured Chinese, I was lucky to get half of what he said. But as Cervantes would have said, that half was profound.

After practicing and being minutely corrected on my form and push-hands, I asked him about breathing. He took my hand and we seated ourselves on his couch.

"It should be natural and must not be forced," he said.

Then, he placed my right hand on his abdomen (he had a small "pot" there that he continually tried to erode with circular massage, but with no apparent success), and I felt it expand as he slowly inhaled. Next he took the index finger of my other hand and placed it under his nose and exhaled. But, try as I might, I felt no exhalation from his nose, though I did feel his belly empty under my right hand. No, put it this way: as I sat there, it struck me that this was utterly impossible, and then I began to think that I felt an extremely light and wire-fine beam of air coming from his nose. But in truth, I may have conned myself into it or simply imagined it. So, I can't really say I felt it. Laughing at my puzzlement—Mrs. Zheng joined in—the Professor repeated it. I still could not feel it nor not feel it. It was a dead end. I don't know which was the most astounding: the fineness of his exhalation or my utter inability to feel it. Either way, it was a most impressive performance.

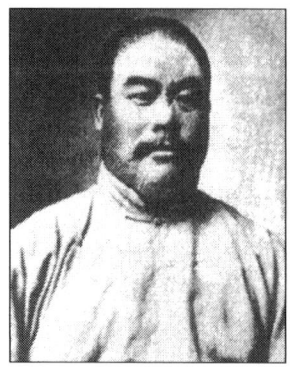 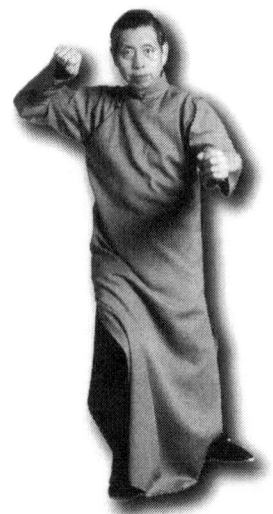

Left: Yang Chengfu. Right: William C.C. Chen "bend bow and shoot tiger" posture.
Photo courtesy of William C.C. Chen.

From this we can confirm Zheng's written record on how he breathed. First and foremost, he breathed *he feng xi yu* (literally, "gentle breeze, fine rain"), that is, in a gentle way. That was natural, not reverse, breathing. The expanding abdomen, not the nose, starts inhalation. The nose is the passage through which air is evenly inhaled and exhaled.[5] With its nasal canals lined with mucous membranes, it filters and cleans inspired air in a way the mouth cannot. The mouth is lightly closed throughout, keeping it from becoming dry. The air is inhaled slowly and exhaled even more slowly. The air fills the belly, but I felt no downward physical pressing of the air by Zheng. Nor did I feel any holding or retention of the breath or any alternation of the nostrils in his natural breathing. Zheng was always direct on holding the breath, telling us not to hold it to resist an attack because it impedes the flow of qi (Full Circle, 1989: 21).

The Breath According to Yang Chengfu and Others

Yang Chengfu, Zheng's teacher, though terse on the subject, also seems to urge natural breathing. "You must not hold your breath which strains your chest and abdomen," he advised (Hsu and Lowenthal, n.d.).[6]

Also, Fu Zhongwen, a nephew of Yang Chengfu and well-known teacher of taiji in his own right, in interviews before his death in 1994 stated that breathing must be natural: it can't be dictated by movements. Because the breathing is done evenly, he said, it can't be made short for some movements and long for others (Smalheiser, 1984: 4).[7]

Chen Weiming, Zheng's classmate under Yang, in his *Questions and Answers on T'ai-Chi Ch'uan*, puts breathing into a functional context: "During inhalation, the [qi] goes inside but does the lifting, and during exhalation, it goes outside but sinks" (Lo and Smith, 1985: 42).

As for Zheng Manqing's seniors, those I know well follow his lead in using natural, not reverse, breathing. They urge that one should not fret over breathing; otherwise, it ceases to be natural. Therefore, one should use breath as one needs it in the form and push-hands. There need be no set pattern for matching breath and movement. The key is to relax and sink without holding your breath: inhale before a push and exhale as you push.[8]

William C. C. Chen of New York City has been the most explicit on breathing mechanics and the most forthcoming on matching breath and form of any of Zheng's seniors. His *Body Mechanics of Tai Chi Chuan* includes the best chapter I have seen on breathing, saying in part:

> Tai Chi Chuan is . . . the natural way of breathing; it is slow, gentle, and deep. Natural breathing increases lung capacity, supplies sufficient oxygen for the body's needs and aids in relaxation during the movements. It also helps to loosen all passages, allowing the distribution of oxygen more effectively and evenly. During inhalation, the diaphragm goes down, which increases the size of the lung cavity and forces more

air to rush in. Exhaling moves the diaphragm up and squeezes waste air out.... The mouth should be kept closed which prevents it from becoming dry. In fighting, keeping the mouth closed will help avoid biting the tongue, breaking the jaw, or becoming exhausted.

– Chen, 1994: xvii

Then, William tells how, in sparring, fighting, or lifting weights, the breathing is different from that of the form. Besides inhaling and exhaling, he writes, we must pay attention to a third aspect called "compression" by which one presses down on the diaphragm while the thigh muscles exert force upward. This pressure on the lower abdomen supports the spine and serves as a connecting link between the root and the fist. This all happens at a brief moment of impact; there is not time for inhaling or exhaling (Chen, 1994: xvii).

Beyond this text, William does more by clearly blending movement with breathing in his photographs. Not too much should be made of this. Those seniors who don't teach the matching have their own good reasons. Whether we teach it or not, after a decade or so of daily form practice, we unconsciously blend breathing in pretty much the same way, making the matter moot.

Another celebrated teacher whose views on breathing mirror Professor Zheng's was Chen Panling, who on the mainland had many esteemed teachers in the internal triad of taiji, xingyi, and bagua. In his *T'ai-Chi Ch'uan*, an eclectic synthesis of the major schools, he scorns rapid, shallow breathing as contrary to good health (Chang, 1995).[9] Abdominal breathing, he writes, is deep and long and naturally stimulates the diaphragm, telling us to breathe deeply and sink our qi to the dantian. Inhale when opening, exhale when closing, he advises, and smoothly blend breathing with movement. There is no reason that Chen's bagua and xingyi breathing differed from his taiji's. Specifically, I find nothing in his writings or in my notes that suggests he contracted the anal sphincter as part of his breathing regimen.

Likewise, Wang Shujin, the great bagua and xingyi expert (he learned taiji from Chen Panling), believed that the breath must be slow and even, like "a cloud floating in the sky" and that the mouth should not be used. If one did use the mouth, it indicated that he or she was over-exerting (Howard, 1995: 25).

Famed Wang Xiangzhai's *yiquan* (Mind Boxing) also has breathing methods close to Zheng Manqing's (Dong, 1993: 30, 34). A student of the inimitable Guo Yunshen, Wang preferred the simple and the natural to the artificial. He urged students to breathe naturally at whatever rhythm pleased them, keeping their mouths closed, tongues against the palate, with all breathing done through the nose. The breath should be sunk to the navel. One should not force it, but should only breathe more deeply, slowly, and quietly. This advice clearly contains the physiology and philosophy of natural breathing.

Ziranmen (Spontaneous Boxing) seems to have had a breathing system similar to that of yiquan. Wan Laisheng writes in his book published in 1929 several details on breathing. Wan, a student of Du Xinwu, says that, though it borrows copiously from Shaolin, Spontaneous Boxing avoided its extreme forms, such as limiting defecation and micturition so as not to exhaust qi. "Ours is the natural way," he writes. Unsurprisingly, he advocates natural breathing, the eyes lightly closed, tongue touching the palate, and the nose inhaling and exhaling (Wan, 1929: 36).

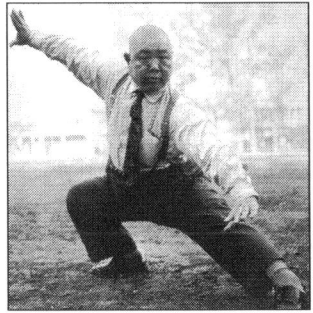 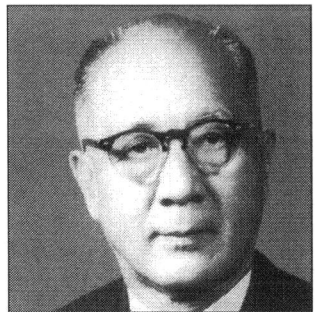 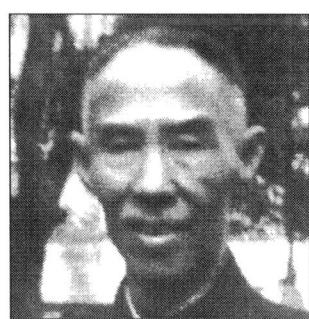

Above: Wang Shujin. Left: Chen Panling. Right: Wang Xiangzhai.
Photos courtesy of R. W. Smith.

Reverse Breathing and Holding the Breath

Before we track breathing back into history, let's look at two aspects of it one meets all along the way: reverse breathing and holding the breath. Charles Luk describes reverse breathing this way: "Inhaling, fill your chest with air but contract your lower abdomen; exhaling, expand your lower abdomen while relaxing and hollowing your chest" (Luk, 1972: 171–172). Apparently, many Chinese boxers use reverse breathing and, if kept gentle and not mingled with extreme holding of the breath and overly muscled manipulations of the diaphragm, the biggest harm it does is to preclude one from doing the more beneficial natural breathing.[10] Ben Lo is not so charitable. He asks (one of Ben's questions says more than five answers by most teachers): "What happens when you blow into a balloon: does it expand or contract?"

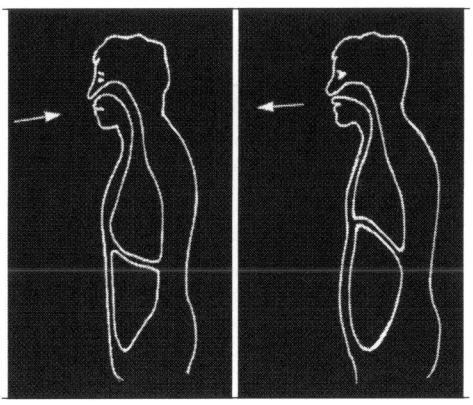 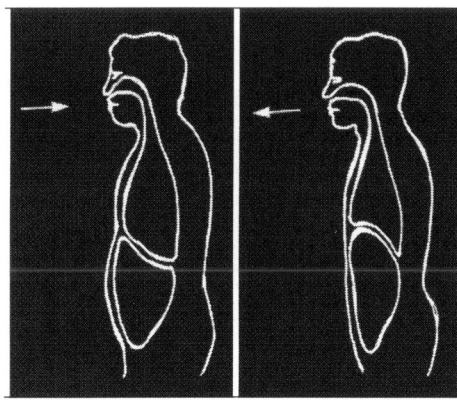

Left: Reverse Breathing. Right: Natural Breathing. Illustrations courtesy of Pat Kenny.

Even Luk, who personally preferred reverse breathing, writes that, because of so many complaints about it from readers, he advises them in later editions of his book to use natural breathing (Luk, 1972: 171–173).[11] West coast karate teacher Joe Svinth describes one version of reverse breathing this way: "Ibuki teaches pupils to inhale into tensed bellies using a series of quick breaths through their noses, and to exhale using a series of slow breaths through partially-opened mouths. While this method allows students to take powerful blows to the midsection, most Daoist, northern Shaolin, and Shorin-ryu authorities decry it as physically dangerous . . . citing evidence linking ibuki breathing with high blood pressure and hemorrhoids" (Svinth, 1995). Researcher K. Cohen, while excoriating reverse breathing recently, dilated on its dangers, pointing out that it is identical to the term used to describe pathological breathing in Western psychological literature (Cohen, 1995: 9).[12] I tried it in Taiwan and quickly discarded it. But even that didn't resemble ibuki, which suggests that the breathing method that Higashionna Kanryo introduced with the basic sanchin kata to Okinawa from south China in the 1890's and that his student, Miyagi Chojun, took to Japan in the 1930's, was either taught them wrong or simply didn't travel well. Or, of course, it could have been changed later by Yamaguchi Gogen or Oyama Masatatsu. Irrespective of this, tyros in Goju-ryu karate are still taught the basic sanchin and tensho katas although some thoughtful teachers are now teaching them more natural breathing.

What harm is there in holding the breath? Some animals do it seasonally. All the thoughts of turtle, Ralph Waldo Emerson mused, are turtle. And one would add, all the breaths—a turtle holds his for five months during hibernation. But humans can't or ought not do this. Yet Indian hatha yoga has a "harmonizing" hold of ten or so counts between every inhale and exhale, a hold, which according to Arthur Koestler, is regarded as more important than either the inhalation or exhalation.[13] On the Daoist side, Scharfstein writes that the ancients tried to hold the air for the length of 1,000 breaths to become immortal (during which some of them found themselves only too mortal) (Scharfstein, 1973: 105).[14]

Good reasons for holding the breath, some Yogi and Daoists believed, were to harmonize the system and to cultivate the qi. This was breathing done with a static body. In a moving body, holding the breath strains the entire body and can produce carbon dioxide poisoning to boot. Hong Yimian, a stellar internal-boxing teacher in Taiwan, said that his two older brothers died of over-exertion in boxing where holding the breath was a prominent feature. Film actor Bruce Lee, ironically, is an instance of a man only pretending to fight who held his breath too much too soon and went early into the shade because of it.

When a man fights, holding his breath is useless at best and injurious at worst. When he is in the thick of it, his blood needs a free flow without artificial manipulation of the abdomen. Even without holding his breath, his carbon dioxide content is already increasing along with his oxygen debt. In sum, gentle holding in static positions for short periods probably poses no great danger.[15] But done hard and excessively or in combat, holding the breath will diminish one's enjoyment of life, if not the life itself. Finally, the only times I can think of to hold the breath are (1) in kissing, (2) when underwater, or (3) when the breath is one's last!

A Historical Look Back

The earliest words on breathing therapy in China were found on twelve jade tablets dating from the sixth century BCE.

> This is how breathing must be done: the breath is retained and collected. When it expands, it goes downwards. When it goes downwards, it becomes quiet. When it has become quiet, it grows firm. When it is firm, it begins to germinate. When it has germinated, it grows. When it has grown, it must be pressed back. When it has been pressed back, it reaches the crown of the head. At the top it presses against the crown of the head, down below it presses downwards. Whoever follows this principle, lives; whoever does the contrary, dies.
> – Palos, 1972: 128–145

The passage states that in sitting or standing meditation one becomes quiet and breathes. The breath spoken of here is air that is inhaled and sunk to the dantian where it is refined and warmed and, with the help of the mind (*yi*), expands throughout the body and up the spine to the *ni huan* point on the crown of the head. This is standard fare, still practiced. It says little on breathing mechanics, however, but words like "retained and collected" indicate that the air was held. What does stand out with exactitude is the denouement in which the lead principles of taiji—an upright body and qi sinking to the navel—are enumerated much as they were when I first was exposed to them in the 1950's.

Both Laozi and Zhuangzi made important allusions to breathing. Laozi, said to be an older contemporary of Confucius (551–479 BCE), hinted that breath control could help one achieve long life and in his *Daodejing* (The Way and the Virtue) advised, "Concentrate your breath and make it supple and you will be like an infant" (Kaltenmark, 1969: 63-4). The other great explicator of Daoism, Zhuangzi, coming along two centuries later, wrote that the Perfect Men of old "breathed deep breaths," not merely from their throats and lungs as others did, but from the whole body (Kaltenmark, 1969: 97).[16] Zhuangzi, whom Zheng Manqing derided as a "storyteller," actually was more than that and could be critical of the old practices. Something of a stoic, he was a philosopher who believed in living the life allotted him (he would have liked H.L. Mencken's window-shattering credo, "We are here and it is now: all the rest is moonshine"). While criticizing Confucians for imposing ethics (probably a key factor in Zheng's disdain) and the hermits' withdrawal from the world, he also scorned the special breathings and gymnastics (*daoyin*) as mere desire for longevity (Needham, 1983: 154).

Joseph Needham's seminal history of China has much to say on breathing. We cited him above on the priority the early Daoists put on holding the breath.

But in the Tang dynasty (CE 618–907), he says, quoting Henri Maspero, this practice of holding external air gave way to an internal respiration (fetal breathing) based on visualization more than lungs (Needham, 1983: 147).

Legend has it that Damo (Bodhidharma) (CE 506–556), the blue-eyed Indian sage with his bundle of Chan (Zen) Buddhism, came to China and sat before a wall at the Shaolin Temple in Henan Province for nine years until he could hear the ants scream. Angry at himself for falling asleep at his meditation, Damo tore off his eyelids and threw them on the ground, whence sprouted China's first tea leaves. Drinking tea and being bereft of eyelids solved his sleepiness. He sought to cure his fellow monks by physical calisthenics said to be outlined in two books, the *Sinew-Changing and Marrow-Washing Classics*. However, Needham believes these books came ten centuries later (1983: 166). Earlier we quoted Zheng Manqing's words on Damo's hard qi method. Though his qi was hard, according to Zheng, there are few hard data on him. He is said to be the founder of Chan Buddhism, a man who rejected sutras and philosophy in favor of mystical faith with intensive prolonged contemplation. In Chinese boxing circles, he is as revered for being the legendary father of Shaolin Temple boxing as for his breathing exercises.

The old manuscript on Shaolin boxing I published as *Secrets of Shaolin Temple Boxing* said this on breathing:

> The lungs are reservoirs of air, and air is the lord of strength. You must learn to breathe properly. Many years ago, the boxers of the north put breathing as a prerequisite for gaining physical power.... Boxers of the south practiced the foothold but few practiced breathing. This was because the internal organs could be damaged through improper breathing. Not until the Ming dynasty (1368–1644) did these boxers learn the secrets of breathing.... The mouth should not be used for exhaling; the prime secret stressed a short inhale and a long exhale.
> – Smith, 1964: 34–35

These words are of interest in the distinction between north and south, but mainly because they veto mouth-breathing, which had a long history among Daoists.

Currently, respiratory therapy (*qigong*) is a prime part of Chinese medicine, practiced widely in hospitals and sanitariums. It has proved effective in treating hypertension, neurasthenia, pulmonary tuberculosis, and other ills. The basic method used is natural breathing. Chinese authorities stress that this therapy won't work if not done "easy and gentle," cautioning those who regard it as work, "Some thrust the abdomen out and purposely suppress the intake of air—so that the patient can neither breathe properly nor control his respiration. Traditional teaching requires the very opposite: the attention should be controlled by the breathing, and not the other way around" (Palos, 1972: 134). The entire automatic nervous system and consciousness participate with respiration to produce qi. According to Pavlov, the cerebral cortex not only controls the equilibrium of the organs; it also affects their regeneration. These breathing exercises, and of course taiji, relax and transform the cerebral cortex into a state of high-degree harmony (protective inhibition).

With the export of Chinese external-boxing breathing methods from Fujian and other southern provinces to Okinawa and Japan in the nineteenth century, we see an expansion in their use in indigenous fighting arts. I don't think the Japanese were dealing with top-drawer sources in borrowing from southern Shaolin. Near the end of his life, Donn Draeger in a lecture (March 30, 1976) freely acknowledged that the Japanese knew relatively little about qi compared with the Chinese. Though he was speaking in the context of using qi to take punishment (I had told him of my kicking Wang Shujin and punching William C.C. Chen and Shi Shufang without result), Donn would include breathing as qi. From my own experience, southern Shaolin seemed deficient in overall boxing technique and breathing compared with northern Shaolin.[17]

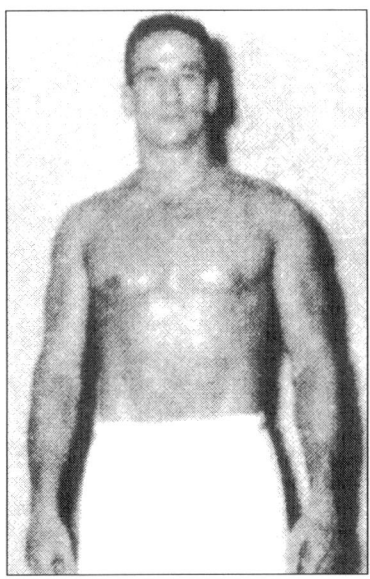 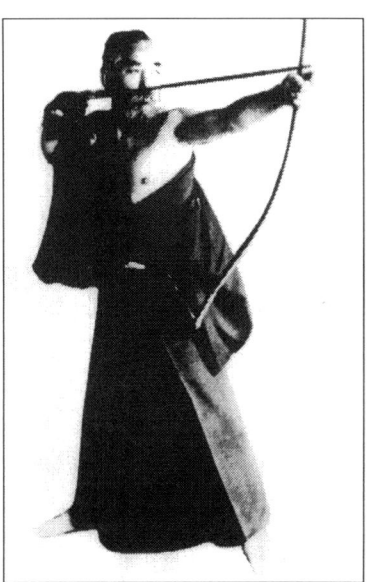

Left: Donn Draeger. Photo courtesy of R. W. Smith. Right: Awa Kanzo who taught Eugen Herrigel Zen and kyudo. Courtesy of Octopus Books, Ltd.

The Japanese Experience

E. J. Harrison's *The Fighting Spirit of Japan* has several excellent passages on abdominal breathing (*fukushiki kokyu*), starting off with famed judoka S. Arima's recollection, "As we went along, Viscount Tachibana told us of the advantage of walking with the abdomen rather than the legs" (Harrison, 1912: 105). "Years later," Arima continued, "the Viscount said to me: 'Whether sitting, or standing, or moving, you must always take care that your lower abdomen is filled with strength'" [inhaled air pressing lightly against the diaphragm] (Harrison, 1912: 105).

Next, Arima quotes an old book: "Stand or be seated facing the rising sun. Then take thirty moderately deep and seven very deep breaths. Close your teeth and exhale through your mouth. Inhale gently from the nostrils. Filling your abdomen with air keeps your center of gravity low for judo" (Harrison, 1912: 105). K. Fukui, a friend of Arima, advises drawing in air gradually until your lower abdomen is full. Hold it as long as you can; then, expel it through your nose (Harrison, 1912: 106).

Harrison wrote that some students would wrap a cotton cloth around the stomach just below the lower ribs and fasten it snugly. Then they would try to inhale 300 to 4,000 times daily through this barrier to the lower belly while keeping the mouth closed and the chin held in (Harrison, 1912: 132).

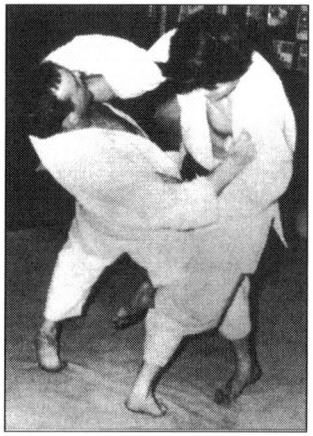

John Osako.
The late John Osako throws author with a small outer reap at the Chicago Judo Club in 1947. Osako (7th dan) was three-time U.S. Judo Champion at 180 pounds. Photo courtesy of R. W. Smith.

Finally, Kunishige Nobuyuki, a towering *kiaijutsu* adept, whom Harrison saw drop a man from a distance with a shout and who could push the rugged Britisher over with one finger, tells of talking with a Zen priest who is overly proud of the swelling belly he has achieved through meditation. Kunishige berates him that his meditation and the development of his *shitahara* would not help him when he descends from his sacred perch and meets a fighter who has developed his *shitahara* not by constant squatting but by constant movement. (In martial arts literature, it is a commonplace that moving meditation is far superior to sedentary sitting or standing meditation.)

The preceding passages from Japan early this century chronicled by an astute judoka—a third-dan then that would equate to a fifth- or sixth-dan now—reflect considerable commonality. All stress or suggest the primacy of deep abdominal breathing over shallow chest breathing. While the old book Arima cites advocates mouth exhalation, it is the only source to do so. Likewise, K. Fukui's advice specifies that the breath must be held as long as possible—again, the only one to do so. But for the most part, these methods are suggestive of natural rather than reverse breathing. Certainly, none use the hard external method (*ibuki*) having loud exhales and tensings seen in some karate schools today.

Let's look further at the Japanese experience, this one from the 1930's. In that little classic *Zen in the Art of Archery*, how does Master Awa Kanzo teach breathing to the German philosophy professor, Eugen Herrigel?

> Press your breath down gently after breathing in, so that the abdominal wall is lightly stretched, and hold it there for a while. Then breathe out as slowly and evenly as possible, and, after a short pause, draw a quick breath of air again—out and in continually, in a rhythm that will gradually settle itself... The breathing in binds and combines... and the breathing out loosens and completes....
>
> – Herrigel, 1953: 37–41

After practicing a while, Herrigel tries to excuse his tension by saying it is because he is trying too hard to be relaxed. Awa tells him that is the trouble—he must not think or make an effort; instead, he should lose himself in the breathing. Herrigel heeds his words and, by the time he finishes his six years of training, he finds that he has mastered the breathing regimen to such an extent that now he has the feeling not so much that he is breathing, but rather "being breathed."

Japanese archery (*kyudo*) is not a sport, and the target is irrelevant to success in it. Instead, one is graded on how relaxedly he draws the bow and releases the bowstring, transforming a tedious task into a highly disciplined expression of selflessness. Direct and deep belly breathing is required so that the archer's chest and upper torso can be left relaxed. Though not reverse breathing, it is idiosyncratic in that it requires some holding of air and a rapid inhalation before the shot.

Psychotherapist K. Durckheim, another kyudo student, wrote of his practice in *Hara: The Vital Center of Man*. Although his slant was more on the psychological than the physical mechanics of breathing, his tome is cogent. What matters in an art, he says, is not what comes out of it but rather what goes into it—that is, into the student (Durckheim, 1962: 39, 42). When he asks a Zen monk how one becomes a master, the response is, by letting the master in us come out. And that master will be "a man with a center" (*hara no aru hito*) (Durckheim, 1962: 49). The texts ending the book brim with good things. T. Okada tells us that the mouth is not used, and that inhaling to the *tanden* (Jp.; Man., *dantian*) is done relatively quickly. However, the exhale is long and enough air is held back so that one can speak a few words. T. Sato writes that one inhales filling, and exhales emptying, the belly. Thus, this appears to be a fairly natural breathing.[18]

Other Methods

Elsewhere, usually in religious settings, one finds other respiration techniques.[19] Perhaps the oldest and one of the most curious breathing methods outside

Asia is the Hesychasm of Eastern Christianity (fourth century to present) that used this method:

> Seated in a cell, off in a corner . . . turn your eyes on your navel, and limit the air that passes through your nose so that you are breathing with difficulty . . . and find in the belly the habitation of your heart.[20] At first you will find darkness and a stubborn density. But if you persevere—felicity unlimited. When the intelligence [the mind] comes to the habitation of the heart, it sees the air there at the center of the heart [the navel] and sees itself wholly luminous and full of discernment.
> – O'Brien, 1964: 96

The similarities with Asian breathing techniques are startling. The breathing is gentle, slow, with no excessive straining or holding of the breath. The Buddhists invoke Buddha; the Hesychasts, Jesus. Both Buddhists and Daoists concentrate on the belly, though unlike the Hesychasts, they don't fix chins to chest and actually watch their navels.[21] The difficulty alluded to probably was due to ennui rather than the breathing itself (they were warned against *acedie*, spiritual listlessness). The prayer demands made on the ascetic seem to have precluded any but the simplest—that is to say, natural—breathing.

The following interesting excerpt from Blundell's *The Muscles and Their Story* (1864), a book drawn largely from Mercurialis' *De Arte Gymnastica* (1595), shows again that there is nothing new under the sun.

> We next arrive at a most singular method of exercise adopted by the ancients, namely, the holding of the breath, as it was called. It is mentioned, and we believe approved, by Galen; and thus it was that the two processes involved in breathing—the inspiration and the expiration—furnished the means of performing this exercise. The old notion was that inspiration was the process by which the air, to temper the heat of the heart and generate the spirit, is drawn into the cavity of the chest. Expiration, on the other hand, was said to take place when the blackness, or soot, generated in the heart is thus led out through the cavity of the chest itself. . . . Under the direction of the gymnasts there were two holdings of the breath in use: one, in which they stretched the whole of the muscles in the chest and relaxed those of the diaphragm, so as the more easily to press downwards upon the abdominal viscera; the other, in which the abdominal muscles were stretched, by means of which the parts of the body below the diaphragm were chiefly affected. In both instances bandages were used, encompassing the thorax ribs, and abdomen, by means of which they more completely effected their purpose.[22]
> – Blundell, 1864: 196–197

Finally, Needham's history shows almost uncanny analogues between Daoist respiratory practices of the first millennium CE with those of Europe and America in the second millennium. He writes of how the cooperative societies that sprang up after 1850 in America (Oneida, Ephrata, and the like) practiced strange breathing without external air to ensure immortality (Needham, 1983: 142–154).[23] He links them through E. Swedenborg with translations of Daoist methods of physiological alchemy (Needham, 1983: 170–173).[24]

Putting Breath to the Test

Breathing's greatest test is in sportive or real combat. The extreme stress of real fighting can rather quickly reduce the most disciplined belly-breathers to shallow chest-breathing, exhaling by mouth, gasping for breath, trying to "catch their puffs," as the British say.[25] But still, the effect of deep-breathing practice pays off. While the breath lasts, it will keep one oxygenated sufficiently to apply the telling techniques in which one has invested untold hundreds of hours. However, once hyperventilation ensues, the rapid, shallow breathing will have difficulty increasing the oxygen content of red blood cells already saturated with oxygen upon passing through the lungs. Simultaneously, the greatly increased amount of expelled carbon dioxide will upset the body's acid balance, causing other physiological and neurological reactions.

Let the well-conditioned karate champion brace a good judoka using judo rules, and try to stay with him standing. In fifteen minutes, the karateka will be exhausted. If the two go to the ground, the karateka's fatigue will be even faster. Next, with wrestling rules, let the karateka try conclusions with a good grappler on the ground, and you'll see a similar outcome. Now, turn it around and let the judoka/wrestler spar with a Western boxer/karateka using their rules, and the breathing advantage shifts. Each man to his own poison or persuasion. Norman Mailer says that a marathoner friend of his lasted with a good boxer for three minutes before he ran out of breath. Every fighting system has a breathing method—learned or acquired—that over time works for its students if they are to succeed. Western boxers and wrestlers don't have a set, or "institutionalized," breathing method. They learn to breathe by doing it aerobically under stress, for the most part through their noses, to a point of fitness and by maintaining that fitness thereafter. In Asia, however, armed and unarmed fighters have a rich tradition of breathing methods drawn from Buddhist, Daoist, and Yoga meditation to help them. Despite the diversity and excess of some of these respiratory methods, most probably produce a measure of fitness that adds to individual fighting skills.

External boxing's mingling of *kiai* (spirit shout) and breath makes for forceful going. In combat, an economical kiai can be helpful initially in centering and adding focus to one's body and psychologically upsetting an enemy. However, I am not persuaded that venting energy and breath in continual kiai during combat will do much beyond speeding fatigue and undermining technique as the kiai become more vocal and less belly.

The kiai that can create an opening (*tsuki*) is indeed valuable so long as it becomes part of the breath instead of all of the breath. And the opening created, even when subtle, often can be exploited by the trained person. There are even those who profess the ability to detect an opponent's emptiness, that is, to divine the point at which he has just finished exhaling or just begun inhaling, and to attack successfully. This is difficult to do in the dojo and even more rare on the street or battlefield.

In the old judo days, I first read and heard about this "detecting an opponent's emptiness" by watching his breathing. I recall during this period a rousing *randori* (free-fighting) with Art Broadbent (fifth-dan). At this point, he was marginally better than I—though the skill difference grew wider with the years. This day I decided to watch for him to become bereft of breath and to get him empty before he could refill. So I watched. And waited and watched. All the while this was going on he was throwing me. Afterward in the shower, puzzled by his success, he asked me what had happened. Why didn't I attack? Ruefully I told him about my "secret." He laughed. "Keep it up," he said, "I'll be a *rokudan* [sixth-dan] in no time."[26]

Those favoring the more extreme external boxing methods, who wince at mention of the word "relax," apparently equating it with "collapse," would do well to consider the infinite variety of athletics. A distance runner relaxes within the physiological requirements of time and space.[27] A sprinter will be more tense but must still relax into his technique or he will fail to get off the starting blocks (in the shorter events, the sprinter is forced to run anaerobically—that is, without oxygen, but the rhythm is still important). The runner, weightlifter, and swimmer all do the same though calibrated differently. Carl Staub ("Dr. Breath") found that most athletes he worked with breathed incorrectly in that they failed to relax their bodies and "gentle" their breaths (Staub, 1970: 53). But he didn't advise them to go beyond relaxation to inertness either. Rather, he espoused a direct natural breathing and regarded involved methods as a waste.

The martial arts are not different on this score from other athletics. A relaxed rhythm is paramount. Karateka Egami Shigeru puts it succinctly: "Never stop your breath, no matter how hectic your movements become. At first, [your breath] will come in gasps, but as you continue, it will return to normal and stay normal, no matter how vigorous your movements" (Egami, 1980: 100). He then advises that no special breathing practice is necessary. Western boxers, if they tensed their bodies as some hard karate and southern Shaolin boxers do, would be immobile and quick work for opponents. Western boxers aren't taught to breathe so much as to keep breathing. They punch to a body rhythm more influenced by the exigencies of the bout—where is the opponent and what the hell is he doing?—than by breath. In this mix, breathing has to adapt to other considerations that can make sometimes for a chaotic business. How the boxer adjusts and moderates his breath so that he maintains a breathing rhythm to movement often determines how successful he becomes.

The extreme boxing systems with their hard breathing can be worse than ugly and embarrassing to see—they can be injurious to do. Most Western boxers, even amateurs, after five years of boxing will have some brain damage from head punches (Guterman and Smith, 1987: 194–210). Add to that what Wang Yannian tells me, that most of the external boxers who won in Taiwan free fight tournaments in recent decades died within six years of their victories. Because, unlike Western boxers, the Chinese external boxers don't box regularly, such deaths may have resulted more from training excesses—particularly breathing—than from actual bouts.

Envois

After a little doing and much rumination for fifty years, I have come to believe that proper breathing combined with relaxation and supple movement can benefit all unarmed and armed martial arts and, for that matter, most everyday activities.[28] All these elements go to make up what we call rhythm. Each of them needs each other and all need a rhythm. Therefore, breathing by itself is no ultimate elixir—it is a part of a parcel. To be proper, breathing ought to be easy, gentle, abdominally deep, and cleansed by the nostrils. Although holding one's breath may have a meditational use, such holding is what one wants to avoid in fighting.[29]

All things considered, this rambling survey concludes that:

- Some breathing methods, such as reverse breathing and holding the breath, are of marginal use for health and self-defense.
- In fact, a few methods—extreme holding and ibuki breathing—probably are deleterious.
- As a general rule, the more complex the breathing system, the less utility it has for fighting.
- There is a method of breathing, largely untaught but learned, proper for a given style of fighting or sport.
- Simple breathing, gently expanding the belly on inhale and emptying it on exhale, will ventilate sufficiently for all physical activity.
- As an important component of rhythm, this gentle breathing can be used in most activities, fighting or otherwise.

To end—and the sigh I hear the reader emit is also a kind of breath—I can do no better than quote from *Judo International* bulletin (1950: 13): "A. Lavoisier said that 'Life is a flame' [and Walter Pater, that we should burn always with a hard gemlike one]. Whence comes this flame? And why should it fail at a given moment? That is the problem. To grow old is to burn badly, and going out is death . . . [The solution is to] always take care of our respiration."[30] The flame is the qi that runs through and animates us and respiration is what fans that flame.

Romanization

PINYIN	WADE-GILES	CHINESE
baguazhang	pa^1 kua^4-chang^3	八卦掌
Chan	Ch'an^2	禪
Chen Panling	Chen^2 P'an^4-ling^3	陳泮嶺
Chen Weiming	Ch'en^2 Wei^2-ming^2	陳微明
Chen Zhicheng	Chen Chih^4-ch'eng^2	陳至誠
Damo	Ta^4 mo^2	大磨
dan tian	tan^1 t'ien^2	丹田
Daodejing	Tao^4 Te^2 Ching^1	道德經
daoyin	tao^4-yin^3	道引
du	tu^1	督
Du Xinwu	Tu^4 Hsin^1-wu^3	杜心五
Fu Zhongwen	Fu^4 Chung^1-wen^2	傅鐘文
Fujian	Fu^2 Chien^4	福健
Guo Yunshen	Kuo^1 Yün^2-shen^1	郭雲深
he feng xi yu	ho^2 feng^1 hsi^4 yü^3	和風細雨
Henan	Ho^2 nan^2	河南
Hong Yixiang	Hung^2 I^4-hsiang^2	洪懿祥
hou tian	hou^4 t'ien^1	後天
jing	ching^1	精
Laozi	Lao^3 Tzu^3	老子
Li Yiyu	Li^3 I^4-yü^2	李亦畬
ni huan	ni^4 huan (wan)	泥洹
ren	jen^4	任
shen	shen^2	神
Shi Shufang	Shih^1 Shu^1-fang^1	施漱芳
taiji	t'ai^4 chi^2	太極
Wan Laisheng	Wan^4 Lai^4-sheng^1	萬籟聲
Wang Xiangzhai	Wang^2 Hsiang^4-chai^1	王向齋
Wang Shujin	Wang^2 Shu^4-chin^1	王樹金
xian tian	hsien^1 t'ien^1	先天
xingyi	hsing^2 i^4	形意
Yang Chengfu	Yang^2 Cheng^2-fu^3	楊澄甫
yiquan	i^4-ch'üan^2	意拳
Zhang Qinlin	Chang^2 Chin^1-lin^2	張欽霖
Zhuangzi	Chuang^1 Tzu^3	莊子
ziranmen	tzu^4 jan^2 men^2	自然門

Acknowledgment

Although it is better to be the bow than to do it, I still must bow to many who helped on this extended chapter. My deepest bow goes to Seattle karateka Joe Svinth who pushed me to finish this piece when I complained that the confusion of voices on breathing would make a sane man leave the subject with dispatch and delight. But Joe thought it worth the candle and provided sufficient source material to light it. Pat Kenny, a veteran booster, did the graphics. Others who contributed include:

- Hunter Armstrong
- Y. W. Chang
- William C. C. Chen
- Warren Conner
- Jay Falleson
- Dr. Tim Geoghegan
- Bob Goodwin
- Bart Ingram
- Dan Johnston
- Harry Johnston
- John Lang
- Peter Lim
- Liu Hsi-heng
- Ben (Pang-jeng) Lo
- Russ Mason
- Pat McGowan
- Paul Nurse
- Allen Pittman
- Kevin Roberts
- Michael Schnapp

Notes

1. Philosophers dispute on what the dying desire most. Is it light (J. Unamuno) or warmth (J. W. Goethe)? We know it is neither. It is breath. One can live in the dark or cold for some time but cannot live for even a few minutes without air. Thus, we should bathe (and revel) in breath while we have it. And we should use it properly. If we breathe too fast or spasmodically, we get too little oxygen and dispose of too little carbon dioxide. Quotidian tensions, even had we zero pollution, can damage the respiratory system as effectively as infection and disease. Many doctors blame incomplete exhalation for a host of troubles in our hurried, hapless society. Most of us inhale sufficiently to function but cut short the exhale at the first vagrant act or thought, thus failing to rid our lungs of stale waste.

2. Professor Zheng placed the dantian 1.3 inches beneath the naval, nearer the abdomen than the spine by a ratio of 3:7.

3. These words of Li Yiyu were from his *Five Character Secret*. Li repeats his first thought in his *Essentials of the Practice of Form and Push-Hands*: "To gather is to close and to release is to open" (Lo, et al., 1979: 82). Another traditional saying amplifies Li's words. He states that in inhalation the outside is open (*wai kai*) [the arms open or rise] and the inside is closed (*nei ho*) [full of breath], whereas in exhalation the inside is open (*nei kai*) [the breath is exhaled or released to the outside] while the outside is closed (*wai ho*) [the arms fall or contract] (William Chen letters to the author, April 14, and September 4, 1996).

4. Despite treating the arcana of taiji in this book (the first time in the literature), in this and his other writing, Zheng Manqing avoided the idea of *xian-tian* (pre-birth) and *hou-tian* (post-birth) breathing. He probably felt that their level

of abstraction was so complex as not to lend themselves to the written word. For this reason, I have shied from getting off on this track here.

5   Hatha Yoga's use of alternate nostril breathing while blocking the other with a finger, though well beyond our enquiry here, is interesting respiration arcana. I remember Hong Yixiang, that Taiwan fighter for all seasons, urging it on me but I resisted, saying that I was having too much trouble absorbing his fistic teachings to take on anything esoteric.

Dr. Tim Geoghegan studied the method in India and sums it this way. The left nostril reflects the moon (*yin*) and is cool, quiescent, and good for sleep, while the right nostril reflects the sun (*yang*) and is hot, active, and good therapy for colds. This jibes with Daoist notions, particularly on sleep.

Professor Zheng advised that one should sleep on the right side, the right arm cradling the head. This left the left nostril uppermost and open while the right was congested and closed by the position of the head.

Debra Werntz showed that lying on one's right side causes the right nostril to become congested while the left nostril opens within a few minutes. She also showed that breathing through the left nostril increased electrical activity in the right cerebral hemisphere while breathing through the right nostril stimulated activity in the left cerebral hemisphere (Rossi, 1988: 121–124).

Dina Ingber (1981: 72–76), while supporting Werntz, goes beyond her research. She states that normal breathing alternates between left and right nostrils every two and a half to four hours, the time increasing as a person ages. In some oldsters there may be eight hours between shifts. Ingber says flatly that there is only one truly efficient way and that is diaphragmatic (belly or natural) breathing.

E. Rossi discusses Werntz's work and also cites Dr. U. Arya's *Meditation and the Art of Dying* (1979) on the relationship between the nasal cycle, sexual orgasm and the bliss of samadhi. The old Yogic tradition held that during orgasm and this form of meditation both nostrils are open and the ecstacy of samadhi is caused by the "upward implosions . . . of kundalini . . . so that celibacy becomes easier and more enjoyable than sex" (Rossi, 1988: 124).

6   Alas, there are difficulties on Yang Chengfu's breathing method. One of the first books on taiji that I read was Yearning K. Chen's *T'ai Chi Ch'uan: Its Effects and Practical Applications*. Professor Zheng told me that Chen knew little taiji but had somehow got hold of Yang's notebooks in the late twenties and used them to produce a book under his own name (Lowenthal, 1994: 110). The theft was worsened by Chen's errors and the whole book became suspect. One of the most devastating was on page 29 where Chen wrote: "When you breathe in, breathe through the nose and contract the abdomen; when you breathe out, breathe through the nose and expand the abdomen." This describes reverse breathing; Chen may simply have garbled the verbs. He is elsewhere credible when he writes that all movements are slow and even, done with no exertion, as one breathes through the nose (Chen, 1947: 9–14).

7   Also Hu Yaozhen, who, like Zheng Manqing, studied under Zhang Qinlin, taught that one should rid taiji and qigong of all breathing rigor. He insisted that natural breathing must be done without interference. In fact, Hu wrote that only by ignoring breathing did one truly achieve natural breathing (Wu, 1984). Lord Dunsany (1911) who wrote germanely, "Genius is to do a thing as a fish swims or a swallow flies, perfectly simply and with absolute ease; genius is, in fact, an infinite capacity for not taking pains..." would have applauded Hu.
8   Late in my career, I taught a matching method to some advanced students with the caveat that it be discarded if it complicated their taiji, an art Zheng Manqing once described as simple to learn but hard to do, and an art that he told Ben Lo was the most difficult of all his "excellences." The demands that taiji made on one were so great in terms of time, energy, and attention (mind) that requiring students slavishly to adhere to a strict regime of matching breath with movement was something he couldn't ask.

    That said, despite Ogden Nash ("Progress is all right, but it went on too long"), some notions on gentle breathing may make for habits that will help one progress. Like blood and bone, breathing is basic but if one can't do it by quiet minding, he or she should not do it. The big principle is that one breathes evenly, fitting the movements to the breathing, not vice versa. Inhale on postures; exhale on transitions. Three-fourths of taiji is transition and one-fourth posture and your breathing reflects that ratio. On "short" postures (such as raise hands, stork spreads wings, and cloud hands), move slowly to accommodate your breath. The rationale is that as you inhale you build a posture that then disintegrates into transitional movement, then builds anew. Most shifting of weight from one fixed foot to another is inhale, most walking (stepping out beyond static feet) is exhale. Thus, most of taiji is transitional and done on exhale. One inhales on all foot separations, the only postures that show final function (besides cloud hands and rollback, which is a yielding done naturally with an exhale). On cloud hands, inhale to the belly, then exhale to the side. Zheng Manqing tried to hide overt function. So one sees that inhaling on posture and exhaling on transition seems to preclude application: this conforms to Zheng's concealing use so that one remained relaxed throughout the form. One simply applies this in a street situation by using the posture already built with an appropriate leg action and short exhalation "and a loud sound [so that the] *chi* [*qi*] will rise up with the energy and discharge (*fafang*)," Zheng writes (Wile, 1985: 42, footnote 10).
9   One of the taiji systems Chen studied was the Wu. As presented by T. C. Lee (Lee, 1982: 19), the Wu breathing style accorded with that of Zheng Manqing.
10 The reverse breathing fashionable in Goju-ryu, Isshin-ryu, Kyoku-shinkai, and Uechi-ryu karate, called *ibuki*, is quite another thing. Though termed abdominal breathing, it is so distant from natural belly breathing that it requires comment. (Some of its own teachers suggest that it is not even traditional reverse breathing but rather a circus-trick, quick-fix aberration sold by southern Shaolin to

the Okinawans and Japanese.) It is an extreme external method which curiosity, piqued by Mas Oyama's books, led me to try for a few days several years ago; I quickly discovered it was nothing I wanted to do. The inhale is done through the nose and the air coiled into a ball in the *tanden* (Jp.; Man., *dantian*) and then exhaled forcefully and audibly through the mouth to the point of using coughs and grunts to expel the last traces of air (Higaonna, 1986: 31). To compound and confound the business, the student does it standing in a short, tensed posture, often contracting the anal sphincter. Besides being inelegant, one questions also its rationale—that it is done to harden one's body to make it impervious to attack. This seems a subversion of breath—to make respiration the agency of hardness—though it probably is no worse in this respect than some extreme Shaolin practices such as inhaling smoke from woodfires.

A tense approach to correct boxing, it stresses the static over the dynamic. While it may work for a while—almost everything works part of the time—the strain from all this tumult and shouting probably cancels any gains in prowess. A hard external boxer using this may become able to absorb body blows with impunity. This is not uncommon. But internal boxers, like William C.C. Chen, Shi Shufang, and the late great Wang Shujin, could do this without such frenetic training. Practical problems occur right off. How does one harden the head? And how can one harden the body so that it can withstand blows one is not expecting? I may be dead wrong on all this. So I hope that Oyama faithful don't, in consequence, get too exercised.

[11] Luk agrees with Zheng Manqing on the characteristics of natural breathing—deep, long, slow, quiet—and puts the tongue on the palate and eschews mouth breathing.

[12] Hunter Armstrong, one of Donn Draeger's seniors, wrote me December 10, 1995, that he had queried Higaonna several years ago about hypertension resulting from forceful breathing under muscular tension. He was told that there was indeed a high blood pressure problem associated with incorrect breathing in sanchin and tensho katas, and few instructors nowadays knew the correct breathing. This made it dangerous at times.

[13] "The main purpose is to suspend the flow of breath by locking in the air . . . to induce trance (*samadhi*)" (Koestler, 1961: 89–90). Although "all yoga are one," Hatha focuses on kinesthetic movement and Raja on meditation. Their purpose is to bring the body, the vital breath (*prana*), and the conscious and subconscious strata of mind under control. But in some exercises and in dynamic practice, for instance, in wrestling, the breath is natural (inhale, stomach out; exhale, stomach in), deep, and regular with conscious thought but without holding (Alter, 1992: 100–107).

[14] Also, Joseph Needham has much interesting data on the subject. The early Daoists, he writes, believed that if they hugged this idea of holding air enough they could become immortal (Needham, 1983: 142–154). We don't know whether Buddha's grand satori came on the inhale or the exhale. But we do know that

satori sidled up only after Buddha gave up his fruitless ascetics and relaxed. A modern author advocates an exhale that can last up to five minutes. Of course, his five-minute exhale is not credible, though certain yogi and other "specialists" hold enormously long.

That exceptional aikido master, Tohei Koichi (who once said that the best way of extending one's ki was in a smile), teaches a 40- to 60-second cycle as a good average. Knowing and respecting his great ability, I believe he might personally double that without strain. But I don't believe, nor does he, that the longer cycle would help his aikido.

15 In fact, I practiced one such method in Taiwan. It had mouth exhalation and an occasional hold, but its relaxation made it pleasant. Liu Chuchiang's "Introversive Centripetal Contraction Physiotherapy," which I learned from Liu's book with that title, had respiration that was the antithesis of aerobic. It was natural and the diaphragm was used gently. One of these methods took the interruptus out of coitus and purportedly let males sustain sex for longer periods. One simply lightly contracted the anal sphincter with the inhale and held for ten seconds or so before exhaling. "Yoga" Chen, so-called doubtless for his esoteric predilections, had taught it to me one Sunday morning at Professor Zheng's house before I found it in Liu's book. In giving me this gift beyond reckoning, "Yoga" asked rhetorically, "Why win all day and lose at night?" Alas, the advertisement proved better than the performance. But it made for mirth at the office where I'd meet a knowing lad ambling down the corridor with his hands clasped over his navel, "holding." Later, the boxing champion of Southeast Asia offered to teach me a similar "secret" technique. I did then what I did later when the same boy, wanting help in coming to America, and offering to "take care of" anyone of my choosing: I refused with thanks.

16 Zhuangzi also recorded these words: "The knowledge of all creatures depends on their breathing. But if their breath be not abundant, it is not the fault of Heaven, which tries to penetrate them with it day and night without ceasing; but, notwithstanding, shut their pores against it" (Legge: 139).

17 The part on breathing in the *Bubishi* is brief but questionable (McCarthy, 1995: 64). It recommends reserving half of your breath as you attack on exhale. What a stew we now have! The old Indians and Daoists held air between inhale and exhale; some modern systems hold the exhale as they try to get it all out; and now we see others holding half of it after exhale. Functionally, some do reserve some *qi* (visualized air) to avoid being countered empty, but holding back 50% of either qi or breath seems excessive.

18 Kenneth Kushner's words are similar to Herrigel's and Durckheim's (Kushner, 1988: 30–32). The air is inhaled into the belly, which protrudes slightly. On exhale, the diaphragm moves up, forcing the air out but simultaneously "thinking" the air into a slightly tensed lower abdomen (below the navel). He calls this natural breathing—the way a body breathes. Close, maybe, but not close enough. The visualization of air into the lower abdomen is beyond the most

precocious baby. To the extent that this is done gently, of course, it becomes more natural. Unlike Durckheim, Kushner does not seem to call for a rapid inhale (writing that the air is "effortlessly drawn into the lungs"), nor does he reserve some air after exhaling.

19. For did not Jesus say to His disciples, "Peace be unto you: as My Father has sent me, so also I send you"? And when He had said this, He breathed on them, and said: "Receive ye the Holy Ghost." We know that Christ bled, and spit, and used breath as a balm. And sometime I know we will find that He also had what the somber Jewish scribes were reluctant to give him—a smile and one little dog.

20. Locating the heart in the belly depends less on anatomy than on scripture. In the Bible, the heart is "the central place in man to which God turns, where religious experience has its root, which determines conduct." By the tenth century, more precise directions included putting the chin on the chest and fixing the eyes on the navel (whence came the word *omphaloskepsis*, belly-gazer) and a prayer intoned every waking moment, "Lord, Jesus Christ, Son of God, have mercy on me a sinner." On this practice, see also, Palmer, 1979; Brianchanivnov, 1965; *The New Britannica Micropedia*, 1990; *New Catholic Encyclopedia*, 1967.

21. In recalling the blessing of old radio compared with television, one wag opined, "At least you didn't have to watch the damned thing!" Regarding fixing the chin on the chest, which must have produced a wryness comparable in pain to what their legs suffered sitting on a tiny stool hours a day, there is a curious nexus with the Chinese. The crane is the Daoist Immortals' bird par excellence. Believed to live a thousand years and to be capable of breathing with its neck bent—a technique for making the breath supple, imitated by the Daoists (Kaltenmark, 1969: 121).

22. E. J. Harrison wrote of the same method using cloth strips in Japanese practice of deep breathing (Harrison, 1912).

23. Members of these sects also tried to restrain the sexual drive by abstinence or coitus reservatus, having sex without climaxing. This aspect, too, derives from ancient Daoist methods.

24. The earliest significant work was the Jesuit P. M. Civot's *Notice du Cong-fou des Benze Tao*. See [Dao-shi] (1799). From such Asian sources, Swedish fencer P. H. Ling (1776–1839) worked out an elaborate system of physical exercise that had a great influence in Europe and America.

25. At the Kodokan in Tokyo, it was not only bone-tired you got stumbling around misfiring on your throws and barely avoiding his, huffing and puffing. But also in groundwork with S. Kotani, now the highest of the high at tenth-dan and the snake-like Shibuyama, neither of whom was above lolling on you till you got feisty, when they'd ratchet it up a notch and cut off your wind as easily as a normal person would turn off a light switch. And then teasingly ease up so you could imbibe a quick breath, all-too-short before they cut it off again, and so on, rationing your air, thoroughly deflating your balloon and you. Good Lord, how good that acrid, sweaty air tasted. As for the struggle—how I'd love to do it one

more time!

26 Which recalls a story about Harry Greb, the famed middleweight boxing champion in the twenties, whom one reporter called "fast as sin and indestructible as rawhide." Harry once fought a boxer who tended to think. Greb said later that all the time the guy was thinking he (Harry) was beating the devil out of him.

27 Paavo Nurmi, "The Flying Finn," between 1920 and 1932 set twenty world distance-running records and won six Olympic events. Dr. Tim Goeghegan tells me that Nurmi, despite the demands on his system, still was able to sustain a deep and slow breathing rhythm while being king of the runners in that period.

28 I know nothing of weapons, but Zheng Manqing believed that any weapon was merely an extension of one's hand and that what held for boxers would hold for armed experts. This is said not to minimize the weapon—indeed, Donn Draeger told me one wet Wednesday afternoon in Tokyo in 1961 that give him a fifty-year-old woman, a broomstick, and six months, and she would whup the best karateka kicking—but merely to state the obvious. Be that as it may, what I've said here on boxers applies equally to weapons experts.

29 This judgment applies to most cases. However, it may exclude those rare recluses (*xian*) or other rare birds (*rara avis*) who eat and breathe and fight in strange and marvelous ways. Some of these probably existed—if they didn't, they should have—but may not now. (I cannot yet reconcile Zheng Manqing with modern physics.) If they did or do, they are beyond our ken. This footnote merely acknowledges their sometime existence.

30 Translated in *Judo International* in 1950, it is unclear who wrote this section on breathing. Most of the preceding section was written by K. Mifune (tenth-dan) and M. Hashimoto (ninth-dan), but since the breathing section glowingly refers to Mifune as forever young, its author is doubtless someone else. Trevor Leggett does a small section elsewhere and the breathing bit could have been his. But, because Henri Plee was the overall editor (and because of the mention of Lavoisier), I believe the breathing section is his.

Bibliography

Alter, J. (1992). *The wrestler's body: Identity and ideology in north India*. Berkeley: University of California.

Blundell, J. (1864). *The muscles and their story*. London: Chapman Hall.

Brianchanivov, I. (1965). *On the prayer of Jesus*. London: Watkins.

Chang, Y. (Ed.). (1995). *T'ai chi ch'uan*. By Chen Panling. Manuscript.

Chen, W. (1994). *Body mechanics of t'ai chi ch'uan*. New York: William C. C. Chen. Revision of the 1973 edition.

Chen, Y.K. (1947). *T'ai chi ch'uan: Its effects and practical applications*. (Chang Kuo-shui, Trans.). Shanghai: Kelly and Walsh, Ltd. Reprinted in Hong Kong.

Cheng, Man-ch'ing. (1985). *New method of self-study for t'ai-chi ch'uan*. (Douglas Wile, Trans.). Brooklyn: Sweet Ch'i Press.

Cheng, Man-ch'ing, and Smith, R. (1967). *T'ai-chi: The "supreme ultimate" exercise for health, sport, and self-defense.* Rutland, VT: Charles E. Tuttle, Co.
Cohen, K. (Fall, 1995). *Hsing I Journal,* 4: 3, 9.
Dong, Y.P. (1993). *Still as a mountain, powerful as thunder.* Boston: Shambhala.
Draeger, D. (March 30, 1976). "The role of sound in Japanese martial arts and ways." Xerox transcript of lecture given at University of Hawaii.
Dunsany [Lord]. (1911). *Gods of Pegana.* London: Peganna Press.
Durckheim, K. (1962). *Hara: The vital centre of man.* London: Allen Unwin.
Egami, S. (1980). *The heart of karate-do.* Tokyo: Kodansha.
Full Circle. (March, 1989). Cheng Man-ch'ing taiji classmates—New York City, August 2, 1973. *Full Circle,* 2: 2, 21.
Guterman, A., and Smith, R. (1987). Neurological sequelae of boxing. *Sports Medicine,* 4: 194–210.
Harrison, E. (1912). *The fighting spirit of Japan.* New York: Fisher Unwin.
Harrison, E. (1982). *The fighting spirit of Japan.* New York: The Overlook Press. Reprint of 1912 edition.
Herrigel, E. (1953). *Zen in the art of archery.* New York: Pantheon.
Higaonna, M. (1986). *Traditional karate-do Okinawa goju ryu.* Tokyo: Japan Publications.
Howard, K. (Sept./Oct., 1995). Wang Shu-jin's ba gua: Principles and practice. *Pakua Journal,* 5: 6, 25.
Hsu, L., and Loewenthal, W. (nd). Yang Cheng-fu's comments on t'ai chi ch'uan. Manuscript.
Ingber, D. (June, 1981). Brain breathing. *Science Digest,* 72–76.
Judo International. (1950). *Judo International.* Paris: Editions A.M.I. Translated from *Judo Monthly* (1950), Tokyo: Kodokan.
Kaltenmark, M. (1969). *Lao Tzu and Taoism.* Stanford, CA: Stanford University Press.
Koestler, A. (1961). *The lotus and the robot.* New York: Macmillan.
Kushner, K. (1988). *One arrow, one life: Zen, archery, and daily life.* London: Arkana.
Lee, T.C. (1982). *The Wu style of tai chi chuan.* Burbank, CA: Unique Publications.
Legge, J. (1962). *The texts of taoism, Part II.* New York: Dover Publications. First published by Oxford University Press in 1891.
Lo, P., et al. (1979). *The essence of t'ai chi ch'uan: The literary tradition.* Berkeley, CA: North Atlantic.
Lo, P., and Inn, M. (Trans.). (1985). *Cheng tzu's thirteen treatises on t'ai chi ch'uan.* By Chen Weiming. Berkeley: North Atlantic.
Lo, P., and Smith, R. (Trans.). (1985). *T'ai chi ch'uan ta wen* (Questions and Answers on T'ai Chi Ch'uan). By Chen Weiming. Berkeley: North Atlantic.
Lowenthal, W. (1994). Book review of Cultivating the ch'i: The secrets of energy and vitality. (Stuart Alve Olson, Trans.). In the *Journal of Asian Martial Arts, 3*: 4, 110–111.
Luk, C. (1972). *The secrets of Chinese meditation.* New York: Samuel Weiser.

McCarthy, P. (1995). *The bible of karate: The bubishi.* Rutland, VT: Charles E. Tuttle Co.

Needham, J. (1983). *Science and civilization in China*, vol. 5, pt. 5. Cambridge: Cambridge University Press.

New Britannica Micropedia. (1990). Chicago: University of Chicago Press. p. 901.

New Catholic Encyclopedia, Vol. 6. (1967). New York: McCraw-Hill. pp. 1089–90.

O'Brien, E. (1964). *Varieties of religious experience.* New York: Holt, Rinehart.

Palmer, G. (1979). *The philokalia.* London: Faber.

Palos, S. (1972). *The Chinese art of healing.* New York: Bantam.

Random, M. (1978). *The martial arts.* London: Octopus Books, Ltd.

Rossi, E. (1988). *The psychobiology of mind-body healing.* New York: W.W. Norton.

Scharfstein, B. (1973). *Mystical experience.* New York: Bobbs-Merrill.

Sebel, P., et al. (1985). *Respiration: The breath of life.* New York: Torstar.

Smalheiser, M. (April, 1984). *The true history of the Yang style. T'ai-chi: Perspectives of the way and its movement.* Los Angeles: Wayfarer Publications, p. 4.

Smith, R. (1964). *Secrets of shaolin temple boxing.* Rutland, VT: Charles E. Tuttle Co.

Staub, C. (1970). *Dr. breath: The story of breathing coordination.* New York: W. M. Morrow.

Svinth, J. (Nov. 11, 1995). Letter to R. Smith.

Wan, Lai-sheng. (1929). *Wu-shu hui tsung* (Essential focus of Chinese martial arts). Beijing: Peking Agricultural College.

Wile, D. (1985). *Cheng Man-Ch'ing's advanced tai chi form instructions.* Brooklyn: Sweet Ch'i Press.

Wu Ta-yeh. (April, 1984). *Ch'i and breathing. T'ai chi: Perspectives of the way and its movement.* Los Angeles: Wayfarer Publications, pp. 6–8.

• 12 •
Conservator of the Taiji Classics: An Interview with Benjamin Pangjeng Lo[1]
by Donald D. Davis, Ph.D. and Lawrence L. Mann*

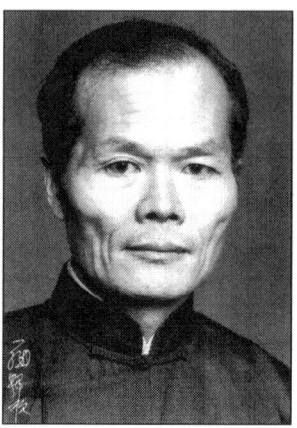

Photo courtesy of Michael Jang.

Taijiquan is one of the most famous and widely studied of the Chinese arts devoted to health, self-defense, and internal development. Its origin is uncertain, due to centuries of reliance upon oral transmission of its principles and traditions. Legend points to Zhang Sanfeng, a Daoist monk who lived in the Wudang Mountains of Hubei Province, as the founder of taijiquan.[2] Zhang allegedly lived during the Yuan dynasty (1271–1368), established by the great khans from Mongolia, although the dates of his birth and death are uncertain. Zhang reportedly combined martial movements based upon those of the snake and white crane with internal exercises derived from his Daoist practice (Yang, 1982b: 10). Taijiquan continues to distinguish itself from other martial arts by its emphasis on softness, internal development, and other Daoist principles.

Today there are many styles of taijiquan. Despite questions concerning its origins, Chen Xing traces the practice of modern styles of taijiquan to the Chen family, in China's Henan Province (Chen, 1919–1964). The style taught by Yang Luchan (1799–1872), a student of Chen Zhangxing (1771–1853), and now known simply as the Yang Style is arguably the most popular style of taijiquan practiced today in the United States, probably due, at least in part, to its being the first style introduced in this country (DeMarco, 1992).

Taijiquan, with its centuries-old history, has had many distinguished teachers. Some, such as Chen Zhangxing, have enhanced the development of taijiquan through their innovation and systemization of principles and practices. Others, such as Yang Luchan and his two sons, Yang Jianhou and Yang Banhou, are famous for their martial skills. Yet others, such as Yang Chengfu, are celebrated as great proponents of the art. Still others, such as Zheng Manqing, are noted for their mastery of collateral cultural arts, such as poetry and painting, in addition to their mastery of taijiquan. Benjamin Pangjeng Lo, one of Zheng Manqing's senior students, continues this tradition.

Mr. Lo was born in April, 1927, in Jiangsu Province, China. He left with his parents for Taiwan in 1948. Mr. Lo graduated in 1953 from National Taiwan University with a bachelor's degree in Chinese literature. After graduation, he passed the civil service examination and began working for the Taiwan Provincial Government. He received a master's degree in public administration from National Chengchi University in 1968. Mr. Lo began his study of taijiquan with Zheng Manqing in 1949. He was Professor Zheng's first student in Taiwan.

Mr. Lo moved to San Francisco in 1974, where he began to teach taijiquan. Together with other students of Professor Zheng in America, he began to popularize the practice of Professor Zheng's simplified thirty-seven-posture version of the Yang form. Mr. Lo is currently retired from teaching in his San Francisco school, although he regularly conducts workshops throughout the United States, Israel, and European countries, such as Belgium, Holland, Norway, and Sweden. Looking back upon his career, Mr. Lo believes that, in addition to his teaching, his most important contributions to the spread of taijiquan have been his translation of Zheng Manqing's *Thirteen Treatises on T'ai Chi Ch'uan* (with Martin Inn), Chen Weiming's *Questions and Answers on T'ai Chi Ch'uan* (with Robert W. Smith), and his editing and translation of the *Taiji Classics: The Essence of T'ai Chi Ch'uan* (with Martin Inn, Robert Amacker, and Susan Foe). Mr. Lo's contributions to taijiquan are recognized in the Ben Lo Cup, awarded to grand champions at the annual A Taste of China, USA All-Taijiquan Championships.[3]

In this article we discuss Mr. Lo's beliefs concerning the history of taijiquan, his experiences studying with Zheng Manqing and his ideas concerning Zheng's shortened version of the Yang traditional form, his teaching experiences, philosophy, and methods, and his advice to teachers and students of taijiquan.[4] This is the first time Mr. Lo has shared these views for publication.

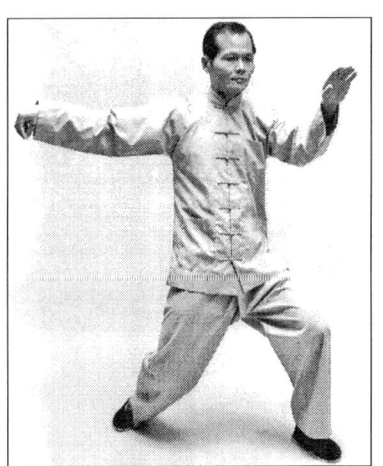
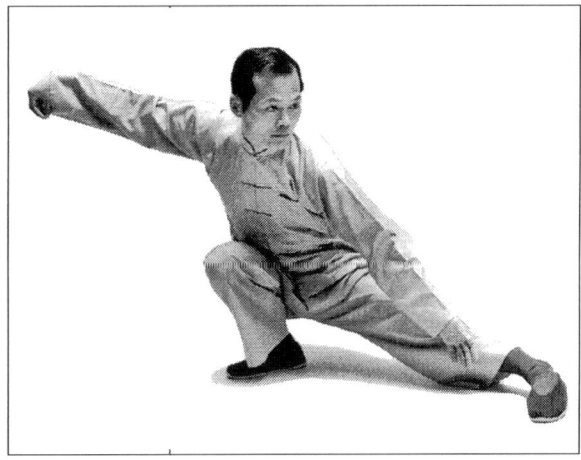

INTERVIEW
On the Origins of Taijiquan

• *Taijiquan skills provided economic and other benefits to the families and clans that possessed this knowledge. This knowledge was transmitted orally to others to maintain secrecy and because of the limited literacy of most Chinese martial artists at the time. As a result, there are few written records concerning the history of taijiquan, particularly its early years. We asked Mr. Lo to give us his thoughts concerning the origin of taijiquan.*

• Some say Zhang Sanfeng; some even say Laozi. These are just stories handed down. There is no evidence because all of the martial arts were secret at that time. We really don't know the origin of taiji. We have to wait for the evidence. Perhaps someday some archaeologist will discover artifacts to show the early history of taijiquan. Then we will know for sure.

Today in China, some believe that the Chen family created taijiquan. How can Chen be the inventor? Some, for example Wu Tunan, even say that the Chen Style is not taijiquan [Wu, 1984]. In the beginning, the Yang family called their style *mianquan* [cotton fist]. That's because it was a soft style. That's taijiquan. The Chen family called their style *paochui* [strike like a cannon]. Also, the Chen family doesn't have the *Taiji Classics*.[5] The *Taiji Classics* are like the taiji bible. Some of the most important principles from the *Taiji Classics* are relax, separate yin and yang, make the waist the commander, keep the body upright and movements slow. The Chen Style doesn't adhere to these principles. Later, when Yang Luchan became famous, the Chen family called their style taijiquan. All styles of taijiquan—Chen, Yang, both Wu styles, Sun, and so forth—should follow the principles described in the *Taiji Classics* if they are going to call themselves taijiquan. If the Chen family invented taiji, why don't they have the *Taiji Classics*?[6]

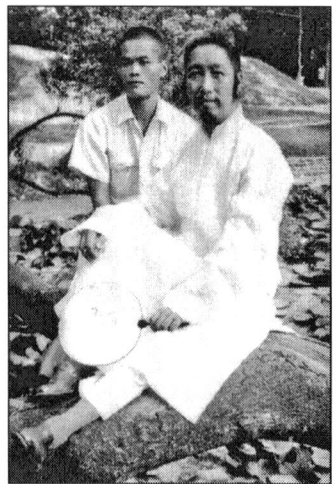 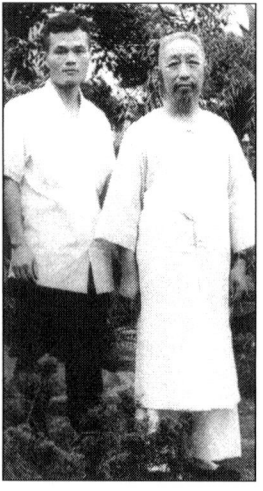

Photographs of Benjamin Lo with Zheng Manqing taken in Taibei, Taiwan.
Photo courtesy of Benjamin Lo.

• *Huang (1979: 61–62) states that Yang Luchan, after studying with the Chen family, probably returned to the original concepts of Zhang Sanfeng and Wang Zongyue to create a new school that took his name. That is, Yang may have changed the style of taijiquan that he learned from the Chen family in order to emphasize these earlier principles.*[7]

⦁ I think that this is an inference based on incomplete information. I do not believe there is any evidence to support Huang's claim. At this point, no one knows for certain from whom Yang Luchan received the taiji principles. Yang may have received these principles from Chen Zhangxing and Wu Yuxiang.

On the Origins of Taijiquan

I first sought out Professor Zheng because I was sick and he was a famous medical doctor and friend of my father. Western-trained doctors I visited said I had neurological problems, but the Professor diagnosed my illness as an internal injury. He gave me some herb medicine to take and suggested I begin to practice taiji to make my body stronger so that it could absorb the medicine he was giving me. I asked him where I could study taiji, and he said I could learn from him. I looked at him and thought to myself that he was not a martial arts teacher. I asked, "You know taiji?" He said he knew a little—enough to teach me! At that time I felt surprised, because I didn't know that he was a martial arts expert. Later on, many famous martial artists came to visit him. They told me how famous he was, but at the time I didn't know. Gradually I found out that he had been head of the martial arts school in Hunan Province. He presented himself quite simply, even to me. That's the Chinese way. After about three months, I began to improve and feel better. After I started to feel better, I became very serious about practicing taiji because it gave me hope of recovery from my illness. Before then, I'd been sick for a long time and had little hope for improvement. At this time I was twenty.

For the first four years of training, I improved rapidly. But after five years, I began to feel frustrated and I thought about quitting. I'd reached a plateau and didn't feel that I was improving. Later, I also felt like quitting after fifteen years and after twenty-six years of practice. Each time classmates would push with me and encourage me. This helped me to maintain my practice. Also, I learned to compare my practice with myself and not with others. For instance, I believed that it was a good achievement if last year I caught a cold, but this year I didn't catch one. Throughout this time, I studied only with Professor Zheng. I have never been able to master everything he taught to me, so it never seemed sensible to me to study other martial arts or with other teachers.

• *Zheng Manqing began his martial arts training as a student of Yang Chengfu, grandson of Yang Luchan, founder of the Yang school of taijiquan.*[8]

⦁ The Professor began to study taiji because he had an advanced stage of tuberculosis [third degree] from which he thought he would not recover. After a while, he began to improve, but he quit practicing because he became too busy.

Then he got sick again. He went through this cycle of practice followed by improvement and quitting practice followed by relapse twice more before deciding never to quit again.

• *Professor Zheng was an accomplished man, the Master of Five Excellences—taijiquan, painting, calligraphy, poetry, and traditional Chinese medicine. For Zheng, the common theme underlying each of these arts was his study and application of the principles of Confucianism and Daoism, and the opportunity to live in harmony with the Way. Sutton (1994) states that Professor Zheng, because of his experience in these other arts, changed his practice of the form enough to merit a new name—the Zheng Style of taijiquan. Lo (1985) and Smith (1995) have rebutted this claim. Mr. Lo wished to explain.*

• Some people say that Zheng Manqing changed the Yang form, but it's not true. What was changed? Which parts of his simplified form aren't the same as the Yang form? His major contribution to taiji was simplification of the Yang form. There is no such thing as the Zheng Style of taiji. Professor Zheng could not create his form because it was already there; it was the Yang form. He explains how he shortened the Yang form and his reasons for simplifying it in his *Thirteen Treatises* (Zheng, 1950/1985). He simplified it by deleting repetitions; the longer Yang form merely repeats the parts that were extracted into the simplified form. He did this because it took too long to learn and master the long form. Today, people and their lifestyles have changed, and they don't have the patience to learn and practice the long form. Also, in the old days taiji was practiced as a serious martial art. People who practiced it were willing to commit the time required to master it. Today many people practice taiji for health and exercise. They aren't so serious and don't have the time to learn and master the long form.

When one states that teachers have changed the way they do the form, it's sometimes due to faulty perception and limited understanding of the form. This problem also occurs when teachers teach the form before they've mastered it themselves. Sometimes when a student observes others doing taiji and their postures seem different, it's the student's fault. Usually when a posture seems changed, it's because the student isn't doing the posture correctly; he isn't following the principles. Even now, when I ask students . . . to do the postures, they can't do them; they can't maintain the taiji principles while doing these postures. If those students teach someday, their students will follow them in doing the postures incorrectly. Then the posture will appear to be changed. The Professor's classmate, Chen Weiming, was asked by his students, "Why does each teacher do the form differently?" Chen answered, "Students change the postures because they did not learn them correctly in the first place." Also, in the old days teachers were very strict; a student wouldn't dare ask a question if he didn't understand what the teacher taught him.[9]

The Professor simplified the form during the Sino-Japanese War.[10] He was in charge of martial arts training in Hunan Province. Martial arts instructors from throughout the province came to be trained by him. After discovering that there wasn't enough time to teach the long form to those who wanted to learn taiji, the Professor shortened the form. He didn't simplify the form with the intention of increasing its popularity, as some people believe. No, he didn't have this ambition when he simplified the form. He merely thought that more people would be willing to invest the time to learn taiji if it didn't take so long to do. Later on, it just happened to become popular.

• *Professor Zheng must have been an extraordinary person with great confidence in his own ability to simplify the form taught to him by Yang Chengfu.*
    • Yes, he was a very special person. At the age of eighteen most people are in high school, but he was already a professor in a university.[11] How many people are expert at painting, Chinese medicine, calligraphy, and poetry in addition to taiji? Around the age of thirty he was president of the National Association for Practitioners of Traditional Chinese Medicine. Every city and province in China had an association and president, yet he became leader of them all at quite a young age. At the same time, he was president of a fine arts college.[12] People followed him because of his achievements. He had exceptional natural gifts as a human being.

• *We were astonished to learn that, during twenty-six years of studying with Professor Zheng Manqing, Mr. Lo never saw him do the form in its entirety during practice or instruction.*
    • The only chance I had to see the Professor do the form was when some organization invited him to give a speech and the audience asked him to do the form. Then he would do the whole thing. But I never saw him do it by himself. Nobody saw that. It's like, if you study singing with Pavarotti, you wouldn't say to him: "Please sing this part for me. Let me see how you sing it." When he taught me, he taught me one posture at a time. First this part, then the next part, and so forth. When I began to study taiji forty-eight years ago, I remember that going from single whip to lifting hands took 120 hours.[13] At this time, Mrs. Zheng observed me doing the form. She was surprised that I hadn't learned more postures. She asked the Professor why he hadn't taught me more, and he said that my leg was shaking like a pipa string.[14] She said that times change, and the Professor shouldn't teach me like Grandmaster Yang taught him. After this, the Professor began to teach me the next postures. Later, he changed his teaching style when he came to the United States. In fact, I was surprised to learn when I visited the Professor's New York school that the students there had seen him do the entire form.

    Professor Zheng taught students in China differently from the way he taught students in the United States. When he taught me, he was very strict, especially when he was younger. My legs would be so sore that, when I went to bed at night, I had to use my hands to lift my legs onto the bed. He was kinder with American students. He got softer as he grew older. The Professor also said in the Thirteen Treatises that practicing taiji made him softer.

• *Zheng Manqing did not practice with weapons often used by Yang Style practitioners—for example, broadsword, spear, and staff—although he greatly enjoyed practicing the taiji straight sword.*

• I know he learned the sword and spear. He really enjoyed the sword. He showed me how to use the spear once in his study. I don't know why he did not use these other weapons. Perhaps Master Yang didn't have time to teach him, or maybe Professor Zheng didn't have time to learn. At that time, when Professor Zheng was twenty-eight or thirty, he was president of a fine arts college; maybe he was too busy.

Professor Zheng wanted to teach me the sword, but I told him I didn't want to learn it. I had trained hard but couldn't do the form perfectly yet, so why waste time on learning the sword?

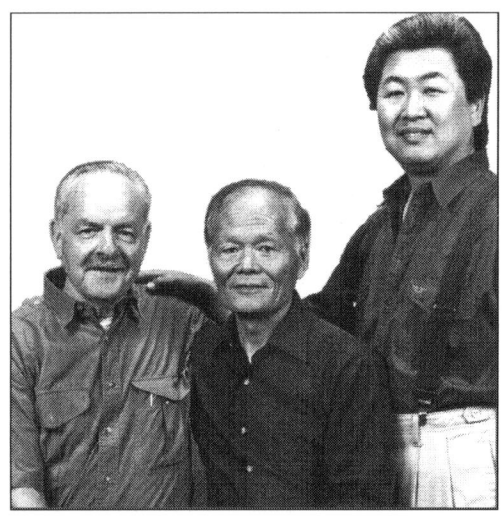

Left to right: Robert W. Smith, Benjamin Lo, and Patrick Cheng, Professor Zheng's son.
Photo courtesy of Tim Barnwell.

• Despite his early resistance, after practicing the taiji form for fifteen years, Mr. Lo learned the sword form at Professor Zheng's insistence. Since coming to the United States, Mr. Lo has taught the sword form only twice to a small group of selected students who already had a good foundation in the taiji form. He also recognized that students in the United States wished to learn more quickly and were not prepared to wait as long as he to learn the sword form.

> **"No burn, no earn; no pain, no gain."**
> —Benjamin Lo

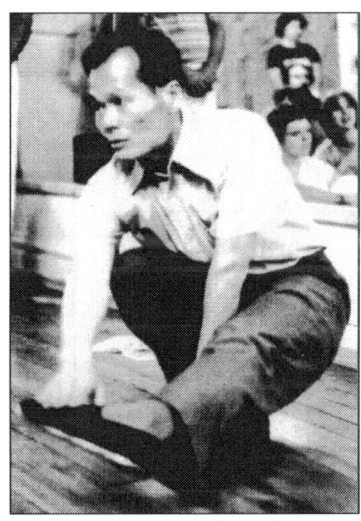

Benjamin Lo in a variation of snake creeps down, also known as squatting single whip. Note that Mr. Lo is utterly relaxed and picking up his front foot.
Photo courtesy of R. W. Smith.

Teaching, Philosophy, and Methods

• *Benjamin Lo is a traditionalist. His teaching emphasizes the Taiji Classics and the proper practice of each posture in Zheng Manqing's simplified version of the Yang form. He teaches in the same manner in which he was taught. Mr. Lo is noted for asking his students to stand still and to sink low in each posture. He often tells students, "Remember my name—'bend low'" (Ben Lo), to encourage strengthening each posture. We asked Mr. Lo to share advice he would give to students and teachers of taijiquan.*

• If a person really wants to learn taiji, he should look for a teacher who follows the principles described in the *Taiji Classics*—for example, relax, separate yin and yang, sink the qi, keep the body upright, and so forth.[15] If the teacher doesn't follow the principles, do you think this is taiji? Real taiji has to follow the principles described in the *Taiji Classics*.

You must practice the form every day, morning and night, and hold the postures. You need to hold the postures to get stronger. To get good, you need to *chikou* [literally, "to eat bitter," meaning to work very hard despite difficulties]. That's why I say, the more you suffer, the more you gain. It's like depositing money in the bank. You can't put one penny in the bank and get a lot of interest. If you put more money in the bank, you'll get more interest. I always tell my students, "No burn, no earn; no pain, no gain." But to avoid injury, you shouldn't overdo it.

To be good, a taiji player requires several things: natural gifts, proper attitude, perseverance, and a good teacher. One natural gift is the ability to comprehend the *Taiji Classics*. This is a type of taiji intelligence. With some people, you explain something a hundred times and they still don't get it. With others, you explain it once and they understand. It's like the bell curve, where most people have average intelligence, and a small number are more intelligent than average, and another small number are less intelligent than average. Some people just comprehend the principles of taiji more easily.

Another natural gift is the ability to relax the body. If you can't relax, taiji doesn't work. Like gymnastics or swimming, where physical gifts provide advantage, some people are more capable of relaxing and therefore of excelling in taiji.

Proper attitude is the second thing required to be skilled in taiji. Attitude refers to whether you are serious about your practice.

Perseverance is the third quality needed for success in taiji. If you have great natural ability but lack perseverance, you can't become very good.

Finally, you need a good teacher. Without a good teacher, you can't learn the proper way to do taiji. A good teacher is like having a compass when you're in the jungle. The compass shows you the correct path to take. Without a good teacher, you can't find the right way to practice.

• *Besides doing the form, Mr. Lo stresses the practice of push-hands (tuishou) to learn the application of taiji principles. In push-hands, the postures from the form are practiced with a partner. The purpose of push-hands is to learn to sense and control a partner's energy. One should learn to be as sensitive as the "feelers of a cricket" (Wang and Zheng, 1983: 188). The ability to sense and control a partner's energy is required to master taijiquan.*

• In pushing hands we learn feeling. Professor Zheng always said, "Know yourself through practicing the form; know others through practicing pushing hands."[16] Through pushing hands, you can tell something about a person's character, for example, whether they're gentle or aggressive. Pushing hands teaches sticking to your partner. In taiji we stay close to the joints, for example, the wrists, elbows and shoulders. In some ways this sticking is like qinna, but it's also different.[17] In qinna, you stay close to your partner's joints like in taiji, but in taiji we use the whole body to break the partner's balance.

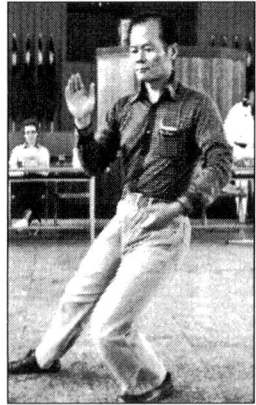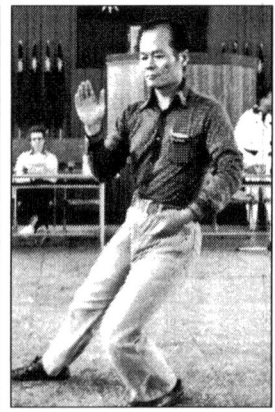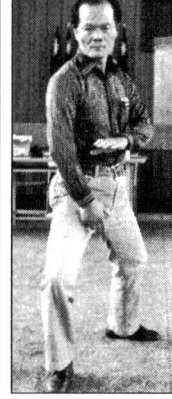

Taijiquan postures photographed in Taiwan: rollback, single whip, and shoulder stroke. Courtesy of Robert W. Smith.

- *Lowenthal (1994: 63) states that one must be aware of three points of contact when practicing push-hands: the partner's two elbows and leading wrist. It is through these three points, he writes, that one senses and controls the partner's energy. Mr. Lo expands on this idea.*
  - The Professor said, "The whole body is a hand and the hand is not a hand." This means the whole body should act at one time. The Professor wrote that he once dreamed that he had no arms, and after awakening he finally understood how to move in taiji. In other words, when doing push-hands one must use the entire body, not just the arms and hands, to sense one's partner and move in response to his actions.

- *Practicing applications and push-hands is required to learn the martial arts aspects of taiji.*
  - The study of martial arts is hard work. Most people can't take it. I always tell people that, although the Hong Kong gongfu movies exaggerate the difficulty of training, they're partly true. You have to work really hard. Holding the postures is important, but you must be relaxed. Your body can't be stiff as a rock. For example, when I teach classes, I tell people to assume a posture and not move, but after one or two minutes they stand up and move around. This isn't the way to excel in the martial arts.

  When the Professor taught push-hands, he said that when you touch people, in one second it should be like a clock—tick, you touch me; tock, you're out. You learn this through practicing push-hands (*tuishou*). But if your form is no good, you can't do anything in push-hands. If you have time, you can learn pushing hands; if you don't have time, you don't have to learn it, especially if you just do the form for exercise.

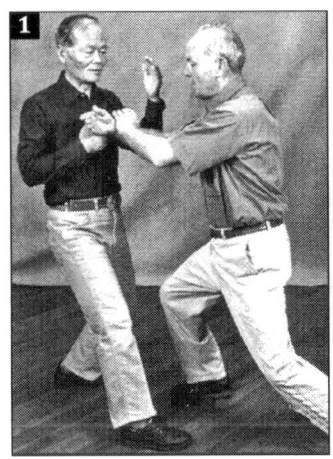 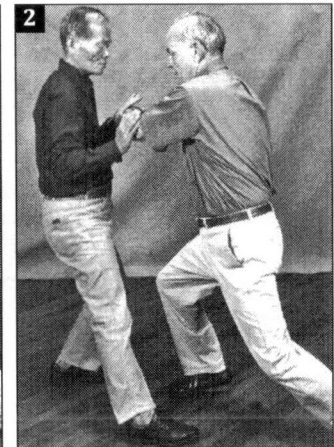 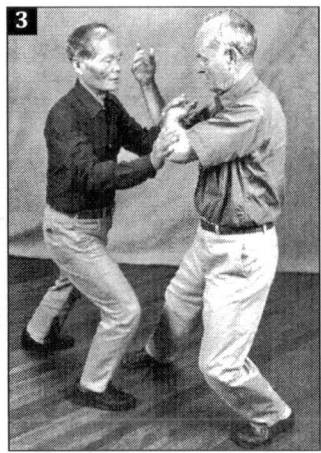

Mr. Lo and R. W. Smith pushing hands.
1) When Lo neutralizes Smith's push with rollback, Smith changes to press.
2) Lo neutralizes Smith's press and begins to push.
3) Smith uses rollback to neutralize. Photographs courtesy of R. W. Smith.

• *Bagua and xingyi are the internal cousins of taijiquan (Smith, 1981a, 1981b). We asked Mr. Lo if studying these or other arts would help one to master taiji.*

• You think Yang Luchan learned bagua or xingyi? You think Dong Haichuan, founder of bagua, learned taiji? Do you think Li Cunyi, a great master of xingyi, studied bagua or taiji? No! If you cannot be good at one thing, how can you learn other things? However, bagua, xingyi and taiji do share certain principles derived from the *Book of Changes* [Yijing], and they all rely on yin and yang.

• *Given taijiquan's historical foundation in Daoism and the fact that throughout his lifetime Zheng Manqing and studied the Yijing and Daodejing (Zheng, 1950/1985, 1981), we asked whether study of these classical texts is necessary for the mastery of taiji.*

• No, no, not at all. If this were necessary, university professors who teach about the *Yijing* would also be taiji masters. Also, some taiji masters, such as Yang Chengfu, were not highly educated. His reputation was strong because his taiji was good. Of course, it's not bad if you read these books, but it's not enough. Other books like Sunzi's are also useful.[18] But we have to know the difference between Daoist philosophy and Daoist religion. Taiji is related to Daoist philosophy but not to Daoist religion. Elements of Daoist philosophy—yin and yang, five elements theory, practices to extend longevity—have something to do with taiji. However, the student of taiji must be careful that he doesn't just study books, that he not become a mere armchair boxer.

The mind is important in taiji. For example, if I tell you to move your hand here, you can do that. Now if I tell you to put your mind [yi] here, what does that mean? It means you have to direct your attention and focus to this spot. If you can't do this, you can't do anything. But you can't force it. You go naturally, little by little. First, direct your mind for a short time, then for a longer time. The way you learn to do this is by practicing the form. When you start to learn the form, of course, you think about each posture. Gradually with practice, you can think about other things because you no longer have to concentrate on doing the postures. But later, after you master the form, you just do it. You forget yourself. You forget everything. You just do the form. It's like going to visit some pretty place. You don't pay attention to any one thing in particular. What's pretty? All of it together is pretty.

• *Related to the use of mind to direct actions is the difference between li (force) and jin (internal strength) as sources of power in taijiquan.*

• *Li* is derived from the bones, while *jin* is derived from the ligaments. Li is used by moving in a straight line, while jin is used by moving in a curve. Jin is also related to the development of the qi and is more powerful than li. That's why in push-hands we try to use jin to neutralize a partner's force. You relax, stick to him, and neutralize him when he pushes you—that's *jin*. But the form is important too. Without the form, you can't develop jin. Practicing the form is like putting money into the bank. When you get more money, then you can spend some (*jin*). However, a lot of people have money, but they don't know how to use it properly. That's the use of jin too. That's why we have to practice push-hands, to learn how to use jin.

• *We asked Mr. Lo to describe the relationship among taijiquan, qigong, and other forms of internal strength training.[19] We first asked if Professor Zheng had ever studied internal strength training with Zuo Laipeng, as stated by Sutton (1994).[20]*
   • The Professor never received any internal strength training from Zuo Laipeng. The Professor never learned any Zuo Style of taiji. The only thing the Professor practiced throughout his life other than the Yang form was *yijin* [muscle/tendon changing]. When he got older, around sixty, he also began to meditate. He did taiji meditation by just sitting and sinking the qi into the dantian.[21] In taiji meditation you don't need to count the breaths or breathe in any special way. When you practice taiji, you gradually learn how to breathe naturally.

   When people do qigong, they repeat one posture. Taiji has a variety of qigong postures. To me, any part of taiji is qigong. So if people do taiji, they also do qigong. Taiji is a form of *neijiaquan* [internal art]; it develops the qi. Now if you have time, you can learn other methods of qigong. They are not in opposition to taiji principles. But if you have extra time, I feel it would be better spent on practicing taiji because taiji uses the whole body. If you are thirsty, you drink a glass of water. Should you drink orange juice too? You don't have to. Also, you can't learn everything. In China there are more than one thousand kinds of qigong. If you learn one every year, or even one every day, there isn't enough time. And you need time to practice every one.[22]

• *Some taiji teachers emphasize the use of music while practicing the form or practicing the mirror image of the form. We asked Mr. Lo to comment on these practices.*
   • The Chinese have practiced taiji for several hundred years without these things. In Confucius's time, we already had classical music. Do you think that the founder of taiji didn't know about or think about using music? As for doing the form on both sides, if you want to do it, why not? Some people are left handed, and some people are right handed. But you don't have to do it this way because in the form we already practice on both sides. Also, the founder of taiji wasn't stupid. If he thought practicing on both sides was necessary, he would have put it in the form.

• *We followed up by asking Mr. Lo if he thought the form was perfect as it is or whether it could be improved.*
   • We can't even follow it as it is. When people can't finish what they are eating, why offer them more food? What I give you, you can't even digest, and you want more? But I would never say no. Nothing is perfect. Maybe in the future somebody like Yang Luchan may improve the form, but this kind of person is very rare. We simply don't know.

• *Taiji schools experience conflict at times. This conflict sometimes exists between teacher and students or, more often, between students themselves. We asked Mr. Lo to share his thoughts regarding proper relationships among those who practice taiji.*

• First, you should respect your teacher. That's ethical. I feel very strongly about this. Even if I learn more and become better than my teacher, he is still my teacher. Without him, I wouldn't know taiji at all. However, if I'm the teacher and you've learned everything I know, then I'd tell you I have nothing more to teach you and then tell you where to go next to study. I would write a letter to introduce you to a new teacher, to recommend you as a good person. This other teacher may then accept you as his student. But you shouldn't sneak to work with this other teacher. That's not right. You have to tell your teacher if you plan to study with someone else. I've refused some students who wanted to work with me. They came from Taiwan, where they were the students of teachers I knew there. I asked for their letter of introduction, but they didn't have one. I knew that they were sneaking to study with me. If they do this now to their teacher, someday they'll do it to me too. It's not honest.

The number one student is the one who has trained with the teacher the longest. If the teacher retires, he usually leaves the school to the number 1 student. But this is not always the best student. Sometimes, a younger student may have more natural ability. If the number 1 student is not the best, then he knows that he will cause the school to lose face, so he may ask the best student to take charge. But this younger student will still have to respect and listen to his senior classmate. This requires good character. But the teacher knows this too. I wouldn't want my school ruined by leaving in charge a student who didn't have good character and a high level of skill.

• *Traditionally, Chinese martial arts teachers are reputed to keep the secrets of their masters until they reach the last hours before their death. Sometimes these secrets die with them. We asked Mr. Lo to share with us a secret learned from his many years of studying and teaching taijiquan.*

• The teacher can only show you how to do it. The rest is all your work. The secret is to practice.

APPENDIX—Transliteration of Chinese Terms

Pinyin	Wade-Giles	Pinyin	Wade-Giles
bagua	pa-kua	Quanzhen sect	Ch'üan-chen sect
Chan Buddhist	Ch'an Buddhist	Sunzi	Sun-tzu (Sun-tsu)
Chen	Ch'en	taiji, taijiquan	t'ai chi, t'ai chi ch'üan
Chen Wangting	Ch'en Wang-t'ing	tuishou	t'ui-shou
Chen Weiming	Ch'en Wei-ming	waijiaquan	wai chia ch'üan
Chen Xing	Ch'en Hsing	Wang Beixing	Wang Pei-hsing
Chen Zhangxing	Ch'en Chang-hsing	Wang Maozhai	Wang Mao-chai
chikou	ch'ih-k'ou	Wang Zhengnan	Wang Cheng-nan
Damo	Ta-mo	Wang Zongyue	Wang Tsung-yüeh
dantian	tan-t'ien	Wudang Mountains	Wutang Mountains
Daodejing	*Tao Te Ch'ing*	Wu Tunan	Wu T'u-nan
Daoism, Daoist	Taoism, Taoist	Wu Guozhong	Wu Kuo-ch'ung
Dong Haichuan	Tung Hai-ch'üan	Wu Heqing	Wu Ho-ch'ing
Fu Zili	Fu Tzu-li	Wu Qiuying	Wu Ch'iu-ying
gongfu	kung-fu	Wu You	Wu Yu
Han Gongyue	Han Kung-yüeh	Wu Yuxiang	Wu Yü-hsiang
Henan Province	Honan Province	xiangyi	hsing-yi
Huang Lizhou	Huang Li-ch'ou	Xu Chen	Hsü Chen
Hubei Province	Hupei Province	Xu Xuanping	Hsü Hsüan-p'ing
Hunan Province	Hunan Province	Yang	Yang
Jiangsu Province	Chiangsu Province	Yang Banhou	Yang Pan-hou
jin	chin	Yang Chengfu	Yang Ch'eng-fu
Laozi	Lao-tzu (Lao-tsu)	Yang Jianhou	Yang Ch'ien-hou
li	li	Yang Luchan	Yang Lu-ch'an
Li Cunyi	Li Ts'un-i	Yang Yuding	Yang Yu-ting
Li Yiyu	Li Yi-yü	Yang Zhenduo	Yang Chen-tuo
mianquan	mien-ch'üan	Ye Jimei	Yeh Chi-mei
Ming	Ming	yi	i
neijiaquan	nei chia ch'üan	*Yijinjing*	*Yi Chin Ching*
Ninbo	Ningpo	*Yi Jing*	*I Ching*
Paochui	P'ao-ch'ui	Ying Lihen	Ying Li-hen
pipa	p'i-pa	Yuan	Yüan
qi	ch'i	Yuwen University	Yü-wen University
qigong	ch'i-kung	Zhang Qinling	Chang Ch'in-ling
qinna	ch'in-na	Zhang Sanfeng	Chang San-feng
Qing Dynasty	Ch'ing Dynasty	Zheng Manqing	Cheng Man-ch'ing
Quan You	Ch'üan Yu	Zuo Laipeng	Tso Lai-p'eng

*** NOTE:** Work on this article was assisted by a Fulbright Fellowship awarded to the first author and by resources provided by Wuhan University, in China, and the Department of Psychology at the University of Virginia, where the first author was a visiting professor.

Acknowledgments

We are grateful to Robert W. Smith for his help. His comments on earlier versions of this article reveal why he is the dean of martial arts scholars. Of course, we accept all responsibility for any remaining errors. We thank Peggy Kinard for her help in preparing transcripts of our taped interviews.

Notes

1. Pinyin, the transliteration system employed today in China, rather than the more traditional Wade-Giles system, is used for all Chinese terms except references published using the Wade-Giles system. We retained existing Wade-Giles titles in our bibliography to make it easier for readers to locate them although we used pinyin for all authors' names to make them consistent with citations in the text. We include in the appendix Pinyin terms and their Wade-Giles equivalents. We used Wu (1979) to choose equivalent terms.

2. Belief in Zhang Sanfeng as the founder of taijiquan is widespread, although there is little historical evidence to support this claim. Chen Weiming (1929/1985: 13) states that, according to the *Ningbo Chronicle*, Huang Lizhou wrote at the end of the Ming dynasty (1368–1644) that Wang Zhengnan's tombstone shows taijiquan was transmitted to Zhang Sanfeng and Ye Jimei. Chen also states that taiji was transmitted to four other people: Xu Xuanping, Fu Zili, Han Gongyue, and Ying Lihen.

    Jou (1981: 2) states that Zhang Sanfeng was born at midnight on April 9, 1247. Lo, Inn, Amacker, and Foe (1985: 9) state that the time during which Zhang is believed to have lived is 1279–1368, although legend has it that he lived more than 250 years. Liao (1990: 10) states that Zhang founded his temple on Wudang Mountain in 1200, decades before the date Jou or Lo and his colleagues cite for his birth. Seidel (1970: 485–487) states that Zhang began his study of Daoism years after the time that Liao says he founded his first temple on Wudang Mountain and that he died around 1393. Differences in these dates demonstrate the uncertainty concerning the facts of Zhang Sanfeng's life.

    Seidel (1970), in a careful historical study, provides the following conclusions. Zhang Sanfeng was a Daoist master who was loosely connected with the Quanzhen sect of Daoism, received imperial honors, and founded several retreats in the Wudang Mountains. She could discover no evidence to demonstrate that he was the founder of taijiquan. The association of taijiquan with Zhang Sanfeng seems instead to represent an attempt to add historical validity to the lineage of internal martial arts (*neijiaquan*), just as Damo (Bodhidharma) has been used to validate the origin of external styles (*waijiaquan*) at the Shaolin Temple.

Records concerning the history of taijiquan become more reliable during the late Ming (1368–1644) and Qing (1644–1912) dynasties. Some evidence points to Chen Wangting (1597–1644) and his family, with influence from Wang Zongyue (1736–1795), as the source of modern taijiquan styles. Seidel (1970: 505) states that Wu Heqing, a student of Yang Luchan, wrote about taijiquan, and that Wu ascribed the origin of his writings to Wang Zongyue to give them more weight. Yang Zhenduo, third son of Yang Chengfu, states that taijiquan was founded at the end of the Ming dynasty, presumably by Chen Wangting, although he does not state this explicitly (Yang, 1988: 1). See DeMarco (1992) for a discussion of the origin and evolution of various taijiquan lineages.

3 Pat Rice, cofounder and director of A Taste of China, USA All-Taijiquan Championships, one of the oldest and largest taijiquan tournaments in the United States, explained why the grand champion trophy is named the Ben Lo Cup. She states that this was done to encourage competitors to maintain proper taiji principles while pushing hands. She says that, because Mr. Lo has such a high level of skill and embodies taiji principles in his practice and teaching, he serves as an exemplar for serious practitioners of the art.

4 We took Mr. Lo's responses from transcripts of interviews conducted in March and June 1995, and April 1996. We have edited his comments, and he has reviewed our editing to ensure accuracy.

5 The *Taiji Classics* are a collection of songs and poems written in classical Chinese that were used to aid in the oral transmission of taijiquan principles. Although some of the writings are alleged to be more than one thousand years old, the evidence for this is inconclusive. The facts seem to be that they were discovered in the middle of the nineteenth century in a salt shop by Wu Qiuying, who took them to his brother Wu Yuxiang (creator of the Wu Style of taijiquan). Wu Yuxiang then showed the manuscript to his teacher, Yang Luchan, who interpreted them for Wu due to their being written in a form of taiji code. From this point, both Yang and Wu incorporated the *Taiji Classics* into their teaching. The compiler of the *Taiji Classics* was reputed to be Wang Zongyue, the eighteenth century visitor to the Chen family village, but this is probably not true. In addition to works allegedly written by Wang Zongyue, the *Taiji Classics* contain writings attributed to Zhang Sanfeng, Wu Yuxiang, and Li Yiyu. Moreover, modern taiji writings by Yang Chengfu and his students Chen Weiming and Zheng Manqing were added later (see Lo et al., 1985). Still other writings were provided by anonymous authors. Liao (1990), Lo et al. (1985), and Yang (1987) provide different compilations and translations. The principles expounded in the *Taiji Classics* continue to provide the foundation for the Zheng Manqing school of taijiquan, as well as other practitioners of the Yang style.

6 Some may say the *Taiji Classics* were written by practitioners of the Yang family style. If this is true, it would be obvious that they would emphasize the Yang

manner of doing the postures. The story concerning the discovery of the *Taiji Classics* manuscripts by Wu Qiuying, who took them to his brother Wu Yuxiang, a practitioner of the Yang family style, supports this claim. On the other hand, the Yang family was illiterate and incapable of writing the *Taiji Classics*. Nevertheless, allegations that the *Taiji Classics* had a more ancient origin would be more believable had they been discovered by someone outside of the Yang family circle.

7 Huang (1979: 62) cites a study of the history of taijiquan written by Xu Chen and published in Hong Kong that states that it was Yang Luchan who first attributed the origin of taijiquan to Zhang Sanfeng.

8 Sutton (1994: 58; also footnote 1) states that Professor Zheng began his martial arts training with Shaolin boxing during his youth, not with taijiquan, as we claim. He cites Zheng's biography engraved on the wall of his tomb and translated and published in English by Tam Gibbs. Mr. Lo states that this was a mistranslation by Gibbs. He states further that Zheng instead studied a set of stretching exercises associated with the *Yijinjing* (Muscle/Tendon Changing Classic) during his youth, not Shaolin boxing. Moreover, Jou (1981: A19), citing the preface to Zheng's 1946 book on taijiquan, says that Zheng practiced *yijin* to cure himself of rickets and rheumatism he suffered in his youth. *Yijin*, a form of qigong employing massage and Chan Buddhist and Daoist meditation practices, was allegedly created by Damo (Bodhidharma) at the Shaolin Temple and later incorporated into various forms of boxing practiced there (Yang, 1989: 11). Given its connection with the Shaolin Temple and some of its forms of boxing, Tam Gibbs apparently confused *Yijinjing* with a Shaolin Style of boxing.

9 Emphasis on family transmission and the "closed door" approach to teaching contributed to the uncertainty concerning the history and teaching of taijiquan and other Chinese martial arts. As a result of this tradition of secrecy, knowledge of different styles was limited and distortions marked the knowledge that was transmitted. Moreover, the emphasis on hierarchy in Chinese society amplified the social distance between teacher and student. This distance prevented students from asking questions to seek correction of mistakes. Even today, many teachers in China feel insulted if a student asks questions because this questioning implies that the teacher did not teach the lesson clearly enough for the student to understand. Questioning also reflects on the student's character by suggesting that the student is not very adept or has not studied very hard. It is hardly surprising that errors occur and remain uncorrected within this type of learning environment. The relative openness of the Western teaching tradition and the greater tendency of Western, especially North American, students to ask questions merely make corrections and discussion of them more salient.

10 Smith (1995) states that Zheng Manqing may have been experimenting with a simplified version of the Yang form in 1938, and that it did not become finalized until 1947, just before he moved to Taiwan. Lo (1985) also states that Zheng adopted the simplified form in 1938.

[11] Zheng taught at Yuwen University in Beijing. He became director of the Department of Chinese Painting at the Shanghai School of Fine Arts when in his mid-twenties. See the short biography written by Tam Gibbs and printed in Zheng (1981).

[12] Professor Zheng was president of the College of Chinese Culture and Arts in Shanghai, which he cofounded when in his late twenties (Zheng, 1981).

[13] Single whip and lifting hands are the eighth and ninth postures in Zheng's simplified form.

[14] A pipa is a Chinese plucked string instrument with a fretted fingerboard, similar to a Western lute or classical guitar.

[15] "Separate yin and yang" refers to the division of weight between one's legs. According to traditional Chinese theories of human physiology and medicine, qi is the energy that travels along a network of meridians throughout the body. Development and use of the qi is a goal of advanced taiji practice.

[16] Wang Beixing (a student of Yang Yuding and his teacher Wang Maozhai), who teaches the Wu Style today in Beijing, states, seek "to know one's own energy through the sequence practice, and the other's energy through push-hands exercise" (Wang and Zeng, 1983: 189). Given that Wang Beixing's teacher—Wang Maozhai—was a student of Quan You (also known as Wu You), founder of the Wu style, who was in turn a student of Yang Banhou, Yang Luchan's son, this teaching concerning sensing energy is clearly part of the Yang Style tradition. It is, therefore, obvious that Zheng Manqing should continue to impart this insight to his students, demonstrating his root in the Yang tradition.

[17] Qinna emphasizes striking nerves and manipulation of muscles, fascia, and joints to subdue one's opponent. It is generally associated with external martial arts (*waijiaquan*) (see Smith, 1996; Yang, 1982a).

[18] Sunzi is the author of the *The Art of War* (Sun, 1988), an ancient treatise devoted to military strategy that is still studied widely throughout Asia.

[19] Qigong is a system of deep-breathing exercises that have associated physical movements. The Chinese have practiced qigong for many centuries to improve Rooster health and increase longevity. Qigong is very popular today in China, more popular than taijiquan, with many instructional programs broadcast on television and published in the popular press.

[20] Sutton (1994) claims that Zheng Manqing studied internal strength techniques under Zuo Laipeng. He cites Wu Guozhong (1985) to support his claim. Lo (1985) and Smith (1995) demonstrate why this claim is false. Lo (1985) states further that there is no such thing as a Zuo Style of taijiquan. Zheng really learned a method of internal energy cultivation from Zhang Qinlin, a senior classmate who studied with Zuo Laipeng.

[21] The dantian is a point in the abdomen about 1.3 inches below the navel and located closer to the navel than the spine. It is a point of focus for many meditative traditions.

[22] This point was stressed repeatedly during all of our conversations with Mr. Lo.

He felt that a lifetime of dedication and practice are needed to master taijiquan, and effort and time devoted to other practices or martial arts merely take away resources needed to master taiji. After one has mastered taijiquan, then one may consider studying qigong or other martial arts.

Bibliography

Chen, W. (1929/1985). *T'ai chi ch'uan ta wen* [Questions and answers on t'ai chi ch'uan] (B.P. Lo and R.W. Smith, Trans.). Berkeley, CA: North Atlantic Books. (Original book published in Shanghai in 1929 and reprinted by the T'ai Chi Ch'uan Research Association of Taiwan, 1967).

Chen, X. (1919/1964). *Chen taijiquan tuishuo*. (Original book completed in 1919 and published by Chengshanmei Books, Taibei, Taiwan, 1984).

DeMarco, M. (1992). The origin and evolution of taijiquan. *Journal of Asian Martial Arts, 1*(1), 8–25.

Huang, W. (1979). *Fundamentals of t'ai chi ch'uan* (3rd. Ed.). Hong Kong: South Sky Book Company.

Jou, T. (1981). *The Tao of t'ai-chi ch'uan*. Warwick, NY: Tai Chi Foundation.

Liao, W. (1990). *T'ai chi classics*. Boston, MA: Shambhala.

Lo, B. (1985, August). Explanation of Tsuo-style tai chi chuan. *T'ai chi ch'uan*, issue no. 40, 8–14. (Published in Taiwan, translated into English by the author).

Lo, B., Inn, M., Amacker, R., and Foe, S. (1985). *The essence of t'ai chi ch'uan: The literary tradition*. Berkeley, CA: North Atlantic Books.

Lowenthal, W. (1994). *Gateway to the miraculous: Further explorations in the Tao of Cheng Man-ch'ing*. Berkeley, CA: Frog, Ltd.

Seidel, A. (1970). A Taoist immortal of the Ming dynasty: Chang San-feng. In W.T. deBary (Ed.), *Self and Society in Ming Thought* (pp. 483–531). New York: Columbia University Press.

Smith, R. (1981a). *Pa-kua: Chinese boxing for fitness and self-defense*. New York: Kodansha International.

Smith, R. (1981b). *Hsing-i: Chinese mind-body boxing*. New York: Kodansha International.

Smith, R. (1995). Zheng Manqing and taijiquan: A clarification of role. *Journal of Asian Martial Arts, 4*(1), 50–65.

Smith, R. (1996). Han Qingtang and his seizing art. *Journal of Asian martial arts, 5*(1), 31–47.

Sun, T. (1988). *The art of wa*r (Thomas Cleary, Trans.). Boston: Shambhala. Sutton, N. (1994). The development of Zheng Manqing taijiquan in Malaysia. *Journal of Asian Martial Arts, 3*(1), 56–71.

Wang, P., and Zeng, W. (1983). *Wu style taijiquan: A detailed course for health and self-defence and teachings of three famous masters in Beijing*. Hong Kong and Beijing: Hai Feng Publishing and Zhaohua Publishing.

Wu, D. (1984). *T'ai chi ch'uan yenchiu*. Hong Kong: Shangwu Books.

Wu, G. (1985). *T'ai chi ch'uan taochi*. Taibei: Shenlong Books.

Wu, J. (Ed.). (1979). *The pinyin Chinese-English dictionary*. Beijing: The Commercial Press.

Yang, J. (1982a). *Shaolin chin na: The seizing art of kung-fu*. Burbank, CA: Unique Publications.

Yang, J. (1982b). *Yang style tai chi chuan*. Burbank, CA: Unique Publications.

Yang, J. (1987). *Advanced Yang style tai chi chuan (vol. 1): Tai chi theory and tai chi jing*. Jamaica Plain, MA: Yang's Martial Arts Association.

Yang, J. (1989). *Muscle-tendon changing and marrow/brain washing chi kung: The secret of youth*. Jamaica Plain, MA: Yang's Martial Arts Association.

Yang, Z. (1988). *Yang style taijiquan*. Beijing and Hong Kong: Hai Feng Publishing and Morning Glory Press.

Zheng, M. (1950/1985). *Cheng Tzu's thirteen treatises on t'ai chi ch'uan* (B.P. Lo and M. Inn, Trans.). Berkeley, CA: North Atlantic Books. (Original book published in Taiwan in 1950).

Zheng, M. (1981). *Lao-Tzu: My words are very easy to understand.* Berkeley, CA: North Atlantic Books.

Sacrifice, Ritual, & Alchemy: Spiritual Traditions in Taijiquan
by Dennis Willmont, B.A., L.Ac.

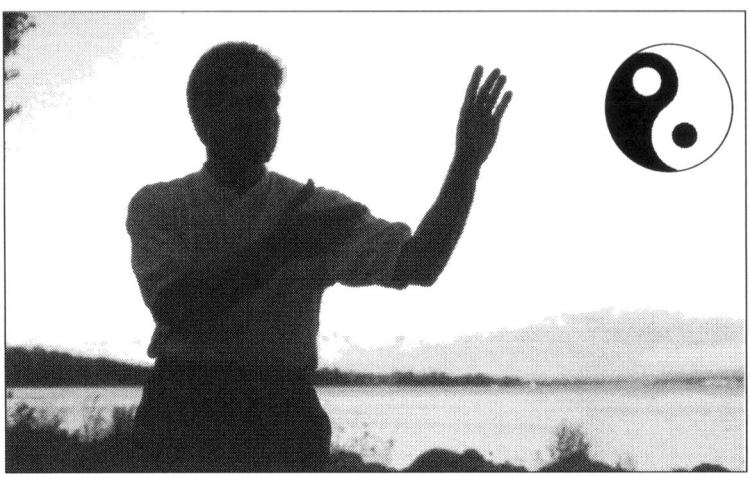

"Wave Hands Like Clouds."
Photograph courtesy of M. DeMarco.

Philosophical Background of Taijiquan

Taijiquan is an internal martial art known for its emphasis on mental and spiritual development. It is further characterized as a predetermined sequence of movements performed in slow motion. Thus, taijiquan is set apart from other martial arts whose movements are always performed at fast speed, as well as forms of sitting meditation and contemplation that place much less emphasis on the body. In contrast to dance as a performing art, which connects to the world externally through the interpersonal and horizontal communication between the artist and his or her audience, taijiquan connects to the world internally through a vertical communication between matter and spirit or, as in the Chinese manner, between heaven and earth (*tian di*). Communication between the heavenly and earthly poles of existence has been of paramount importance to the Chinese throughout their long history, of which taijiquan is but a comparatively recent development.

Although legends say taijiquan was created by Zhang Sanfeng in the Song Dynasty (960–1278 CE), its philosophical roots go back to the beginning of recorded history in China encompassing the development of Chinese thought as well as men's relation to one another and the natural universe. These roots include ancestor and spirit worship in the Shang Dynasty (1766–1154 BCE), the development of Confucianism in the Zhou Dynasty (1122–255 BCE), the origination of Daoism in the Warring States period (403–222 BCE), the development of alchemy in the Han Dynasty (206 BC–189 CE), and beyond. To understand important concepts in taijiquan, such as *xu* (emptiness), *wuwei* (effortlessness), and *zuran* (spontaneity), as well as the internal purpose of taijiquan itself (i.e., connecting to the source of the universe within the core of one's being), it is necessary to view taijiquan in this cultural and historical context.

To begin with, the very name "taijiquan" denotes a process that is simultaneously physical, mental, and spiritual. The word *quan* etymologically depicts a hand (*shou*) flexing (*quan*) into a fist (Weiger, 1965: 710). Superficially, this refers to taijiquan as a style, but on a deeper level *quan* refers to the embodiment of the spiritual and philosophical realms, i.e., "grasping" the relevance and deeper meaning inherent in the term "taiji."

"Taiji," or Great Ridgepole (sometimes called Great Ultimate), is a very ancient philosophical term referring to the gateway to the universe's origin. The term "taiji" first appears in the Great Appendix of the *Yijing* (Book of Changes), where eight stages are described in the creation of the physical world. According to the *Yijing*, taiji (stage 1) is what produces the two principles (*yi*) of yin and yang (stage 2) from the Great Void, which is considered the nondifferentiated, empty (*xu*) source (*yuan*) of all things (stage 0). Yin and yang, then, begin an energetic process of interpenetration and incubation through which the physical embryo is fashioned, and birth takes place. The third stage produces the first level of this interpenetration in what are called the "Four Symbols" (*si xiang*), which describe this interpenetration in four different polar aspects: yin, yang, yin within yang, and yang within yin. The following four stages describe this continuing interpenetration in more detail. To avoid the confusion that would result by naming each of these stages according to the linguistics of yin and yang, especially on the seventh level, where there are six levels of yin-yang interpenetration, more easily understood visual symbols were used by ancient philosophers instead. Thus, this yin-yang interpenetration was conveyed by them through a system of solid and broken lines, in which the solid lines represented yang and the broken lines represented yin. Stage four resulted in eight different groups of three-lined symbols called the eight trigrams. Stage seven resulted in sixty-four different groups of six-lined symbols called the sixty-four hexagrams (Sung, 1935: 229).[1] Each trigram and each hexagram was further associated with names and symbols derived from the natural and social worlds. In this way, they were more readily distinguished from one another. The trigrams were named according to symbols from the natural world: heaven, earth, water, fire, thunder, wind, mountain, and lake. The hexagrams were named according to symbols mostly from the social world: "the Return," "Difficulty at the Beginning," "Before Completion," etc. All complexities aside, this creation sequence begins with the void and then progresses through seven stages of yin-yang polarization in which the physical process of creation is completed evolving from: (1) void, through (2) yin-yang (3) Four Images, (4) Eight Trigrams, and then (5) sixteen, and (6) thirty-two continuing subdivisions of yin and yang until (7) the sixty-four hexagrams are reached, which represent the completion of the yin-yang archetypal image preceding (8) the physical manifestation of the world (Dhiegh, 1973: 73).

Yin-Yang Interpretation								
8 →	Materialization							
7 →								
6 →								
5 →								
4 →	Earth	Mountain	Water	Wind	Thunder	Fire	Lake	Heaven
3 →	Yin-in-Yin		Yang-in-Yin		Yin-in-Yang		Yang-in-Yang	
2 →	Yin				Yang			
1 →	Taiji							
0 →	Void							

In Chapter 7 of the *Zhuangzi* (350 to 222 BCE, one of the three major early Daoist texts including the *Daodejing* and the *Huainanzi*), a legendary version of these seven stages is recounted in the myth of Hundun. Hundun, whose name means "chaos," was a "cosmic-egg" type creature with no orifices in his body. He was also called the Emperor of the Central Region and, when visited by the two Emperors of the North and South (symbolizing water and fire, see chart), treated them so generously that, to repay his kindness, they said (Yu, 1981: 481; Schipper, 1978: 360):

> All men have seven openings so they can see, hear, eat, and breathe.
> But Hundun doesn't have any. Let's try to bore him some! Everyday
> they bored him another hole, and on the seventh day Hundun died.

In this story, the seven openings symbolize, not only the seven sensory orifices of the head and the opening of the unmanifest source to the external world, but also the seven polar stages of creation developing from the central void. It is interesting to note that this legend signifies that the birth of creation implies the death of, or disconnection from, the Source, a plight that, as we shall see, becomes fundamental to the Daoists.

The idea of creation emerging from a nondifferentiated void is also reflected in the *Daodejing* (Classic of the Source and Its Power), China's oldest Daoist text, generally believed to have been composed after Confucius sometime during the Warring States period (Feng, 1952: 170). Here the process of creation goes through four stages. The second chapter posits the origin of this sequence in Dao: "The origin of Heaven and Earth (*Dao*) is the mother of all things" (Wu, 1961: 3). In chapter 42, it describes the order of this sequence in symbolic detail (Wu, 1961: 60):

> Dao engenders the One, One engenders the Two,
> Two engenders the Three and the
> Three engenders the ten thousand things.[2]

In the *Daodejing*, Dao is equated with the void space of the *Yijing*; One is equated with Taiji; Two refers to yin and yang; Three is equated with the five levels of yin-yang interpenetration through the binary sequence (2, 4, 8, 16, 32, 64, etc.), which leads from the "Four Images" to the Eight Trigrams and sixty-four hexagrams; and Four is associated with the material world. The *Yijing* and *Daodejing* traditions are somewhat unified in the *Lu Shi Chun Qiu* (third century BCE), in which the term Taiji is replaced by *Taiyi* (the Supreme One), one of the divinities esteemed by the magical practitioners (*fangshi*) of this period (Robinet, 1990: 381–382).

Inherent in these early maps of creation was also the reverse path for returning to the Source. It was believed that, since the creation path led, in its extreme, to disharmony, disconnection from the Source, disease, and death, the "return" path led to renewal, healing, longevity, and, according to the ancients, immortality as well. The key to both maps is none other than the philosophical term taiji, the invisible gate between the unmanifest and the manifest. Ancient shamans travelled through this gate in their rituals to connect heaven and earth and harmonize these two paths. This shamanistic activity is depicted etymologically in the word *ji* of taijiquan, which depicts a cosmic tree (*mu*) in this axis mundi function, through which the human supplicant (*ren*), or shaman, connects heaven and earth (*er*) through his words (*kou*, or chanting), and deeds (*you*, ritual actions), as signified by the moving of the arms (*you*) (Weiger, 1965). These shamanistic rituals were the earliest aspects of Chinese religious function, and their most important aspects (the ritual connection of heaven and earth, matter and spirit) were incorporated in highly significant ways in the historical development of later Chinese tradition of which Confucianism and Daoism were the most important. A thousand years later, all of these aspects came together in the formation of taijiquan.

	Stage	Yi Jing	Dao De Jing	Lu Shi Chun Qiu
THE CREATION SEQUENCE: PATH OF MANIFESTATION	0 →	Tai Xu (Great Void)	Dao	Taiyi (Great One)
	1 →	Taiji	Taiji	Taiji
	2 →	Yin and Yang	Yin and Yang	Yin and Yang
	3 →	Yin-Yang Interpenetration ("Four Images"; Eight Trigrams; 16, 32, 64 Hexagrams)	Yin, Yang and Balance	Yin, Yang and Balance
	4 →	The Material World	The Material World	The Material World

The ideographic component of *ji*, from which *tian* and *di* (heaven and earth) are likewise derived, can symbolize a building's ridgepole from which the eaves spread out on either side. In Chinese temples, the most striking and unmistakable feature is the roof. "Instead of sitting simply on walls like the typical Western roof, it looks to be, as it structurally is, independent of the building itself; and therefore, one has the impression that it is light and free despite its relatively massive proportions" (Thompson, 1989: 70). From this apparently immaterial ridgepole, the eaves extend, as if generating yin and yang as well as heaven and earth from the void, and ultimately sheltering the birth and death of the human activities carried out below.

Both Confucian and Daoist philosophers frequently cite that human activities as well as the creation of the world emerge from a common center to an increasingly complicated and diverse periphery. This emergence is frequently symbolized by the root, branches, stems, and flowers of a tree.

Creation and its activities are symbolized by the flowers, whereas the source of creation, the Great Void, Dao, or Taiyi, is symbolized by the root from which these flowers spring. Around 1130–1200 in the time of the legendary creation of taijiquan, Zhu Xi, the greatest neo-Confucian synthesizer, said: "Taiji is like a tree growing upward, it divides and becomes branches and stems... flowers and fruit... and continues until it produces seed" (Meyer, 1976: 32). The more one's consciousness becomes entangled in the flowers, the more one is cut off from the root. In as much as the expansion of the lifeforce (*qi*) naturally tends toward its own dissipation as it reaches its periphery, all the great traditions of China have recognized in some form or another that for the life of the spirit to be maintained there must be some accompanying attention or even devotion to the periphery's corresponding center and source. These two directions give rise to the two paths of "creation" and "return." When the outgoing path of creation reaches its extreme in the devotion to material impulses, such as greed, lust, pride, etc., there is a tendency to lose the connection to one's immaterial or spiritual source (*dao*) as well as the internal power or virtue (*de*) that it generates. Confucius called this materialistic path the path of the petty person or "small man" (*xiao ren*). In contrast, he called the more inner-directed path, even when it was connected horizontally through human relations, the path of the "great person" (*da ren*). The recognition and idealization of the "great person" gave rise to many other names, e.g., the sage (*junzi*) in Confucianism and the realized person (*zhen ren*) in Daoism. In effect, these were the saints of the ancient Chinese and were characterized, in essence, by their constant relation with *dao* and *de* through the connection of *dao* and *de* to taiji. The main difference was that in Confucianism, the sage applied the knowledge of these two paths horizontally in the social domain, while the realized person in Daoism applied them vertically to the natural and spiritual world.

Philosophy in Practice

The Daoist path of "return" is symbolically traversed by following the focus of one's intention in the reverse order of the creative path, i.e., from flower, to stem, to the small and then the large branches, and finally to the trunk and root. If we relate this metaphor, as well as the metaphors given in the *Yijing* and *Daodejing* creation maps cited above, to the most basic yin-yang aspects of taijiquan training, such as those found in the taijiquan sequence and described in the *Taiji Classics*, we will then be able to see how the return path of regeneration applies to taijiquan as a practical expression of these philosophies. To do this, we must substitute for the abstractions mentioned in the philosophical texts four of the most basic yin-yang aspects of taijiquan training. The *Taiji Classics* describe these four as (1) the in and out, opening and closing, movement of the breath including its connection to the joints; (2) movement itself with its corresponding yin stillness (*jing*) and yang action (*dong*); (3) the shifting of weight from substantial (*shi*) to insubstantial (*xu*, note that this term is the same word "empty" used for the Great Void itself); and (4) movement in the six directions (up/down, left/right, and forward/ backward) through a seventh neutral or pivot space (recall the seven stages of creation in the *Yijing* and the seven openings or movements of Hundun, the Emperor of Center). To incorporate these yin-yang principles into practice, we must begin with the basics of taijiquan standing postures, which are represented by Horse Stance, Bow Stance, Embrace the Pillar, and each of the thirty-seven postures of the taijiquan sequence on both the right and left sides. In the standing postures, external movement is reduced to the absolute minimum. In effect, there is no external yin-yang or outward motion except for the opening and closing of the breath and the joints. This simple opening and closing represents the taiji principle, prior to that is the nonbreathing, totally unmoving source that the philosophers call *wuji*, dao, or void, and following which is the sequence of the taijiquan form.

With this void space established, we begin to add the most basic movements (slow movements, of course) to our basic taijiquan sequence. In the *Taiji Classics*, it says that this movement is rooted at the feet, is generated from the legs, directed by the waist, and expressed in the fingers (Yang, 1987: 213). This movement begins by shifting our weight either from side to side in a medium to upright Horse Stance, or from front to back in Bow Stance. In this first aspect of shifting our weight, we have gone from point (*taiji*) to line (simple left, right, forward, or backward movement).

Now, from this simple shifting of weight from foot to foot, let us progress to the third stage, which is a circle. Focusing specifically on the origin of movement in the feet (done slowly), notice that the linear movement of weight, shifting from the substantial to the insubstantial foot, "grows" from a straight line to a curved line that "circles" under the feet in two directions when the movement shift to substantial has become complete. For example, when the weight on the right foot (substantial) shifts, the substantiality of that shifting should be perceived as the bottom of a circle traveling under the floor until it reaches the left foot, which then becomes substantial again. When the left foot starts to shift its substantiality back to the right, the top aspect of the circle moves up the left leg to the waist where it is then directed into the right leg, which then becomes substantial. This circle, then, continues throughout the exercise (right to left). At the same time, however, there is a circle rotating in the opposite direction (left to right). In other words, any time the substantial leg changes to insubstantial, there is a downward circle moving under the floor to the other leg and a corresponding upward circle moving up the substantial leg to the waist and down the other leg to the foot, where the two circles meet when the other leg becomes substantial. One must keep the structural integrity of the body to experience these circles. This means that the feet, ankles, knees, and hips must be in alignment. The knees should be held at the same height throughout the exercise. They should also be bent, but not poking out over the front or sides of the feet. This structural integrity allows the muscles to relax and the tendons and ligaments to be strengthened so that the body weight can be supported more by the skeletal system, which is designed specifically for this purpose.

The fourth stage of our progression now moves from circle to sphere by involving the expression of movement through the fingers (level 4 of the *Taiji Classics*). This fourth stage of progression from circle to sphere also corresponds to the fourth stage in the *Daodejing*, in which the "three begets the ten thousand things" (*wan wu*) or the created universe. At this stage, we add the motion of the arms and hands in, for example, any of the more complex thirty-seven postures of the Yang Style form. Picture any one of these postures being performed repeatedly in a continuous sequence as they would be if they were linked together by doing them on both the right and left sides, one following the other. This sequence can be visualized more easily when the right and left versions of the postures follow one another in the sequence such as brush knee twist step, repulse monkey, cloud hands, etc. At this fourth stage, we have completed the "materialization" of our basic yin-yang principles through the taijiquan sequence as well as the creation path of materialization into the three-dimensional realm or sphere.

At this stage of movement, breath, as well as the shifting of weight from substantial to insubstantial, completes the top and bottom polarity of directions and becomes much more complex as the shift now includes the shoulders, arms, and fingers moving in relation to the waist, legs, and feet and encompasses the entire sphere of activity. Now, with the mind focused on these principles, imagine continuing through not only the rest of the thirty-seven postures but all the movements of the taijiquan form. When one learns taijiquan in this manner, these yin-yang aspects are incorporated into the taijiquan sequence in the order following the creation path. Therefore, as in the *Yijing*, when the development of polarity reaches completion in the sixty-four hexagrams, all the archetypal yin-yang aspects are now in place. The final materialization of the creative path here would be to apply this development either in a martial or healing situation or to use these principles in daily life. At this point of completion, the return path begins to establish these yin-yang aspects within the sequence on a deeper level in which each of these basic aspects, from the most basic to the most complex, is understood as the basis within the next level. This process connects the expression of the entire sequence to its most basic foundation. The focused mind (*yi*) and body (*shen*) then discovers that the sequence is founded upon more and more basic principles.

Image	Stage	Weight Shift	Movement in Classics	Substantial/ Insubstantial			
No-thing	Wuji	None	None	None	← 0	Three-	
Point	Taiji	None	Breath-Joints	None	← 1	Dimensional	
Line	Yin-Yang	In the feet	Rooted in Feet	Horizontal	← 2	Weight Shift	
Circle	Yin-Yang Interpenetration	To the waist	Directed by the waist	Horizontal & vertical	← 3		
Sphere	Manifestation	To the fingers	Flowers in the hands	Horizontal, vertical, & forward	← 4		

This process of discovery changes the performer into an observer deeply anchored in the still center of a heart now in resonance with the universe and at "one with the Dao." By practicing the choreographed and conscious sequence of taijiquan, our minds become aware, not so much of the peripheral phenomenal world, which is the realm of the "small person," but the perceiver of the whole of motion itself that lies within as our immortal spirit. We now have a map for mind and body that can act as a ritualized procedure with which we can, at any moment, return to where we started. By keeping the heart/mind on the polarities of yin-yang instead of the periphery of the external world, it is easier for the heart/mind to become aware of itself where, in the empty stillness of its center, the cosmic Source is found.

Alchemy, Rooting, and the Development of Jing

In their observations of heaven and earth's permutations, the ancient Chinese became aware of the polarity between transience and long life, the nurturance of which has been an overriding concern of the Chinese, especially the Daoists, since antiquity. There have been many phrases over the centuries that depict this fascination, including: *bao shen* (preservation of the visible individual); *nan lao* (to retard the advance of old age), which implies the retardation of senility; *que lao* (warding off old age); and *wu si* (deathlessness), all of which are "exemplified ... in the common greeting and toast *wansui* 'May you live 10,000 years!'" (Knoblock, 1988: 114). The practices associated with these concepts, including alchemy (*jin dan*), a term first seen in Ge Hong's *Baopuzi* (265–419) (Barnes, 1936: 453), were the forefathers of both taijiquan and modern-day qigong.

Chinese alchemy consists of both exoteric (*waidan*) and esoteric (*neidan*) aspects. Exoteric alchemy works with chemical substances in the laboratory to refine what is called the "elixir," which supposedly confers immortality upon those who take it. Esoteric alchemy, also called inner alchemy, works to refine the elixir within the human body through meditation. Both types of Chinese alchemy are fundamentally concerned with blending the polarities of matter and spirit so that each contains something from, and is transformed by, its opposite. This process not only spiritualizes, or vitalizes, matter, but also materializes, or concentrates, the spirit as well. Central to this idea is what the alchemists called the "three treasures": *jing, qi,* and *shen*, which are three different polar states of the life-force. *Jing* corresponds to earth, is the most material, and is stored in the kidneys and bones; *shen* corresponds to heaven, is the most spiritual, and is stored in the heart; and *qi* is in between, corresponding to man, and associated with the spleen and pancreas. Heaven, earth, and man were considered the cosmic triad in which heaven and earth come together, due to the man's participation, to form what is known as the "three powers" (*san cai*) (Bodde, 1991: 112).

The system of correspondence between the three treasures and the three powers also integrates with the system of the "five phases" (fire, soil, metal, water, and wood), which adds an additional dynamic to the three powers system in the same way that the equinoxes add a harmonizing dynamic to the more extreme polarities of the summer and winter solstices in the seasonal cycle.[3] These three systems blend so that the three treasures and three powers connect with the five phases and their more comprehensive associations, e.g., the primary organs of the body as well as specific emotions, psychic counterparts, and virtues. Thus, earth, representing matter, is associated with water, the kidneys, fear, will, and wisdom. In contrast, heaven, representing spirit, is associated with fire, the heart, elation or giddiness, spirit (*shen*, conscious awareness), and the ritualization of social relations and behavior. Between heaven and earth, the central harmonizing level of man is associated with soil, the spleen and pancreas, worry, intention, and trustworthiness.

Qualities of the Three Powers & Five Phases					
Three Powers	Phase	Organ	Emotion	Psychic Counterpart	Virtue
Heaven	Fire	Heart	Elation	Consciousness	Ritual
Man	Soil[3]	Spleen	Worry	Intention	Trustworthiness
Earth	Water	Kidneys	Fear	Will	Wisdom

When the ancient Chinese examined the creation path (*sheng dao*) of the "small man," they realized that this path naturally reaches an extreme in which its very manifestation becomes worldly attachment. At this point, psychic loss as well as the loss of virtue prevail and the connection to the Source wears thin and breaks. In contrast, the return path (*fu dao*) of the "great man" embraces the void at the heart of Self, in which one's virtue and psyche are regenerated through a spontaneous process. The *Daodejing* describes the spirituality of the great man thusly (Wu, 1961: 9):

> Heaven lasts long, and Earth abides. What is the secret of their durability? Is it not because they do not live for themselves [i.e., worldly pursuits] that they can live so long? Therefore, the Sage (*sheng ren*) wants to remain behind, but he finds himself at the head of others; reckons himself out but finds himself safe and secure. Is it not because he is selfless [i.e., in his non-pursuit of the world] that his Self is realized?

It appears the creative process itself, especially the separation of heaven and earth from the Great Void, automatically contains within it the seeds of its own dissolution. According to the *Huainanzi*, a Daoist text of 139 BCE (Girardot, 1983: 148):

> The pure yang (*qi*) drifted up and became heaven; and the heavy and turbid congealed downwards and became earth.... Heaven and earth

unified their essence (*jing*) making yin and yang. Yin and yang blended and circulated their essence and produced the four seasons; and the four seasons in scattering their qi produced the ten thousand things.

In as much as yin and yang continue to blend with each other in the ongoing creation of life, the initial seed of separation continues to occur as well. After all, life and death are both aspects of yin and yang. This happens because the yin and yang, light and heavy, elements (meaning especially *jing* and *shen*) reach an extreme point at which they simultaneously recycle and interpenetrate to maintain the life form and separate from the body to maintain their connection with the Dao. After a period, the amount lost is more than that regained so that the spirit and body separate and death results.

The *Huainanzi* explains how the loss of spirit occurs (Roth, 1991: 643):

When perception comes in contact with external things, preferences are formed.... When preferences are formed, perception is enticed by externals, and one cannot return to the self [which is, then,] destroyed.

The progression of perception to preference ultimately leads to lust, greed, pride, fame, fortune, and pleasure, and becomes the ancient formula describing the path of the "small man." The ancients thought that the loss of *jing* (physical) and *shen* (spirit) through this progression was automatic unless there was some conscious intention to rectify it. The dissolution results in the water phase through the abuse of will so that *jing* leaks out below in the form of urinary incontinence, loss of sexual vitality, and senility. The dissolution results in fire when the spirit burns itself out above in direct proportion to one's indulgence, creating insomnia, heart disease, and loss of self through the ego's attachment to deluded thoughts, attitudes, and beliefs. Chapter 12 of the *Daodejing* admonishes (Wu, 1961: 15):

The five colours blind the eye.
The five tones deafen the ear.
The five flavors cloy the palate.
Racing and hunting madden the mind.
Rare goods tempt men to do wrong.
Therefore, the Sage takes care of the belly, not the eye.[4]
He prefers what is within to what is without.

And again, in Chapter 52 (Wu, 1961: 73):

All-under-Heaven have a common beginning [the Source].
This Beginning is the Mother of the world.
Having known the Mother, we may proceed to know her children

[the flowers of creation], we should go back [return]
and hold on to the Mother [renew ourselves in the Source] . . .
Block all the passages!
Shut all the doors!
And to the end of your days, you will not be worn-out.
[This refers to sense perception in pursuit of worldly desires.]
Open the passages! Multiply your activities!
And to the end of your days you will remain helpless
[The plight of the small man indeed].

The alchemists realized that if they could recycle more of their yin-yang elements, they could prolong life, perhaps even to the extreme state of "deathlessness" that they so ardently sought and attain the Dao. Thus, they needed to ensure that yin and yang continued their immortal interplay and that *jing* and *shen* did not leak away. Therefore, the exoteric alchemists came up with the idea of a closed container in which they would bury alchemical ingredients underground so that they could not leak away and, therefore, be completely transformed in their interactions with one another (Needham, 1956: 4–6). The internal alchemists followed the same idea but used their intention (*yi*) to contain the alchemical process within the human body. We can also see this idea at work in Chinese herbalism in the most important kidney-strengthening formula, the "Six Flavor Rehmannia Decoction." This important formula uses only six herbs and focuses on the lead herb, Rehmannia, to create the physical and mental stillness so important for the kidneys and the water phase as well as for the practice of taijiquan. The ancient herbalists recognized that even the absolute stillness produced by Rehmannia could leak away so they included the astringent herb Cornus to contain Rehmannia's stillness (Kaptchuk, 1996).

We can also find this idea of containing the *jing* and *shen* in the *Taiji Classics*, in which the *yi* (psychic counterpart of the "power man," the phase soil, and the organs spleen and pancreas) takes on the function of container (Yang, 1987: 214):

Up and down, forward and backward,
left and right, it's all the same.
All of this is done with the Yi....
Elsewhere, the *Classics* build on this same idea (Yang, 1987: 228):
[Throughout your] entire body,
your mind [*yi*] is on the Spirit of Vitality
[*jing shen*],[5] not on the [*qi*].

In taijiquan, it is easier to understand how intention (*yi*), as a closed container, can preserve and develop the *jing* and *shen* through the standing postures in which movement is reduced to its extreme slowness. Whereas the taijiquan sequence is characterized by continuous and repetitive motion through its thirty-seven basic postures, the standing postures are characterized by holding any one of these postures for an extended period (five to sixty minutes). What is most readily perceived while doing any of these postures is that they are difficult, if not impossible, to hold for more than a few minutes with muscular force alone. And yet a common, traditional way is for a beginner to hold these postures for up to an hour before any further work involving movement in the sequence is to be done. To achieve this, it is necessary to let go of muscular strength to go deeper in the body to the tendons, ligaments, and finally into the bones. In Chinese medicine, the bones are associated with the kidneys, the "earth power," and the water phase. The kidneys are the source of *jing*, which is stored, among other places, inside the bones in the marrow. The *Taiji Classics* say: "Condense (*lian*, literally draw together, *qian*, with the breath, *qian qi*) the qi into the marrow (*sui*) [or center of the bones]" (Yang, 1987: 234). The process of "condensing" *jing* into the bones in the standing postures is like storing more and more energy in a battery. At a certain point the *jing* and bones resonate with the earth's qi and one's deep root is established (Clay, 1996).

The containment of fire revolves around what in alchemy is called the fusion of *kan* and *li*. Kan and li are the names of the *Yijing* trigrams for water and fire and represent the third stage of manifestation, after the initial interpenetration of yin and yang as heaven and earth, but prior to the creation of the hexagrams or even tangible things. In the body, *li* is in the top, heart region and *kan* is in the kidney region below. According to the *Yijing*, hexagram 64, "Before Completion" (Wilhelm, 1967: 249):

> When fire, which by nature flames upward, is above,
> and water, which flows downward, is below,
> their effects take opposite directions and remain unrelated.

The opposing directions of water and fire in this position is that of dissipation and separation. The archetypal stages of the creation path are characterized by yin-yang interpenetration, but once materialization has been achieved, the yin-yang principles gradually lose their attraction for each other and tend to go their separate ways, leaving one's existence "in a rather dubious state" (Wilhelm, 1967: 15). The purpose of the *kan* and *li* method is to return the opposing tendencies of water and fire to their original interpenetration. It does this by bringing the fire essence below that of water so that fire can steam the water essence into qi, which can then later become spirit, while bringing water to bear on fire so that the volatile spirit is subdued. Through this interpenetration, the opposing energies of water and fire, heaven and earth, are "returned" through the taiji gate to their central Source (e.g., *Dao*).

If the storage of *jing* in the bones is like the charging of a battery, then its transformation into spirit is like a generator. In the standing postures, while one sinks the *yi* and qi into the bones to concentrate the *jing*, one's conscious awareness is lowered automatically into its associated water realm. The result is that the heart/mind is stilled while the *jing* is increased. Stilling the mind and increasing the *jing* is also typically achieved through acupuncture and Chinese herbal medicine. As such, these practices are, along with these standing postures, an introduction into the alchemical *kan* and *li* procedures.

Placing the bones into the earth, if you will, to attract the *shen* is also a practice found in ancestor worship, especially in *feng shui* and its utilization in the ancient Chinese grave-siting practices. The ancients practiced both primary and secondary burials. The primary burial involves a process of one to two years, the purpose of which is to rot the flesh. After the flesh decays, the bones, which contain the ancestor's essence, are then dug up and placed in a container and reburied in a place where the bones are kept dry (Granet, 1930: 332). After they were placed in jars for secondary burial, the ancestors' bones were called "yellow gold," a name referring to alchemy and the transmutation of matter to spirit (Freedman, 1966: 29).[6] According to the *Zang Shu* or *Burial Book of Qiu Bu* (276–324 CE), the bones of the ancestors resonate with heaven and earth qi as well as with Dao itself. This resonance is then directed toward the living descendants, who thereby receive various benefits from both the ancestral spirits and their connection to the cosmic source (March 1978: 29).

Chinese alchemy is derived from these much older practices of ancestor worship in which the interrelation between matter and spirit in relation to longevity and immortality practices first became important. To understand these interrelationships more completely regarding the development of *shen* in taijiquan, we will now explore the connection of these ideas to sacrifice and ritual in the context of not only ancestor worship, but also the later development of Confucianism and Daoism, and finally the connection of each to the development and practice of taijiquan some thousand years later.

Sacrifice and Ritual in the Development of Shen

The practice of ancestor worship involves making an earthly and tangible offering, usually in the form of food and drink served in sacred vessels, to the spirits and ultimately their connection to *Dao* to secure *de* (i.e., their wisdom, blessing, and protection). Therefore, sacrificial offerings symbolize man in his mediating role between heaven and earth for the purpose of securing blessings.

Chinese ancestor worship attempts to contain the spirit(s) (bring them down) through the sacrifice of earthly, material things that alchemically represent the *jing* in the human body. Alchemy reiterates the earlier idea of external sacrifice found in Chinese ancestor worship but does so internally within the body and mind through the conversion of *jing* to spirit via the intermediary level of qi and intention (*yi*). Whereas in alchemy what "contains" the spirit(s) is *kan* and *li*, in Chinese ancestor worship it is what the ancient Chinese also called *li* but signified with a different character meaning ritual. Both *li*, the trigram and the ritual, relate to fire in the five-phase system of correspondence that associates them both with the heart and spirit. Whereas the sound and association with the five phases of these two *li*'s is similar, there are also relevant differences. *Li*, the trigram, also carries the meaning of separation, leaving, and distance (Weiger, 1965: 617), which reflects the inherent scattering tendency of fire as discussed above, whereas ritual (*li*) connotes the containment of fire through sacrificial activity. In the Shang Dynasty, enormous attention was given to every conceivable detail of the royal sacrifice. These details were carefully orchestrated to correspond to seasonal and cosmic (astrological) events as well as to the ancestor or spirit to whom the sacrifice was directed. Thus, tremendous significance was given to the colors one wore, the kinds of nourishment one ate and drank, as well as to the specific actions and words that were used at specific times (recall the definition of the *ji* of "taiji" where the *wu* [shaman], to make life meaningful enough to bring the spirit[s] down, had to make his words and actions congruent).

Later, in the Zhou Dynasty (1122–255 BCE), Confucius made ritual into a virtue and, in so doing, made *li* (and *shen*) available to the common person by defining it as one of the three main aspects in the development of the "great man." For Confucius, it was not enough to simply perform the mechanics and technique of ritual, however perfectly that could be done. For ritual to truly qualify as Confucius' *li*, it had to be performed with great intention, but even more importantly, with the conscious awareness and feeling that characterize *shen*. Even though ritual contained aspects of mechanical actions, true ritual (*li*), required the presence of spirit. The intention behind Confucius' *li* was to create a symbolic learning situation, not unlike taijiquan, that would prepare his disciples for life in the everyday world by bringing something sacred to the mundane.

If you think about it, most of life is concerned with mechanical activity, and in the mundane world it is easy to become preoccupied with these affairs. You must up, get dressed, brush your teeth, cook your food, wash the pots, get to and from work, say hello, say good-bye, and on and on before any otherwise "meaningful" activity ever takes place. In his emphasis on *li*, Confucius was the first to realize the importance of a Zen-like "presence of mind" in the simple activities of daily life, e.g., chopping wood, carrying water, etc. Everyone has probably noticed that, in times of emotional stress (such as in great joy, grieving, anger, fear, worry, or even boredom), it is sometimes difficult to be fully present. Instead, the heart/mind (locus of the *shen*) drifts off toward an external image that may or may not correspond to what is happening. If one becomes traumatized into, or by, one of these emotions, one will then develop attitudes and beliefs about life that will make one prone to react to these attitudes and beliefs about life instead of responding directly to life itself. These false images spend the *jing* as the will chases illusory goals down wasteful paths that bear no return. According to Confucius, in times like these, *li* is what creates the container for spirit, keeping it linked to its surroundings, so that it can appropriately respond to the external world and thereby receive the blessings and protection (*de*) that Dao has to offer without losing itself either to the external world or one's imagination of it.

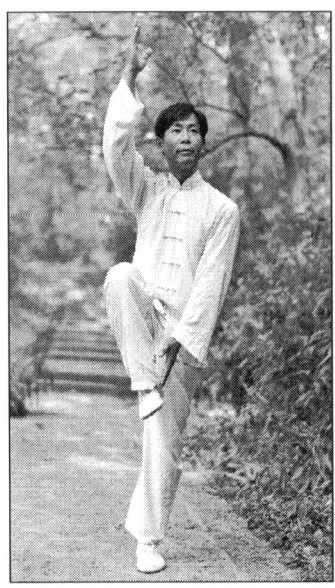
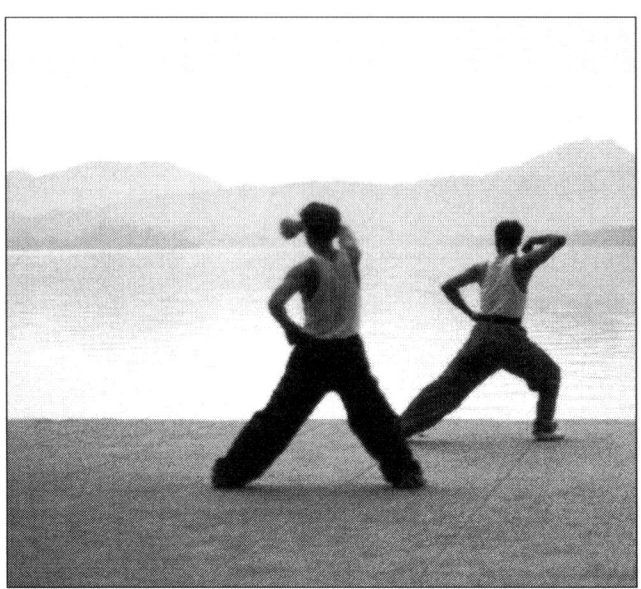

Left: Xia Tao, President of the Hangzhou Wushu Association, practices a variety of taijiquan styles. He embodies the spiritual traditions of each style. Photography courtesy of D. Mainfort. Right: Taijiquan in Hangzhou, China. People gather along West Lake every morning before dawn to practice taiji and other exercises. The approach is holistic, combining traditions conducive for the mind, body, and spirit. Photograph by M. DeMarco.

Like alchemy, ritual contains spirit (*shen*) in the process of its transformation from *jing* and qi. If in the standing postures we build up a great quantity of *jing* and qi only to squander it away again in the transformation to spirit because there is nothing to contain it, then we not only lose the spirit, but the *jing* as well. This is a dangerous situation because the *jing* is the essence of material existence. If the heart's spirit is not trained to identify with its greater source in emptiness, external cravings will arise that lead one out to squander the *jing* in even greater amounts than before training because there simply is more power to waste. The irony is that, in doing so, what should become empty (the heart) now becomes full, whereas what should have been full (the kidney *jing*) becomes empty.

There is a fail-safe to this drawback built into the taijiquan sequence due to its embodiment of ritual. After all, taijiquan is a ritualized performance. Not only must one repeat the same sequence each time it is performed but do so with intention and spirit. This means that one must coordinate the opening and closing of the breath with the opening and closing of the joints, the three-dimensional movement from substantial to insubstantial and back again in the six directions throughout the progression of the thirty-seven postures and 108 or so movements. Performance on this level, as a starting point, certainly transcends mechanical action. The mind is unified with the body, the right (creative) and left (structured through ritual) sides of the brain are brought into balance, spirit and matter are coordinated, and heaven and earth are reunited through the return to the Source via the taiji (ridge) pole. In the *Taiji Classics*, it says that where the heart/mind goes the qi will follow (Weiger, 1965: 617).

(Throughout your) entire body, your mind [*yi*]
is on the Spirit of Vitality [*jing shen*], not on the [*qi*].
[If concentrated] on the [*qi*], then stagnation.
A person who concentrates on [*qi*] has no *li* [strength];
a person who cultivates [*qi*] [develops] pure hardness [power].

"That which goes against the Way will come to an early end."

– Laozi, Ch. 55

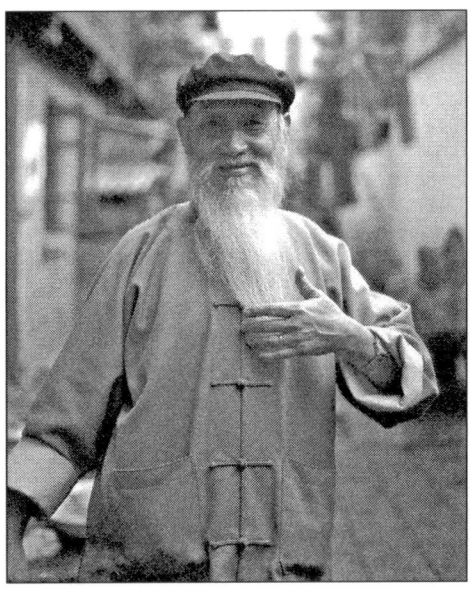

In Yunnan province, a man on the streets of Kunming city
proudly displays his long white beard. A long beard,
like long noodles, is a symbol of longevity.
Photograph by M. DeMarco.

This means that when one keeps the intention focused on the *jing shen* (an aspect of spirit) instead of the qi, or any other phenomena that may occur in practice, what develops is spirit.

At this point, taijiquan practice turns into play as the spontaneous movement of qi expressing itself naturally from its source is experienced. The *Taiji Classics* speak thusly of this spontaneity (Yang, 1987: 232):

The true nature of the Heart [*xin xing*] as well as the Intention [*yi*] should be calm [*jing*], and then spontaneity [*zuran*] will miraculously [*ling*] appear from nowhere [*wu*].[7]

This calmness (*jing*), or quiescence, is a Daoist technical term used to refer to the root state preceding birth. According to the *Zhuangzi* (Rickett, 1960: 227),

From emptiness comes quiescence; from quiescence comes movement; and from movement comes attainment. From quiescence comes non-activity [*wuwei*, stillness] and when [the ruler] [Heart] is non-active, those in charge of affairs may assume their responsibilities.

There are several paradoxes at play here through which apparently simple things turn to their opposite. Turning away from the outward directed path of life to the path of return creates not death, but an everlasting spiritual life. Turning away from the fire-like, externally directed movement of spirit to embrace the earthliest energy of *jing*, provides the foundation and perpetuation of spirit. Placing one's spirit in a "container" through the ritualization of the taijiquan sequence results in the deepest and most comprehensive level of spontaneity revered by the ancient masters and saints. Perhaps these paradoxes are symbolized in the legendary creation of taijiquan through the battle between the bird and the snake. After all, these are, in fact, the traditional Chinese symbols of the water and fire interaction discussed above.

Notes

1. This progression follows what is called the binary sequence, in which each level multiplies itself by two, i.e., 1, 2, 4, 8, 16, 32, etc.
2. Translation is mine.
3. The wood and metal phases fit here in their association with man but are, however, irrelevant to this discussion.
4. The Chinese word "belly" (*fu*) rhymes with "return" (*fu*) and is also etymologically similar. The belly, or *dantian* (literally "elixir field"), is the locus classicus of Daoist meditation (Weiger, 1965).
5. I prefer translating the term *jing shen* as "concentrated awareness."
6. Alchemy was often called the art of the "yellow and white," with yellow referring to gold and white to silver. Gold and silver were two of the main symbols for yang and yin respectively.
7. Translation is mine.

Pinyin	Wade-Giles	Chinese
bagua	pa^1 kua^4	八卦
bao shen	pao^3 shen^1	保身
can	ts'an^1	參
da ren	ta^4 jen^2	大人
dantian	tan^1 t'ien^1	丹田
dao	tao^4	道
de	te^2	德
di huang	ti^4 huang^2	地黃
dong	tung^4	動
er	erh^4	二
feng shui	feng^1 shui^3	風水
fu	fu^4	復
fu	fu^4	腹
fu dao	fu^4 tao^4	復道
gen	ken^1	根
gua	kua^4	卦
huang jin	huang^2 chin^1	黃金
hundun	hun^4 tun^4	混沌
ji	chi^2	極
jin dan	chin^1 tan^1	金丹
jing shen	ching^1 shen^2	精神
jing	ching^1	精
jing	ching^4	靜
junzi	chün^1 tzu^3	君子
kou	k'ou^3	口
li	li^3	禮
li	li^2	離
lian	lien^4	斂
ling	ling^2	靈
mu	mu^4	木
nan lao	nan^2 lao^3	難老
nei dan	nei^4 tan^1	內丹
qi	ch'i^4	氣
qian	ch'ien	欠
qian	ch'ien	僉
quan	ch'üan^2	拳
que lao	ch'üeh^4 lao^3	卻老

Pinyin	Wade-Giles	Chinese
ren	jen^2	人
san cai	san^1 ts'ai^2	三才
shen	shen^2	神
sheng ren	sheng^1 jen^2	聖人
sheng dao	sheng^1 tao^4	生道
shi	shih^2	實
shou	shou^3	手
sui	sui^3	髓
taijiquan	t'ai^4 chi^2 ch'üan^2	太極拳
tai ji	t'ai^4 chi^2	太極
tai xu	t'ai^4 hsü^1	太虛
tian di	t'ien^1 ti^4	天地
tu	t'u^3	土
wai dan	wai^4 tan^1	外丹
wan sui	wan^4 sui^4	萬歲
wan wu	wan^4 wu^4	萬物
wu	wu^1	巫
wu	wu^2	無
wu ji	wu^2 chi^2	無極
wu si	wu^2 ssu^3	無死
wu wei	wu^2 wei^2	無為
xiang	hsiang^4	象
xiao ren	hsiao^3 jen^2	小人
xin	hsin^4	信
xin xing	hsin^1 hsing^4	心性
xu	hsu^1	虛
yang sheng	yang^3 sheng^1	養生
yi	i^2	儀
yi	i^4	意
you	yu^4	又
yuan	yüan^2	元
zhang sheng	chang^3 sheng^1	長生
zhen ren	chen^1 jen^2	真人
zhi	chih^4	志
zhi	chih^4	智
zhu	chu^3	主
ziran	tzu^4 jan^2	自然

Bibliography

Barnes, W. (October 1936). Diagrams of Chinese chemical apparatus. *Journal of Chemical Education*, 453.

Bodde, D. (1991). *Chinese thought, society, and science: The intellectual and social background of science and technology in pre-modern China.* Honolulu: University of Hawaii Press.

Clay, A. (August 6, 1996). Personal interview.

Dhiegh, K.A. (1973). *The eleventh wing: An exposition of the dynamics of the i ching for now*. New York: Dell Publishing Company.

Feng, Y.L. (1952). *A history of Chinese philosophy, vol. 1*. (D. Bodde, Trans.). Princeton: Princeton University Press.

Freedman, M. (1966). *Chinese lineage and society*. London: University of London, The Athlone Press.

Girardot, N. (1983). *Myth and meaning in early Taoism: The theme of chaos (huntun)*. Berkeley: University of California Press.

Granet, M. (1930). *Chinese civilization*. (K. Innes and M. Brailsford, Trans.). London: Kegan Paul, Trench, Tribner and Co. Ltd.

Kaptchuk, T. (1996). A course in Chinese herbalism. Unpublished course notes. Arlington, VA.

Needham, J. (1956). *Science and civilization in China, Vol. 5*. Cambridge: Cambridge University Press.

Knoblock, J. (1988). *Xunzi: A translation and study of the complete works, vol. 1, books 1–6*. Stanford: Stanford University Press.

March, A. (1978). The winds, the waters and the living qi. *Parabola* 3/1: 29.

Meyer, J. (1976). *Peking as a sacred city*. Taipei: Oriental Culture Service.

Rickett, W. (1960). An early Chinese calendar chart: Kuan-tzu, Book III, Chapter 8. *T'oung Pao Archives*, 48: 227.

Robinet, I. (1990). The place and meaning of the notion of taiji in Taoist sources prior to the Ming dynasty. *History of Religions*, 29/4: 381–382.

Roth, H. (1991). Psychology and self-cultivation in early Taoist thought. *Harvard Journal of Asiatic Studies*, 51: 643.

Schipper, K. (1978). The Taoist body. *History of Religions*, 17: 360.

Sung, Z. (1935). *The text of the Yi King* (and its appendixes). Shanghai: The China Modern Education Company.

Thompson, L. (1989). *Chinese religion: An introduction*. Belmont, CA: Wadsworth Publishing Company.

Weiger, L. (1965). *Chinese characters: Their origin, etymology, history, classification and significance*. New York: Paragon.

Wilhelm, R. (1962). *The secret of the golden flower: A Chinese book of life*. New York: Harcourt, Brace and World, Inc.

Wilhelm, R. (1967). *I ching or book of changes*. (C. Baynes, Trans.). New York: Bollingen Foundation.

Wu, J., (Trans.). (1961). *Lao Tzu: Tao te ching*. New York: St. John's University Press.

Yang, J. (1987). *Advanced Yang style tai chi chuan, vol. 1: Tai chi theory and tai chi jing*. Jamaica Plain, NY: YMAA Publications.

Yu, D. (1981). The creation myth and its symbolism in classical Taoism. *Philosophy East and West*, 31: 481.

Chen Weiming, Zheng Manqing, and the Difference Between Strength and Intrinsic Energy
by Robert W. Smith, M.A.

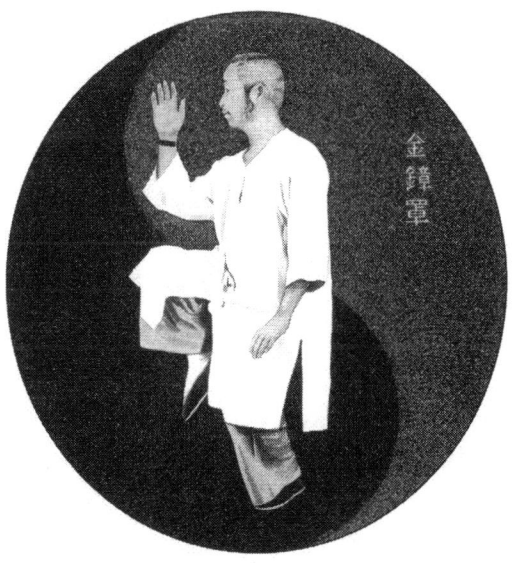

Zheng Manqing in rooster stands on one leg. Illustration by Michael Lane.

When Zheng Manqing began learning taiji from Master Yang Chengfu in Shanghai during the early 1930s, he was a quick study. He had been practicing taiji with another teacher for two years and had conquered the tuberculosis that had been dogging him. At the same time, he learned to acquit himself well during push-hands with larger and more experienced students. This background provided him the impetus to soak up Master Yang's teaching like a sponge. Zheng's rapid progress accelerated even more after he treated and cured Mrs. Yang of a chronic malady, causing Master Yang to give him additional personal instruction.

During this early period, one of the most formidable of Master Yang's senior students, the scholar and writer Chen Weiming, was absent for a time on business. On his return, Master Yang introduced Chen to Zheng and suggested they try conclusions. Chen soon found the meaning of frustration. Every move he made, every push he tried, was unavailing. Newcomer Zheng neutralized him easily: Chen could touch Zheng but couldn't "find" a place on which to use his energy. This astounded the other students, who had stopped to watch, but not Master Yang, who knew young Zheng's ability even then. For his part, Chen Weiming, then near fifty, was impressed and immediately became fast friends with Zheng. The pair then became the intellectual leaders of Master Yang's group, cementing it and spreading the good news of taiji to the populace.

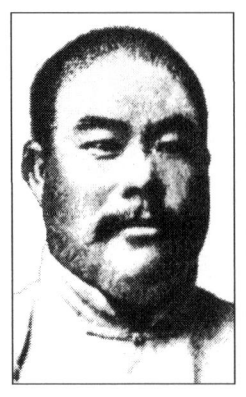 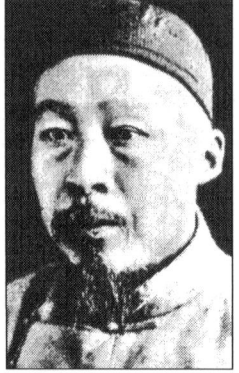 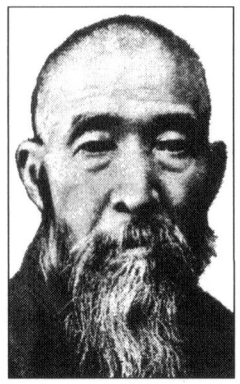

Left: Yang Chengfu, the taiji master.
Center: Chen Weiming, taiji "older brother" of Zheng Manqing.
Right: Sun Lutang, Chen's bagua teacher. Photos courtesy of R. W. Smith.

Chen Weiming Trains under Master Yang

Of all the great boxers Professor Zheng met during his life, none was closer to him than Chen Weiming (1881–1958). Chen came from a gifted family: his father was an intellectual, his mother was a calligrapher, and three of their sons passed the provincial examinations with high marks. Chen was employed by the Qing History Office and was esteemed by all who met him.

After moving north to Beijing from his home in Xishui, Hubei Province, in 1915, Chen began studying xingyi and bagua from famed Sun Lutang. Around 1918 he traveled to Hebei, where he went to the home of Yang Chengfu in Guangping County to ask Master Yang why, if his style of taiji were so good, he didn't teach it more.

Yang replied that he wanted to spread taiji and, since his grandfather Luchan had learned it from the Chens of Chenjiagou in Henan Province, he, Chengfu, would now repay the Chens by teaching Chen Weiming (Chen, 1925: preface).

Chen Moves to Shanghai

After training under Master Yang for seven years, Chen Weiming moved south to Shanghai. In 1925 he started the Achieving Softness Boxing Association (*Zhi Rou Quan She*) and wrote a book called *The Art of Taijiquan* [Taijiquan shu], which was a compilation of Master Yang's taiji teaching.

Chen's move to Shanghai was the first significant appearance of taiji in the south. Just as Yang Luchan had been the first to take the art to Beijing, Chen was the first to take the art to Shanghai. Qian Chongwei, who became one of Chen's leading students, describes his first meeting with Chen:

> Soon I saw a fair, elegant man enter the practice hall and sit on a couch at the side and watch everyone doing their postures. After a while he calmly got up and corrected them. I learned that this was Chen Weiming, the head of the society. I was surprised because I . . . expected

that the head of a boxing group would be strong and vigorous, but Chen appeared to be an intellectual with a leisurely manner.....

—Chen, 1927

Another of Chen's students, Hu Yunyu, learned taiji and sword from Chen for fifteen years. In a preface to Chen's *Taiji jian* [Taiji Sword], Hu admits to having learned a little, saying, "I am now past fifty and my body has gradually stiffened, a fact my heart and mind know, and my tongue can say but, because of taiji and Teacher Chen, one that my body doesn't acknowledge" (Chen, 1927).

By 1929 taijiquan was well known in Shanghai and Chen's society prospered. After a time, he invited Master Yang to visit. Whereas Yang previously had taught in a private or semiprivate venue, here he gradually opened taiji instruction to the public.[1] That same year Chen Weiming also helped his xingyi and bagua mentor Sun Lutang to relocate to Shanghai.[2] Meanwhile, Chen worked on books that stimulated the spread of taiji. Chen's *Art of Taijiquan* (1925) was followed in 1927 by *Taiji Sword*, and in 1929 by *Questions and Answers on Taiji Boxing* [Taijiquan da wen].

Once, while Master Yang was on a trip south, Chen's association brought Master Yang's "older brother" Yang Shaohou to teach for three months.[3] He taught the same large form as his "younger brother" during this time, but privately taught his idiosyncratic, small, trigger-force form too.[4]

Chen Recounts Stories of the Yang Family

In an appendix to his 1927 book *Taiji Sword*, Chen Weiming recorded the following:

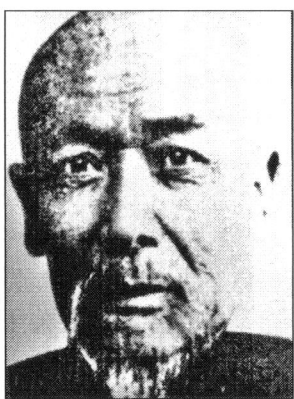

The painstaking and pains-giving Yang Shaohou.
Photo courtesy of R. W. Smith.

There are many schools of boxing, but only the Wudang school is pure *neijia* [inner family] handed down from Zhang Sanfeng.[5] One should use *qi* [internal energy], but not the slightest external force. Yang Luchan, a native of Guangping County in Hebei Province, first learned it from Chen

Zhangxing of Chenjiagou in Henan Province. Yang later taught his sons Banhou and Jianhou. Later, Jianhou taught his sons Shaohou and Chengfu.

It came about this way. Yang Luchan first learned *weijia* [outer family]. But when he heard of the taiji skill of Chen Zhangxing, he sold everything and moved to Chenjiagou in Henan Province to study with him. For several years he practiced with the other students and was beaten soundly by many of them. But late one night, rising to go to the toilet, he heard a noise outside the wall. Peering through the window, he saw some of his classmates being taught secretly by Master Chen. After that, he covertly watched the class every night. The upshot was that one day the students asked him to push-hands, and he was able to roundly defeat them. They told Chen of this, and he approached Yang, saying, "I've watched you for several years. You are honest and diligent. I will teach you the principles of real taiji. Come to see me tomorrow."

When Yang went the next day, Chen sat in a chair, apparently asleep or sick, his head lolling uncomfortably to one side. Yang, with his hands, supported Chen's head for a long time, and after a while, his arms ached from the effort. Finally, Chen appeared to awaken, noticed Yang, and told him to return the next day, as he was too tired to practice. Next day, Yang came again to find Chen apparently still asleep. When Chen awoke, he told Yang to return the next day. When Yang returned on the third day, Chen capitulated. "Very well, I'll teach you now. But you must practice in your room also." After this training, no one could stand before Yang.

Later, Chen assembled his students and scolded them. "I wanted to give my skill to you, but you couldn't get it. Yang was stronger and I didn't want him to get it, but he did. Now he is leaving."

From Chenjiagou, Yang went to Beijing to teach at the home of a rich family. The incumbent teacher there became angry at this intrusion and wanted to fight. Yang agreed but insisted that the master of the house should know first. When told, the master agreed but insisted that the bout be kept sportive rather than mortal. There was to be no killing.

They began. Yang took several steps and stood stock still. The other boxer quickly attacked and, just as quickly, was pushed several meters away. He acknowledged defeat by saluting Yang with a fist salute and they ate together. Immediately afterward Yang decamped, refusing to deprive the other of his job. He taught elsewhere in Beijing, being the first to introduce taiji there.

While gaining fame teaching others, Yang's real vigor was expended on his sons. He taught them many hours daily without stint. Both sons tried to escape, one to become a monk. Neither succeeded and by age twenty both were great experts. A member of the royal family invited Banhou to teach at forty dollars a month, a huge salary then.

In Song County of Hebei, there was a strong boxer surnamed Liu with over a thousand students. Some of these students started a friction between Liu and Banhou, and Liu challenged Banhou to . . . combat.[6] The whole city heard about it and thousands flocked to see the fight. Liu fiercely seized Banhou's wrist. (Yang later said it was like the bite of a dog.) Banhou used *jie jing* (a form of "receiving energy") and snapped his arm out of Liu's vise, causing Liu to fall heavily to the ground. Liu rose and hurried from the arena, while Banhou proudly strutted home to his father.[7] When he told his father of the bout, Yang Luchan smiled coldly and observed, "You did all right, I suppose, but your sleeve is torn off. Do you call this taiji energy?" After that, Banhou's fame spread but he was no longer proud.

Senior Fu Tells of His Experience

Yang Banhou's chief students in Beijing included Chen Xiufeng and Senior Fu. While Chen Weiming never met the former, he was able to visit Fu in Beijing. Though over seventy at the time, Fu looked fifty. In fact, his son, who was fifty, looked like his brother. Nevertheless, he told Chen that he could not teach Banhou's art because he had not taught or practiced it for more than forty years. Of his experiences, Fu said,

> My older brother was a good wrestler, and he taught me some moves every day. Before he joined the army and went off to Gansu Province, he asked me to study wrestling diligently while he was away. Years later he returned and asked me if I had kept up my practice. I responded no, that I was studying taiji from Yang Banhou and that it would not be good to mix the strength of wrestling with the subtle energy of taiji. This so angered my brother that he struck at me powerfully. I quickly countered him with deflect downward, parry, and punch [*ban lan chui*] from taiji, and he fell out the door and into the yard. He couldn't get up for a while and took several weeks to recover. My father berated me and forbade me to practice taiji again. This was unfortunate but I had to obey.
>
> When I was young, Yang Luchan liked me for my hard work. Even after he was past eighty, he practiced taiji every day. He often sat around smoking his long pipe and talking. I remember once he came to my door when it was raining and muddy. When he entered my house, though he had walked through the mire, his shoes were clean as new with no mud on them. This gongfu we called *ta xue wu hen* [to step on snow with no trace]. His son Banhou also had this ability, but few knew this and I saw him do it only once.
>
> The day came when Yang Luchan wrote to all his disciples telling them that he was going on a trip and that he would like to see them before departing. They went to his house, but their suspicions were

aroused when they saw no carriage outside. Yang sat in the middle of the room so all could see and let each man take a turn at trimming his long pipe. For some time, he advised and encouraged them in their pursuit of taiji principles. After a while he wiped his sleeve and passed away while sitting straight.

Yang Banhou also had "floating" gongfu. Away when his beloved seventeen-year-old daughter died, he hurried home to find her coffin nailed shut. He cried and became so agitated that he soared and was suspended eight feet up in the air, much to the astonishment of his disciples. I witnessed him do this gongfu, which we called *fei teng* [flying and soaring].

Chen Weiming Resumes

Banhou and his younger brother Jianhou were reluctant to show the art, believing that trouble follows fame. They were polite and never bellicose. One day a famed southern boxer came to visit Banhou, who was then past sixty. The boxer paid his respects and then, after some friendly words, asked if it were true that Banhou had sticking energy [*zhan*]. Modestly, Banhou said, "My father had this skill. I know a little about it but certainly don't have his skill." The boxer would not be put off and persisted. Banhou asked how he wanted to test him. The visitor suggested that they put bricks two feet apart in a circle and [said], "I will get on the bricks, and you follow with your right hand attached to my back. If your feet leave the bricks or your hand leaves my back, you lose."

Banhou agreed: "Very well. I am old and apt to get dizzy, but since you ask, I will do my best." On the bricks, the boxer began slowly and Banhou followed, concentrating his spirit. The man accelerated and suddenly his body became like a swallow, exquisitely light, and Banhou had to use his "flying" skill to keep up. But try as he might, the man couldn't rid himself of Banhou's hand. Finally, with one quick movement, the man jumped to the roof and turned around to find Banhou gone, leaving no trace. The boxer turned again and there was Banhou, his hand still on the boxer's back. "Let's get down," Banhou said. "You've made me very tired."

Yang Luchan's youngest son, Jianhou, once taught taiji at a military compound. One day, returning there from town, a local strongman attacked him with a club from behind. Jianhou easily deflected the attack and pushed the man ten feet away. Indeed, Jianhou was so skilled he would let a swallow stand on his open hand and prevent it from flying off. Incredibly, Jianhou would "hear" its tiny energy and yield so that the bird would not have the needed base from which to initiate flight.

Yang Luchan's disciple, Wang Lanting, also had great ability, but, alas, died early. Li Binfu, Wang's senior student, inherited a part of his art. Once a robust young boxer from the south visited Li and challenged him.

The boxer had qigong skill and could move chairs and tables without physically touching them. Li, holding a small dog in his left arm, tried to refuse, but the boxer attacked him, giving him no time. He did have time, however, to deftly knock the youth down while not relinquishing his gentle hold on his dog. The southern boxer cried bitterly and left.

I learned taiji from Yang Chengfu for several years. He said: "One must distinguish the pure from the motley. Many practice taiji nowadays, but it is not the real taiji. The real has a different taste and is easily distinguished. With real taiji, your arm is like iron wrapped with cotton. It is soft and yet feels heavy to someone trying to support it. You can feel this in push-hands practice. When you touch an opponent, your hands are soft and light, but he cannot get rid of them. When you attack, it is like a bullet penetrating cleanly and sharply [*gan cui*], yet without using any force. When he is pushed ten feet away, he feels a little movement, but no strength and no pain. In touching him, you don't grab him. Instead, you lightly adhere to him so that he can't escape. Soon his two arms become so sore he can't stand it. This is real taiji. If you use force, you may move him. But it will not be clean and sharp. If he tries to use force to hold or control you, it is like trying to catch the wind or shadows. Everywhere is empty. It can be likened to walking on gourds on the water. You cannot get to where the substantial is. Put simply, real taiji is marvelous.

A Word on the Photographs in Chen's First Book

Because the taiji form photos in Chen Weiming's *Art of Taijiquan* raise questions, let me venture some modest opinions. These photos include fifty pictures of Masters Yang and Chen doing postures, four of Master Yang doing push-hands and *dalü* (large rollback) with Xu Yusheng, and nine of Chen Weiming doing push-hands and dalü with Chen Zhijin (Chen, 1925).[8]

Obviously, not too much can (or should) be made of still photos, and I have chided some westerners for using them to draw sweeping conclusions. But perhaps this needs saying anyway, since these photos puzzled me greatly when I first saw them in Taiwan in 1960. When I asked Professor Zheng about them, he replied that photography was a new and rare thing in China during the twenties and that it took a while for taiji teachers to understand how to use the medium correctly.[9] One senior even suggested Yang and Chen had purposely posed incorrectly so casual readers would not get the real taiji as personal students did. While the same things are said about masters of karate and many other martial arts, I personally doubt this.

Therefore, let's look at these graphics in which both Yang and Chen are doing the same form but, shall we say, differently. First, Yang and Chen both do exceptionally long and deep postures. This is especially noticeable for the smaller Chen, who would have had trouble separating his weight in such low stances. Often both of their backs appear slightly bent, their rear legs fairly straight, and their wrists "broken." Yang often thrusts his chin out, and though better, Chen's head is also awry at times. In bow posture, both turn their rear toes only slightly inward from ninety degrees.

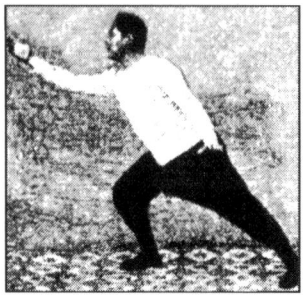 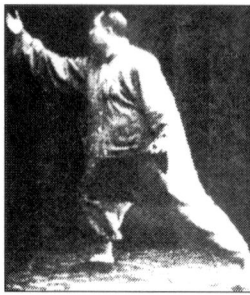

In the early photo (ca. 1918) of diagonal flying,
Yang is not erect, and his rear leg is locked.
In the later photo (ca. 1932), Yang stands straighter,
his left knee is bent a bit, and he appears more relaxed.

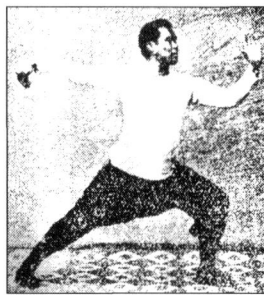 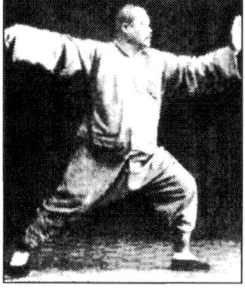

In single whip, Yang's posture is longer—and stiffer—than the relaxed later one.
Although deeper, Yang in the early shot turns his rear foot slightly inward
from ninety degrees but keeps it at ninety degrees in the later one.

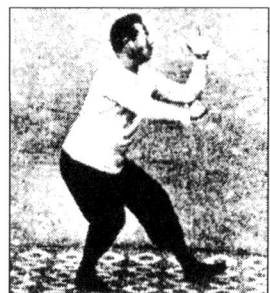 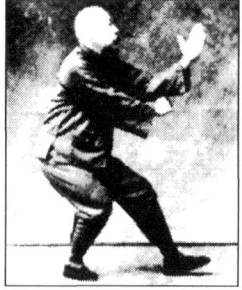

In fist under elbow, Master Yang (ca. 1918) and Chen Weiming (1932)
reflect long, low postures. Yang's head is awry, and neither
is erect nor as relaxed as he could have been.

Some of these postures may not be stiff—though they appear to be so—but they are not quite accurate. Zheng Manqing stressed accuracy. Ben Lo, who was Zheng's first student in Taiwan, has said he was taught privately, posture by posture. That is, Zheng would not teach him a new posture until he had the current one down pat. As part of this training, Zheng taught that the postures had to be done both outwardly and inwardly yin. This confirmed the *Classics* and concealed the function of the form.

This may explain, at least partly, the seeming inaccuracy of some of the Yang/Chen photos. (Though the book was published in 1925, the photos may have been taken as much as a decade earlier.) In other words, they may have posed in the yang aspect, showing function, while Zheng's yin forms deliberately obscured this use. Either that, or they tried to pose the postures just as they did them daily—that is, with more of a yin emphasis—but were then made self-conscious by the camera.

By the time of the photo session for Master Yang's 1934 book (Yang, 1934), his form looks much better (or at least more like we do it now). Yang himself admitted his form had improved much in the interim, even though he had gained ninety pounds. However, the added bulk cost Yang some flexibility, notably on bow postures, in which he is unable to turn his rear foot inward from ninety degrees. While Yang was just too obese to make it, one wonders if this impediment has led many Yang Style teachers unknowingly to teach the bow posture without the turn-in to this day (Yang, 1983; Dong, 1948, 1953).[10]

Where We Come Out

Later in the thirties, Master Yang died (1936), Japan invaded (1937), and the Chinese government retreated westward to Chongqing in Sichuan Province. After the Japanese surrender, Professor Zheng returned to Shanghai from Sichuan and met up with his old friend Chen Weiming, who had also survived the war. Zheng showed Chen the manuscript of his *Thirteen Chapters*, which he had written during the war. Chen was pleased with it, writing in his preface to the published work that it was excellent, kept strictly to Master Yang's original principles, and gave students a fine path to follow. In every respect, he wrote, it accorded with his own *Questions and Answers on Taijiquan*, written in 1929.

In the same preface, Chen stated that Master Yang had given Zheng Manqing all the secret oral transmissions, and that "no one else had ever heard them." He also mentioned that, in Sichuan, Zheng had met "an extraordinary man, studied with him, and made great progress" (Wile, 1985: 1–2).

From the evidence, we know Chen Weiming was exceptional in both the theory and practice of taiji. We've seen his appreciation for the real taiji versus the normal taiji (which is to say the abnormal), and we've seen how he impressed his students. For example, the popular writer Xiang Kairan (Hsiang K'ai-jan), who often used martial art themes in his fiction, recalled Chen's push-hands skill during the twenties in Shanghai. Xiang, who had pushed with such adepts as Master Yang, Xu Yusheng, and Liu Ennuan, wrote of Chen Weiming that, like Master Yang, he liked ward off and press but didn't use power. Instead, he "merely insinuated me lightly into a position from which I could neither dodge nor neutralize" (Hsiang, 1987).

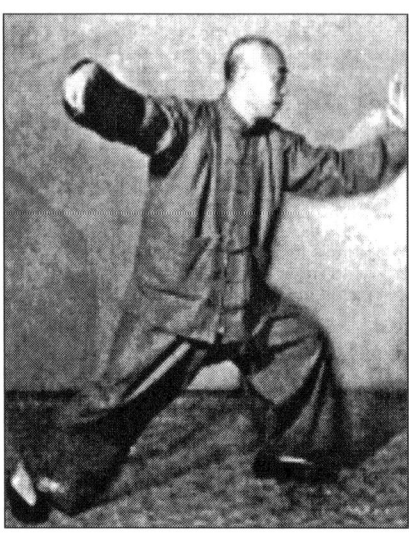

Dong Yingjie in single whip.

Notwithstanding Chen's great abilities, he lacked one thing. Professor Zheng, honest almost to a fault, disclosed it in his *Manran san lun* [Three treatises of Manran], published in Taibei in 1974. In the context of using *jin* (intrinsic energy) from the sinews instead of *li* (strength) from the bones, the Professor wrote, "My classmate Chen Weiming studied taiji for several decades, but when it came to the difference between strength and intrinsic energy, he was not able to get to the bottom of it" (Wile, 1985: 148).

Some may think Zheng's words gratuitous, particularly about such a close friend as Chen. I think he wrote them, however, because principle and truth precede conventional courtesies. The principle of resilient intrinsic energy was so important as to demand it. After all, if his dear friend, Chen Weiming, one of the finest boxers in China,[11] failed to fully understand the difference, then it must be doubly hard for the rest of us.

The idea of intrinsic energy from the sinews is not hard to understand intellectually, but to practice it and express it with your body, that is a far different thing. Zheng Manqing was not gloating over the shortfall of his old friend so much as commiserating over the struggle. Two friends had sought the knowledge, but only one had achieved it.

Acknowledgments

Thanks go to several persons who helped with this article. Warren Conner, Barbara Davis, Russ Mason, and Joe Svinth reviewed the text, Dan and Harry Johnston aided on graphics, and Ben Lo provided much substance. Barbara Davis translated parts of Chen Weiming's works (1925, 1927) that appear with my modifications in this article.

Notes

1. Although more sustained in Shanghai, studio teaching had occurred somewhat earlier in Beijing. The man spearheading it there was Xu Yusheng (1879–1945). A student of Yang Jianhou, Song Shuming, and other greats, Xu was an intellectual greatly respected in Beijing. In 1912 he became vice-director of the Beijing Physical Education Research Association, teaching mainly taiji. In this venue, he was able to invite famed colleagues such as Yang Shaohou, Liu Caijen, Yang Shao, and Wu Jianquan to teach taiji there at least occasionally. In 1921 Xu published a book called *Diagrammatic Explanations of the Taijiquan Postures* [Taijiquan shi tujie]. We can see him in photographs in Chen Weiming's *The Art of Taijiquan* (Chen, 1925: 48, 50).
2. Also in 1928, Wu Jianquan moved with his family from Beijing to Shanghai, where he taught his idiosyncratic Wu style, further establishing Shanghai as a center for taiji. Wu's father, Wu Quanyu, had been a direct student of the famed Yang Banhou (Zee, 1992: 15).
3. Besides Shanghai, Yang also spent periods teaching in Nanjing, Hangzhou, Hankou, and Guangzhou. On these trips, he took along as assistants such men as Wu Huiquan, a 250-pound ex-wrestler, Dong Yingjie, Yang Kairu, Zhang Qinlin, and Fu Zhongwen.
4. When young, Shaohou had been given to his somewhat irascible uncle Banhou as a foster son and acquired some of that man's fiery temperament. This fieriness was reflected in Shaohou's teaching, which many regarded as so harsh that he couldn't keep students. Elsewhere, I've told of Shaohou's suicide in 1929 (Draeger and Smith, 1980: 39). Sources in Taiwan told me he took his life by nailing scissors to a table and then impaling his throat on them. The reason was that one of his students, a high government official, had left him for another teacher. (Doubtless Shaohou's harshness played a part in this departure.) Since then, I've heard a less credible story in which Shaohou, while fencing with his beloved daughter, ran her through. This caused him such grief that he exited with the scissors. As I said, I prefer the more quotidian version to the sensational one and only mention it here to quash the latter with skepticism.
5. Although the story of Zhang Sanfeng as the creator of taiji has little historic weight, both Chen Weiming and Zheng Manqing openly subscribed to it, perhaps in deference to Yang family belief. If so, this seems too much of a kowtow.
6. "T'was ever thus," sayeth the Bard. More frictions and fights were (and are) caused by gossiping students than directly by teachers.
7. If true, it seems significant that Luchan hadn't even bothered to attend the match. This may speak more loudly than the match itself.
8. A longer set of 118 photographs done by Chen is appended at the back of the book. Since he has aged appreciably in these pictures, this set may not have been a part of the 1925 first edition but added in a later edition.
9. Similarly, as far as I know, there were no films made of Vaslav Nijinsky, the greatest dancer of all time. All we have of this artist, who could fly onto the stage

through a window, leap head down with his feet straight up, and soar and hover before descending, are descriptions, posed photographs, and legends. "I am God in the body; everybody has this feeling. Only nobody uses it; I do use it," Nijinsky wrote before dancing his last dance in 1919 and going mad at the age of twenty-nine (Hallander, 1996: 9). I do not mean to compare Nijinsky with Yang but say only that still photographs are inadequate for capturing the movement, look, or essence of either man.

[10] Yang Zhenduo turns in slightly on bow posture, as does Dong Yingjie. However, neither man turns his foot to forty-five, as Zheng taught (Yang, 1983; Dong, 1948, 1953).

[11] Wang Yannian and several other leading lights in Taiwan told me that, excluding Zhang Qinlin and Zheng Manqing, the most skilled of Master Yang's seniors was Chen Weiming. In 1973 Zheng, a man not given to lavish praise, told the New York City class that his elder brother under Master Yang, Li Yaxuan, had extraordinary skill unapproached on the mainland. Ben Lo remembers Zheng speaking glowingly of Li and rating Li's skills higher than Zheng's own.

Bibliography

Chen, W. (1927). *Taiji jian* [Taiji sword]. Shanghai: Self-published.

Chen, W. (1925). *Taijiquan shu* [Art of taiji boxing]. Shanghai: Self-published.

Dong, Y. (1948, 1953). *Taijiquan shi-yi* [An explanation of taiji boxing]. Hong Kong: Commercial Press.

Draeger, D., and Smith, R. (1980). *Comprehensive Asian fighting arts*. Tokyo: Kodansha.

Hallander, A. (25 Jan. 1996). God in the body. *London review of books, 18*(2): 9–10.

Hsiang, K. (Sept.–Oct. 1987). Push-hands. (K. Cohen, Trans.). Bubbling well journal.

Wile, D. (1985). *Cheng Man-ch'ing's advanced t'ai-chi form instructions*. Brooklyn: Sweet Ch'i Press.

Xu, Y. (1921). *Taijiquan shi tujie* [A diagrammatic explanation of the taijiquan postures]. Shanghai: Self-published.

Yang, C. (1934). *Taijiquan ti yong quan shu* [Complete principles and function of taijiquan]. Shanghai: Self-published.

Yang, Z. (1983). *Yang style taijiquan*. Hong Kong: Hai Feng Publishing Co.

Zee, W. (April 1992). *Wu Ying-hua on Wu style. T'ai chi.* Los Angeles: Wayfarer Publications.

Zheng, M. (1974). *Manran san lun* [Three treatises of Manran]. Taibei: Zhonghua-shuju.

Romanization

Pinyin	Wade-Giles	Chinese
bagua	pakua	八卦
Beijing	Peiching	北京
Chenjiagou	Ch'en chia kou	陳家溝
Chen Zhangxing	Ch'en Chang-hsing	陳長興
Chen Weiming	Ch'en Wei-ming	陳微明
Dong Yingjie	Tung Ying-chieh	董英傑
feiteng	fei t'eng	飛騰
Fu Zhongwen	Fu Chung-wen	傅鍾文
Guangzhou	Gaung-chou	廣州
Henan	Honan	河南
li	li	力
Li Yaxuan	Li Ya-hsuan	李雅軒
qigong	ch'i kung	氣功
Sichuan	Szechuan	四川
Sun Lutang	Sun Lu-t'ang	孫祿堂
Wang Lanting	Wang Lan-t'ing	王蘭亭
Wu Huichuan	Wu Hui-ch'uan	武匯川
Wu Jianquan	Wu Chien-ch'üan	吳鑑泉
Wu Quanyou	Wu Ch'uan-yu	吳全佑
xingyi	hsing-i	形意
Yang Banhou	Yang Pan-hou	楊班侯
Yang Chengfu	Yang Ch'eng-fu	楊澄甫
Yang Jianhou	Yang Chien-hou	楊健侯
Yang Luchan	Yang Lu-ch'an	楊露禪
Yang Shaohou	Yang Shao-hou	楊少侯
Yang Zhenduo	Yang Chen-tuo	楊振鐸
Zheng Manqing	Cheng Man-ch'ing	鄭曼青
Zhang Qinlin	Chang Ch'in-lin	張欽霖
Zhang Sanfeng	Chang San-feng	張三丰

• 21 •

Dalü and Some Tigers
by Robert W. Smith, M.A.

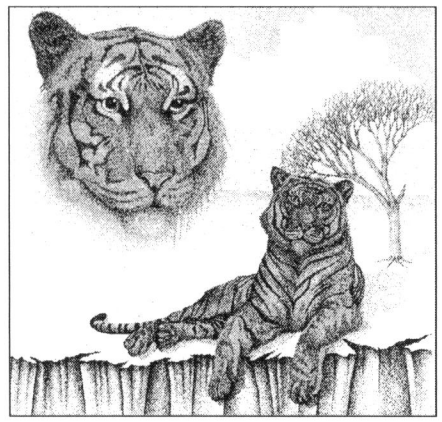

Illustration by Gene Scott.
All photographs courtesy of Robert W. Smith

Other than weapons play, taiji comprises four categories:

- **Basic Solo Form** (*gongjia*, literally "task framework")—having twenty-four, thirty-seven, 108, 128, 150, or more individual postures, depending on the system.
- **Push-Hands** (*tuishou*)—done with a partner in either a fixed–or free–step atmosphere, featuring ward off, rollback, press, and push; oriented largely to the cardinal directions.
- **Large Rollback** (*dalü*)—a set routine with a partner, emphasizing the use of pull (*cai*), split (*lieh*), shoulder strike (*gao*), and elbow strike (*chou*); oriented to the four corners or diagonals.
- **Dispersing Hands** (*sanshou*)—a mock fighting set with a partner in which both use a prearranged series of hand and foot techniques for attacking and defending.

Of these, only the form, the crucible of the art, is done slowly and by oneself. The rest are practiced at a normal or appropriate speed in pairs. The form requires slowness and evenness.[1]

Here I want to dilate on dalü, the shortest of the set exercises. The name is one of those special terms that crept into the taiji patois at an early date. It does not translate very well.[2] Some call it push-hands of the four corners. Close maybe, but not close enough. Sensing hands, which I prefer to push-hands, is a fairly free practice and softly (a word that needs shouting, not murmuring) competitive. It is a disciplined balance, in fact, of the competitive and the cooperative. However, while the play in dalü involves two people, one competes only with oneself. In cooperating and moving in accord with the *Taiji Classics*, both players gain immeasurably.

While Professor Zheng Manqing devoted a few pages to dalü in his seminal *Thirteen Chapters* (1950), he used only five photographs to illustrate the concept (he posed with Li Shoujian).[3] For our book, *T'ai-chi: The "Supreme Ultimate" Exercise for Health, Sport, and Self-Defense* (1967), Professor Zheng provided text and photos done with Liang Dongcai. Because of space constraints, these dalü photos and text were never used. I have incorporated them here. The basic set is done here by Benjamin Lo and me.[4]

Directions and Explanations of Photographs
Directions correspond to Mr. Lo's movements.
The attacker and defender swap roles in photo 11.

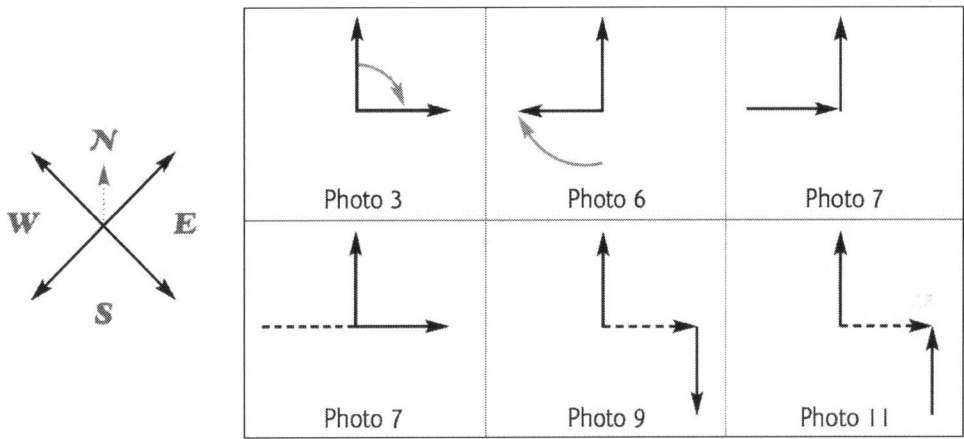

About Dalü

Dalü is usually done at normal speed, but for variety it can be done slow or fast. You and your partner start with your right hands joined, and later round the set out by starting with your left hands joined.

As in push-hands, quantity is less important than quality. Stand upright and relaxed. Though rooted, move lightly with celerity in absorbing, sticking, neutralizing, and countering. Be soft and pliable. No resistance and no letting go. Yield a little and then turn. Breathe naturally through your nose. Most importantly: keep your mind at your navel. The techniques used during dalü include pull (*cai*), split (*lieh*), elbow strike (*chou*), and shoulder strike (*gao*). These four were part of the original taiji set of thirteen postures and supplement the four basic techniques of push-hands, namely ward off (*peng*), rollback (*lu*), press (*ji*), and push (*an*). The remaining five techniques of the original thirteen are associated mainly with "dispersing hands" (*sanshou*), and have to do with the "attitudes" of advancing, retreating, looking left and right, and maintaining one's center.

Doing Dalü

Smith and Lo face each other on the cardinal direction (photo 1). Next, they ward off with their right wrists, the hands forming press (photo 2). Each shifts his weight to his left foot, leaving his right foot empty. (This is the conventional beginning. In real use, Smith has struck at Lo, who blocks the attack with ward off.) Now Smith shifts his weight to his right foot and steps forward with his left while Lo shifts his weight to his right foot and pivots on his left to the right (photo 3). In photo 4 Professor Zheng, right, and Liang Dongcai show Zheng's press unfolding so that his left hand is on Liang's forearm to prevent him from using his elbow strike. In photo 5 Zheng pivots on his left foot while Liang steps forward with his left.

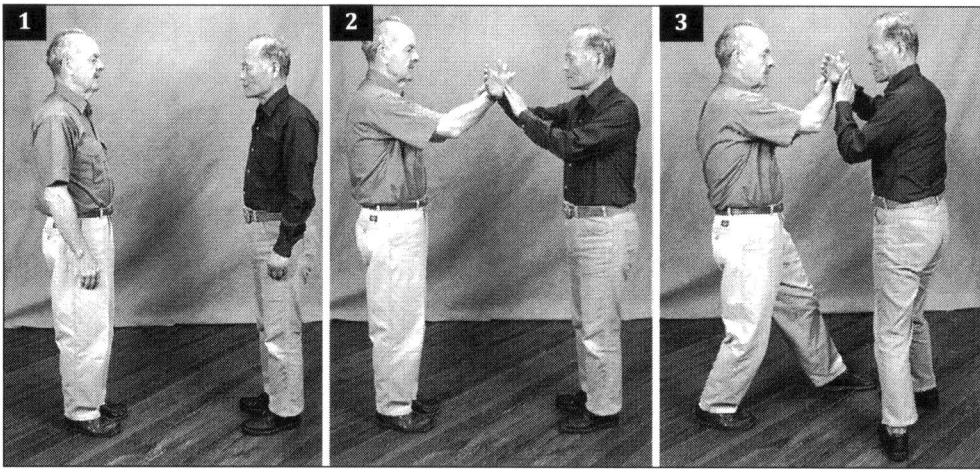

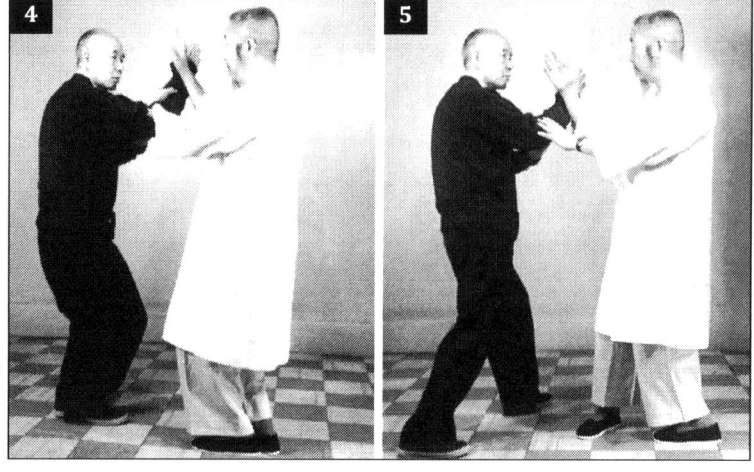

Smith next steps forward with his right foot near Lo's groin, causing Lo to circle his right leg to the rear right corner. Rolling back with his left elbow on Smith's right elbow while pulling Smith's right wrist with the thumb and middle finger of his right hand (photo 6a; 6b is a rear view of the same action).

Next, when Smith neutralizes Lo's pull, Lo circles his right hand rearward and counterclockwise, then back to the front in an attempt to slap Smith's face with his right palm (split) while simultaneously stepping forward with his right foot. As Lo steps forward with split, Smith steps backward with his right foot, bringing his feet together, and warding off Lo's split (photo 7a; 7b is a reverse shot).

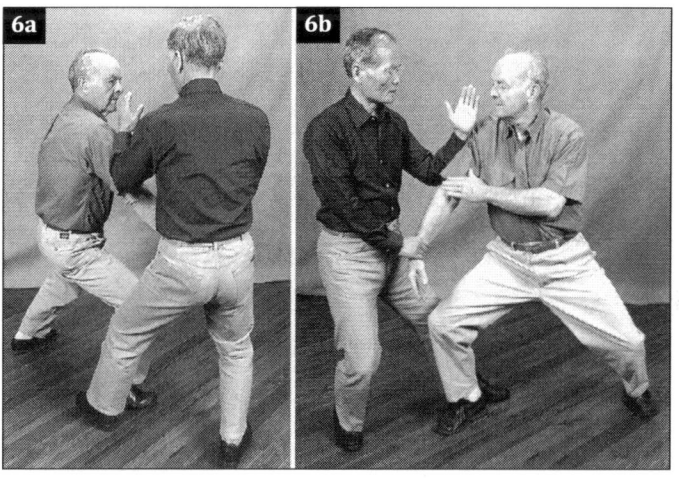

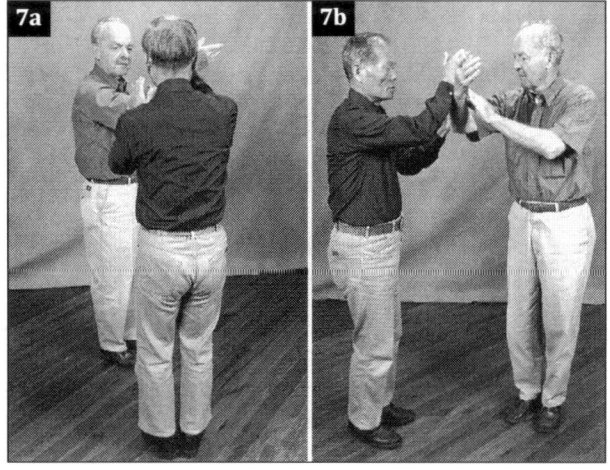

Next, Smith toes his left foot inward and begins to withdraw his right foot to the rear (photo 8) while clasping Lo's right wrist lightly with the thumb and middle finger and pulling him forward using his left elbow on Lo's right elbow in rollback. While this is occurring, Lo is stepping with his left foot and then placing his right foot forward, near Smith's groin, using shoulder strike (photo 9a). Although oriented to a different corner, I have juxtaposed Liang's rollback opposing Zheng's shoulder strike to show Liang's vertical left arm here (photo 9b). In photo 9c, a reverse shot of photo 9a, Smith has neutralized Lo's shoulder strike and is folding down from rollback.

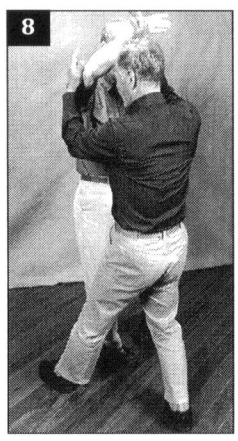

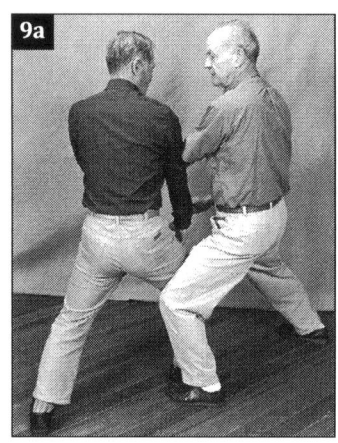

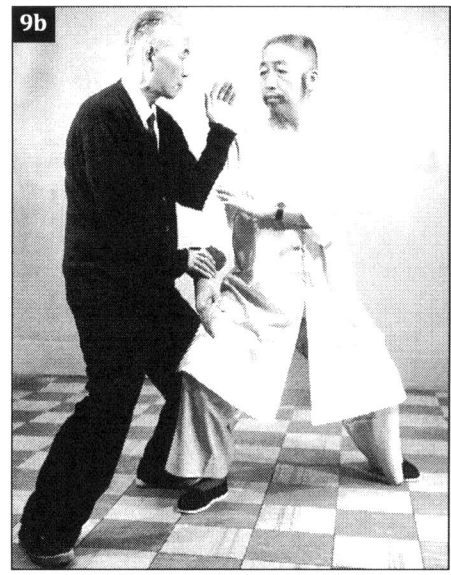

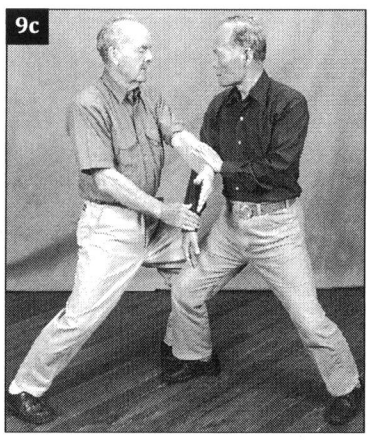

Resuming the proper orientation, Smith takes his right arm back, circling it counterclockwise to the front, attempting to slap (split) Lo's face. Smith's right foot accompanies his strike with a right ward off while stepping back with his right foot to join his left (photo 10; photo 11 shows this posture frozen for function with Zheng in Lo's role and Liang in Smith's but oriented toward a different corner).

In photo 12 Smith steps forward with his left foot and then with his right near Lo's groin. Lo uses rollback, pulling Smith's right wrist lightly with his right thumb and middle finger, and putting his left elbow on Smith's right elbow. This neutralizes Smith's shoulder strike. Lo then withdraws his right hand (photo 13). Now, with Zheng in Lo's role and Liang in Smith's in the correct orientation, Zheng circles his right hand counterclockwise to the rear and then to the front in split, striking Liang's face (photo 14). (Note that their splits, Liang's in photo 11 and Zheng's in photo 14, are frozen to show use, while in the splits done by Lo and Smith, the legs accompany the strike to show form.)

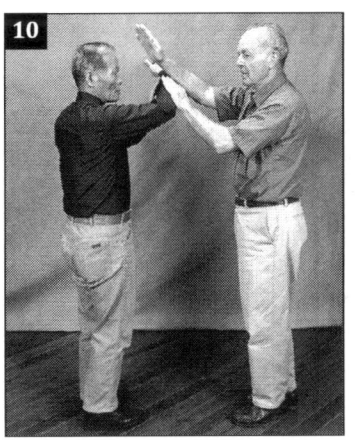
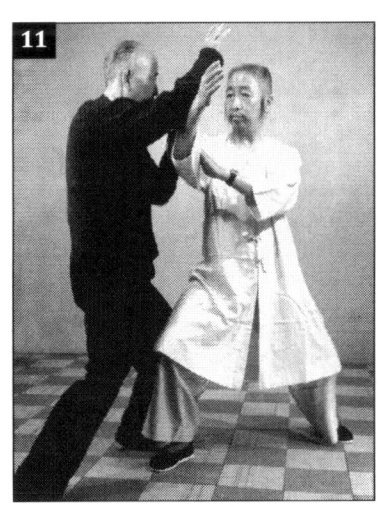
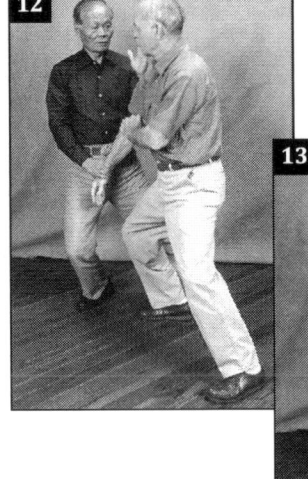
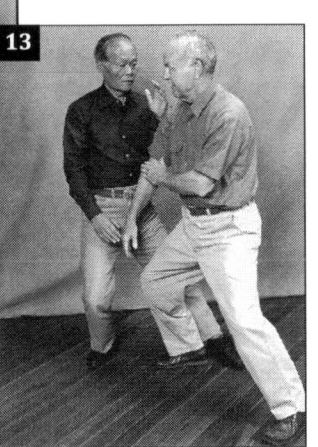
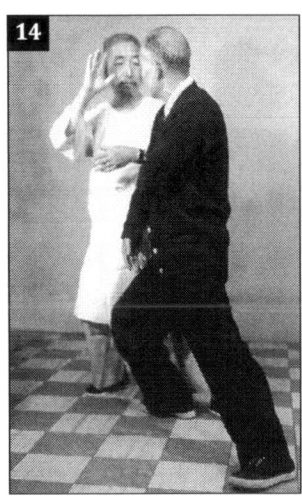

Concluding, as Lo splits, stepping forward with his right foot to join his left, Smith steps back with his right foot to join his left while intercepting Lo's right slap with right ward off (photo 15).

Confucius once said, "If I give you one corner [of a square of a handkerchief, for example], and you cannot find the other three corners for yourself, am I obliged to find them for you?" Here, I have given you dalü done to three of the four corners. You can find the last yourself. And finding, do. And doing, learn. And learning, enjoy.

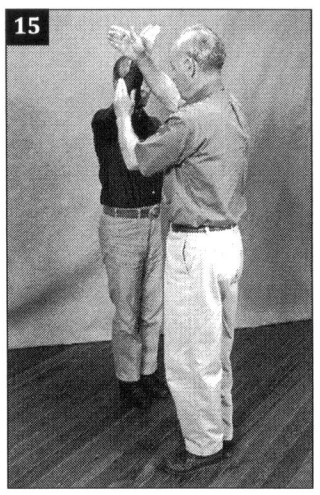 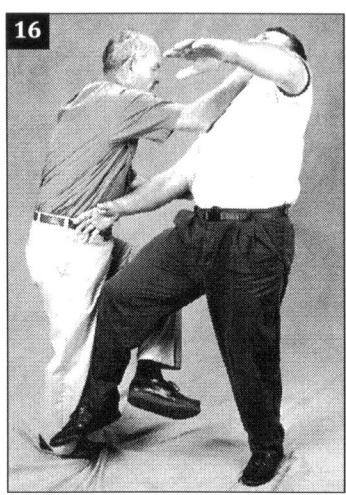

The Uses of Dalü

Like the solo form, dalü is awash with function. In pull, you use the thumb and middle finger to hold your partner's wrist lightly and throw him out. In this regard, it is like brush knee, in which it is contained. In split, when he pushes my elbow, I yield, follow, and neutralize his strength by slapping his head with my palm. One can see this technique in the posture step back and ride the tiger. Elbow strike can be used in step forward, deflect downward, parry, and punch, at the outset of dalü following the initial joining of hands, and in many other postures. Shoulder strike follows lift hands and is applicable whenever the opponent pulls on you.

I mentioned above that split is like step back and ride the tiger. In the latter, however, your left foot is empty, whereas in split it can be full, depending on the circumstances. If empty, your left foot can be used to sweep your opponent's approaching foot in concert with your split (photo 16, step back and ride the tiger). Another tiger posture is embrace tiger and return to mountain. Zheng's short form has three tiger postures that can be used against someone whose split or punch has miscarried. In photos 17 and 18 Zheng ducks Liang's strike, wraps his right arm around Liang's back, and grabs his right knee. He then stands up and upends Liang by pulling sharply upward with both hands to the left.

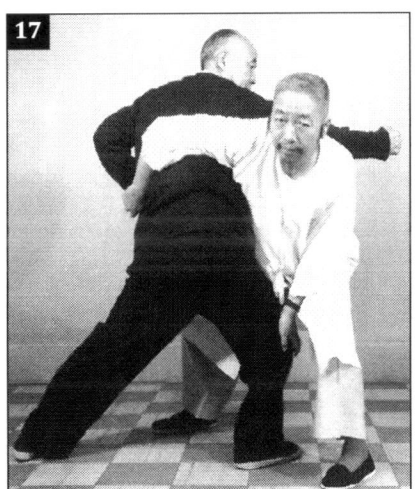 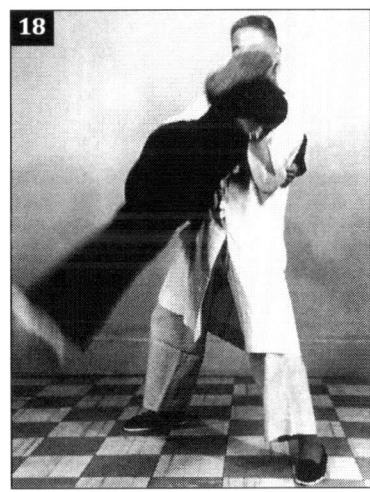

Function of embrace tiger and return to mountain
(Professor Zheng and Liang Dongcai).

Speaking of tigers, let me tell you of one.
It was a special tiger—the only one Zheng ever met.

Zheng Meets a Tiger

In an introduction to the translation of *Cheng Tzu's Thirteen Treatises on T'ai-chi Ch'uan* (1985: 13–15), Min Xiaoqi (Min Hsiao-chi), a celebrated authority on Chinese literature, stated that he met three extraordinary men in his lifetime. One was an eighty-year-old monk with a child's face who gathered rare herbs in the mountains of Zhejiang Province by climbing and jumping through pines and vines like a monkey. Later, Min met and was awed by a seventy-year-old Daoist priest with a young appearance and a resonant voice who had meditated for forty years. Zheng Manqing was the third outstanding man he met. In enumerating Zheng's excellences, which included medicine, painting, calligraphy, and taiji, Min mentioned that Zheng liked to climb mountains that had deep gorges. "Danger did not deter him," Min wrote. "Once he met a tiger but was not frightened because he was internally strong and his mind was calm" (Lo and Inn, 1985: 12).[5]

Professor Zheng told Tam Gibbs of his encounter with the tiger, and Tam recounted it to me years ago. Zheng was walking on a meandering path up a mountain, probably in Zhejiang, when he met a tiger coming down. Because the path was narrow, there was no way for the two to pass without incident. So when Zheng saw the huge animal coming around a turn toward him, he slowly retreated to the outside of the path until he came to the edge of the cliff overlooking the gorge below. Just as he noticed his plight, his hand touched a sapling growing from the cliff edge. Keeping his eyes steadily on the tiger, Zheng pulled and bent the pliable sapling back for its full length, ten feet or so, and held the leafed top in the face of the tiger in the taiji movement step back and repulse the monkey. Note well: he did not shake the tree to scare the tiger. A tiger is unlikely to be frightened by either a man or a small tree, but he may become excited by a tree brandished in his face. No, Zheng merely put it near the tiger's nose and held it there. After a time, the tiger broke off his baleful look into Zheng's eyes, shook his head slightly, and sauntered on past Zheng down the mountain path. Zheng stood up and released the tree, and in a rush, the cool, imperturbable face he had shown the tiger disappeared and his whole body shook uncontrollably. After a while, the shakes subsided and, with an occasional look over his shoulder, he continued up the path.

Some readers will not believe this story, a quite understandable reaction given the state of truth in media. However, I think it probably happened. For starters, Professor Zheng was not given to "terminological inexactitudes," as Winston Churchill called lies. He was no politician. He would sometimes forget details, but deceit was alien to his nature. Nor did he make himself a hero by bare-handedly killing the tiger as the Tiger Swami in P. Yogananda's *The Autobiography of a Yogi* (1948: 67–68) reportedly did. Professor Zheng was no hero, merely a survivor. Given the tightness of the passage and the fact that Chinese tigers are presumably as hungry as Chinese people, it was a close thing. Perhaps the tiger had eaten recently and when he met no antagonism from the small man he chanced upon, with only a focused desire to be left alone, the tiger gave him his space. Instinctively, Zheng made the right choice. If he had panicked, the animal would have picked up on his fear; if he had shaken the sapling aggressively, the tiger probably would have mauled him grievously.

Curiously, in Taiwan many years before I heard this story from Tam Gibbs, Zheng and I had been discussing function and he spoke of the ferocity of a tiger as being short lived. If one could survive the first charge, he said (and his "if" was a beaut), one might have a chance to escape. The tiger does not economize; his attack is total, and thus he tires quickly. Biologists agree on this. Like all cats, the tiger cannot maintain exertion for long because of its narrow chest and relatively small lungs. Did Zheng's focused mind have room for this contingency? I doubt it.

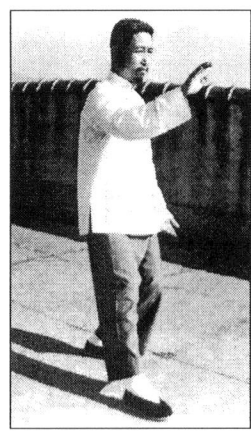 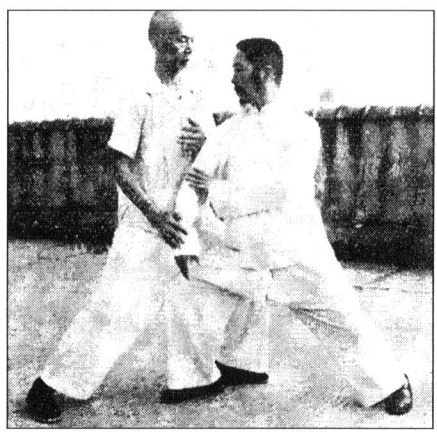

Zheng in repulse monkey and with Li Shoujian doing dalü.

So much for the tiger. During his exposition of his three great men, Mr. Min ranked Zheng Manqing above the other two by saying Zheng "was a great man compared with those who stayed in old temples and remote mountains, who preferred to seek quietness and protect themselves rather than participate in the country's destiny or the rise and fall of the world" (Lo and Inn, 1985: 15). Mr. Min makes an insightful point. Perhaps Professor Zheng's greatest gift was that in an always eventful, sometimes tumultuous life, he remained rooted and relaxed while living and raising a family in the real world. In letting the world go past instead of through him, he minded his center and never left off meditating. And according to the ancients, this moving meditation is superior to the static meditation done in monasteries.

Notes

[1] Yang Shouting reportedly had a "small frame" taiji set he taught privately comprising seventy-three postures (two hundred, counting repetitions) that was done in two to three minutes (Lim, n.d.: 36). If true, this was racing with a vengeance. In the black and white film we made of Zheng in Taibei in 1960, he did the thirty-seven postures (sixty-five, counting repetitions) in about three minutes. Though impatient that morning and running late, he still did it correctly, separating all the way. Hurried, his form still effused beauty. However, Mr. Lim would double the number of postures and triple the total with repetitions. I do not think it could be done and still fall under the rubric of taiji, as such speed defies, if it does not defile, the *Classics*, where Li Yiyu writes, "In practicing the form we want slowness not speed"; and Wu Yuxiang advises that one should "outwardly exhibit calmness and peace" (Lo, 1979: 47, 82). Physiologically, taiji works by relaxing the cerebrum. Without slowness, this will not happen (China Sports, 1980: 78). Mr. Lim is stingy on sources. Here is one to confound him. Yang Chengfu's nephew (and a famed taiji adept in his own right), Fu Zhongwen, said in an interview a few years back, "There is none nor was there ever a fast set in the Yang Style traditional system. People who practice a fast set and call it the Yang style are not practicing the traditional Yang style taijiquan. Any fast set was developed by students of the Yang style. The form takes normally twenty to thirty minutes to practice, and it is practiced in a slow, evenly paced manner" (Yu and Sharp, 1993). Even Dong Yingjie, a senior under Master Yang, often practiced an auxiliary short "flying form." The late Kuo Lienying showed me his normal speed "Guangping" form, said to be derived from Yang Banhou, in Taibei in 1962. However, there was little separation of weight evident. Some other schools do taiji at normal speed, a prime example being Sun Lutang's *houbujia*, or "lively pace form." Other schools, such as the Chenjiagou style, sporadically exceed even normal speed, or create a variant fast form as a break from the ennui of doing it slowly. However, none of the fast forms

I have seen separates the weight into one leg as required by the *Classics*. There is no great harm in these quickie steps, if they do not distract from or become confused with real taiji.

2. As Bix Beiderbeck, our finest jazz cornetist, said of the prose of the noted French novelist Marcel Proust.

3. Though I cannot recall meeting Li Shoujian during my stay in Taiwan (1959–1962), I heard about him. One Chinese friend told me that he had seen Li do taiji on the lawn on a windless day and his indescribably beautiful postures made the grass move.

4. Ben Lo was Professor Zheng's first student when Zheng relocated to Taiwan from the mainland in 1949. I met Laoshi ("teacher") a decade later, and both Lo and I are still trying to decipher and live life by practicing taiji (it is difficult, but it beats working). Modest to a fault, Lo has forgotten, if you will forgive the cliché, more taiji than most so-called masters know. We are old friends, having been born within four months of each other in 1926–27, and I bow deeply to him for his help with this article.

5. In his translation (1982), Douglas Wile has Min, whose given name he misspells as Hsia-chi, say that Zheng "often encountered tigers." If Zheng had met tigers often, we would never have heard of him . . .

Bibliography

China Sports Series. (1980). *Simplified taijiquan*. Beijing: China Sports Series 1.
Lim, T. (n.d.). The origins and history of taijiquan. Singapore: n.p.
Lo, B., et al. (1979). *The essence of t'ai chi ch'uan*. Richmond, CA: North Atlantic Books.
Lo, P., and Inn, M. (1985). *Cheng Tzu's thirteen treatises on tai-chi ch'uan*. Berkeley, CA: North Atlantic Books.
Wile, D. (Trans.). (1982). *Master Cheng's thirteen chapters on t'ai-chi ch'uan*. Brooklyn, NY: Sweet Ch'i Press.
Yu, W., and Sharp, G. (April 1993). Fu Zhong Wen: A family legend. *Inside Kung-fu*, pp. 44–46.
Yogananda, P. (1946). *The autobiography of a yogi*. New York: The Philosophical Library.
Zheng, M. (1950). *Zhengzi taijiquan shisan pian* [Master Zheng's thirteen treatises on taijiquan]. Sections 1 and 2. Taibei: n.p.
Zheng, M., and Smith, R. (1967). *T'ai-chi: The "supreme ultimate" exercise for health, sport, and self-defense*. Rutland, VT: Charles E. Tuttle, Co.

Taijiquan as an Experiential Way for Discovering Daoism
by Michael A. DeMarco, M.A.

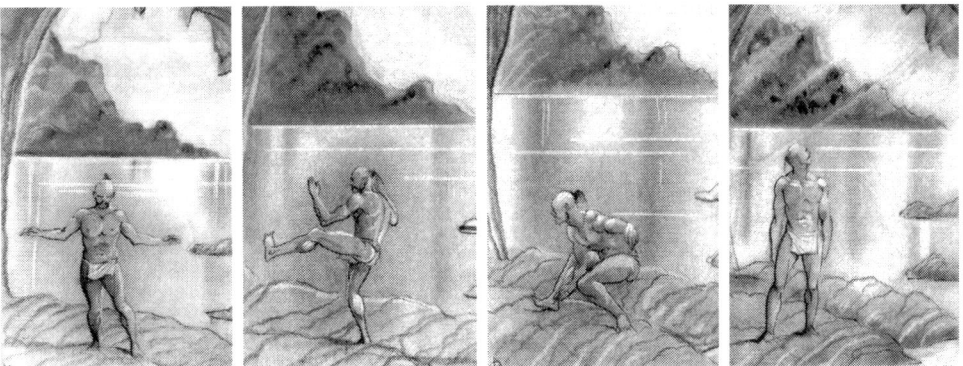

As the alleged founder of Daoism, Laozi retired from his worldly occupation and departed westward on an ox. Legends give many fanciful embellishments to the story. However, the artistic renderings by Oscar Ratti accompanying this chapter invite the reader to create a personal interpretation. All illustrations courtesy of © 1997 Futuro Designs and Publications.

Introduction

If someone without any previous exposure to Daoist philosophy began to study taijiquan, what would he or she learn regarding taiji's fundamental principles? And how closely would the resulting philosophical insights concur with Daoist tenets? —The following presents a way of directly discovering taiji boxing's philosophical principles through experiential involvement in the art itself. There certainly is no real need for delineating historical roots with footnotes here, but only rooting our feet in taiji.[1]

We will first look at the learning process involved from a student's viewpoint. The philosophical insights gained through this practice will be indicated as they arise during this learning process. A summary of these philosophical principles can then be compared to those found in the Daoist tradition.

Learning Taijiquan's Solo Form

Regardless of the taiji style being taught, a new student begins by learning a solo routine that contains a series of movements which, depending on its length and tempo, takes five to forty minutes to perform. While learning the solo routine, the student's main objective is to become aware of how the body moves. During this initial stage, martial applications are usually not taught so that the student may focus on himself without distraction.

The instructor simply demonstrates a movement and lets the student repeat it. Consecutive movements are shown one-by-one according to the student's readiness until the complete series of movements is memorized. The learning process here involves little or no discussion between teacher and student. A student learns by copying the master's techniques and repeating them thousands of times. The understanding of how the techniques are executed is gained largely through intuition and awareness resulting from hours of devoted practice. What is learned through this practice gives an evolving definition of "taijiquan," a definition which changes with time according to one's ever-deepening insights into the art. However, practice of the solo form should demonstrate all the fundamental principles for which taijiquan is noted.

To simplify a presentation on taijiquan practice, the following material focuses on the Yang-style, but similarities would be found in other branches as well. Traditional Yang taiji is composed of over one hundred movements strung together in three sections. From the beginning posture comes the first step, then the second step, and the form continues in a flowing sequence of movements which closes with a posture that is exactly like the beginning posture. The compositional structure of the sequence itself is very similar to a symphony with its own melodic flow of changing passages held together by repetitive bars to form an overall unity. Even though a symphony may contain a highly complex inner structure, its unity can be recognized as a singular "masterpiece."

After many months, regular practice brings a familiarity with the solo form and the practitioner becomes more and more comfortable with the routine.

The movements seemingly begin to flow of their own accord, releasing mental and physical stress found in students at the beginning level. By the time the complete routine is learned, the student can enter the door of discovery that allows an experiential sensing of taiji's philosophical core.[2]

Principles Derived from the Solo Routine Practice

Upon first observing the traditional Yang routine, most new students are apprehensive of the number and complexity of movements. They ask, "How is it possible to remember all those movements in sequence?" They later realize that the movements are not as difficult to learn as they first appeared, especially when learning only one movement at a time. Within the routine itself, many movements are repeated in whole or in part.

By the time the student has completed learning the routine, he has a distinct sense for the three sections. Furthermore, he sees individual movements as parts of sequences. Where there was once "brush knee, twist-step left, twist-step right, twist-step left," there is now simply the "brush knee sequence." The same, for example, can be said for "the three kicks," "four corners," or "cloud hands." As the practitioner gains greater familiarity with the routine, he sees such sequences as forming parts of even longer sequences.

Analyzing the individual taiji movements, we find that each movement is brought about by a simple change in body posture, with one simple change leading to other changes. Shifting of body weight in the legs and feet is easily sensed, particularly in taiji routines which are practiced in a very slow manner. As one leg becomes "full" with weight, the other is "emptied" and capable of moving in any chosen direction. The body's trunk remains in balance over the legs as the hands follow the waist in deflecting left or right; striking, pressing, or pushing forward; rolling-back or "repulsing monkey." These horizontal movements are coupled with vertical movements as well. This is particularly noticeable in "snake creeps downward" and "rooster stands on one leg," since these are extremes of low and high following one another. But vertical movement should be equally sensed throughout the routine, commencing with "taiji beginning."

Whether we look at the complex composition of the complete Yang routine or the individual movements which form it, there develops an underlying sense of flow that unites all the movements. The taiji solo routine is often compared to the slow, steady flow of a long river. It is this flow which provides the continuity and wholeness of the routine. All the movement from "beginning" to "conclusion" is performed in smooth even tempo with no clear demarcation to signify where one technique begins or ends.

Reflecting on the learning process involved in taiji, the student becomes aware that taiji's complexity is simplified by grouping certain movements into sequences. In turn, these small sequences form part of larger sequences, often simply referred to as the traditional "three sections" for convenience. However, all taiji movements find their source in the most basic principle of change. At an advanced level, the practitioner finds himself changing effortlessly from one movement to another. An observer cannot tell where one technique ends and the next begins. The sequence of movements connects as a single thread and the exercise feels like a unified routine.

Taiji as practiced by an accomplished master looks easy to do, but the necessary skills take years to hone. For the beginner, practice is characterized by tenseness, staccato movements, and off-balanced postures. How do these evolve into taiji characterized by balance, smoothness, and relaxed grace? Taiji body mechanics can be summed up in one word: naturalness.

The slow-motion Yang Style routine magnifies the awareness of each movement, which, in turn, allows the practitioner to feel what makes his movements cumbersome and offers direction for making appropriate corrections within each movement. Consciously and subconsciously, the movements can be transformed from a rustic set of physical exercises into a true martial art routine.

Solo Routine Principles and Daoist Tenents

The preceding section outlines a typical mode of learning Yang Style taiji and presents some of the common psychological insights associated with the practice. These insights are gained through the practice itself, but what of the Daoist flavor is expressed, if any? Any similarities or differences between the two we can find by comparing the contents of the preceding section with principles long held as the most fundamental to Daoism.

Ten Thousand Things in the Way

The Chinese have traditionally viewed the world as composed of "ten thousand things." Things, infinitely numerous in shapes and sizes, dazzle our senses with an ever-changing kaleidoscope of colors, sounds, aromas, tastes and textures. From birth, we are forced to find our place within this ever-turning world. The philosophy we develop can provide the wisdom and skills that determine how successful we will be. It is our means for survival.

During the formation of early Chinese culture, it was recognized that, to solve any complex problem, the "ten thousand things" surrounding the matter must first be simplified. What is the most important aspect of the problem? What roles do other factors play which are significant? Through such questioning the Chinese were developing a highly sophisticated mode of logic and reasoning. They found it useful to categorize the "ten thousand things" to better adapt to their environment.

A parallel can be found in taijiquan practice, in which the student is initially confused by the "ten thousand" movements. Here the student is challenged to find a way to properly master the complexity of all the movements. A step along this path involves the discovery of categories by which the taiji movements can be better understood and performed.

The Ways and Means of Five Forces (*wuxing*)

Stopping to contemplate the world, insightful Chinese viewed the "ten thousand things" that appeared between Heaven and Earth. They looked closely in every direction. As a person peers outward, he realizes that he himself forms the center of his existence, the center of the universe. Perhaps this orientation between man and his universe led the Chinese to the idea of *wuxing*. Likewise, a taiji practitioner is the ever-present center of the moving art form of taiji.

An analysis of the characters *wu* and *xing* helps us clarify the general meaning usually given to the compound term as Five Forces. *Wu* simply stands for the number five. In ancient times, it was written like an "X," where four lines indicated the directions from a common central focus. Later, a line was placed above and another below the "X," symbolic of Heaven and Earth. This is like man's position on Earth. Only from his own viewpoint can he look out into all directions under Heaven.

Xing carries with it such meanings as to go, operate, conduct or set into motion. Combined with *wu*, we have five active forces, or movers. They represent five basic phases through which matter continuously transforms itself. As a concept, *wuxing* stands for abstract forces, five movers which keep the "ten thousand things" in operation.

Besides being associated with the five spatial directions (north, south, east, west, and center), the *wuxing* concept was conveniently and suitably applied to other aspects of nature. A partial list indicates its significance as a comprehensive tool for understanding the "ten thousand things." It often was associated with the seasons, animals, weather, bodily organs, numbers, musical notes, colors and even flavors.

How do the Five Forces work? According to Daoist philosophy, they work quite easily! Just as one season naturally follows another, any one phase is connected to the next. Plus, all phases are interrelated in some way, each having its own characteristics and influences. In short, each plays its part in an overall process of construction and destruction that keeps the "ten thousand things" in movement. Due to cause and effect, they flow in cycles, passing from one phase to the next until completing a circuit. By an intimate understanding of the laws involved in such changes, man can better adapt himself to the continual changes in the world.

The Five Forces theory became so important that an independent school of philosophy arose under its name during the fourth and third centuries BCE. In the third century BCE, a strategist named Zou Yan made it a regular feature of political theory. Kingdoms, under the influence of a given *wuxing* phase, rose and fell in predictable order much like earth produces wood, which in turn is destroyed by fire.

The theory of Five Forces was applied to all fields of study, including astronomy, divination, medicine, agriculture, politics, art, and religion. It served as a valuable schematic upon which subjects could be analyzed and understood within their specialized sphere of changing relationships. Thus, within their changes, an underlying order and permanence could still be found.

China's ancient philosophers were seeking the wisest way to obtain the insight and skills necessary to master life. Although the *wuxing* theory proved very practical, its application was still so complex that only the most gifted of sages could successfully employ it to advantage. It is too easy to become entangled by five ever-changing variables. Laozi was clearly aware of this, writing:

> The five colors cause one's eyes to go blind . . .. The five flavors confuse one's palate. The five tones cause one's ears to go deaf. Therefore, in the government of the Sages: He is for the belly and not for the eyes. Thus, he rejects that and takes this.
> – Henricks, 1989: 64 (Ch. 12)

The *wuxing* were understood to be the simplified basis of the "ten thousand things." To be more workable, would it be possible to simplify further? Chinese sages did just that—they categorized the world into two: yin and yang. In so doing, the *wuxing* became easier to understand and, therefore, so did the "ten thousand things."

In a similar manner, the taiji practitioner eventually finds order within the complexity of movements comprising the routine. Some practitioners become so infatuated with individual techniques that they miss the overall importance of the system! They do not heed Laozi's advice and get lost in the "ten thousand" movements. Others focus on the complete routine. After the routine is categorized into sections and sequences become familiar, the routine is performed with less difficulty. From the starting movement the practitioner feels as if he is moving through sections of the routine rather than many individual movements, until the end which completes the cycle.

The Bi–Ways of Yin and Yang

We walk a road with two feet, view the world through only two eyes. In the fourth century BCE, at roughly the same time the *wuxing* theory developed, the Chinese also formulated a polar view of the world with the theory of yin-yang. By the Han Dynasty (202 BCE–220 CE), this Yin-Yang School absorbed that of *wuxing*. Together they offered a comprehensive system useful not only for analysis, but also in the control and manipulation of all areas to which they were applied.

There are earthy roots to the yin-yang theory. It is believed that the ancient characters derived in part as symbolic images of the daily fluctuation between day and night, or more precisely, light and dark. The yang character shows the sun on the horizon, radiating its brilliance down on the earth. Yin is composed of *jin*, meaning "now" and *yun* meaning "cloudy." As a result, yin became associated with cloud-like characteristics, including cold, night, shade, dark, and water. Similarly, yang came to imply a varied list of sun-like attributes, such as hot, day, clear, bright, and fiery. The written characters have changed over the centuries into their simplified modern versions. However, the implications do remain the same as those of the original characters. Oddly enough, no written character can fully express the meaning with which yin-yang became associated.

Since the symbolism of language failed to convey the meaning of yin-yang, a more appropriate symbol was required. All of the cosmological diagrams invented in China, the taiji symbol is no doubt the most famous. It also remains the most useful symbol for expressing the yin-yang theory. The characters for taiji should first be analyzed before discussing the symbol itself.

When the characters for *taiji* are broken down, the individual character *tai* we find refers to something "very big" or "extreme." It resembles a stick figure who is stretching his limbs out to their limits in four directions. *Ji* is more complicated. It also has a significance of "extreme," but more importantly a "pole," the extreme of any axis. In ancient times, *ji* was a common word for "ridgepole" upon which the structure of a house would rest. With reference to cosmology, taiji is the "Supreme Ultimate Principle," the cosmological ridgepole which supports the whole universe.

In philosophical terms, the taiji is the Absolute. It is the most basic principle upon which *wuxing* and the "ten thousand things" rest. An Absolute is so limitless and pervasive that it does not have any visible signs to be perceived. For this reason, yin-yang became its first visible attributes.

The symbol for the taiji, or Supreme Ultimate, is the intertwining of yin and yang. The parts are not static, but are constantly in movement, varying their relationship in fluctuating percentages or even transforming one into the other. Through the varied interactions of yin-yang, the universe is kept in motion. No aspect of creation exists without their signature. Laozi wrote:

> The ten thousand things carry yin on their backs and wrap their arms around yang. Through the blending of *qi* (their energies) they arrive at a state of harmony.
> – Henricks, 1989: 11 (Ch. 42)

The yin-yang interplay is the foundation of taiji's boxing routine. It is the impetus of the flowing movements. Throughout the taiji routine, practitioners experience the fluctuating pulse of yin and yang. How this categorization functions in taiji is shown through the following examples:

YIN	YANG
closed	open
inward	outward
hidden	shown
slow	fast
soft	hard
mind	body
sinking	rising
down	up
low	high
passive	active
back	front
inside	outside
light	heavy
north	south
empty	full
defensive	offensive
receiving	giving
curved	straight
round	square
pull	push
retreat	advance

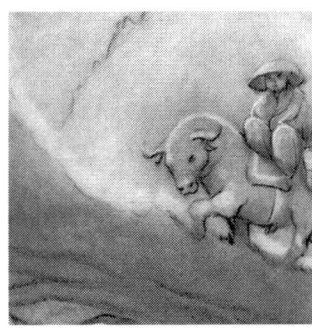
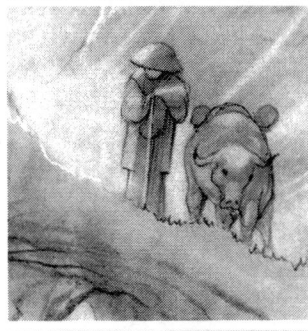
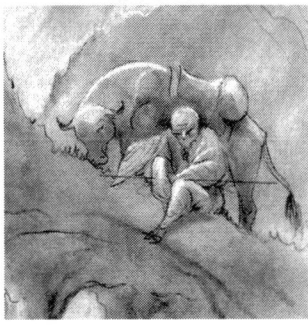

In Daoism, *wuxing* and yin-yang serve to categorize the "ten thousand things." This helps one to understand the universe in its varied aspects. *Wuxing* and yin-yang also demonstrate how the universe operates. The experience of taiji boxing likewise illustrates the flow of movement through positional phases and fluctuations between yin and yang. On an even more subtle level, movement is brought about from stillness. Stillness is found in the Dao.

Dao: The High–Way of Daoism

The *Daodejing* states:

> There was something formed out of chaos,
> that was born before Heaven and Earth.
> Quiet and still! Pure and deep!
> It stands on its own and doesn't change.
> It can be regarded as the mother
> of Heaven and Earth. I do not know
> its name: I style it "the Way."
> – Henricks, 1989: 77 (Ch. 25)

Carl Jung said that the "value of Dao lies in its power to reconcile opposites on a higher level of consciousness" (Chang, 1970: 3). We find this in the highest levels of taijiquan practice.

It is made known when the practitioner transcends the complexity of the "ten thousand" movements, transcends the arbitrary groupings of sequential techniques, transcends even the mind-body duality. This is a mystic state which does not limit itself to taiji boxing.

A dominant thought existing in Laozi's time is found in the *Book of Odes*: "Heaven in producing mankind annexed its laws to every faculty and relationship. Man possessed of this nature should strive to develop his endowment to perfection." A "Heavenly Identity," or Dao-realization, comes to one through polishing the mirror-like mind, cleansing away its mundane dust. Zhuangzi called this a process of "purifying the mind." Laozi further advised one to rid himself of desires to observe the Dao's secrets (Lau, 1963: 57).

Dao realization is of great importance because whoever attains this state takes on all the attributes of the eternal Dao. Why this is important in taijiquan and other martial arts can be discerned from a quote from the *Daodejing*, Ch. 16: "If you're one with the Dao, to the end of your days you'll suffer no harm" (Henricks, 1989: 68).

The Dao is described in Chinese literature as being complete and whole. As such, it is the abode of stillness and tranquility. It is the "mother of the ten thousand things." "The Way [Dao] gives birth to them, nourishes them, matures them, completes them, rests them, rears them, supports them, and protects them" (Henricks, 1989: 20).

Daoism	Taijiquan
"10,000 things"	Over one hundred movements in the Yang Taiji routine.
Five Elements	Three sections into which the Yang Taiji routine is divided.
Yin-Yang	Duality inherent in each taiji movement.
Dao	The oneness of the unified taiji routine.
De	The virtue/power expressed in taiji movements.

Conclusion

A student of taiji boxing passes through various psychological stages in experiencing the complexity of the routine. At first a mysterious hodgepodge of techniques, the numerous movements within the routine become easier to understand and perform as regular practice brings a familiarity with the set. The *wuxing* and yin-yang concepts help one understand the underlying process of change within the routine. We also learn the inherent relationship that exists within the unity of all body parts as utilized in the movements.

However, at the highest level of practice the completeness and wholeness of the taiji routine find a parallel in the oneness of Dao. When the dualism of mind and body are transcended, the taiji routine seems to flow of its own accord. It is as spontaneously natural as a flowing river. This is taiji in the state of "non-doing" (*wuwei*). A solo performance in this state is characterized by tranquility and freedom from thought, which for the martial artist has other implications as well. It makes the power (*de*) of Dao available, for in self-defense it is necessary to move spontaneously with the accuracy and strength possible only through the complete unification of human thought and movement.

What we have analyzed in this chapter is the discovery of Daoist principles in the taijiquan routine. Here, the inner workings of the individual are found, presenting the physical and mental operations as they are seen in the solo routine. There are also other taiji practices, such as push-hands and a paired form. These practices seek to let the individual discover his relationship with others.

For the Daoist, this may be the ultimate reason why the name "taiji" was chosen for this boxing style.

Notes

[1] An earlier version of this chapter was presented at the 73rd annual meeting of the Central States Anthropological Society on March 21–24, 1996, in Covington, KY. Laozi writes: "Throw away knowledge, and the people will benefit a hundredfold" (Henricks, 1989: 71). In Daoist fashion, I have tried to minimize the academic documentation in this present version to focus on actual experience.

[2] There is a strong tradition among Western scholars to categorize Daoism according to its use in Chinese society, with philosophical and religious Daoism forming the two major categories. Again, I have chosen to ignore the standard approach

in favor of the Daoist unitary vision. This holds true even with the philosophical concepts mentioned in this chapter, since they may fall under other philosophical schools of thought as well, e.g., Confucianism.

Acknowledgments

Appreciation goes to Barbara Davis, Michael Davis, and Douglas Wile for reading and making suggestions for improving this chapter. As I did not heed all these suggestions, I will bear the burden for any faults found in the final draft. An appreciative salute is given to Oscar Ratti for his appropriate artwork. He brings to life the essence of the Chinese proverb: "What is accomplished in the mind, is made known by the hand."

Bibliography

Blofeld, J. (1978). *Taoism: The road to immortality.* Boulder, CO: Shambhala Publications, Inc.

Bodde, D. (1978). *Harmony and conflict in Chinese philosophy. Studies in Chinese Thought.* (A. Wright, Ed.). Chicago: University of Chicago Press, 19-80.

Breslow, A. (1995). *Beyond the closed door: Chinese culture and the creation of t'ai chi ch'uan.* Jerusalem: Almond Blossom Press.

Chang, C. (1970). *Creativity and taoism.* New York: Harper and Row Publishers, Inc.

Chen, Y. (n.d.). *T'ai-chi ch'uan: Its effects and practical applications.* Hong Kong: n.p.

DeMarco, M. (1983). The mirror-like mind of taoism and its implications for the individual and society. Ann Arbor, MI: University Microfilms International. Master's thesis for Seton Hall University, 1981.

Finazzo, G. (1968). *The notion of tao in the Lao Tzu and the Chuang Tzu.* Taipei: Mei Ya Publications.

Fung, Y. (1966). *A short history of Chinese philosophy.* (D. Bodde, Ed.). New York: The Free Press.

Henricks, R. (Trans.) (1989). *Lao-Tzu te-tao ching.* New York: Ballantine Books.

Huang, A. (1993). *Complete tai-chi: The definitive guide to physical and emotional self-improvement.* Rutland, VT: Charles E. Tuttle Co.

Jou, T. (1981). *The tao of tai-chi chuan: Way to rejuvenation.* Warwick, NY: Tai Chi Foundation.

Kaltenmark, M. (1969). *Lao Tzu and taoism.* (R. Greaves, Trans.). Stanford, CA: Stanford University Press.

Kuo, L. (1994). *The t'ai chi boxing chronical.* (Guttmann, Trans.). Berkeley, CA: North Atlantic Books.

Lau, D. (Trans.). (1963). *Lao Tzu tao te ching.* Baltimore, MD: Penguin Books Inc.

Maspero, H. (1981). *Taoism and Chinese religion.* (F. Kierman, Trans.). Amherst, MA: The University of Massachusetts Press.

Needham, J. (1956). *Science and civilization in China. Vols. I and II.* Cambridge: Cambridge University Press.

Waley, A. (Trans.). (1962). *The way and its power: A study of the tao te ching and its place in Chinese thought.* New York: Grove Press, Inc.

Watts, A. (1975). *Tao: The watercourse way.* New York: Pantheon Books, Inc.

Welch, H. (1965). *Taoism: The parting of the way.* Boston, MA: Beacon Press.

Welch, H., and Seidel, A. (Eds.). (1979). *Facets of taoism.* New Haven: Yale University Press.

Wile, D. (1996). *Lost t'ai-chi classics from the late ch'ing dynasty.* Albany, NY: State University of New York Press.

Wong, K. (1996). *The complete book of tai chi chuan: A comprehensive guide to the principles and practice.* Rockport, MA: Element Books, Inc.

Internal Training:
The Foundation for Chen Taiji's Fighting Skills and Health Promotion
by Adam Wallace

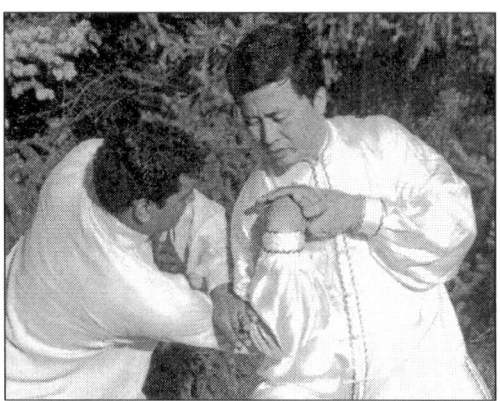

Reversal of a qinna technique by Ren Guangyi.
All photographs courtesy of Adam Wallace.

Today in the Western hemisphere *taijiquan* (also abbreviated as *taiji*) for combat is really something of a contradiction in terms. It has become a "moving meditation" or a martial arts dance at best. The fact that taiji boasts a comprehensive fighting system for self-defense and full-contact offense when there are so few practitioners of the art aware of this fact is a great anomaly. The explanation for this discrepancy, and how it has come to be, can be found within taijiquan's evolution.

Taijiquan's Origins and History

In the 1930's an eminent martial arts master and historian named Tang Hao (1897–1959) concluded after thorough research that taijiquan had originated in Chenjiagou (Chen Village), Wen County, Henan Province, over three hundred years ago. Its founder, Chen Wangting (c. 1600–1680), was a knight and scholar and a ninth-generation ancestor of the Chen family. He was chief of the civil troops around 1640 at the end of the Ming dynasty (1368–1644). According to the genealogy of the Chen families, he was renowned as a "born warrior, as can be proven by the sword he used in combat," and a "master of martial arts having defeated over one thousand bandits in Shandong province." In 1644, after the Qing dynasty came to rule China, Chen Wangting returned to his village where, in addition to working in the fields and teaching disciples and children to become worthy members of society, he began creating his new "Grand Ultimate Fist." He invented this system as a means of training warriors in a healthy, well-rounded manner from his lifetime of researching, developing and experiencing martial arts.

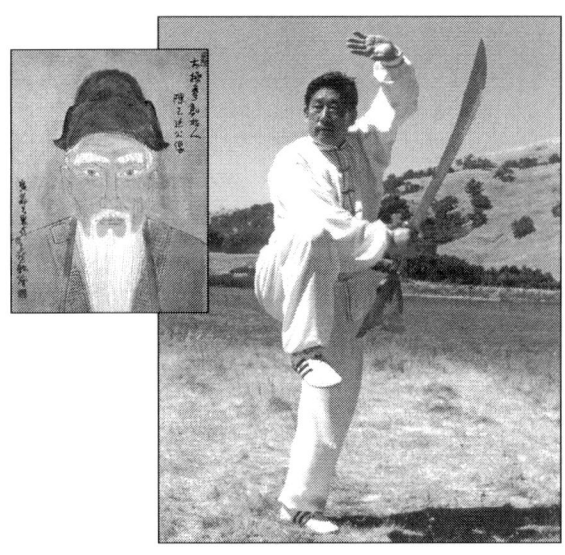

Painting of Chen Wangting, probable creator of taijiquan.
Chen Xiaowang in sword posture Golden Roosters Stands Alone.

The original Chen taiji was created as an eclectic martial art embodying the most empirically tested techniques from General Qi Jiguang's *The Canons of Boxing*, an effective and powerful repertoire which covered sixteen different martial art schools. Qi Jiguang (1528–1587) lived some fifty years prior to the advent of taiji. From *The Canons of Boxing*, Chen Wangting created five sets of taiji shadowboxing, one set of Longboxing (108 forms) and one set of Paochui combat boxing. These incorporated skills from Shaolin Fist, the Red Fist in particular, Shaolin Staff, and "Buddha's Warrior Eighteen Grasping Techniques" in addition to other boxing and staff techniques. He added to this foundation special techniques from other famous masters of the time, such as Li Bantien's legwork, "Eagle Claw" Wang's grasping, "Thousand Falls" Zhang's takedowns, and Zhang Baijing's striking. These individuals, all masters of their respective arts, were equally as celebrated as General Qi Jiguang.

Historically, Chen family boxers were essentially bodyguards required to protect valuables and transport them across neighboring provinces, especially Shandong province, which had endured a long history of turmoil. The Chens relied on their martial skills, specializing in the sword and spear, not only for their survival but also for their livelihood. Their skill was a closely guarded secret, and for five generations it had remained intact within the family and village.

Chen Changxing (1771–1853), the fourteenth-generation patriarch, was the first to teach it to an outsider, Yang Luchan (1799–1872), who came to Chenjiagou for the sole purpose of learning taiji. Yang had previously only studied external gongfu but his tenacity impressed Chen Changxing. He was taught under the condition that he would vow never to teach the art to the public or use its name. After a time, he traveled to Beijing, where he become known as "Yang the Invincible," and true to his oath, formulated his own shadow boxing. His Yang Style taiji was based on Chen's *laojia yilu* (old frame first routine). He omitted the stamping, explosiveness, low postures, and changes in tempo characteristic of Chen taiji, as well as the more difficult motions, to make it easier to learn and perform, and to suit it more for keeping-fit purposes. This style soon became popular and was embraced by the masses.

After several revisions to the original Yang forms, Yang Chengfu (1883–1936), Yang Luchan's third grandson, adapted and created the large frame of Yang family shadowboxing. This is the most popular form in China and the world today, with its slow tempo and extended, graceful and circular movements.

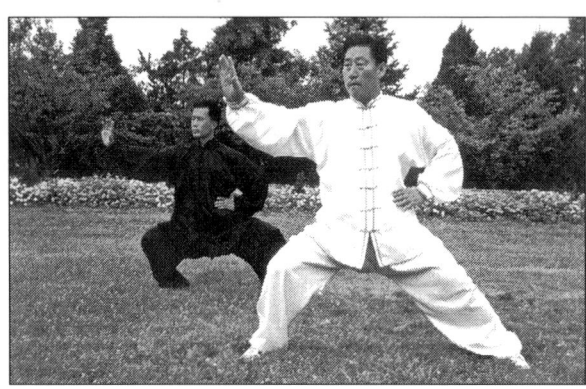

Ren Guangyi and Chen Xiaowang perform
Lazily Tying Clothes (*lanzhayi*) from Chen's old frame routine.

Wu Jianquan (1870–1942), having learned small frame Yang taiji from his father (who studied under Yang Luchan), taught this style, which became known as Wu Style. The frame is very compact, performed with uniform slowness, and contains none of the leaps and jumps that exist in the Chen school. It is the second most popular style, next to the Yang style. Another Wu school evolved around 1850, unrelated to the first mentioned Wu clan, with their own brand of taiji, which derived from Chen Style laojia (Yang Luchan's version and the Chen's new frame from Chen Qingping [1795–1868]). Its emphasis was on body structure and inner power. This was adopted by Sun Lutang (1861–1932), already an expert in *xingyi* (form-mind) boxing and *baguazhang* (eight trigram palm), who combined the best of these three styles and formed Sun Style taiji. These five styles comprise the largest and most noted styles of taiji in the world today. Directly or indirectly, Chen's new frame, Yang, Wu, Wu, and Sun all have their origins in Chen's laojia yilu.

Due to the simultaneous advancement of firearms, the function of martial arts on the battlefield gradually became obsolete. Yao Hanchen, a scholar and a student of Yang Luchan, questioned the role of taiji and proposed that it was to "enhance longevity and extend radiant good health into old age." This view brought the transformation of fighting art into health exercise.

In China, "shadow boxing" is a valuable health exercise and has had remarkable success as a curative for neurasthenia, neuralgia, high blood pressure, heart disease, tuberculosis, arthritis, and diabetes, among other conditions, due to its deep regulated natural breathing, relaxed frame of mind, and smooth circular movements (*chansijing* or silk reeling energy) which contribute to dredging the acupuncture channels and collaterals (*jingluo* and *jingmai*), as well as to improving the functions of the skeleton, muscles, and lymphatic and digestive systems. Taiji, in having diluted the martial aspects, has lost its original essence over the generations. Chen taiji, however, has seen the least amount of change as a martial art, yet through standing pole training (*zhanzhuang*) and silk reeling exercises (*chansigong*), detailed in this article, it offers one of the most comprehensive systems of qigong, or internal training for health, available.

Until very recently, Chen taiji was perhaps the least known of the major styles, largely because it remained within Chenjiagou. Ironically, when Chen Fake (1887–1957) was invited to Beijing in 1928 (after Yang Luchan had introduced his Yang taiji to the public) and performed Chen taiji, it was scarcely recognized as taiji, with its intense focus, release of power, stamping, etc., as the public was already familiar with the slow and gentle form suited for the elderly practitioners of the art.

Now that it is being more widely spread around the world by masters directly from Chen Village, interest in taijiquan's roots is booming. While many of the other styles have almost completely lost their combat capability, Chen taiji has always remained a martial art. But it should be noted that even within Chen taiji there are relatively few teachers who have a high enough level of proficiency in the combat arts to teach them.

One such teacher exists in the United States. His name is Ren Guangyi (b. 1965), and he studied directly under Chen Xiaowang (b. 1946, the nineteenth-generation standard–bearer for Chen family taiji) full-time for ten years, to become Chen's top disciple. Chen Xiaowang now has thousands of students all over the world and travels ten months of the year giving seminars, but there were only four main disciples studying together in the beginning. When Chen Xiaowang left China and emigrated to Sydney, Australia, Ren headed West and brought the genuine high-level skills of Chen taiji with him to America.

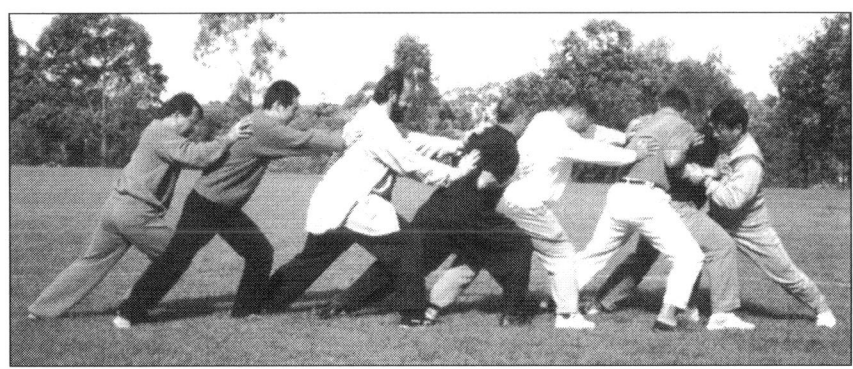

The rooting power of Chen Xiaowang as he withstands the push of seven men.

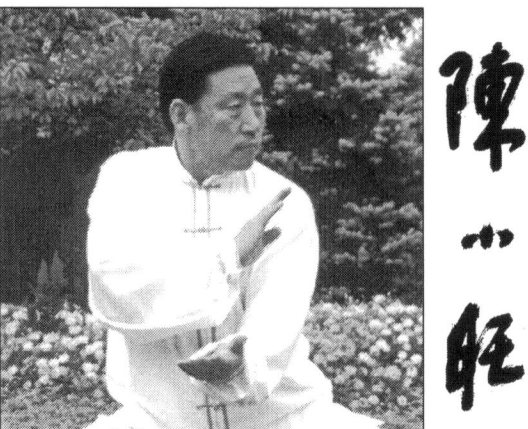

Chen Xiaowang and his signature.

Evolution Within the Style

Chen Changxing, the fourteenth-generation master, created the two barehanded sets, *yilu* (first routine) and *erlu* (second routine). Yilu is a fusion of the first three routines created by Chen Wangting. Yilu provides the foundation and prepares the student for push-hands (*tuishou*), joint-locking (*qinna*) techniques and some light wrestling.

Yilu is considered eighty percent internal and twenty percent external, with its use of "issuing power or explosive energy" (*fajing*), which is to say that the form is intrinsically more soft than hard. Erlu is a synthesis of the earlier Long Boxing and Cannon Fist routines and prepares the student for free fighting. This form is eighty percent external with its emphasis on increased fajing, speed, footwork, leaping, dodging, elbow and shoulder strikes, foot sweeps or leg takedowns, and sudden changes of direction. The first form is to build up the practitioner's vital energy (*qi*) and concentrates on developing stability, with focus on silk reeling energy (*chansijing*) and the eight skills or energies (*bafa*):

1) *peng*: "inflate/ward off," used to intercept and control an opponent's advance.
2) *lu*: "rollback/pull downwards," to deflect and control an advancing opponent.
3) *ji*: "press/follow," dropping and rotating in contact with the opponent.
4) *an*: "push," pressing one's weight into the opponent.
5) *cai*: "pluck," or grasping and twisting an opponent's joints and extremities with maximum force.
6) *lie*: "split," creating a torque of two opposing forces within the opponent's body, such as stepping in and throwing from behind, or trapping the opponent's body between the practitioner's leg and a pivoting arm or shoulder.
7) *zhou*: "elbow strike", and

8) *kao*: lean, or striking with the shoulder, knee, or hip.

Pinyin	Wade–Giles	Chinese
an	an	按
cai	ts'ai	採
ji	chi	擠
kao	k'ao	靠
lie	lieh	挒
lu	lü	履
peng	p'eng	掤
zhou	chou	肘

In tuishou and combat, these energies are frequently used in combination.

The second routine is for total combat and vast amounts of energy are expended performing it. Traditionally it was believed that one's training was not complete unless one studied both bare-handed forms, as the emphasis in each is quite different.

The legendary seventeenth generation master Chen Fake (grandson of Chen Changxing and grandfather to Chen Xiaowang) created *xinjia*, or new frame, which is widely practiced in China and the West today. This too comprises an yilu and erlu, and laojia was used as its blueprint. Xinjia was created to enhance the family's fighting skills. Chen Fake added more detail, making both forms longer, and designed his new frame to be more compact, and to contain more complex *chansijing*, more *fajing* (with more places from which it can be issued) and more qinna techniques, rendering it more useful in practical application and combat situations.

In addition, there are other subtle differences between the two renditions. For example, the stepping in laojia tends to be more forward on a straight line while in xinjia the stepping is more at oblique angles. Xinjia has become the more prevalent of the two and is certainly the preferred form in competition in mainland China, due to its more flowery, expressive style, and dynamic nature. Laojia and xinjia are the same style and share the same root, with the same principles, but the latter is more difficult to learn and perform, and so the former is generally taught first.

A common mistake with many practitioners of the new frame is that they tend to exaggerate the spiraling movements, which results in the appearance of excessively large, flaccid circles and loops, causing the individual parts of the body to become separated from the waist. Those practicing taiji in this manner fail to grasp the principles of chansijing, which are far more subtle, and more internal than external.

The most recent addition to Chen family taiji is Chen Xiaowang's simplified thirty-eight-movement solo form, a combination of laojia and xinjia which contains many of the fundamental movements, but less of the more difficult ones and less repetition of movements. It takes a shorter time to learn and perform (between four and five minutes) than laojia (approximately ten minutes) and xinjia (approximately fifteen minutes). The thirty-eight-movement form has become very popular throughout China and is hailed as something of a triumph by taiji beginners.

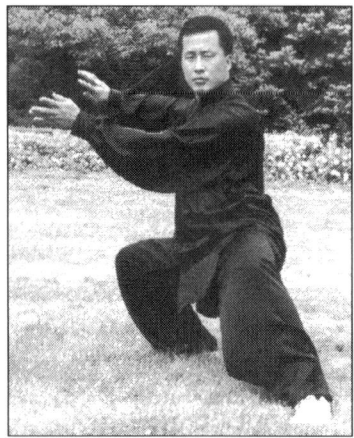 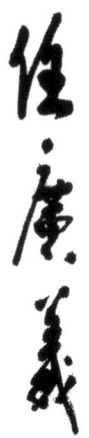 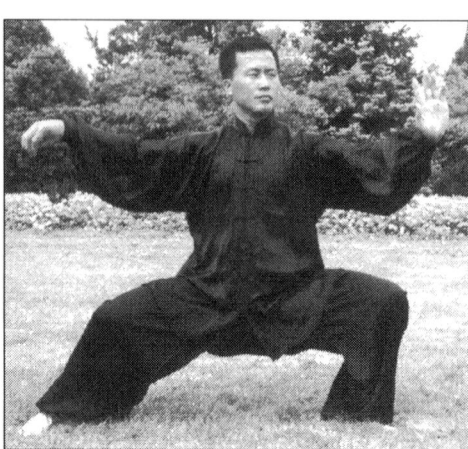

Ren Guangyi in Buddha's Attendant-Warrior
Pounds the Mortar (left) and Single Whip.
His name brushed by Chen Xiaowang.

The Main Sources of Chen Taijiquan

Taiji was intended to be more than just a fighting art. Chen Wangting combined the external martial techniques with the ancient methods of *daoyin* (guiding qi down to the dantian or lower abdomen) and *tuna* (deep breathing exercises from the dantian). Both of these health preserving skills, which date back to fourth century B.C.E., later combined and evolved to become what is today's qigong.

Chen Wangting developed his martial art with careful attention to the *jingluo-jingmai* channels through which qi flows. The purpose of this is really two-fold. On the one hand, knowledge of *jingluo-jingmai* theory enables the practitioner to effortlessly attack the qi of the opponent's internal organs. On the other hand, the spiraling, twining, and arcing movements (characteristic of Chen Style taiji) which originate from the *dantian* (or lower abdomen) are primarily for opening these channels and encouraging the natural flow of qi, to cultivate the health of the practitioner. If the dantian is strong and open, the individual will be healthy and possess vitality.

It is because taiji is trained with the knowledge of the workings of the inner body and combined with breathing that it is often referred to as an "internal" martial art. The taiji boxer's consciousness, movements, and breathing are all interrelated. Many people do not really understand the concept of "internal" so it is generally assumed that because taiji is an internal art it must be soft. This is a mistake. By definition, "taiji" must embody both soft and hard. This is why Chen taiji has an external set—*erlu*, better known as *paochui* or cannon fist. When one has witnessed this form performed correctly there can be no doubt as to whether taijiquan is wholly "internal."

In addition to the eclectic fighting techniques, deep breathing, and jingluo-jingmai theory, Chen Wangting also incorporated the ancient Daoist yin-yang concept, the universal principle of complimentary opposites, which forms the foundation of Chinese culture and philosophy. Within the scope of taijiquan, yin and yang refer and relate to: opening and closing, firm and yielding, hard and soft, expanding and contracting, fast and slow, ascending and descending, solid and empty, etc.

Regarding the legs, yin and yang are most important. The weight must be clearly distinguished to avoid double-weighting. This is not the same as balancing the weight or having the weight equally distributed throughout the limbs (as in zhanzhuang or the preparing form in any of the routines). "Double weighting" means that one's body is in a position that is not readily mobile because the weight is not properly placed. To develop a strong root, one leg must be full and support the body while the other leg is empty and can move in any direction. When stepping one must move like a cat; the weight should not be transferred until it is safe to do so. If one needs to retreat, one should be able to withdraw the leading leg without any disturbance to the balance or any shift in position or height to counterbalance the movement. According to Ren Guangyi, many taiji practitioners do not transfer their weight properly, therefore limiting their self-defense skills.

Yin and yang also applies to the upper and lower body. If the legs are firm, strong, and solid, then the upper body must be correspondingly relaxed, loose, and empty. This softness is needed for developing sensitivity which is necessary for the fostering of "listening or awareness energy" (*ting jing*) needed to sense the opponent's intentions. The slightest movement by the opponent after contact has been made with the arms should be read by the taiji practitioner, as his body is like a scale. With the legs providing the base, the upper body is light, with a feeling that the head is suspended from above. Light and heavy or rising and falling should be measured to the slightest degree. When the practitioner's silk reeling energy is good, he will react with just the right amount of energy, which means that he will not break his own energy and lose balance. Too little in counterattack will be rendered ineffective and too much may cause the practitioner to lose his root by over-extending. The right amount requires great subtlety. If the opponent does not move, then one should remain still. One should feel the opponent as he shifts his position, no matter how slightly, and uproot him while his weight is in transition, i.e. yin and yang are unclear. Through the practice of chansigong, one's energy becomes more refined and one's sensitivity increases. Eventually, one's reaction to the opponent when he advances or retreats will never be premature or too late, and one's neutralization skills will be honed to perfection.

Understanding yin and yang in defense is paramount. If the opponent resists a qinna technique (a major feature of Chen taiji) for example, it is no use to resist his will and struggle for domination. Instead, adhere to him where contact has been made and when he moves follow and borrow his energy to collect and strike. If he is yang, then become yin and change direction or revolve. If the opponent pushes, one needs to pull, and vice versa. If he attacks with the left fist, all the qi is concentrated in the left arm, so it becomes yang, or strong. This means that his right shoulder, arm, and fist will be yin (weak or empty), so that is where one's attack should be directed. Knowledge, understanding, and application of these principles leads to the ability to spontaneously implement the famous taiji principle "four ounces deflects a thousand pounds" and to taijiquan mastery. Ren Guangyi explains: "It is like trying to move a bull. Push it. It will not move. But tie a rope through its nose and pull, then it will come quite peaceably. It is a matter of reading energy, which comes through repeated practice of the forms and push-hands." Form and push-hands practice are dependent on the basic training exercises called standing pole and silk reeling, both explained in detail below.

The Poem of Chen Wangting

It is ironic that today taiji is generally thought of only as a "gentle martial art." The earliest recorded taiji poem is Chen Wangting's "Song of the Canon of Boxing." Within the verse he outlines many techniques and fighting tactics. It may astonish many people that he writes, "Two round kicks smash the face, then with left and right side kicks" and "Covering the face to attack the body is known to everyone but striking the heart and elbowing the ribs are uncommon." This type of aggression may seem barbaric to those who practice taiji solely for relaxation and health or to those who appreciate only the aesthetics of the art, as a form of self-expression or an expression of Chinese culture. However, one's thoughts must always return to the simple fact that it was created as a martial art. It is undeniably a healthy exercise, but it was not created solely for this purpose. Those who are interested in taiji for health only may eventually receive greater health benefits through the practice of qigong, which is purely for health and longevity and has been in existence several millennia before taiji.

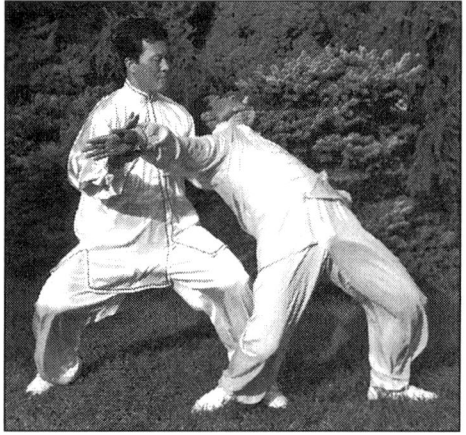 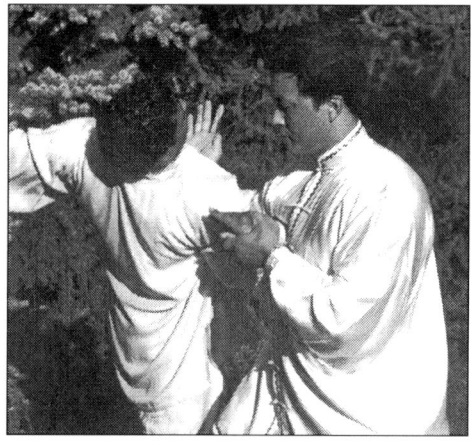

Left: Split (*lie*), creating a torque of two opposing forces within the opponent's body. the photograph shows Master Ren, after stepping in behind his opponent, throws him from behind. Right: Ren's left hand locks the opponent's wrist while his right arm coils under the opponent's elbow, which then acts like a fulcrum.

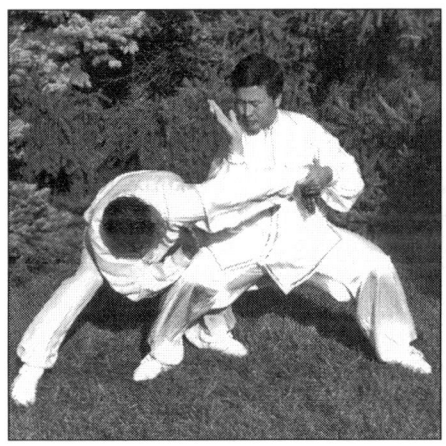 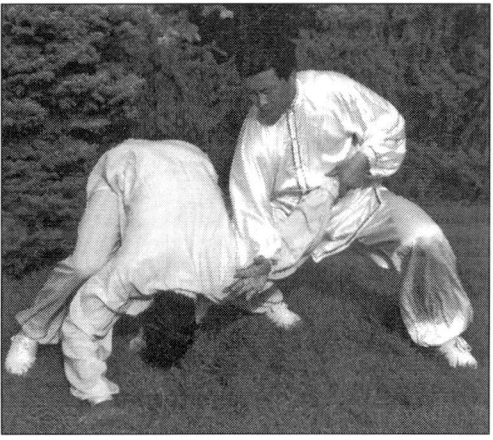

Left: Pluck (*cai*); grabbing and twisting the opponent's arm with force.
Right: Completion of the cai technique.

Chen Wangting advocated using every part of the body in attack, or whichever part was in contact with the opponent's body at any given time. In his poem, he refers to "attacking (feinting) to the left and striking the right," and the element of psychological surprise, such as feigning retreat only to suddenly change direction and stop the enemy in his tracks (breaking the enemy's rhythm). This is in addition to techniques such as "chopping, punching, pushing and pressing, dropping, blocking, grasping, hooking, opening, closing, dodging, rolling, tying, sweeping," etc.

There are five groups of sparring techniques within Chen Style taiji:

1) leg techniques, which include kicking, hooking, linking, sweeping, and stamping.
2) striking, namely with the hand, elbow, and shoulder.
3) fajing, which includes *cunjing* or 'inch energy,' short-range power.
4) joint locking, often used in combinations with the other techniques, and
5) wrestling.

So, while taiji develops sensitivity and is generally thought of in connection with yielding and redirecting, it can also be extremely aggressive, a characteristic not typically associated with this martial art.

Most of the experienced and seasoned (non-Asian) taiji practitioners in America today are the "old guard" who grew out of the 1960's and early 1970's "peace movement" (when taiji became popularized here). Many of them were fueled by antiwar sentiment and/or under the influence of illegal substances. As a result, they did not possess the "warrior spirit" which belonged to their Chinese predecessors and is needed to fully develop the skills to become an indomitable fighter. Many also dislike Chen taiji for this reason and are not willing to readily accept that the art they practice descended from a pure fighting style. This attitude reflects that of many practitioners and instructors today. This generation has further contributed greatly to the dilution of taiji, as a combative art.

Basic Skill

Excellence in taiji comes only from daily repetitive internal training. To practice correctly and achieve the results of a firm unshakable root, heightened sensitivity, the ability to neutralize from any position, internal strength and explosive power, takes hours of hard practice every day for many years. The work involved does not merely refer to sweat but also to pain. It would be a delusion to think that a high level can be attained any other way.

Generally Western students of martial arts differ from those in China. The majority do not have the time, patience, or the inclination to put in the hours needed. Many are either too lazy or too content to spend even minimal time practicing, and often basic skill is omitted in favor of forms. As a result, few achieve levels of mastery. Hence the overall standard of Western practitioners is not as high as in China, and this only strengthens the case against taiji as a combat-oriented art today.

The following describes some of the basic training techniques for Chen Style taiji, namely the standing pole (*zhanzhuang*) and two methods of silk reeling (*chansigong*). Standing pole is a very common form of static qigong, usually practiced as if holding a ball with the eyes closed. However, Chen Style standing pole can be practiced with the eyes closed or open. This exercise enables the practitioner to gather qi and strengthens the muscles and bones. The silk reeling methods within the Chen repertoire, some practiced stationary and some moving, are too numerous to be listed here. The following are the first two basic stationary skills as taught by Chen Xiaowang. The first trains single-hand silk reeling while the second trains double-hands. No matter what style of taiji one may practice, these exercises will only enhance one's level of skill.

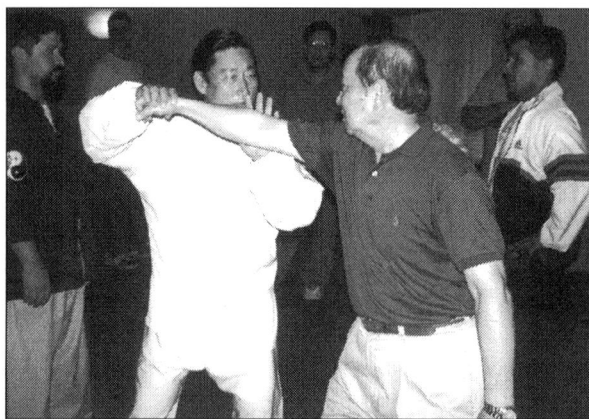

Chen Xiaowang demonstrating application
of laoji yilu at recent seminar in New York.

Standing pole and silk reeling are essential to taiji's practice for health, but also to its martial capability. Both are superb exercises for health, especially the standing pole, practiced by millions of Chinese, many of whom do not practice any martial art. In Chen taiji training, even though standing pole and silk reeling constitute the basis of forms training, they are never to be disregarded, even later when the practitioner becomes advanced. The principles adhered to during standing relate directly to the form's practice, i.e., head kept upright, shoulders relaxed, chest concave, hips sunk, etc. and are retained throughout the routines. Standing pole and silk reeling are integral to developing a stable root, powerful legs, and relaxed and sunken hips (needed for an open, low, and comfortable stance), as well as a relaxed and calm frame of mind.

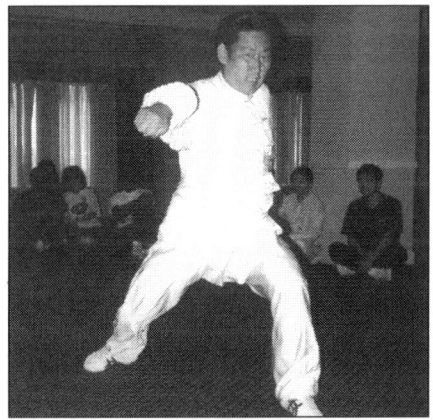
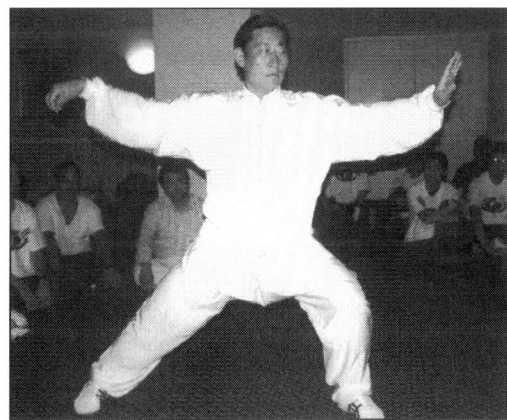

Left: punching with fajing. Right: Single Whip posture.

Practice of all these above characteristics leads to the proper development of fajing. True fajing is not mere brute strength but internal power—a sudden, relaxed and fluid explosion of force. Many attempt to imitate it, either through making excessive noise exhaling while striking, or by simply vibrating the fist upon full extension of a weak punch. In these cases, either too much external force is used, or there is no power at all. Those that rely solely on their might only become stiff. Fajing is only possible through the correct alignment of the body, proper relaxation in the posture, and the sudden transference of weight from one leg to the other.

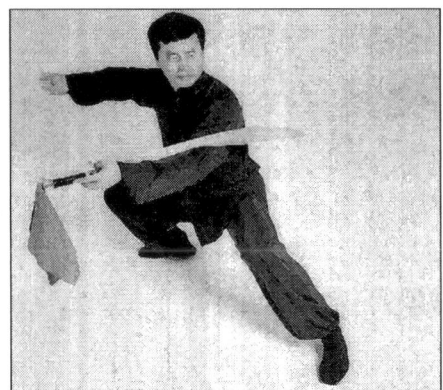
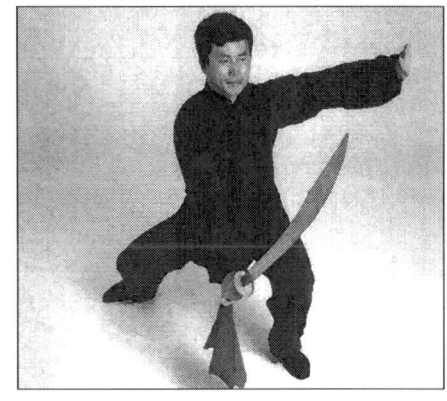

Ren Guangyi practicing a Chen Style sword routine.

Standing

Standing in the manner described below is really a dynamic tension exercise for the legs and is crucial for qi development. For health, the practitioner does not need to stand very low, but to develop taiji as a martial art one must sink lower. Leg power becomes fortified as the practitioner learns to sink and relax. Mastery of this exercise comes from learning to relax with a painful pressure placed on the legs. As the legs are solid (yang), the upper body must become empty and relaxed (yin) to achieve balance. In the beginning stages this is difficult to achieve, but the more time one spends 'standing' the easier it becomes to relax. The intense pressure comes from within and is, therefore, completely under the practitioner's control. It all depends on how low he is prepared to sink. When he feels too tired or has endured too much pain, he can simply raise his posture until such time when he is ready to sink again. To the casual observer this exercise may not look beneficial, but internally circulation is increased, hormones are stimulated, and he may well wonder why the practitioner who appears to be doing nothing perspires so profusely, despite no shortage of breath. The object is to assume control of the internal pressure, strengthen the internal organs, calm the mind, and develop strength without physical effort by the musculature.

As the body sinks and the degree to which the knees bend increases, the tendency is for the knees to extend forward beyond the toes or for the upper body to lean forwards. This is common among practitioners, especially beginners, or those who have no teacher to correct them. This bad posture removes the burden from the thighs, where it should be, and places it squarely on the knees, which can result in damaged ligaments. To compensate for this, one must sit slightly backwards. (However, this does not mean to lean backwards.) The problem then becomes one of balance. It may seem awkward and uncomfortable in the beginning but eventually this becomes easier through correct practice. The key is to relax and open the hips.

In the beginning, the main difficulty with standing pole is disciplining oneself to sink more and increase the pain threshold, and to stand still for increasingly longer periods when the mind is used to activity and constant stimulation. The idea is eventually to relax completely and forget everything and enter a mild meditative state. Thus, the qi will sink to the dantian and flow more strongly, passing through the entire body, causing the practitioner to feel calm, clear, and energetic. Once the body is still, the mind neutral and balanced, the spine relaxed, and the dantian's qi balanced and strong, the body internally becomes like a "taiji painting," according to Chen Xiaowang.

Wuji and Taiji

Standing pole is also known as wuji standing. The Chinese believe everything comes from wuji or "nothing" (an infinite void) and then becomes taiji or "something." When it does become something, we have the One (taiji). The famous Chinese yin/yang symbol embodies this concept. Taiji is the circle, the One, the condition before yin and yang. It is a common Western misconception that taiji and yin/yang are one and the same. Taiji is moving, dynamic and chaotic. Only when taiji settles does it separate to become Two (yin and yang). Once One becomes Two, this gives birth to the Four Dimensions which divide to give the eight situations (*bagua*), which provide the sixty-four hexagrams (*pa*) as detailed in the *Yijing* (Book of Change), which holds the formula for divination. It is believed that everything in the universe is symbolically represented within this book and can be divined by understanding the hexagrams. Taiji is the principle or concept on which the eight trigrams and the *Yijing* are based.

Taiji is the martial art based on this philosophy. Thus, following the Dao (nature), wuji should be practiced before taiji. In other words, stillness is developed before movement. We follow nature by practicing wuji first and then when the qi is strong from having been accumulated, we can begin to use it in preparation for silk reeling and the taiji forms. Thus, balance is maintained between yin (stillness) and yang (movement).

Chen taiji is physically very demanding and consumes vast amounts of energy because of its low postures and especially the use of fajing. This is even more apparent in *erlu* (second routine), also called the cannon fist. Erlu, which is geared more towards full combat boxing, is the antithesis of *yilu* (first routine) and is predominantly an internal form. Chen family taiji is the only style of taiji boxing which has a second empty-hand routine. This tremendous energy must first be cultivated and stored to be used, otherwise the practitioner would become exhausted. This is the purpose of standing pole and silk reeling. In fact, many practitioners of erlu who have failed to follow the principal safety rules concerning internal development have injured themselves and suffered many unpleasant side-effects, such as nausea, fainting, retching, and, in worst cases, some have even coughed blood. Taiji without internal training would cease to be a health-giving martial art.

When one stands still long enough, focuses internally, and closes the door of the senses to all external stimulation, one will develop an increased awareness of the body, and eventually come to gain sensitivity to movement inside. Externally the body is static but internally the heart is beating, and the qi is flowing. This is the condition known as "motion in stillness." During the practice of forms, externally there is activity, but internally one should be very calm relaxed and centered, and the mind should be still. This is the condition known as "stillness in motion."

Stillness in Motion and Sensitivity

Internal sensitivity is only possible through becoming yin: internally focused, mentally still, relaxed, calm, and receptive. If the posture is not correct, the flow of qi will be impeded and one will be unable to relax, which will inhibit not only the sensitivity of the individual to his own internal workings, but also to the energy of his opponent. In Chen Wangting's 'Song of the Canon of Boxing' is contained the line, "Nobody knows me, while I know everybody." This refers to the practitioner's sensitivity to an opponent's energy and intentions and the simultaneous ability to conceal his own intentions. The way to know the enemy is to know oneself first.

Chen Wangting also created the two-person training exercise known as push-hands, whereby practitioners' arms make contact and press mutually with the idea being to conceal one's own movements so that the opponent has no way of knowing whether one is opening or closing, to be wholly unpredictable, as through twisting and coiling together one uses sensitivity to read the opponent's movements and foretell his next move. This is a high level of martial art because one is not required to merely block incoming force with force but to follow the opponent's energy to defend oneself.

The fighting skills are raised to a higher level through silk reeling where, according to the poem, "power comes from within" and "inner energy becomes outward power." In the early stages one should aim to stand for a minimum of ten minutes. The time spent on standing pole should be increased gradually. According to Ren Guangyi, serious taiji students should spend between thirty minutes and one hour. For the first six months of his preliminary training, all Ren did was this painful standing. His teacher has been known to 'stand' for two hours. The longer one can accomplish this task, the stronger one will be and the better one's taiji will become.

The principle of taiji is not to force anything, so a weak person should practice building up slowly. For many people who practice taiji solely for health purposes, ten minutes may be sufficient. But to develop taiji as a high-level martial art, standing must be done for long periods and this can be painful. As the object of push-hands and combat is conquering an opponent, it could be said that standing pole is for conquering oneself.

Silk Reeling

Chansijing (silk reeling) actually takes its name from the silkworm itself, as it manufactures silk in a coiling motion. The external movements of the taiji form resemble the work of the silkworm as it creates silk. The purpose of silk reeling as health exercise is to strengthen the body and open the dantian through the turning of the waist and to smooth the jingluo/jingmai. In taiji all the energy is generated from the dantian. Silk reeling prepares the practitioner for forms practice and strengthens the body through its coiling motions.

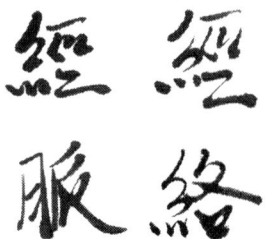

Left: jingmai; right: jingluo.

The martial application of the silk reeling exercises comes through teaching the student to move in circles until this becomes instinctual. The jingmai jingluo first half of the circle is used to neutralize or redirect an opponent's attacking force and the second half is for counter-attacking the opponent, using (borrowing) his own force against him. When the silkworm first ejects the silk from its body the single strand of silk is very fragile, but after it's wound around a branch numerous times it becomes extremely durable and resilient as it has been amply reinforced. This same principle is applied to the human body. For his efforts, the dedicated practitioner will achieve the physical quality most often associated with the great taiji masters, that of "steel wrapped in cotton."

The silk reeling practice involves a flow of uninterrupted sets of movements. The purpose of this is to keep the qi flowing, to prevent it from becoming blocked. In martial usage, this capacity enables the practitioner to flow and regain his center when he is pushed. This is the neutralization capability of silk reeling.

Most people become stiff when they are pushed and their qi becomes blocked, causing the body to lose its connection with its center and waist. If the incoming force is greater than their root, they will lose their balance because the ability to neutralize has been lost due to the dantian and back having become tight. When the center of gravity or the centerline is struck or pushed, the individual tends to lose equilibrium. Repetitive practice of reeling silk prevents the qi from becoming blocked so the center can always be preserved. High-level skill involves the sensitivity to be able to change jing internally and reposition the body so that the center is never in this vulnerable position. The dantian is constantly shifting, or at very least, it is always in a stable position where it can change when the need arises.

On the health level, according to traditional Chinese medicine the body's healthy functioning depends on naturally free flowing qi. When the qi becomes blocked along a specific organ network the corresponding organ will be adversely affected, causing the whole body to become ill. The channels need to be dredged and kept open. Silk reeling keeps the qi flowing and opens the channels. This is the exercise's primary goal.

The main principle when practicing silk reeling exercises is to be natural and relaxed. Turn the waist and allow the hands to follow. It is a grave mistake to use force to push the qi along. This will only arrest the development of the looseness needed to reach a high level. All silk reeling movements originate from the waist and involve the dantian and the *mingmen* acupoint (on the lower back directly opposite the dantian) and require the cooperation and coordination of the whole body. When the waist spirals, this creates spiraling movement through the shoulders, elbows, and wrists to the fingers. As the hips, knees, ankles, and feet are connected to their upper counterparts, silk reeling movements pass down through these joints to the toes and return to the dantian.

There are millions of taiji practitioners throughout the world. Not all practice silk reeling. Those that do not are only able to use up to fifty percent of their body's capacity to accomplish any individual movement or strike. This also means that when they need to use power or fajing they will only be able to use fifty percent or less of their power. Mastery of silk reeling enables the practitioner to utilize his entire body into a concentrated, focused strike with an effortlessness that most practitioners of taiji can only dream of ever achieving.

The Requirements of Standing Pole

The head should feel as if suspended from above. One can imagine that there is a light object on top of the head and to prevent it from falling one must remain very still. The chin must be slightly tucked in so that the *baihui* point (crown of the head) is facing the sky and connects with the *huiyin* point (inside the legs, between the reproductive organs and anus). The hearing should remain concentrated behind so that the qi will sink to the dantian. In this situation the mind should be very clear. The chest should feel loose and relaxed, which will make the dantian feel full. If the abdominal muscles are tight and the dantian is tense it will close. This means that the qi cannot pass through the dantian. In this case it will become lodged in the chest and cause a feeling of tightness or oppression in the chest which, in turn, will increase the burden on the heart. This situation can be remedied by a simple readjustment of the posture.

The fundamental goal of standing pole is for the entire body to support the existence of the dantian and not the stomach muscles. When the arms are held at shoulder height peng energy is developed. This is an important quality, used for warding-off and for maintaining distance or space between oneself and an opponent. The effect of this should be like an inflated tire. *Peng qi* is best described as the power of resilience and flexibility. Of all the eight methods (*bafa*) associated with taiji, it is the most important essential energy. A taiji practitioner should always have peng energy. It is the energy of defensive attack, used to evade and adhere. This energy is used when moving, receiving, collecting, and striking. With peng qi, the body reacts like a spring which rebounds when pressed. If an opponent applies pressure and one's arm folds, peng qi has been lost, and so has ones best line of defense. Often during standing the arms begin to feel tired and ache. In this case, you can lower the arms to waist height but keep them extended (see photo 5 in the silk reeling double-hands exercise #2 in the technical section) which develops the qi at the dantian, or just bring them closer to the body at shoulder height, making the circle smaller. When the shoulders and arms once again feel comfortable, return them to the original position.

In the beginning stages, it is common for the legs to shake and burn. In fact, there is a traditional saying in Chen Village, "Whosoever drinks the water of Chen Village, their legs will shake." As the legs become stronger, standing in this manner becomes more comfortable and one may even come to enjoy the sensations that accompany standing pole practice. When the strain on the legs becomes unbearable, slowly raise the posture, but do not stand up completely. The hips should always maintain a degree of relaxation. Then, when the pain finally disperses and strength has been regained, sink down once again to a low posture. Pay careful attention that the knees do not push outwards, fold inwards, or extend beyond the toes. The toes, heels, balls and sides of the feet should all contact the ground except for the *yongquan* point on the sole of the foot (in the center of the arch) which should be kept hollow.

In the beginning to intermediate stages of taiji practice, one needs a teacher to check the body's alignment and make the necessary corrections. It is common for a student to feel intense heat consuming his body when the teacher corrects his posture ("fixes his frame") or even occasionally when he does so himself. This is merely the qi flowing freely once again after having been obstructed, like dammed water after a hole has appeared in the wall. It is the result of the acupuncture channels' having been opened and the blockages of qi removed as the body's posture is allowed to become more natural. This sensation, which is quite pleasant, disperses after a time when the qi becomes balanced.

The time one spends on this exercise depends on the individual's standard. The first ten minutes are always the hardest. After this, time appears to pass at an increasing rate. Suddenly one day one may discover that forty minutes or even an hour has flown by.

ZHANZHUANG
How to Stand Like a Mountain

1) Stand naturally. Feet together. Hands at the sides. Hips slightly relaxed. The ears, shoulders, hips, knees, and ankles should all be in a straight line to maintain body balance (photos 1; 1a sideview). In this instance the musculature surrounding the dantian is not needed, so the dantian can relax and open which means that more qi will flow through it and be available to the rest of the body. The more qi which can return to the dantian from the internal organs, the more vitality one will have.

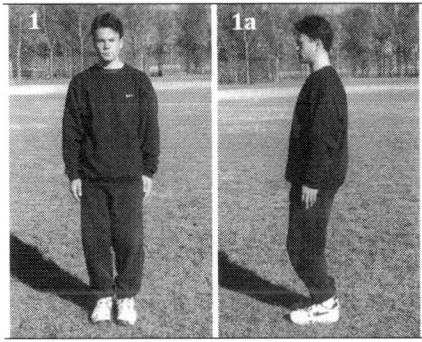

2) Close the mouth with the tongue resting lightly on the upper palate to facilitate the flow of qi downwards and close the eyes (or if you prefer you can allow them to remain open).

3) Repeat the following words to yourself as a mental checklist: "Weight balance. Mind balance. Listening behind. Dantian qi balance."
4) Slowly bend the knees and relax the hips to lower the center of gravity and allow the qi to sink more.
5) Transfer the weight onto the right leg. Sink down. Lift the heel of the left foot and then the toes (photo 2). Step out to a position shoulder-width (with the weight still solid/firm on the right leg) placing the toes to the ground first and then the heel (photo 3), slowly shifting the weight to the center so that it is balanced between both legs (photo 4; 4a sideview). Do not transfer the weight as you step out. This leads to "double weighting."
6) Again, repeat silently, "Weight balance. Mind balance. Listening behind. Dantian qi balance." Relax the spine from the neck down to the coccyx. As you mentally relax each vertebrae, count from one to nine. As the qi sinks the dantian becomes stronger and should feel very comfortable. Internally, the body becomes like the taiji image.

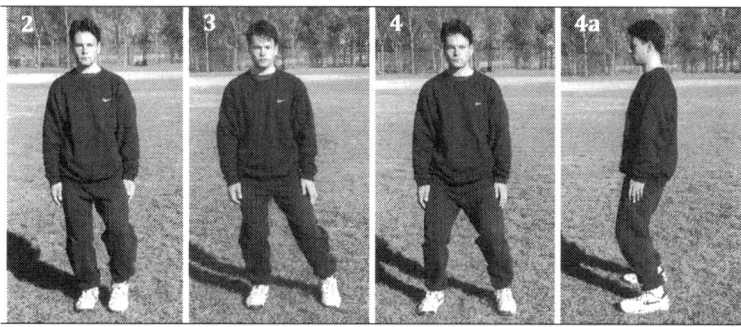

7) Very slowly rise the hands to a position shoulder height and shoulder width (photos 5, 6 and 6a). The arms can be slightly wider than the shoulders to open the chest and allow more qi to sink to the dantian. As the hands raise, simultaneously sink the hips more deeply and relax. It is imperative that the shoulders and elbows be relaxed and sunk and the wrists loose. In other words, do not fully extend the arms, straightening the elbows and fingers.
8) When the arms are at the correct position, repeat again "Mind balance. Weight balance. Listening behind. Dantian qi balance."

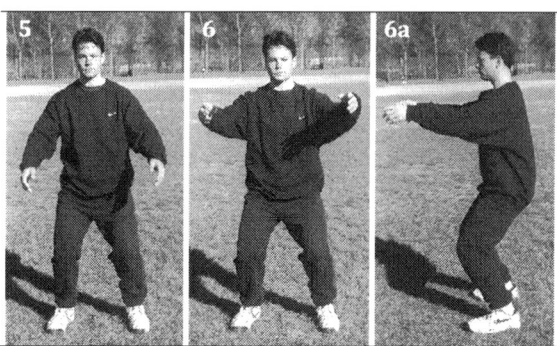

9) Now find the most comfortable position (i.e. check that the chest is concave, and shoulders and hips are as relaxed as possible). You may need to make slight adjustments if any part of the body feels stiff or tense. When you feel comfortable hold this position. Stand firm "like a mountain" for as long as possible (photos 7).
10) When you decide to finish the exercise, repeat again: "Mind balance. Weight balance. Listening behind. Dantian qi balance."

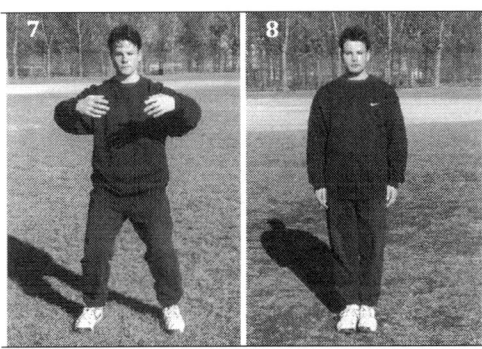

11) Very, very slowly, lower the hands down to the sides. At the same time stand up slowly, though not completely. The hips should still maintain a degree of relaxation (photo 5).
12) Repeat once more: "Mind balance. Weight balance. Listening behind. Dantian qi balance."
13) Slowly transfer the weight back to the right leg. Lift the heel and then the toes of the left foot and replace the left leg next to the right (photos 3 and 2). As the foot lands, plant the toes first and then the heel. The hips are still relaxed at this point.
14) For the very last time repeat the words: "Mind balance. Weight balance. Listening behind. Dantian qi balance." Count silently, one through nine.
15) Then slowly stand all the way up. The hips are now straight. You are back to the original position (photo 8).
16) Relax and slowly open the eyes. This completes standing pole or wuji standing. After cultivating stillness, one is ready to begin taiji movement. It is generally best to follow this exercise with silk reeling exercises prior to forms practice.

SILK REELING

Exercise #1 Single-Hand

This exercise requires the practitioner to work both left and right sides of the body. The number of times that silk is reeled should be equal on both sides. You can begin with ten times and go to fifty or more on each side. The eyes should focus lightly on the hand (the middle finger especially) and follow as it moves in wide circles. Technically the hand should not pass higher than the eyebrows or lower than the chin, though some teachers claim no higher than the top of the head or lower than the shoulders. The size of the circles described by the hand are directly related to the width of the stance.

Beginning with the left side first, the procedure for the opening position is as follows:

1) Stand naturally. Feet together. Hands by the sides. Relax the hips and bend the knees slightly (photo 1).
2) Place the right hand on the hip. Left hand by the side. The weight should be balanced between the legs (photo 2).
3) Bend the knees more deeply and sink down. Transfer the weight to the right leg. Lift the heel of the left foot followed by the toes (photo 3) and step out to the side in a wide stance landing with the heel first and then the toes. At the same time as the left leg steps out, turn the waist towards the right with the left hand following the waist, palm pushing to the right (without force) to a position above the knee and opposite the dantian (photo 4).

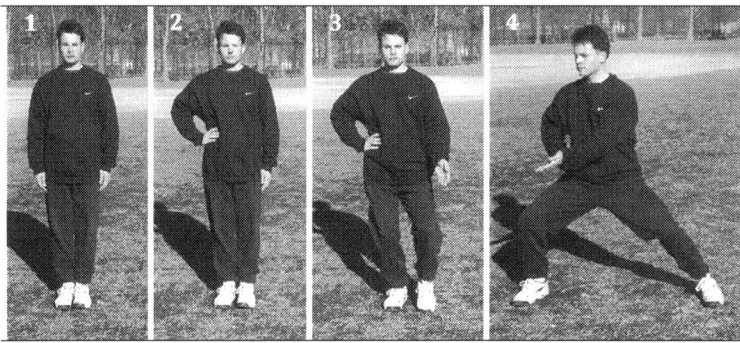

4) Relax the wrist and raise the hand to approximately shoulder height, turning the palm outwards (photos 5 and 6).

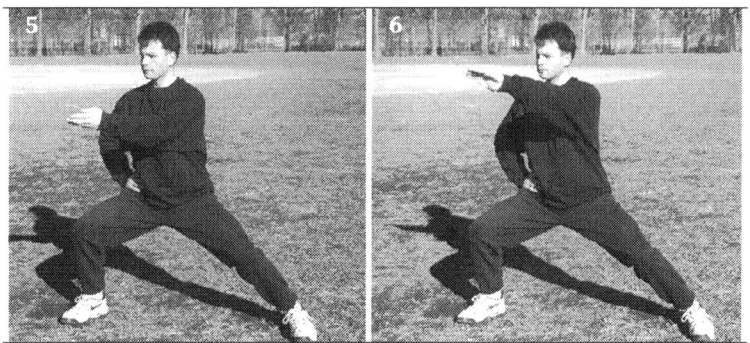

5) Transfer the weight to the left leg and turn the waist to the left. The left hand follows the waist and describes an arc, to a position shoulder-height but wider than the shoulders in front of the body (photos 7, 8, and 9). Relax the shoulder and keep the elbow sunk (lower than the shoulder), otherwise the shoulder will become tense, and the qi will become blocked.

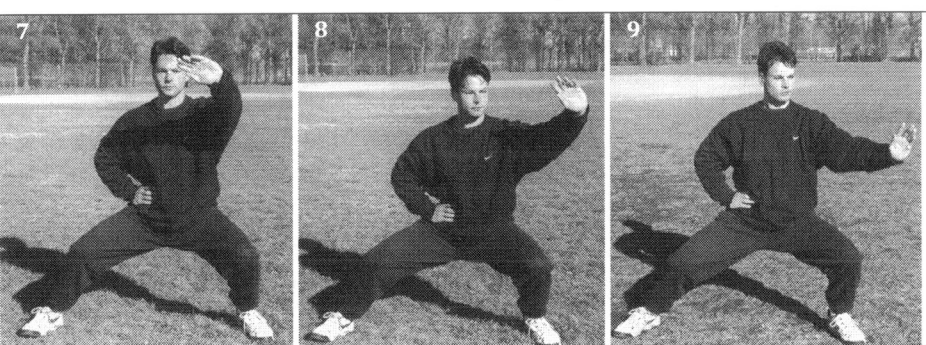

Without pausing, follow the proceeding steps:

Step 1: With weight on the left leg, drop the left elbow as the hand spirals inwards in a circular motion down to waist-height to the left of the hips, with the palm facing right (qi travels to the waist) (photo 10).

Step 2. Transfer the weight to the right leg and turn the waist to the right. The hand follows the waist to a position opposite the dantian above the right knee—as in opening movement (qi passes to the dantian) (photos 11 and 4).

Step 3. With the weight still on the right leg, relax the wrist and raise the arm to a position opposite the right shoulder, turning the palm outwards as in opening movement (qi travels up the back and to the shoulders) (photo 6).

Step 4. Transfer the weight to the left. At the same time, turn the waist and move the hand in a circular motion to a position outside of the left shoulder in front of the body—as in opening movement (qi passes through the arms to the fingertips) (photo 7). This completes one cycle. After Step 4 repeat the process 1 through 4 and continue for a minimum of ten cycles each side to a maximum of fifty. To close on the left side, follow the proceeding steps:

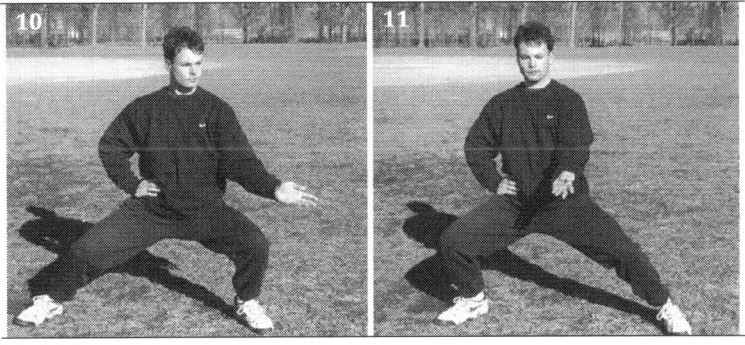

Step 5. On the last cycle follow steps 1, 2, and 3, and on the 4th step, as you turn the palm outwards and transfer the weight to the left leg, close the right leg by lifting the heel and then the toe and replacing the toe and then the heel next to the left foot. The weight is still sunk with the knees bent (photo 12).

Step 6. Raise the right hand until it comes to a position opposite the left hand, about shoulder height (photo 13).

Step 7. Lower both hands together down the center (fingers facing inwards) and straighten the legs at the same time (photo 14). The hands come back to a position at the sides of the thighs, as in the natural opening position (photo 1). To begin the right side, follow the preceding steps from the opening position to the closing position, but reverse all instructions so you have a mirror image. When you close the right side, this completes the single hand silk reeling exercise.

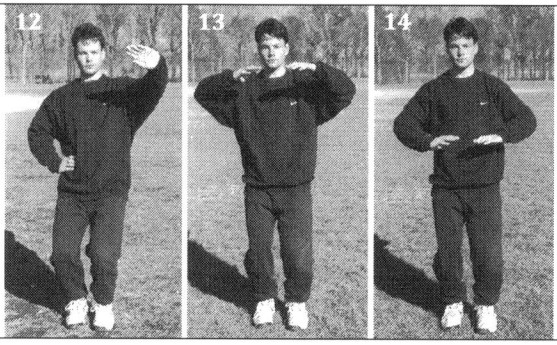

SILK REELING - Exercise #2 Double-Hand

This exercise also works both the left and right sides. Begin with the left.

1) Stand naturally with arms by the sides and feet together. The weight is balanced. The hips are relaxed and sunk, and the knees slightly bent (photo 1).

2) Pivot on the right heel and turn the right toes out at a ninety-degree angle (photo 2).

3) Bend the knees and sink down more. Transfer the weight to the right (rear) leg and lift the left heel. At the same time turn both palms to face the rear, waist height—the left hand is carried more forward, opposite the dantian, and the right hand is outside of the right hip (photos 3–4).

4) Lift the left toes and step forward into a deep stance at forty-five degrees, landing with the heel and then the toes. As you step, turn the waist to the rear; hands follow. The toes of the front leg are turned slightly inwards to maintain a line with the knee (photo 5). Twine hands clockwise to face the front (photos 6–7).

5) Transfer the weight to the left (front) leg (photo 8). Turn the waist to the left. The hands follow with the left hand parallel to the left knee and the right hand opposite the dantian (photo 9). The left hand is carried naturally slightly higher than the right. This is the opening position. Throughout the proceeding cycles the eyes follow the hands.

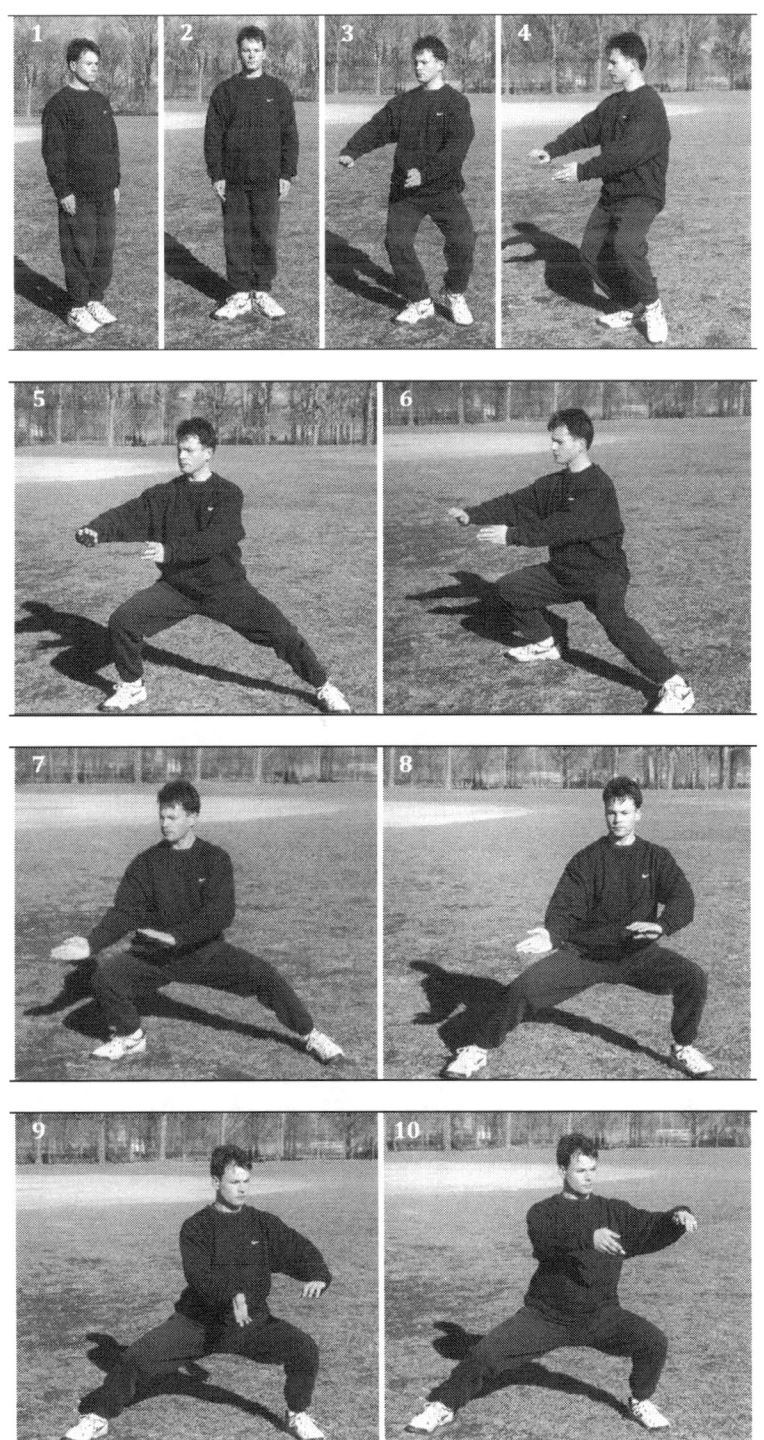

Step 1. Weight on the left leg. Relax the wrists and raise the arms together turning the palms to face outwards, hands approximately shoulder height, elbows sunk, and shoulders relaxed (left hand, qi to the waist; right hand, qi to the back) (photos 10–11).

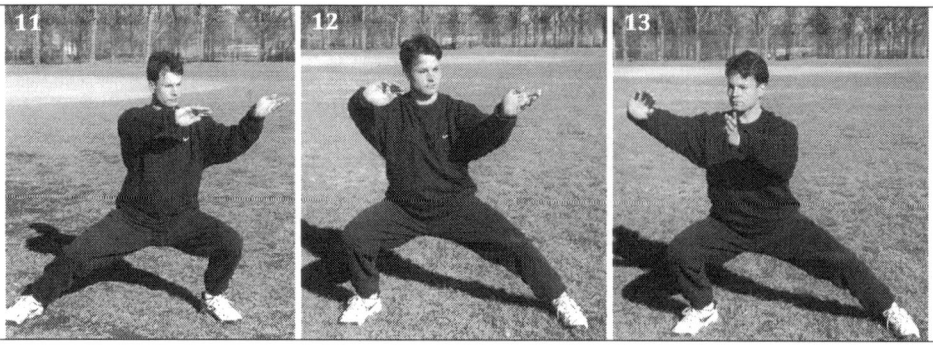

Step 2. Transfer the weight to the rear (right leg) and turn the waist to the right with the hands following. The left hand comes to a position opposite the left shoulder with the right hand carried outside to the rear with both palms facing outwards (left hand, qi to the dantian; right hand, qi to the fingers) (photos 12–13).

Step 3. While keeping the weight on the right, move the arms downwards in an arc to a position waist height. The left hand is in front of the right hip, palm facing downwards, and the right hand is carried to the rear, outside of the right hip and palm facing slightly forward (left hand, qi to the back; right hand, qi to the waist) (photo 5).

Step 4. Transfer the weight to the front (left leg). Turn the waist to the left and front with the hands following, left hand in front of the left hip and right hand in front of the dantian (left hand, qi to the fingers; right hand, qi to the dantian) (photos 6–9).

This is one complete cycle. Repeat as many times as you feel comfortable, being sure to balance the number of repetitions on both sides.

When you decide to finish the left side and begin the right, on the last cycle follow steps 1, 2, 3, and on the 4th step, as you transfer the weight to the front (left leg) and the hands follow the waist to the dantian, close the right leg next to the left (photo 14).

In a closing position raise the arms in an arc to shoulder height (photos 15–16) then lower them down the center to the sides and straighten the legs, returning to the natural beginning position (photo 1).

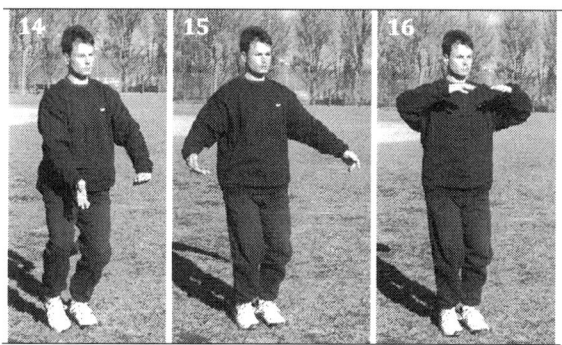

To work silk reeling on the opposite side, follow the instructions above but reverse the instructions, i.e. begin with turning the left toes out at a ninety-degree angle and step out with the right foot, etc. Reverse the directions for steps 1 through 4. Close in the same manner as before.

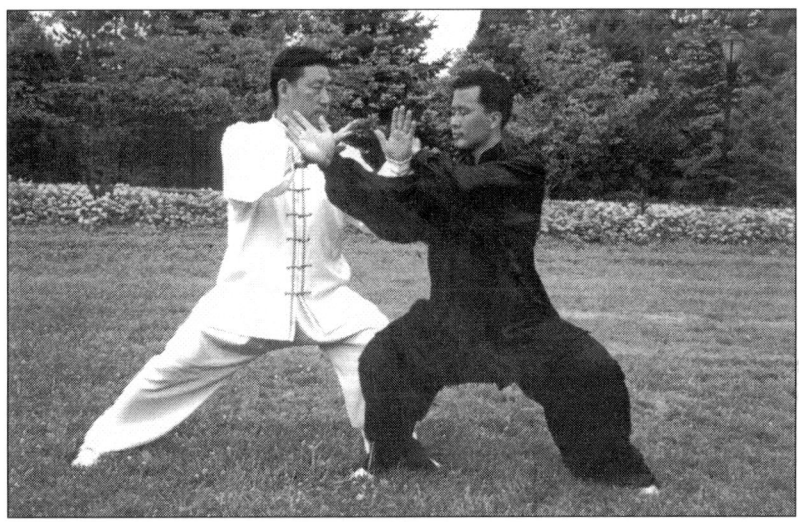

Push-hands: Chen Xiaowang and Ren Guangyi demonstrating.

With both of these exercises, don't step too wide. Chen stylists are noted for their low stances, but these should not be forced. You must know yourself, your strength, body structure, and range of motion. Then you can determine the width of your stance, how low you can sit, and which posture is right for you. The general rule is to be natural. Otherwise, the qi will not flow freely, and your movement will be restricted.

All silk reeling exercises should be performed in a very relaxed and comfortable manner. A common mistake is to use too much energy or force. In this case the arms will become stiff. The movements should be slow, fluid and continuous, without interruption. Through both standing pole and silk reeling the mass of the practitioner's thighs increases dramatically, making his gait stronger and steadier. The sinking and rooting achieved through these skills opens the hips and increases the mobility of the waist, necessary in neutralizing an opponent's energy. There are no mystical powers in taiji. The seemingly impossible, or "super-human" ability to throw an opponent twelve feet away, is all accomplished through correct gongfu (time and energy spent) and understanding and applying the taiji principles.

Most real confrontations on the street are concluded on the ground with both parties struggling for control through wrestling and grappling. The winner is invariably the stronger person. However, one who is well trained in standing pole is extremely hard to push as his root is so strong (through relaxed sinking, not the use of raw muscle power). He is, therefore, master of his own balance and can dissolve the greatest force from any direction because his waist is like an axle, having been forged through the training of silk reeling. Without silk reeling, the spiraling necessary for advanced qinna techniques (the ability to follow the opponent as he attempts to escape or to escape from them oneself) and body strikes are extremely difficult to accomplish. Ren Guangyi is quick to point out that one can learn qinna without learning taiji silk reeling, but his level will not be as high. Qinna is not applied using force against force, but with "listening skill" combined with good technique and coordinated waist power.

To apply qinna one must be very quick, using the element of surprise by feinting one direction and then switching or following the opponent. The latter requires sensitivity to know in which direction the enemy is heading and to beat him there. Also to escape qinna requires one first to relax and sink the hips, in other words to be rooted, and then to use the subtle coiling motion developed through intensive silk reeling training. The internal energy travels and changes in the chest and waist, and passes through the shoulders and elbows; when the strength has reached the wrist, one can escape. Only when the shoulders and elbow joints are clear and unobstructed can the internal energy reach the fingers. The shoulders connect with the hips (the elbows with the knees and the hands with the feet), so unless the hips can relax, the shoulders will be stiff. It is extremely difficult, if not impossible, to escape qinna once one's feet have already been lifted off the ground by a painful joint lock, or after one has already been forced to the floor.

The object of standing, silk reeling, and form practice is to achieve balance, fifty percent hard and fifty percent soft, yin and yang. In this situation Man and Nature become One. Generally, in push-hands people are naturally tense, so yang (hardness) comes easier to them than yin (softness). When one uses physical strength, the tendency is to strain and become stiff. In this case it is very difficult to attain softness through relaxation when it is needed. Therefore, this should be the primary intention when practicing foundation training. On the other hand, if one has attained relaxation and softness, one can achieve hardness at will and there will be more internal strength at one's disposal.

To reach a high level of taijiquan, repetitive daily practice of bare-handed forms is, of course, imperative. But many practitioners only concentrate on these and disregard the foundations. If the ability to perform the taiji forms spontaneously in demonstration and the ability to apply them in a free-style manner in real life situations (the purpose for which they were designed) is the fluent language of the art, and the forms (routine training) contain the vocabulary and sentences, then the practice of standing pole and silk reeling provides the sounds upon which the language is based. They cannot be disregarded.

Pinyin	Wade-Giles	Chinese
bafa	pa fa	八法
bagua	pakua	八卦
bai hui	pai hui	百會
chansijing	ch'an szu ching	纏絲經
Chenjiagou	Ch'en chia kou	陳家溝
dantian	tan t'ien	丹田
dao	tao	道
daoyin	tao yin	導引
erlu	erh lu	二路
fajing	fa ching	發勁
gongfu	kung fu	功夫
gua	kua	卦
Henan	Honan	河南
huiyin	huiyin	會陰
jingluo	ching lo	經絡
jingmai	ching mai	經脈
lanzhayi	lan cha i	懶扎衣
laojia	laochia	老架
ming men	ming men	命門
Paochui	P'ao ch'ui	炮捶
qi	ch'i	氣
qigong	ch'i kung	氣功
qinna	ch'in na	擒拿
Shaolin	Shaolin	少林
taiji	t'ai chi	太極
taijiquan	t'ai chi ch'üan	太極拳
tingjing	t'ing ching	聽勁
cunjing	ts'un ching	寸勁
tuishou	t'ui shou	推手
wuji	wu chi	無極
xinjia	hsin chia	新架
xingyi	hsing i	形意
Yijing	I-ch'ing	易經
yilu	i lu	一路
yongquan	yong ch'üan	涌泉
zhanzhuang	han chuang	站樁

Pinyin	Wade–Giles	Chinese
Chen Fake	Ch'en Fa-k'o	陳發科
Chen Zhangxing	Ch'en Chang-hsing	陳長興
Chen Wangting	Chen Wang-t'ing	陳王廷
Chen Qingping	Ch'en Ch'ing-p'ing	陳青萍
Chen Xiaowang	Ch'en Hsiao-wang	陳小旺
Li Bantian	Li Pan-t'ien	李半天
Qi Jiguang	Ch'i Chi-kuang	戚繼光
Ren Guangyi	Jen Kuang-i	任廣義
Sun Lutang	Sun Lutang	孫祿堂
Tang Hao	T'ang Hao	唐豪
Wu Jianquan	Wu Chien-ch'uan	武鑒泉
Yang Chengfu	Yang Ch'eng-fu	楊橙甫
Yang Luchan	Yang Lu-ch'an	楊露禪
Zhang Bojing	Chang Po-ching	張伯敬

References

Berwick, S. (1997, October). The five stages of Chen combat training. *Inside Kung Fu*, 106–111.

Berwick, S. (1997, October). Chen combat training. *Inside Kung Fu*, 106–111.

Berwick, S. (1997, December–January). Chen combat. *Wushu Kung Fu*, 23–25; 40–41.

Bissell, G. (1993, February). Chen style taiji changquan and the five routines of taijiquan. *The Journal of the Chen Style Taijiquan Research Association of Hawaii*, *1*(1), 7–9.

Chen, X. The lectures and teachings of Chen Xiaowang: New York seminars July 20–21, 1996, and September 27–28, 1997, sponsored by Ren Guangyi; Rutherford, New Jersey, Mountain View Martial Arts, April 22, 1996, and September 30, 1997, sponsored by Greg Pinney.

Chi, J. (1993, October). Training techniques for Chen style skills. *Tai Chi, 17*(6), 8–11.

Gu, L. (1984). The origin, evolution and development of shadow boxing. In Zhaohua Publishing House (compilers), *Chen style taijiquan* (pp. 1–12). Hong Kong: Hai Feng Publishing Company.

Kuo, L. (1994). *The t'ai chi boxing chronicle* (Guttman, Trans.). Berkeley, CA: North Atlantic Books.

Liang, B. (1993, August). Sparring techniques in Chen style. *The Journal of the Chen Style Taijiquan Research Association of Hawaii, 1*(4), 1–3.

Ren, G. Personal instruction from Ren Guangyi, New York, 1992 to 1997.

Tse, M. (1994, June). Wuji and taiji. *Combat*, 80–81.

Tse, M. (1995, January). The martial art of Chen Wangting. *Combat*, 74–75.

• 24 •

Immortality in Chinese Thought and Its Influence on Taijiquan and Qigong
by Arieh Lev Breslow, M.A.

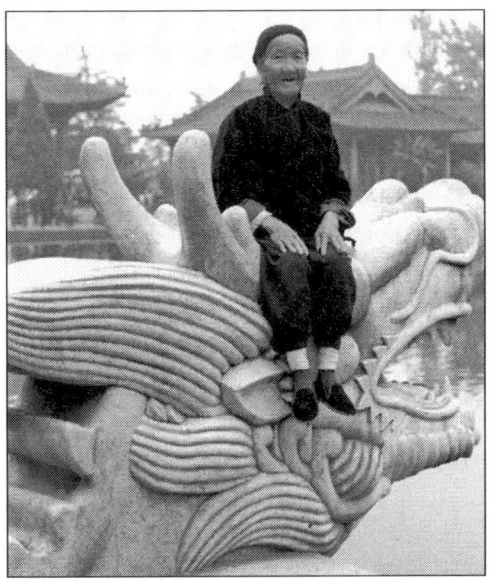
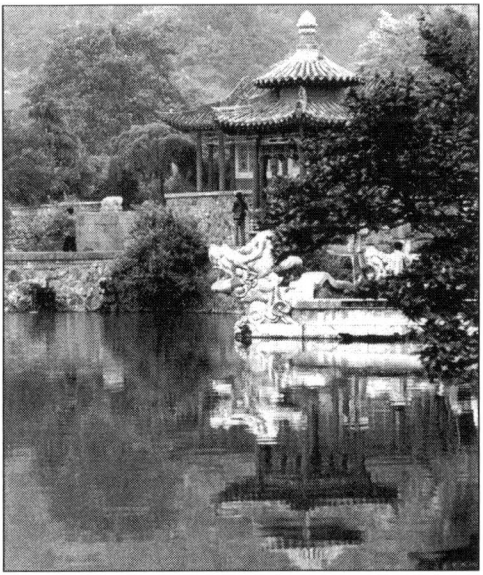

The Nine Dragon Pond within Hua Qing (Glorious Purity) Hot Springs. The springs were first used for medicinal purposes and became the site of a Daoist monastery in 936. Located just outside of Xi'an city, the area served as a resort for emperors and royalty for over a thousand years. Photographs by M. DeMarco.

Immortality is an age-old dream of human beings. Ancient and modern people, East and West, have confronted the same dilemma: the absurdity of death and the loss of personal ego. For most of us, it is an unsettling thought that we will grow old, become infirm, and eventually die. Western traditions have dealt with death in many ways. Judaic-Christian teachings promise the resurrection of the dead in the Messianic age. Against the specter of death, modern science has marshaled the technologies of cloning and cryogenics. In both the East and the West, there are an infinite number of products on the market that promise youth and vitality.

Chinese philosophers have always concerned themselves with immortality. Ge Hong and the religious Daoists believed that they could manufacture a pill that would keep them forever young and transform themselves into immortals. Through meditation and special exercises like qigong and more recently taijiquan, Daoists wanted to purify their coarse bodies into subtle spirit and merge with the infinite and eternal *Dao* (Way). This chapter will examine the origins of immortality in Chinese thought and introduce its influence on qigong and taijiquan.

Religion and Immortality in China

Throughout the centuries, religious attitudes and feelings have played a powerful role in Chinese society. In addition to Confucianism, Daoism, and Buddhism, other native philosophies and superstitions existed. Various powerful gods—each with his or her own turf—required prayers and offerings as payment to safeguard family and home. In his classic study on Chinese religion, C.K. Yang (1961: 28) describes the result of this attitude on the environs of a traditional Chinese dwelling:

> The influence of religion on the Chinese family life was everywhere visible. Upon entering any house, one saw paper door gods ... painted on the doors for protection ... On the floor was an alter to [*tudi*], the earth god ... [*Tian Guan*], the heavenly official, was in the courtyard, and the wealth gods, who brought well-being and prosperity to the family, were in the hall in the main room of the house.....

In addition to the gods and the various religious movements, ancestor worship exerted its towering presence over family life. This form of homage was the one universal and unifying Chinese religious institution. Ancestor worship fostered a binding relationship between the living and the dead, the former to offer sacrifices and the latter to bestow blessings. With such a powerful institution whose figures lived on in heaven and wielded their authority on earth, it is no wonder that the idea of immortality found fertile ground to grow.

The belief in immortality cut a wide swath across the various philosophical, religious, and social camps in Chinese history. Emperors, peasants, merchants, and soldiers could share a belief in and the possibility of attaining eternal life. This was possible because religion in China encouraged a dynamic flow between its multitudinous sects and groupings that was unknown in the West. In Europe, one was a Catholic, a Protestant, a Jew, or a Moslem. An individual could not claim allegiance to more than one religious persuasion simultaneously. In contrast, the Chinese usually did not belong to a specific group nor were they required to profess loyalty to a particular article of faith. Professor Laurence Thompson (1989: 2) observed:

> Except in the case of the professional living apart in monasteries, religion in China was so woven into the broad fabric of family and social life that there was not even a special word for it (religion) until modern times, when one was coined to match the Western term.

Even the strict and uncompromising Confucians were not immune to the lure of immortality. Only the Buddhists, whose faith contained the doctrine of achieving nirvana or ego extinction, were unsympathetic to the transfiguration of the ego-self. Nevertheless, the Buddhists also allowed for a kind of immortality in the doctrine of reincarnation.

Of the many religious ideas, beliefs, and superstitions, the notion of immortality held a prominent and inspirational position in Chinese society, much like heaven in Western religions. Chinese folklore is filled with the stories of immortals who live forever and obtain supernatural powers such as walking through walls, flying through the air, and communing with the dead. These immortals often returned to earth to right wrongs and play tricks on the unwary. The Daoist sage Zhuangzi (third century BCE) drew a vivid portrait of one such immortal:

> There is a Holy Man living on faraway [*Gu-She*] mountain, with skin like ice or snow, and gentle and shy like a young girl. He doesn't eat the five grains, but sucks the wind, drinks the dew, climbs up on the clouds and mist, rides a flying dragon, and wanders beyond the four seas. By concentrating his spirit, he can protect creatures from sickness and plague and make the harvest plentiful. — Watson, 1964: 27

The following tale is a typical tale of immortality, with a moral to boot:

> There once lived a man who claimed to have discovered the secret of immortality. A Daoist priest decided to seek him out to be his disciple. When he reached the immortal's abode, he discovered that the man was dead. The priest was greatly disappointed and left immediately in great despair. Why was the priest disappointed? Was it because the man had departed from this life? But to become immortal, one must first die. — adapted from Van Over, 1984: 197

Significantly, the influence of immortality spilled over into the martial arts. The immortal and Daoist priest, Zhang Sanfeng, is the legendary founder of taijiquan. One tale recounted that he was meditating in a cave when the principles and postures of taiji came to him in a dream. Another version claimed that the postures suddenly appeared on the wall.

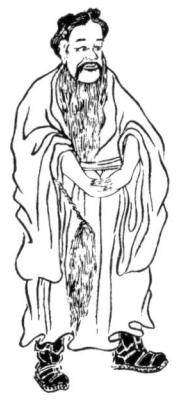

Ink rubbing of the legendary founder of taijiquan, Zhang Sanfeng.

Zhang Sanfeng reputedly lived two hundred years in his physical body and then flew off to heaven as an immortal. It was said that a Daoist monk taught him the techniques of immortality when he dwelled and meditated in the Wudang Mountains, probably the site of his cave experience. During his mortal life, he performed many miracles and feats of strength that grew out of his knowledge of the shamanistic arts (Breslow, 1995: 200–209).

The Origins of the Immortality Cult

The Chinese cult of immortality differed from the way people in the West generally viewed immortality. In Western religions, one lived forever and earned the reward of heaven by, for example, believing in the Divinity; performing good deeds; and, in some cases, through predetermined selection. In China, those who sought immortality had to harmonize their mental and physical lifeforce with the eternal lifeforce of the cosmos. To achieve their goal, they developed a vast array of spiritual practices and alchemical formulas.

Historically, the example of the legendary Yellow Emperor (*Huangdi*) became the paradigm for attaining immortality. While presiding over China's legendary Golden Age (2852–2255 BCE), not only did he teach the people how to use fire, plow their fields, and harvest the thread of the silkworm, but he also devoted his considerable talents and resources to acquiring the secret of eternal life. By virtue of his interest in medicine and in nourishing his own vitality, it was a logical step for the Yellow Emperor to seek immortality.[1] He reputedly experimented with metals and herbs and eventually found the formula for the golden elixir of immortality. After taking the drug, he mounted a dragon and flew away to the world of the immortals. Some legends note that he took his entire household of seventy people with him. Because such a revered figure as the Yellow Emperor was linked to immortality, it was difficult for later philosophers to deny its existence outright.

Following in the wake of the Yellow Emperor, the *fangshi* (magicians) were the keepers of the secret of immortality. These shamans practiced many mystical arts, such as astrology, spiritual healing, and divination. The general populace believed in their powers to achieve immortality, heal the sick, and perform miracles. Occasionally, the fangshi obtained the patronage of the ruling class. One famous emperor, Qin Shi Huangdi (259–210 BCE) sent a famous fangshi on a quest to find the "Isle of Immortals" and to bring back the elixir of immortality. He equipped a seafaring expedition of three thousand men and women with ample supplies to accompany the shaman. They never returned. One legend recorded that they found the isle of immortality and decided to remain there as immortals. Another tale averred that they found the Japanese islands where the shaman crowned himself king and established a kingdom with his retinue. As for the hapless emperor, he used to wander along the shore, gazing at the eastern horizon in the hope of spotting the returning expedition.

Laozi and Immortality

From the third century BCE, several streams of Daoism flourished. While certain later branches of Daoism became identified as seekers of eternal life, other Daoists did not focus their efforts on achieving immortality. On the other hand, all Daoists shared a reverence for the Yellow Emperor and the heritage of Laozi (sixth century BCE) as their historical sources. Daoists were often called Huang-Lao because they were followers of both the Yellow Emperor and Laozi.

Fung Yu-lan, the great twentieth-century philosopher and historian, wrote that the best way to understand Daoism is to divide it into two distinct movements: philosophical Daoism (*Dao jia*) and religious Daoism (*Dao jiao*). Philosophical Daoists accepted certain ideas of Laozi, such as Dao being the creative lifeforce of the universe, a love of nature, and a rejection of war. On the other hand, religious Daoists transformed Laozi's ideas into an all-inclusive belief system, with the *Daodejing*, his masterpiece, as their bible (Fung, 1966: 3).

If the Yellow Emperor was the mythical inspiration for Daoism, Laozi was its intellectual progenitor. Writing in his enigmatic, and at times indecipherable, style, Laozi advocated that the sage must strive to comprehend the mysterious workings of heaven and earth, that is, the Dao. Then, once these laws were understood as well as humanly possible, the sage must bring himself into harmony with them.

Laozi was aware that knowing the Dao was no easy task. In the first chapter of the *Daodejing*, Laozi informed his reader that the Dao cannot be named, that it is mysterious, and that it is "darkness within darkness."[2] Yet this mysterious Dao held within it the secret of life, for it was life itself. Furthermore, the Dao was "eternal." Thus, later seekers of immortality claimed that the sage who unraveled the secrets of the Dao secured for himself the possibility of merging with it and attaining the gift of eternal life.

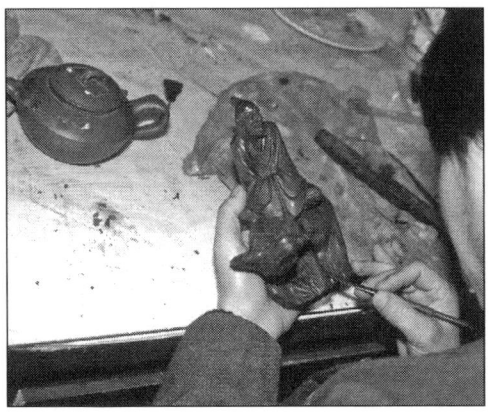
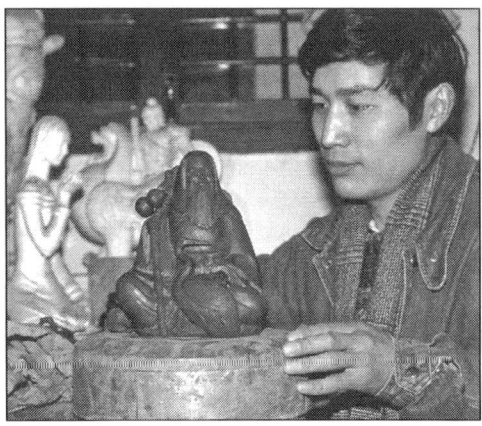

At the Hui Shan Clay Figure Workshop in Wuxi city craftspeople create Daoist images, such as Laozi on a water buffalo (top) and the figurines adorned with longevity symbols such as the medicinal gourd, crane, and long beards. Much of the art reflects ideas associated with immortality. Photos by M. DeMarco.

In the *Daodejing*, Laozi did not speak explicitly on the subject of immortality. Nevertheless, his words, often closer to poetry than a cogent philosophy, profoundly influenced those Daoists seeking immortality. They interpreted his work to show that he indeed believed in immortality, pointing to several passages to support their claim. In Chapter 33, for example, Laozi declared:

> He who stays where he is endures.
> To die but not to perish
> Is to be eternally present.

According to religious Daoists, proper cultivation of the Dao would allow a sage to live eternally, even after death. However, many other commentators, like the great taiji master Zheng Manqing, interpreted this phrase differently. According to Professor Zheng, even though the sage dies, his contribution to humanity (his Dao) lived on.[3] In other words, his reputation and good deeds remained as his living testament.[4]

Another example where the religious Daoists uncovered the idea of immortality was found in Chapter 50. Laozi wrote:

> Rhinoceroses can find no place
> To thrust their horns,
> Tigers no place to use their claws,[5]
> And weapons no place to pierce.
> Why is this so?
> Because he has no place for death to enter.

It is noteworthy that Fung Yu-lan argued that the doctrine of immortality contradicted the spirit of Laozi and his writings (Fung, 1966: 3). Laozi believed that human beings should follow in the "natural" course of things (Feng and English, 1972: ch. 25). Life was followed by death and the sage should calmly accept this reality with cold indifference. On the other hand, religious Daoists focused their efforts on achieving immortality, which was the avoidance of death and, therefore, unnatural.

The Daodejing also provided the intellectual and inspirational wellspring for taijiquan practitioners. The book elaborated on the themes of yin and yang, *wuwei* (no unnatural action), and the relationship of hard and soft.[6] In Chapter 43, Laozi postulated: "The softest thing in the universe overcomes the hardest thing in the universe." This idea forms the pivot on which the entire system of taiji stands. Without this principle, one is not practicing taiji but something else. As the Buddhists were fond of saying: "Do not be fooled. A brass monkey may look like a gold monkey, but it is still made of brass."

Significantly, in Laozi, it is possible to see the confluence of taiji principles with the ideas of immortality. In Chapter 76, he observed:

> . . . the stiff and unbending is the disciple of death.
> The gentle and yielding is the disciple of life.

Both practitioners of taiji and seekers of immortality focused on the positive value of life as opposed to death. Each required a gentle touch; patience; sensitivity; and, at times, a merging of one's personal ego with the greater Dao.

While Laozi's words were easily interpreted in various ways, he remains a seminal figure in the historiography of immortality and taiji. His pithy insights formed the intellectual framework for both the cults of immortality and the soft styles of martial arts that followed him.

Public Morality Versus Immortality

Not everyone wholeheartedly accepted the doctrine of immortality. Its opponents often cloaked their dispute in evasive language, seldom attacking the popular precept head-on. In this debate, what was not said was of equal importance to what was. This was the case with Confucius, the most influential of all Chinese teachers.

Like Laozi, Confucius (or Kongfuzi in Chinese-Mandarin, 551–479 BCE) did not speak about immortality directly. Rather, he focused his attention elsewhere on the Dao of humanity. He was concerned about public morality in the here and now. This meant that he stressed the principles of righteousness, justice, and benevolence; and urged his students to weave these teachings into the moral fabric of normative society. Essentially, he was a social reformer, a radical conservative who wanted his followers to return to the traditional ways of the Chinese classics. The following represents his down-to-earth view of the spirit world:

> [Ji Lu] asked about serving the spirits of the dead.
> The Master said: "If you are not able to serve men,
> How can you serve their spirits?"
> [Ji Lu] added, "I venture to ask about death?"
> He was answered, "While you do not know life,
> How can you know about death?" — Legge, 1971: 241–42

and

> The subjects on which the Master did not talk were —
> extraordinary things, feats of strength, disorder,
> and spiritual beings. — Legge, 1971: 201

The fact that he did not speak about "spiritual beings" and immortality suggests that, at the very least, he found the ideas problematic. His silence would be something like Thomas Jefferson refusing to comment on an important article in the Bill of Rights. Yet, in an interesting twist of logic, some later Daoists claimed that Confucius knew more about the spirit world than anyone else precisely because he did not speak about it (Fung, 1966: 219).

Other philosophers, who followed Confucius, also preferred to ignore the issue of immortality. Yang Xing (53 BCE–18 CE), a philosopher who combined Daoism with Confucianism, was asked to expound on the "actual truth" about immortals. He observed: "I shall have nothing to do with the question (of immortals). Their existence or nonexistence is not something to talk about. What should be asked are questions on loyalty and filial piety" (Chan, 1973: 290). In public, like Confucius, Yang believed that the sage should teach the Dao of humanity, presumably to establish a just and benevolent society. Notice that he did not deny the existence of immortals. Rather he preferred to deflect the question while emphasizing the Dao of humanity.

The Outer Elixir

The path to immortality was divided into two streams with different emphasis and methods: the outer elixir (*waidan*) and the inner elixir (*neidan*). The two were not mutually exclusive, although the inner elixir gradually became the method of choice for the vast majority of Daoists. It is interesting to note that the inner and outer method is the same classification used in defining the two major schools of qigong

To understand the mechanism of immortality, we must grasp the following important concept. The seekers of both the outer and inner schools believed that a person's qi, or lifeforce, was composed of the same stuff as the "eternal" cosmic qi of the universe. According to most Chinese thinkers, everything had its origins in the cosmic qi of Dao, which was something like the mountain water source of a great river (Feng and English, 1972: ch. 42).[7] The great Neo-Confucian Zhang Zai (1020–1077) explained the unity of qi in this manner:

> When it is understood that the Vacuity, the Void, is nothing but material force (qi), then existence and nonexistence, the hidden and the manifested, spirit and eternal transformation, and human nature and destiny are all one and not a duality.[8]   — Chan, 1973: 502

Outer school followers sought to produce the pill of immortality from metals and herbs through alchemical processes.[9] Their goal was to bridge and unify the apparent duality of human qi and cosmic qi. The difference between the two qis was one of appearance, such as water, steam, and ice: their essence, or qi, was the same—H_2O. These pioneers of the modern laboratory scientist believed that a pill of gold and cinnabar combined with other ingredients, such as lead and water, would restore, balance, and harmonize an individual's personal qi with the cosmic qi. Cinnabar (red mercury ore) and gold were touted as the key ingredients of the elixir because they contained unique qualities of indestructibility and endurance.

The best-known alchemist of the outer school was Ge Hong (284–364). He wrote the *Baopuzi*, a how-to book detailing specific techniques and practices for attaining immortality (Breslow, 1995: 132–33; Cooper, 1990; Schuhmacher and

Woerner, 1989: 183). Ge Hong believed that only the pill of immortality could fulfill the promise of eternal life. Physical exercise, sexual yoga, breathing techniques, and meditation could prolong life but could not bestow the gift of immortality. Moreover, the pill could grant supernatural powers such as the ability to walk on water or to commune with the spirit world.

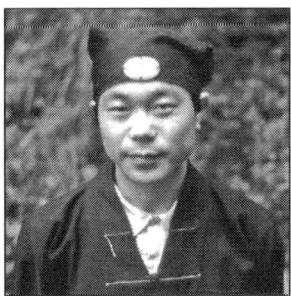

A monk descends Geling Hill which overlooks Hangzhou city. Here, near a Daoist monastery, alchemist Ge Hong was believed to have made pills for attaining immortality. Photo by M. DeMarco.

However, the pill alone could not produce immortality. Despite his belief in the elixir's magic, Ge Hong was also a committed Confucian. To achieve immortality, the practitioner had to practice the Confucian virtues of filial piety, good deeds, loyalty, trustworthiness, and sincerity. This is an interesting point because Ge Hong viewed immortality differently from Confucius and Yang Xing who refused to talk about immortals. It also highlights a Chinese worldview that emphasized the unity of mind and body. The wholeness of the person—spiritual, physical, and moral—was required to achieve immortality. A thief, for example, could imbibe the elixir of immortality and not achieve eternal life due to his character deficiencies.

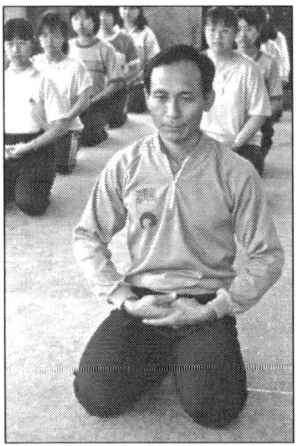

Internal gongfu, including meditative and qigong practices, are now practiced worldwide. Photo courtesy of the Government Information Office, Taiwan, Republic of China.

The Inner Elixir

By the Song dynasty (960–1279), the quest for the elixir of immortality became increasingly understood in spiritual rather than physical terms. In part, this evolution might be attributed to the lack of verifiable success regarding the outer school's approach.[10] Then, too, Neo-Confucian rationalists, such as Cheng Yi and Zhu Xi, who came to dominate Chinese thought from the tenth century CE, did not take kindly to the notion of immortality. The rise of Buddhism was another factor. Because of its highly sophisticated meditation techniques, Buddhism challenged both Daoism and Confucianism to develop their own equally skilled methods of contemplation, which many seekers then applied to achieving immortality.

The objective of Daoist spiritual yoga was the liberation of the yang soul (*shen*) from the hindrance of the yin or gross physical body. Traditionally, the Chinese understood that this separation occurred with death, but the Daoists came to believe it could happen while one lived. Taking their cue and terminology from the outer school, they sought to transform the body into an alchemical laboratory. For example, one early spiritual alchemy master explained that the semen corresponded to lead, blood to mercury, kidneys to water, and the mind to fire. By mixing these elements together, the meditator created the elixir of immortality in the fiery cauldron of his own body.

Gradually, the inner school rejected the outer school's terminology and developed its own framework known as the three treasures: *jing* (essence), *qi* (vitality), and *shen* (spirit). Each of the three treasures had two parts, an abstract and a concrete dimension:

	Concrete	**Abstract**	**Body**
Jing (essence):	male sperm and female sexual fluids	creativity as the seed of life	genitals
Qi (vitality):	air and breath	internal energy and life force	stomach, dantian
Shen (spirit):	ordinary conscious, thoughts and feelings	spiritual consciousness	lungs, head, and heart

To preserve life and to attain immortality, the three treasures had to be conserved and blended into a balanced harmony. Through daily nourishment, seekers of the inner elixir sought to cultivate the natural growth of the three treasures. For example, the breath was not merely a means for maintaining life. If it was not regulated properly, the person's lifeforce would be used up. Conversely, correct breathing techniques would greatly increase the lifeforce in the body.

Ejaculation was another example of body ecology and conservation. Daoists seeking immortality believed that the semen represented a major source of qi and had to be preserved within the body, particularly as one grew older.[11] During the act of lovemaking, the male would prevent ejaculation through various techniques, thereby sending the semen (*jing*) back through the spinal passage as refined lifeforce (*qi*) and to the brain, where it nourished the spirit (*shen*).

Daoist seekers of immortality believed that the bodily processes and functions normally leading to death could be "reversed" by concentrating and purifying the three treasures.[12] By reversing the life-to-death process with various meditation and visualization techniques, one could return to his or her "pre-birth" state and transform the coarse body into subtle energy. This was the same principle utilized in sexual yoga: the transmuting of jing into qi and then qi into shen.

Qigong exercises and taijiquan were important vehicles to improve health and, for some, to attain immortality. These kinds of exercises were highly valued because they conserved and strengthened the body's lifeforce, allowing the qi to flow evenly and freely along the spine to the head.

The *Taiji Classics* adopted the same principle used in immortality, which became a hallmark in its concept of self-defense. The *Taiji Classics* extolled the principle of the "suspended head top" to promote a light and responsive body: "When the ching shen [*jing shen*] (spirit) is raised, there is no fault of stagnancy and heaviness" (Lo, et al, 1985: 47). In other words, the body reacts quickly and appropriately to the attack of an opponent because mind and posture have allowed the jing and qi to flow freely and to become shen (Breslow, 1995: 282–83, 299).

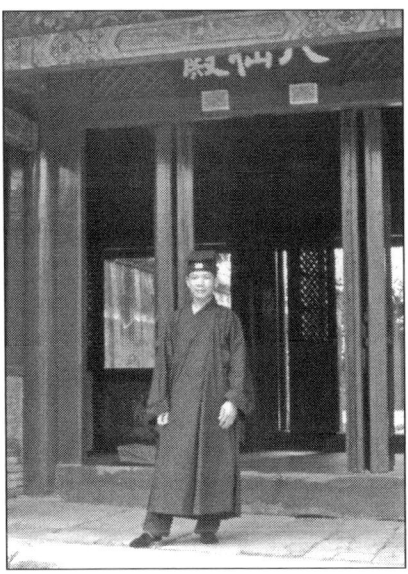

A monk stands in front of the Hall of the Eight Immortals.
He is a native of Guangzhou but came to live in Beijing's
White Cloud Monastery, a leading center of Daoism in China.
Photo by M. DeMarco.

Generally, to conserve their qi and prepare themselves for immortality, Daoists followed the Middle Path whereby they avoided excess in all things. Moderation was their by-word. Even Daoist exercises like qigong were kept within the bounds of common sense. One of my taiji teachers often reminded us to do our best but don't overdo it. The following is a Daoist checklist on maintaining moderation:

> 1) excessive walking harms the nerves
> 2) excessive standing harms the bones
> 3) too much sleep harms the blood vessels
> 4) sitting too long harms the blood
> 5) listening too much impairs the generative powers
> 6) looking at things too long harms the spirit
> 7) talking too much affects the breath
> 8) thinking too hard upsets the stomach
> 9) too much sex injures the lifeforce
> 10) eating too much damages the heart
> — adapted from Cooper, 1990: 104

Taiji masters also recommended that their students should follow the path of moderation. The *Taiji Classics* state:

> It is not excessive or deficient.
> Accordingly, when it bends,
> It then straightens.
> — Lo, et al, 1985: 31

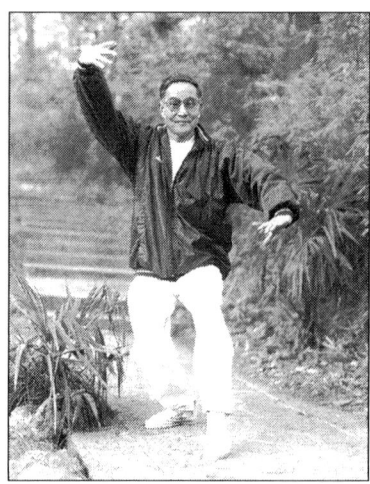

Mr. Jiang Jialun, a member of the Hangzhou Wushan Taijiquan Association, in "Stork Spread Wings." This movement is found in taijiquan and qigong. Because it is associated with long life, many believe it is beneficial to move and breath like the bird. Photo by Donald Mainfort.

In practical terms, this meant that, whether practicing the taiji form or sparring with an opponent, one must hold to the center. "Excessive" indicates that one should not bend over too far and "deficient" means not to lose contact with the opponent (Wile, 1983: 117–18).

Pre-natal Breathing: A Practical Lesson

To understand the inner school theory, it might be helpful to examine a breathing technique called "pre-natal" or "reverse" breathing. This technique is characterized by contracting the lower abdomen on the in-breath and expanding it on the out-breath. According to the Daoists, each baby is born with pre-natal qi, which is the lifeforce it receives before birth. Some babies are endowed with more qi than others, depending on the health of the parents, genetics, and other factors. Before the baby is born, he takes in his nourishment and oxygen through the umbilical cord and stores the energy in his dantian. Once the baby is born, breathing from the nose and mouth begins, which is known as "post-birth" breathing. This transition marks the end of pre-natal breathing.

However, if we closely observe a baby breathing, we will see that, while he breathes through his nose, he still uses his stomach in the breathing process. We can observe the abdomen moving rhythmically with the breath. The Daoists noticed that, as one grows older, the diaphragm and abdomen are employed less and less. The breath gradually moves higher in the lungs until it flies out of the mouth, culminating in death.

The Daoists hoped to accomplish two goals with pre-natal breathing. They wanted to reverse the upward pattern of the breath so that it would remain deep in the lower stomach, that is, in the dantian. In this way, it was thought that a person would not "expire." They accomplished this goal by harmonizing the movement of the abdomen and the breath.

Secondly, the Daoists believed that when one's qi was depleted the person died. Thus, if one could conserve, strengthen, and nourish the pre-natal qi stored in the dantian, then he or she would never get sick and die. The Daoists hoped to accomplish this by mixing the qi from the air outside the body, a never-ending source, with the pre-natal qi inside the body. This was done by simultaneously contracting the dantian and inhaling fresh air, joining them together around the diaphragm, and then sending the revitalized qi back to its storage place in the dantian.

Immortality At Last

One who attained immortality became a *xian*. The modern pictogram for a xian is made up of the pictograms for a man and a mountain, suggesting the correlation between the recluse and immortality. The earlier pictogram for *xian* showed a man ascending toward heaven. The best-known immortals in Chinese mythology were the Eight Immortals (*ba xian*), who are often depicted in Chinese art. They represent the eight conditions of life: youth, old age, poverty, riches, nobility, common people, woman, and man.

Ge Hong divided immortals into three categories: celestial, terrestrial, and those who had given up the body. Celestial immortals fly to heaven with their bodies intact like the Yellow Emperor. Terrestrial immortals dwell in mountains or forests. Ge Hong's death was reputedly an example of the third kind. When he died, he was placed in a coffin. Later when the coffin was opened, only his clothes remained. This passing to the spirit world represented a cross-cultural, archetypal image, as it closely resembles the resurrection of Jesus of Nazareth in the New Testament.

In Chinese folklore, the types of immortals appear less clear than Ge Hong's definitions of the xian. Did the immortal one remain the same after achieving immortality, his or her qi having reached the point of indestructibility? Or did he or she die, dropping the physical body while the body/mind was transfigured into subtle energy? The answer was that the immortal could do and be just about anything he or she pleased. Whatever occurred, the immortal was viewed as a power technician of the highest rank. This meant that he could transform his body and environment to the shape of his will. The immortal often performed magic and miracles. This ability came from great personal power and a deep understanding of the way energy worked.

The following legends illustrate the above point and demonstrate the convergence of immortality with personal power and martial arts. When Zhang Sanfeng, the father of taijiquan, was on his way to the capital at the invitation of Emperor Huizong (1092–1135), he had to pass through mountains populated by dangerous bandits. That night, Yuandi, one of the semidivine immortals, visited him in a dream and taught him certain self-defense techniques. The following day, Zhang was attacked, and he reputedly killed more than a hundred bandits.

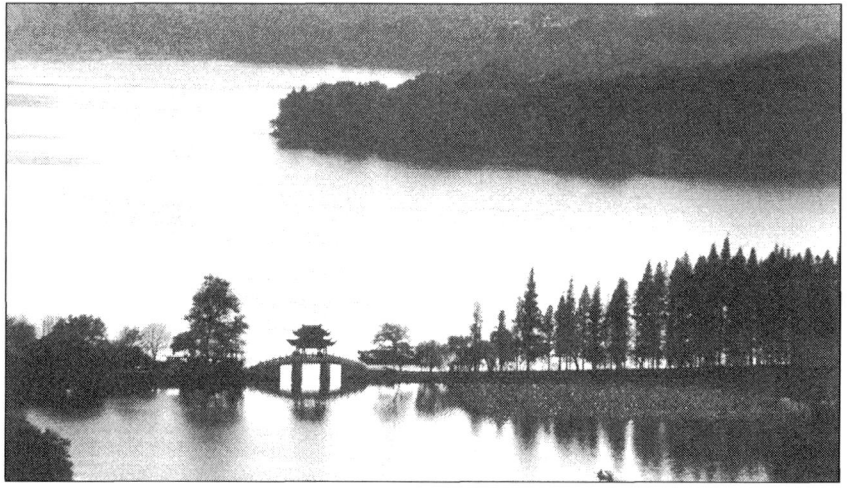

A scenic wonder in any season, Hangzhou city's West Lake has long inspired poets, emperors, and martial artists. People come daily to the shores to "run like tigers," hang upside down like bats from trees, and practice other assorted techniques in a quest for health and long-life. Photo by Donald Mainfort.

Another story about Zhang describes his great personal power. Apparently, in winter, Zhang would walk out of the monastery to enjoy the hoary landscape. It was said that he left no footprints on the snowy paths. The legend does not say whether he flew or stepped down without leaving an indentation. Presumably, he could do either.

Immortality in the Modern Age

In the modern world, belief in the elixir of immortality has fallen by the wayside. Yet we have much to be thankful for its existence and those seekers who aimed for the stars but only reached the moon. For example, Fung Yu-lan praised religious Daoism as heralding the spirit of modern science. Daoist alchemists accumulated a massive body of medical lore and laid the basis for modern chemistry, metallurgy, botany, herbology, and zoology. Traditional Chinese medicine was also greatly beholden to the seekers of immortality.

The search for immortality gave impetus to the belief that human beings can live healthier, longer, and happier lives. It offered an ancient and well-tested structure of exercise, meditation, and visualization that enabled ordinary people to dramatically enhance the quality of their lives. While promising no guarantees regarding death and sickness, the Daoist health systems postulated that it is best to follow the Dao, to "walk like a cat" so that one might live as a lion in winter.[13] The *Taiji Classics* sum it up best: "Think it over carefully what the final purpose is: to lengthen life and maintain youth" (Lo, et al: 66).

In 1935 John Blofeld met a Daoist monk at his monastery in the mountains. This was what that monk had to say about immortals:

> Immortals not only break wind or belch like other people, they die... Becoming immortal has little to do with physical changes, like the graying of a once glossy black beard; it means coming to know something, realizing something—an experience that can happen in a flash! Ah, how precious is that knowledge! When it first strikes you, you want to sing and dance, or you nearly die of laughing! For suddenly you recognize that nothing in the world can hurt you.   — Blofeld, 1979: 180

Notes

1. *The Yellow Emperor's Classic of Internal Medicine*, made up of the Yellow Emperor asking questions regarding health from his minister, Qi Po, forms the basis for traditional Chinese medical practices.
2. All translations of the *Daodejing* come from Feng and English.
3. Tam Gibbs translated the verse differently: "One who does not lose what he has gained is durable. One who dies yet remains has longevity" (Cheng, 1981: 119).
4. This idea is echoed in other cultures. In Judaism, there is this adage: "The right-

eous live through their deeds even though they are dead while the unrighteous are dead even though they live."

5. This phrase should be compared with the wonderful story Robert Smith (1997: 66–68) told when Professor Zheng encountered a tiger. Then, read the Professor's commentary on Laozi (the one we quoted in the text) in Wile (1985: 25).

6. I am often surprised how few practitioners of martial arts, particularly students of taiji, have studied Laozi's masterpiece in depth. It should be read and reread along with the *Taiji Classics* and Sunzi's, *The Art of War*.

7. The *Taiji Classics* also state this principle: "T'ai Chi [taiji] comes from Wu Chi [wuji] and is the mother of Yin and Yang" (Lo, et al, 1985: 31).

8. Many great martial artists drew on their harmony with cosmic qi for their spiritual inspiration and physical power. Witness the words of Ueshiba Morihei, the founder of aikido:

> Regardless of how quickly an opponent attacks or how slowly I respond, I cannot be defeated ... As soon as the thought of attack crosses my opponent's mind, he shatters the harmony of the universe and is instantly defeated regardless of how quickly he attacks. Victory or defeat is not a matter of time and space. — Stevens, 1987: 112

9. We should be misled into thinking that the pill is part of the Inner School merely because it is ingested.

10. How one verifies the existence of immortals or the success of such an endeavor is an interesting problem. Few mystics, East or West, are willing to put themselves to the test. Besides, spirits and immortals are known to be notoriously shy. Furthermore, the Daoists of both the Inner and Outer Schools were not interested in proving anything. They were simply doers, striving to achieve immortality, often recluses who were unconcerned with the cares of the world. They had nothing to prove.

11. Su Nu, the Yellow Emperor's female advisor, suggested the following approach:

> When a man loves once without losing his semen, he will strengthen his body. If he loves twice without losing it, his hearing and vision will become more acute. If three times, all diseases may disappear. If four times, he will have peace of mind. If five times, his heart and blood circulation will be revitalized. If six times, his loins will become strong. If seven times, his buttocks and thighs may become more powerful. If eight times, his skin may become smooth. If nine times, he will become immortal.
> — Chang, 1977: 44

12. Today, taiji and qigong teachers are more modest in their claims and tend to use the words "halting" or "arresting" the process of old age instead of "reversing it." Nevertheless, in some cases, I have seen people drop ten years by strengthening their qi.

Bibliography

Blofeld, J. (1979). *Taoism: The road to immortality*. Boulder: Shambhala Publications, Inc.

Breslow, A. (1995). *Beyond the closed door: Chinese culture and the creation of t'ai chi ch'uan*. Jerusalem, Israel: Almond Blossom Press.

Chan, W. (Trans.). (1963). *A source book in Chinese philosophy*. Princeton: Princeton University Press.

Chang, J. (1977). *The tao of love and sex: The ancient Chinese way to ecstasy*. New York: E. P. Dutton.

Cheng, M. (1981). *Lao tzu: My words are very easy to understand*. (T.C. Gibbs, Trans.). Berkeley, CA: North Atlantic Books.

Cohen, K. (1997). *The way of qigong: The art and science of Chinese energy healing*. New York: Ballentine Books.

Cooper, J. (1990). *Chinese alchemy: The Taoist quest for immortality*. New York: Sterling Publications.

Schuhmacher, S., and Woerner, G. (Eds.). (1989). *Encyclopedia of eastern philosophy and religion*. Boston: Shambhala Publications, Inc.

Feng, G., and English, J. (Trans.). (1972). *Tao te ching*. New York: Vintage Books.

Fung, Y. (1966). *A short history of Chinese philosophy*. (D. Bodde, Ed.). New York: The Free Press Edition.

Legge, J. (Trans.). (1971). *The Chinese classics, vol. 1: Confucian analects, the great learning, the doctrine of the mean*. New York: Dover Publications.

Lo, P., Inn, M., Amacker, R., and Foe, S. (Trans.). (1985). *The essence of t'ai chi ch'uan*. Berkeley, CA: North Atlantic Books.

Smith, R. (1997). Da lu and some tigers. *Journal of Asian Martial Arts, 6*(2), 56–69.

Stevens, J. (1987). *Abundant peace: The biography of Morihei Ueshiba, founder of aikido*. Boston: Shambhala Publications, Inc.

Thompson, L. (1989). *Chinese religion*. Belmont, CA: Wadsworth Publishing Company.

Van Over, R. (Ed.). (1984). *Taoist tales*. New York: Meridian.

Watson, B. (Trans.). (1968). *Chuang tzu: The inner chapters*. New York: Columbia University Press.

Wile, D. (Trans.). (1985). *Cheng Man-Ch'ing's advanced tai-chi form instructions with selected writings on meditation, the I Ching, medicine and the arts*. Brooklyn, NY: Sweet Ch'i Press.

Wile, D. (Trans.). (1983). *T'ai-chi touchstones: Yang family secret transmissions*. Brooklyn, NY: Sweet Ch'i Press.

Yang, C. (1961). *Religion in Chinese society*. Berkeley, CA: University of California Press.

• 25 •
Chen and Yang Taiji Converge in Hangzhou City
by Donald Mainfort, M.A.

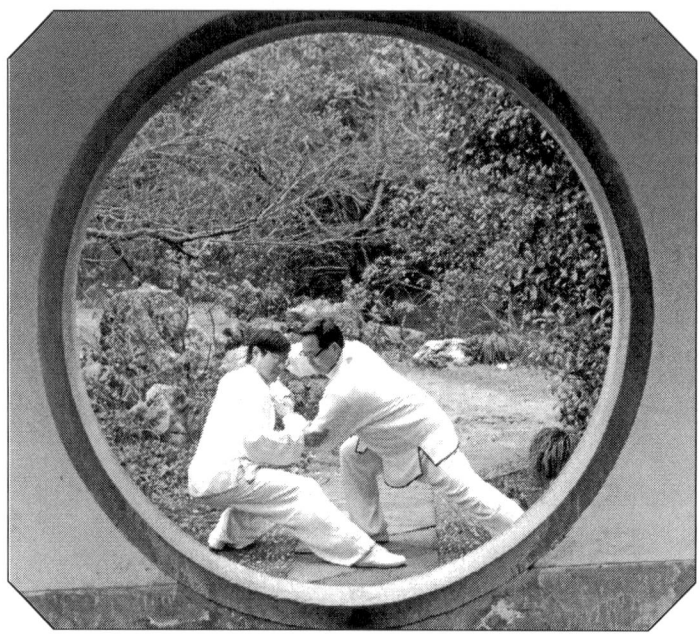

All photographs courtesy of D. Mainfort.

Introduction

Many people practice taiji as a form of gentle exercise or meditation but lack an understanding of the martial principles upon which the art was designed. However, there are several pockets of taiji enthusiasts in China where serious investigation of taiji's martial art applications is still to be found. Hangzhou is a city rich in culture and scenic beauty. There are various taiji organizations and experts in Hangzhou, but one organization in particular places great emphasis on the research and development of taiji applications. Mr. Dai Peisu and Mr. Zhang Youquan, two of the senior members of the Hangzhou Wushan Taijiquan Society, have offered to introduce their findings thus far.

Hangzhou Wushan Taijiquan Society

Mr. Dai Peisu and Mr. Zhang Youquan have been friends for many years and have exchanged information and experiences with fellow members of the Hangzhou Wushan Taijiquan Society in Zhejiang Province. Mr. Zhang is the vice president. Both he and Mr. Dai initiate contact with other practitioners and attempt to compile and evaluate the information obtained. The membership consists of approximately sixty-eight regular local members and a handful of overseas practitioners, mostly from the U.S. and Germany. Among the more noteworthy associates who have influenced or shared their knowledge with the group are Wang Peisheng, Yu Zhijun, Yu Tonghe, and Gao Zhuangfei, all from Beijing; Liu Chengde from Shandong; and Lin Mogen from Sichuan. Dai Peisu, Zhang Youquan, and the society's president, Mr. Xia Tao, believe that these men all have genuine skill and understanding of taiji.

Dai Peisu's Taiji Studies

Dai's primary teachers were Wang Zhuocheng and Wang Xianggen. Wang Zhuocheng, who worked as a bodyguard in his youth, went on to establish a good restaurant business in Hangzhou and live a comfortable life. His neighbor, Tian Zhaolin, relied entirely on teaching taiji for his livelihood and frequently had trouble making ends meet. The two became close friends and shared their martial arts information. Wang Zhuocheng taught bagua to Tian and saw to it that his friend never went hungry.

Although Tian Zhaolin was widely rumored to have been a student of Yang Chengfu, and there are some published photos of them together, Tian's real teacher was Chengfu's father, Yang Jianhou. Tian spent some time with Yang Chengfu after Jianhou's death. Although he was remotely linked to Jianhou through his teachers, Dai said that his form was not a hand-me-down from this relationship. Rather, he said that it evolved because of many different teachers and influences, including bagua (also learned from Wang Zhuocheng) and xingyi. Dai learned xingyi from a master who came to Hangzhou from Shanghai who was known to him only as "Master Lin." Dai said that Lin had a deep affect on his approach to martial arts. He said that with gongfu, as with math or physics, it really doesn't matter where you get information; the principles are pretty much the same.

Wang Xianggen was born in Suzhou but has spent the latter half of his life in Hangzhou. He studied with Huang Yuanxiu, a prosperous and affable Hangzhou martial arts aficionado whose long list of friends included Yang Chengfu. Huang Yuanxiu was an intellectual and imparted some important points to Mr. Wang on how to issue power. Mr. Wang also learned Chun Yang Style Wudang sword from Huang Yuanxiu, who learned it from Kuomintang General Li Fangsen (also known as Li Jinglin). The two of them published a book entitled, *How to Exercise Wudang Sword* (1931) in Shanghai.

Although Dai Peisu views Yang Taiji as his major focus, he considers his form to be somewhat of an amalgam. People viewing his form sometimes remark: "That's not Yang Taiji! He's using a function from Wu Style there, and that's an application from Chen Style!"

Mr. Dai explains that, as most students realize, the Wu family learned taiji from Yang Banhou, so if you practice Wu Style, you are, in effect, practicing a version of Yang Taiji (DeMarco, 1992: 23; Ma and Zee, 1990: 8; Wile, 1996: 35; Wong, 1996: 27, 248). Also, because Yang Luchan learned taiji from Chen Changxing, there must be a strong relationship to Chen taiji (DeMarco, 1992: 20; Zhaohua, 1984: 7–8). Before the popularity of Yang Chengfu's form (now in common use as an exercise), more of the older influences were apparent. Dai said that Yang Chengfu came to Hangzhou (Wile, 1983) and that Yang's form was deceptively simple in appearance. In fact, he was using some of the waist movement seen in earlier forms (vertical circling as well as horizontal) but did so in a less obvious manner.

Xingyi uses vertical circling to generate force and Dai Peisu incorporate this into his actions as well. When asked what form of taiji he practices, he smiled broadly and replied: "Dai's taiji!"

Dai strongly suggests that every serious student of Yang taiji should also look at the Wu Style. He feels that many subtleties that seem to have disappeared in the modern teaching of the Yang Style can still be found in the Wu. The small and concentrated circling actions in the Wu form were derived from the Yang's. After students practice for some time on a large frame, they should refine and concentrate their movements. He feels that Wu taiji might be difficult for beginners, though, and suggests learning the larger Yang form first until you begin to get the idea of the applications. After you see how taiji is used in self-defense, the meaning of this idea of smaller movements becomes clear.

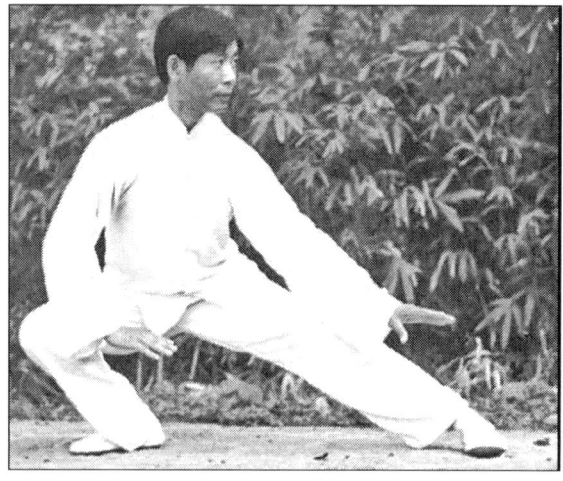

Xia Tao, President of the Hangzhou Wuchan Taijiquan Society.

Zhang Youquan's Taiji Studies

Mr. Zhang's primary teacher was Hong Junshen of Shandong, from whom he learned the silk reeling method and Chen Taiji. Earlier Zhang had learned *Xiao ia* (small frame) Chen Taiji from Chen Liqing, a descendant of the Chen family from Xi'an. Zhang's first teacher was Jiang Yukun, from Beijing. Zhang says his major focus is silk reeling along with the concept of "hardness contained in softness." Using small and compact movements to initiate explosive *fajing* and *doutan* ("trembling energy"), Mr. Zhang's form appears nebulous, and it is difficult to recognize any of the set patterns that Chen Taiji practitioners are familiar with. You can see an example of this (as well as Dai's form) demonstrated in the videotape, *Taijiquan at West Lake* (1993).

Zhang approaches taiji movement as that of a clock mechanism: the small activates the larger, generating from the center, with each part following a circular pattern of hand and body. His hands are the key, and they activate a chain of relationships: hand to wrist, wrist to elbow, shoulder, back, waist, legs, and finally feet. Using many joint-locking techniques (in taiji, not Shaolin Style), Zhang can cause an opponent to lose his balance, which will leave him vulnerable to a whole host of explosive attacks. Zhang uses the method of *yin dao shu*, or "imaginary pathway." Here, you imagine your root of power to be somewhere else. For example, if you want to use power in your wrist, you imagine that you are using your elbow. If you want to use force from your elbow, you focus attention on your shoulder, and so on. The very subtle circling actions of his fingers exert astounding torque and leverage when he applies them in qinna-type situations. Zhang used the image of wringing water out of a wet towel to describe this procedure. The ease and power are much greater than those of the Shaolin qinna that I have experienced with many other practitioners around China, which were also effective, but not nearly as efficient.

Taiji Synthesis

Although he can use the explosive force of Chen taiji to do great harm, this is used only for demonstration and then only with care. Mr. Zhang prefers to use the torque of his silk reeling to control an opponent using the smallest amount of force and causing the least amount of pain necessary. Zhang and Dai never try to hurt people, or to throw them to the ground. In practice, when they "bounce someone out," they always maintain contact so that the person does not fall. Also, they never issue harsh *fajing*, except in controlled situations with advanced warning—never suddenly during friendly practice. Although Dai is known to be very expert in the issuance and neutralization of *fajing*, he differs from Zhang in that he considers this to be more in the realm of regular gongfu and not sophisticated taiji, which emphasizes soft power. Both evaluated my own attempts at issuing *fajing* and explained that most of my force was being directed into the ground, rather than into my hands. If you are making a lot of stomping noise with your feet, then you are losing your force, and you will not be able to get the electrifying whip-like blast from your hands. When Zhang demonstrates it, I can barely see any movement in his waist and practically none in his knees. The movement should be small and compact, and the upper body should be very relaxed. It takes a proper understanding of relaxation and much practice to get good at it.

Dai said that while it is easy to become relaxed practicing the taiji solo form as a type of meditation, the goal of taiji is not just to become relaxed, but to most effectively resolve conflict in the real world. His taiji uses relaxation to enable the whip-like speed and economy that is impossible if the muscles are tight and stiff due to the "fight or flight response."[1] He said that taiji is not a process of thinking about your own relaxation, but rather one of sensing and responding to another person's actions in a creative way. In fact, it is incorrect and in violation of Daoist philosophy to become too relaxed—there must be strength contained within the softness. Sometimes when I practiced push-hands with Dai, he appeared to be less than relaxed. When I attacked his "hardness," I found that he was simply giving me an empty target and therefore my attacks fell on nothing. He also demonstrated for me how it is not good to be too relaxed on the outside in neutralizing, and that knowing this can prevent a spontaneous counterattack. Sometimes I find that when practicing with them, I am unable to move and they are just standing there, seemingly motionless, smiling at me. Then I will gradually and incrementally be set off-balance. "How do you do this?" I asked. They directed my attention to an area known as the *ming men*, in the lower back.

Both have highly developed musculature in this area that they can control in an undulating motion. It was very odd to see this and to feel the effect of power channeled in this way from the waist, shoulders, and out through the hands. Both Zhang and Dai advise that people breathe naturally when practicing taiji. After a while, your breathing (*tuna*) becomes naturally coordinated with certain actions. This can be taught by a proper teacher, but they warn that today most of this knowledge has been lost and they do not know anyone who has a real understanding of it. According to them, there is a lot of false information being disseminated that can be harmful. The last time I spoke with Dai, he was experimenting with a method of "gulping" in air during a very fast neutralize and pull-down defense.

Mr. Dai and Mr. Zhang are close friends, yet a typical encounter with the two always results in heated debate regarding various aspects of taiji: What is practical in a real encounter? What is the role of fajing? How does the action in question reflect the principles of taiji philosophy? Are some famous classic quotations about taiji true, or are they merely clichés? There is usually a conclusion reached regarding the point in question. Many times, I have heard them discuss how aspects of the form are merely gross exaggerations that are far removed from any practical, spontaneous response to an opponent. The bottom line is always "what works." They say that constant debate and critical evaluation are useful to continued discovery and improved understanding. Their debates are always accompanied by much practice, with each attempting to demonstrate the validity of his position. They are always open to new ideas or opinions and are eager to put them to the test. They feel that openly exchanging knowledge will lead to higher levels of understanding.

They encourage students to meet as many different teachers as possible and gain from varied perspectives. I attended several of the Hangzhou Wushan Taijiquan Society meetings and it was really inspiring to be able to see a variety of experts exchanging ideas and holding up their skills and abilities to peer review.

Dai once told me that Mr. Zhang was more experienced and knowledgeable about taiji than he was. Zhang responded by saying that when he first met Dai years ago, he found that Dai didn't have a clear understanding of how to maximize power from the feet. "After I explained it to him, he combined it with what he already knew and now he is better than me.... I don't care, though, because we are good friends!" Zhang said that some teachers wish to maintain an air of authority by not revealing all their information to their students. He feels that this attitude contradicts Daoist philosophy and is harmful to taijiquan's future.

Conclusion

What I have noticed about Dai Peisu and Zhang Youquan is that although they have different styles, they are equally effective. As two accomplished painters approach the same scene in different ways, each serious taiji practitioner must determine what is effective, what works for them. Serious practitioners should eventually develop their own "style." Otherwise, taiji loses its meaning and degenerates into a kind of synchronized dance performance. For those who wish to practice taiji for health, it is necessary to understand some of the theory and practice of the applications so that your posture will be correct. Good gongfu equals good health.

Dai and Zhang both seek the balance of defend and attack (yin and yang), all in the same motion with minimum force. Each uses a different style to accomplish this, but both adhere to taiji's general principles.

What effect are you trying to achieve? Is there a lighter, more efficient way? The classics tell us that we should practice taiji by using our minds. Dai and Zhang say that the form and tuishou practice are not ends in themselves, but merely training exercises that people should not follow blindly. They are constantly seeking more sophisticated methods, and they are not satisfied with ideas that cannot be proven, or that contradict Daoist philosophy.

Wang Xianggen says that the principles of Daoism and taijiquan are simple physics and should not be made complicated by mysticism. Although they say that in the beginning it is necessary to understand "hard" force (they recommend a study of Shaolin for this), the eventual aim should be to avoid any direct conflict or "meeting force with force," and that this idea has deep cultural roots in China. Mr. Zhang also points out that if you really wish to understand taiji, it is necessary to learn about some of the other traditional arts of China, such as brush painting; music; poetry; and his specialty, literature.

Both men cherish the martial art applications contained in taiji and view them as a unique part of the cultural and historical heritage of China. They also view taiji as a form of self-cultivation and to reduce conflict and anxiety in daily life. Dai Peisu and Zhang Youquan say that they still have many questions regarding taiji and that taiji is a never-ending process of discovery and self-realization.

•••

TECHNICAL SECTION
Three Examples of Yang Taiji

Xie Fei (diagonal flying)

A1: Dai Peisu's right hand uses *lu* (neutralizing action) and *chai* (pull-down action) to break his opponent's balance in such a way that his body inclines forward. Simultaneously, Dai cross steps with his right foot half a pace so that it becomes vertical to his opponent.

A2: Dai steps forward with his left foot in a circular manner until it reaches behind his opponent's back, while at the same time Dai's left-hand rolls forward along the opponent's chest. Strength is directed outward though the index finger, creating the action known as *peng* (ward off). As a result, the opponent bends his back, and his center of gravity is elevated.

A3: When Dai's left arm has become tightly stuck to his opponent's body, Dai utilizes *kao* (shoulder-strike action). Remember that "shoulder strike" is an expression and the power generates from the feet, legs and waist. In the fraction of a second in which this is accomplished, Dai's right hand quickly exerts *an* (push downwards) in a backwards, arching motion and Dai's legs subsequently assume a "bow and arrow" stance.

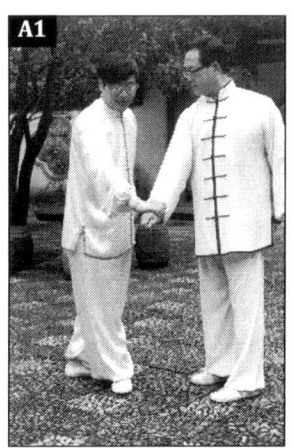
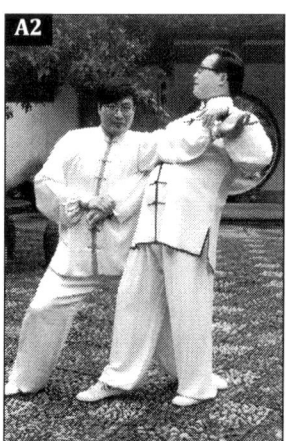
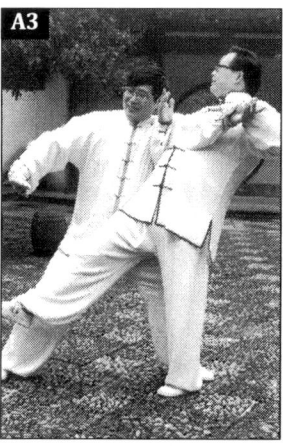

Xie Fei method is now completed and as a result, the opponent loses his balance and falls. Either that, or he stumbles backwards in such a way as to cause his arms to "flap," like the wings of a bird. This is the reason for the name of this form. Those practicing this form should not have the sense of flying—they should have a feeling that their imaginary opponent is sent flying!

One very important point to remember is that the action of the "empty arm" —it's downward, arching motion—is a key to this technique. The "empty arm" activates much of the force generated here. It creates the momentum needed to send the opponent back, along with a short, swift opening of the thighs of about an inch or so, also triggered by the action of the "empty arm."

Shan Tong Bei (spread the fan)

B1: Using *peng* (ward off action), Dai raises the incoming hand upwards and forwards.

B2: His left hand passes beneath the opponent's arm pit as Dai steps forward with his left foot in the same manner as seen in A2.

B3: Dai's right hand quickly moves forward using *ji* (pressing action) and weighs down using *an*. This completes the form known as *Shan Tong Bei*. Note that Dai is holding the "opponent's" hand to prevent him from falling and hitting his head. In dealing with a real opponent, you must also be careful to control the hand and arm because your head is vulnerable to his possible attack.

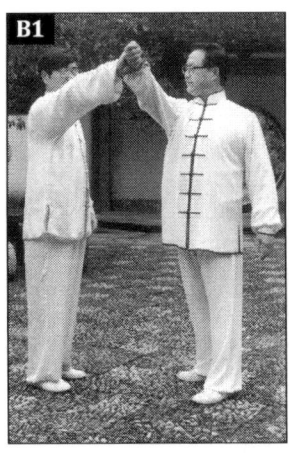

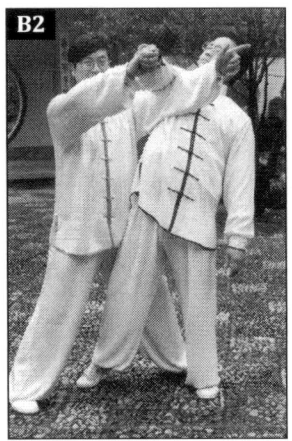

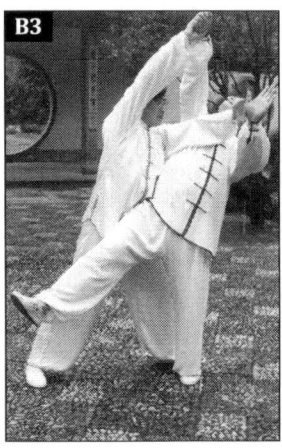

Ban Lan Chui **(step forward, deflect downwards, perry and punch)**

C1: Mr. Dai's forearm rolls inside-out using *peng* to deflect the opponent's attacking hand.

C2: Using *lu*, Dai neutralizes the attacking hand and cross-steps half a pace, forming an angle that is perpendicular to the opponent's feet.

C3: Dai steps forward with his left foot in the same manner as seen in photos A2 and B2. At the same time, his left arm is brought straight across the opponent's chest and Dai's left hand then exerts *peng* and *ji* into the opponent's chest, locking him into position. Note that strength is extended from the index finger of the attacking hand.

C4: Dai's right hand quickly forms a fist and strikes forward, while his legs form a "bow and arrow stance." Note that he is not attempting to strike the opponent's body with his fist. Instead, he strikes the air. There are two reasons for this. The first is that he will not receive resistance and counteraction. Second, the momentum generated from striking into the air will magnify the strength that Dai wishes to use from his waist in the form of *ji* and *kao*. This will cause the opponent to deflect and fall.

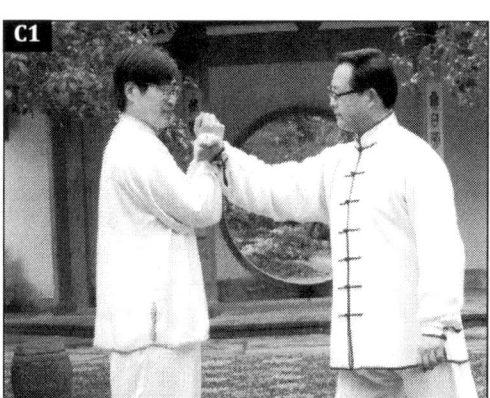
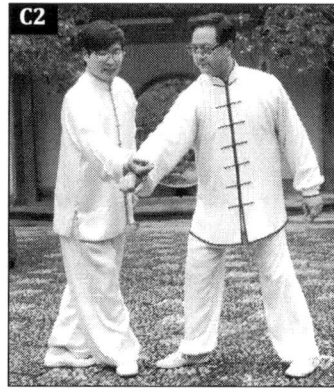
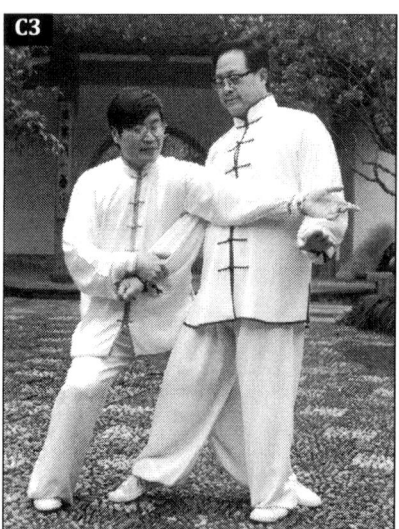
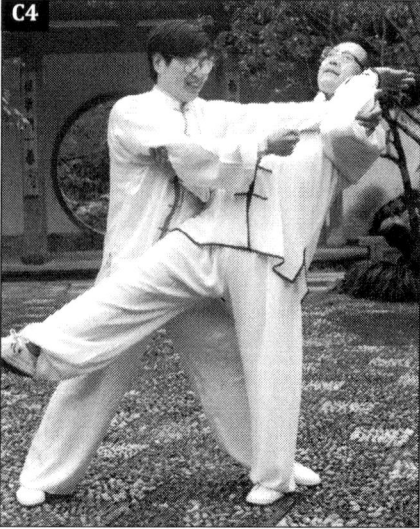

In the three forms illustrated above, Mr. Dai avoids the hard attack, while striking the invisible, thus weak, points. His strength is not directed at the opponent's body. Instead, it aims at weak points which his opponent cannot easily protect, using strength from different sources in his body.

THREE EXAMPLES OF CHEN TAIJI

Jin Gang Dao Dui (immortal pounds mortar)

D1: The opponent grabs hold of Mr. Zhang's wrists.

D2a: Zhang keep his hands still, while at the same time loosening his shoulders and allowing the opponent to do as he pleases. Zhang then rotates his body clockwise and transfers the strength to both his hands.

D2b: Zhang's right hand forms a fist, which is then placed in his left palm.

D3: Zhang raises his hands up towards the opponent's head, raising his own left foot at the same time.

D4: Zhang's hands stick to his opponent's hands, and he steps with his left foot beside the opponent's left foot.

D5: Zhang circles his arms upwards and toward the left (counterclockwise) and as a result, the opponent is under control. If he continues turning, the opponent will stagger and fall backwards.

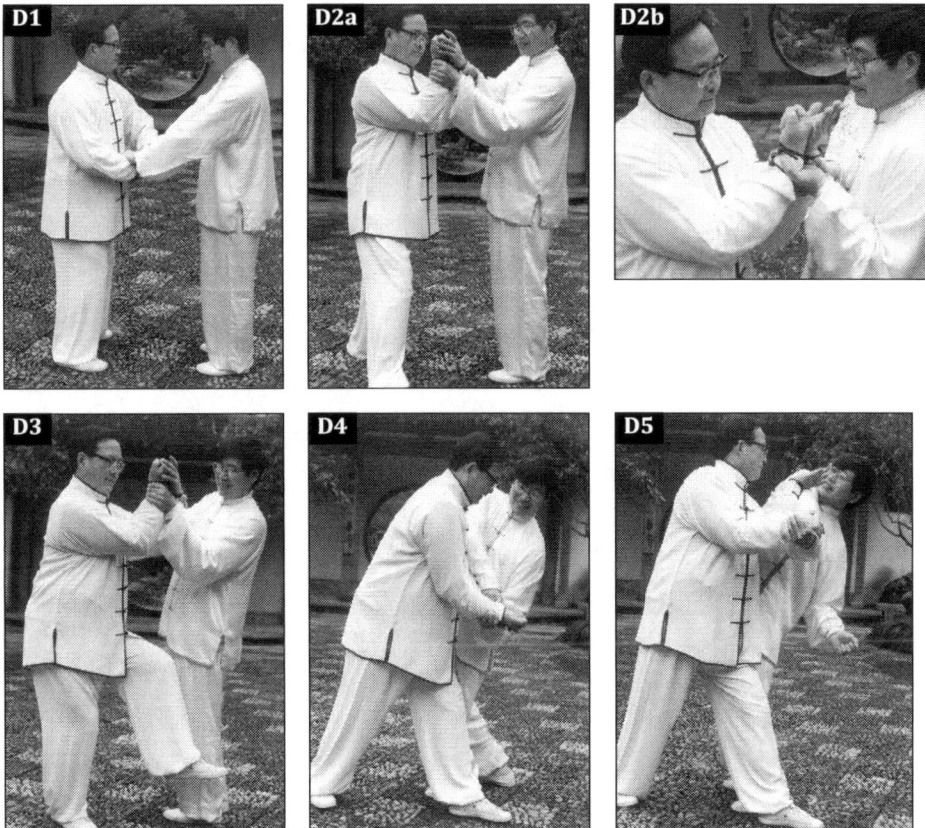

Liu Feng Si Bi (six seal, four close)

E1: The opponent seizes Zhang's right wrist with his right hand.

E2a: Zhang's right hand circles upward (clockwise) while his left hand gently covers the opponent's right elbow.

E2b: Detail of hand positions.

E3: Zhang continues circling his right hand while revolving his left hand along the opponent's right elbow (counterclockwise) then steps forward one pace with his left foot, placing it beside the opponent's left foot. The opponent's right arm is now stuck and under Zhang's control.

E4: Zhang continues circling his right hand clockwise until the palm is downwards while at the same time his left hand continues to circle counterclockwise, so that the opponent is unable to move.

E5: If Zhang continues to circle his body to the right, then the opponent's body will be twisted, and he will fall down.

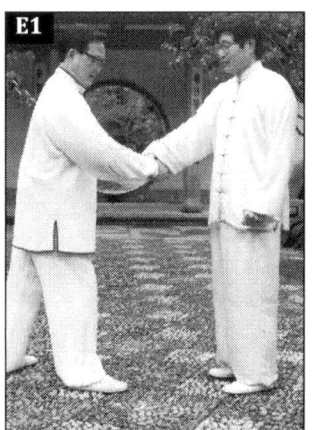
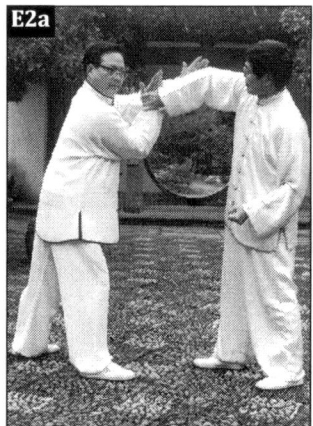
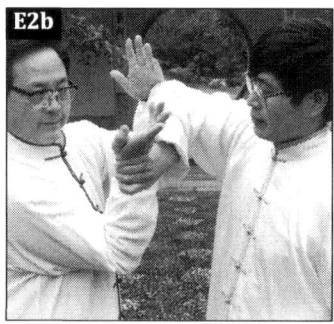
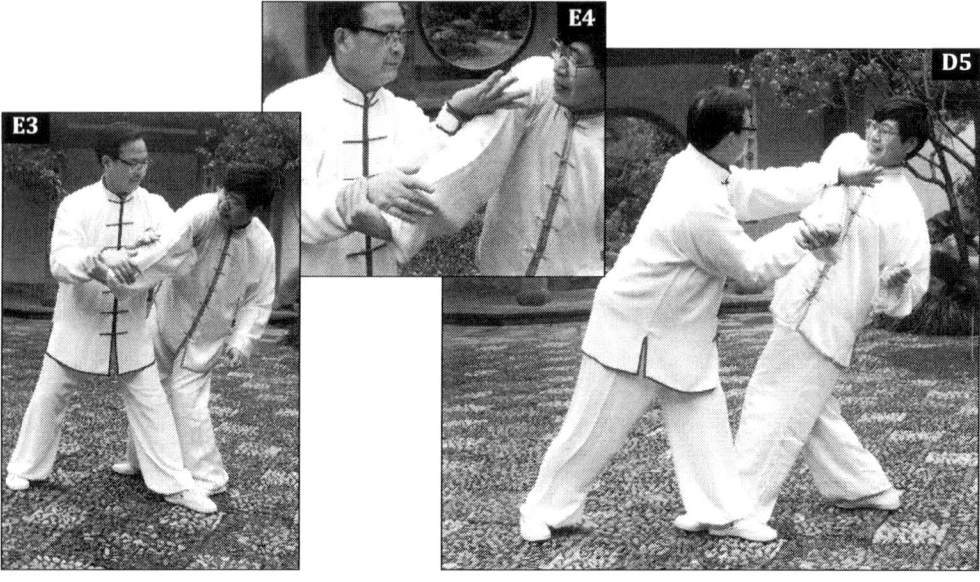

Shan Tong Bei (spread the fan)

F1: The opponent catches Zhang's right wrist with his right hand, or he forms a right fist and strikes towards Zheng's chest.

F2a: Zhang loosens his shoulders and puts weight down on the opponent's wrists while his right hand revolves clockwise towards the right and the left hand secures the opponent's wrist from underneath.

F2b: Detail of hand position.

F3: Zhang's hands continue to revolve and raise the opponent's right hand.

F4: Zhang keeps his hands still and turns his body clockwise to the right by turning on his left foot while stepping backwards with his right foot, placing it to the side and slightly behind the opponent's right foot.

F5: As a result of Zhang's repositioning, the opponent's arms are twisted toward his back and his body bends backwards while his feet "float." If Zhang keeps his hands still, loosens his waist, and adjusts the rotation of his body, the opponent will remain under his control.

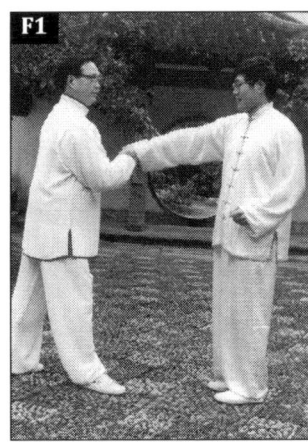
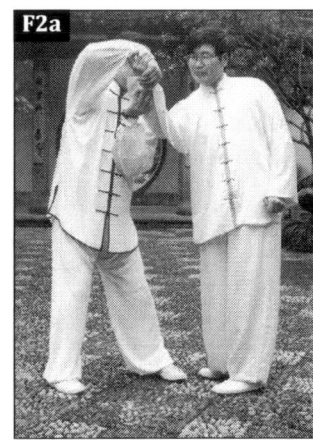
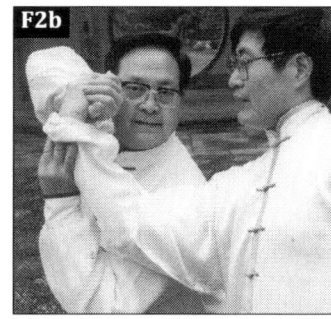
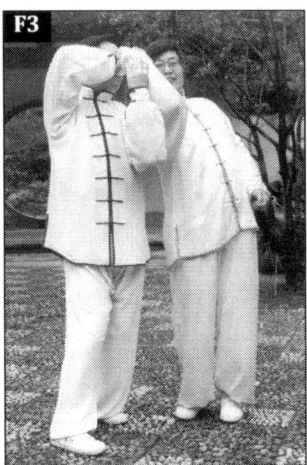
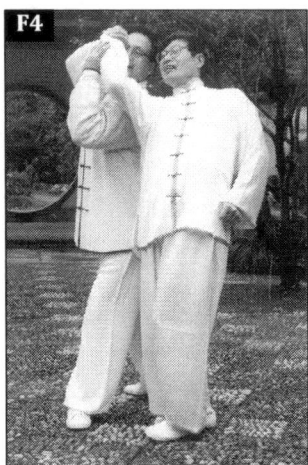
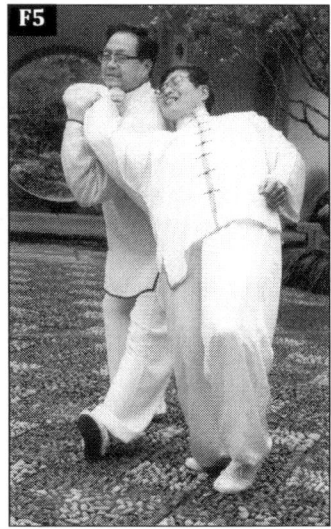

GLOSSARY

Pinyin	Wade-Giles	Character
an	an	按
cai	ts'ai	採
Chen Changxing	Ch'en Chang-hsing	陳長興
Chen Liqing	Ch'en Li-ch'ing	陳立清
Dai Peisu	T'ai P'ei-su	戴培粟
doutan	tou t'an	抖彈
fajing	fa ching	發勁
Gao Zhuangfei	Kao Chuang-fei	高壯飛
Hong Junsheng	Hung Chün-sheng	洪均生
Huang Yuanxiu	Huang Yüan-hsiu	黃元秀
ji	chi	擠
Jiang Yukun	Chiang Yü-k'un	蔣玉坤
kao	k'ao	靠
Li Jinglin	Li Ching-lin	李景林
Liu Chengde	Liu Ch'eng-te	劉成德
Lin Mogen	Lin Mo-ken	林墨根
lu	lu	捋
ming men	ming men	命門
peng	p'eng	掤
Tian Zhaolin	T'ien Chao-lin	田兆麟
tuna	t'u na	吐納
tuishou	t'ui shou	推手
Wang Peisheng	Wang P'ei-sheng	王培生
Wang Xianggen	Wang Hsiang-ken	王祥根
Wang Zhuocheng	Wang Chuo-ch'eng	王卓誠
Xia Tao	Hsia T'ao	夏濤
Yang Banhou	Yang Pan-hou	楊班候
Yang Chengfu	Yang Ch'eng-fu	楊澄甫
Yang Jianhou	Yang Chien-hou	楊健候
yin dao shu	yin tao shu	引導術
Yu Tonghe	Yü T'ung-he	余桐和
Yu Zhijun	Yü Chih-chün	于志均
Zhang Youquan	Chang Yu-ch'üan	張幼泉

Note

[1] The "flight or fight response" is a natural response in humans and animals. In times of danger the response is automatically activated and hormones, including adrenaline (epinephrine), are released into the blood stream. These hormones help the body prepare either to stay and fight the danger or to run away from it. This is the body's normal response to danger (Benson, 1990).

Bibliography

Benson, H. (1990). *The relaxation response.* New York: Avon.

DeMarco, M. (1991). The origin and evolution of taijiquan. *Journal of Asian Martial Arts, 1*(1): 9–25.

Ma, Y., and Zee, W. (1990). *Wu style taichichuan push-hands.* Hong Kong: Shanghai Book Co.

Mastadon Productions. (1993). *Taijiquan at West Lake.* Chicago, IL: Mastadon Productions. Video series in four volumes.

Wile, D. (1983). *Tai-chi touchstones: Yang family secret transmissions.* Brooklyn, NY: Sweet Ch'i Press.

Wile, D. (1996). *Lost tai-chi classics from the late Ch'ing dynasty.* Brooklyn, NY: Sweet Ch'i Press.

Wong, K. (1996). *The complete book of tai chi chuan: A comprehensive guide to the principles and practice.* Shaftesbury, Dorset: Element Books, Ltd.

Yang, C. (1974). *T'ai-chi ch'uan shih-yung fa* (Self-defense applications of tai-chi ch'uan). Taipei: Chung-hua wu-shu ch'u pan she. First published in 1931.

Zhaohua Publishing House (compilers). (1997). *Chen style taijiquan.* Beijing: Zhaohua Publishing House.

Body-Mind Connections in Chen Xin's *Illustrated Explanation of Chen Style Taijiquan*

by Miriam O'Connor, M.A.

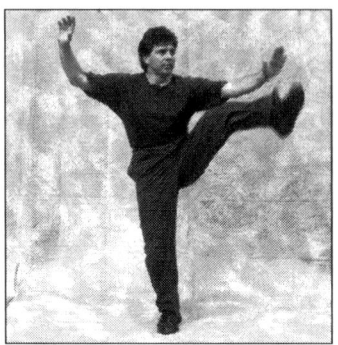

Chen-Style Left separate base.
All photographs courtesy of Michael A. DeMarco.
Photography by Pete Gool.

Introduction

The philosophy underpinning taijiquan practice is a fascinating but elusive field of study. If it is hard for researchers to record or analyze the physical dimension of a moving art, it is harder still to capture the movements of the mind and spirit that inspire these physical movements.

Since the mental world of practitioners cannot be studied directly, their writings naturally appear as the next best source of research material. Thus, my own foray into this research area began with a search for a practitioner's text in classical Chinese, which I would need to translate and discuss in my thesis.[1]

Two obviously valuable texts had already been translated: *Master Cheng's Thirteen Chapters on T'ai Chi Ch'üan* by Zheng Manqing (Cheng Man-Ch'ing) and the short texts, some at least a century old, generally recognized as expressing the essence of taijiquan, and known as the *Taijiquan Classics*.[2] A literature survey of the field of taijiquan also turned up a huge number of superficial introductions in European languages, some more substantial accounts of personal experience, a few useful translations or adaptations from the Chinese, and the historical research in Chinese of Gu Luxin, Tang Hao, and Matsuta Takimoto.

Another work, Chen Xin's *Chenshi Taijiquan Tujie* (Illustrated Explanations of Chen-Style Taijiquan), was recommended to me by both Chinese and Westerners. This book is particularly associated with the Chen family transmission of taijiquan and discusses the art's conceptual background. First published in 1931 or 1933,[3] but written between 1908 and 1919 (later date given in the author's preface), the work seemed to be a promising source of abstruse philosophy with its multitude of abstract yin-yang diagrams.

However, as my research progressed, the *Illustrated Explanations of Chen-Style Taijiquan* appeared more problematic. Many writers on taijiquan referred to the book, and several credited it as valuable for the study of taijiquan.[4] However, none ventured any explicit interpretation of what apparently was a profound exposition of taijiquan's conceptual framework. It seemed that the *Illustrated Explanations* was not merely imposing but also intimidating, and somewhat obscure.

Some twenty years ago, a doctoral thesis entitled Tai-ki K'iuan: Technique de Longue Vie, Technique de Combat[5] included translations into French of some texts from Chen Xin's book (Despeux, 1976; 1981). Even that author, French sinologist Catherine Despeux, did not give an overall account of the work but gave the most attention to the sections listing postures, sequences, and the paths that the qi (vital energy) takes through the body in taijiquan practice. While Dr. Despeux's later research covers corporal and meditation practices other than taijiquan, she was able to inform me that current doctoral research by a Chen Style practitioner Jean-Pierre Bonpied (under the direction of Professor François Jullien at Paris VII) was addressing some of the Chen Xin texts that interested me, namely those dealing with body-mind and micro-macrocosmic connections. Mr. Bonpied was kind enough to supply me with a summary of his research, which helped in my selection of texts from Chen Xin's book for my own study.

Overview of the Book's Contents

Though my own research focused on just a few pages of the philosophical texts, I include here a summary of the contents of the *Illustrated Explanations of Chen-Style Taijiquan*, which appears to be a heterogeneous compilation rather than an original synthesis. The first and most imposing section, which had initially attracted my interest, constitutes some seventy pages (vol. 1, pp. 17–87) of philosophical discussion and graphic representations of the Taiji (Supreme Ultimate).

The subsequent forty-four pages of the *Illustrated Explanations* (pp. 97–140) detail qi circulation in an orthodox account of the traditional medical theory used in acupuncture, moxa, or *qigong* (energy work), information that was all widely available early this century when Chen Xin was writing. While perhaps unfamiliar to the Western eye, this section makes little direct contribution to an understanding of taijiquan itself.

Chen Xin does mention briefly martial applications of qi circulation theory, but without explicit detail. For example, he gives the "classic eight intersections of the meridians," mentioning that the meridians can be blocked by an attack to these points, and that the time of the attack is significant. Dr. Chen Shing-pok, a Chinese acupuncturist working in Hôpital St. Louis in Paris, and who is also a Chen Style practitioner, was able to shed some light on this vague reference. In Chinese medical theory, the different organs correspond with set hours of the day, and each organ has its own meridians. At a said hour, an attack can thus target the meridian corresponding to the organ then dominant in the body: thus, in a midday combat while the heart is dominant, the heart meridian might be attacked.

Did Chen Xin hesitate to publish explicitly such dangerous techniques? He does include (juan shou, pp. 137–140) the traditional list of "mortal points" or "vulnerable points" (*dianxue*). These points are well known to martial artists, who protect them, for example, by preventing the opponent from touching the central axis of their bodies (front and rear), and thus protecting their two main meridians.

Whereas Chen Xin does not explicitly link meridian theory to martial application, his book does go on to set out another theory concerning the movement of energy in the body. In this case it is the spiraling *nei jing* (internal force) or *tan jing* (elastic force) that accumulates and uncoils like a spring. *Chansijing*, Chen Xin's formulation that the Chen Family tradition subsequently adopted, alludes to the coiled silk (*chansi*) of a cocoon. Some contemporary practitioners consider this spiraling aspect of jing important for understanding and training the jing. For example, some seek to strengthen the jing by training the *yi* (intention) along such spiraling paths before following on with the physical movement. With its diagrams, Chen Xin's book provides the most explicit account of this spiraling characteristic, with an overview (juan I, pp. 92–94) and applications to particular movements (e.g., juan II, pp. 16 and 27).

The most voluminous part of the book gives detailed and illustrated instructions for the new style (*xinjia*) Chen individual form. The movements are divided into thirteen groups, symbolizing the Five Elements and Eight Trigrams (vol. I, pp. 172–174). The postures are also described in their correspondence to the sixty-four hexagrams of the *Book of Changes* (Yijing).

The *Illustrated Explanations of Chen-Style Taijiquan* ends with some ten pages of biographical and genealogical material that documents and promotes the Chen taijiquan tradition. These annals celebrate the Chen ancestors' martial prowess, rectitude, and loyalty to the government. For example, the pages devoted to Chen Zhongshen (1809–1871), Chen Xin's father, seem to be the product of filial exaggeration, and were omitted from the 1991 Xi'an edition.[6]

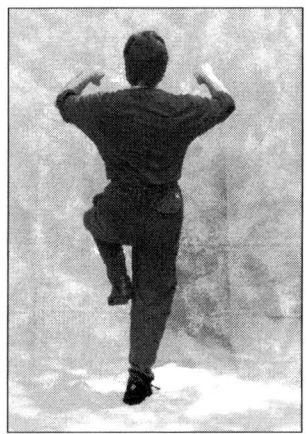 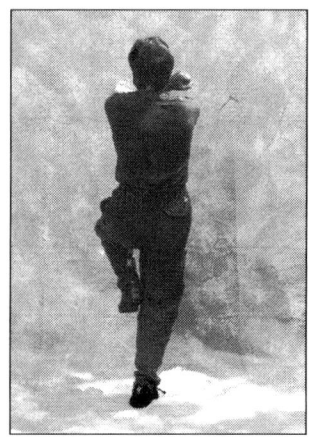 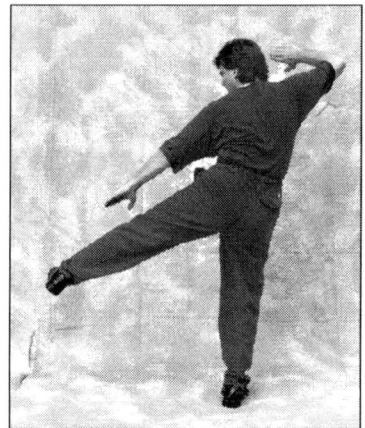

From old Chen Style first routine: transition from double gusts penetrate the ears to kick with left heel.

**Extrinsic Motivations for Chen Xin's
Synthesis of Philosophy and Family Boxing**

I soon discovered that Chen Xin's interest in philosophy was more established than his credentials as a taijiquan practitioner. Indeed, one Wu stylist, Wu Tunan, has had no hesitation in dismissing Chen Xin's work as irrelevant and purely theoretical speculation. In his *Taijiquan Zhi Yanjiu*, Wu (1986: 51) quotes at length a meeting he says the two men had in 1917 (some sixty-five years previous). Chen Xin, then a village schoolmaster, spoke of his regret that his father had made him an academic, unlike his elder brother(s) and his cousins who were able to study boxing and became heroes in the local militia. In fairness, one must note that Wu Tunan tends to minimize the contribution of the Chen clan transmission to the taijiquan's overall development. Within the Chen tradition, however, Chen Xin is generally acknowledged as a skilled practitioner and is credited with disciples in the "genealogies" of taijiquan transmission (Chen, Z. 1991: 9).

However sincere his interest in philosophy and in Chen Style boxing, Chen Xin's melding of the two probably also reflects a concern for "face," both in terms of family prestige and in terms of his own role within his clan. Competition with his clan from the flourishing rival Yang school and his own exclusion (however partial) from the martial prowess that forged his family's identity were both factors encouraging him to validate his family's art. He did this by attempting a detailed synthesis of the martial art of taijiquan and the scholarly art of philosophy.

Throughout the second half of the nineteenth century, the popularity of Yang Style taijiquan had grown steadily, and it was even taught at the Manchu imperial court (Liao, 1990: 13–14). The founder of this style, Yang Luchan, also known as Yang Fukui (1799–1872), had served the Chen family and studied for several years with the Chen Style master Chen Changxing (1771–1853).[7]

According to one source (Ly, 1990: 89–90), it may even have been Yang who, abandoning the earlier names of "supple boxing" (*ruanquan*) and "transformation boxing" (*huaquan*), first adopted the name "taijiquan" (supreme ultimate boxing) after studying Wang Zongyue's *Taijiquan Jing* (Taijiquan Classic).[8] As Yang's sons and grandson also became well-known figures in the martial arts world, Chen Xin's use of the term "taijiquan" in the title and the body of his book might thus have reintegrated into the older Chen boxing the newer Yang branch. More importantly, the ancient term "taiji", which appeared in an appendix to the *Yijing* (Book of Changes) perfectly suited his project of harmonizing boxing techniques with Yijing principles.

Surprises in Terminology and Authorship

As I deciphered the few pages of classical Chinese I had selected, I realized that in Chen Xin's text the term "taiji" was no longer the *Book of Changes* symbol of the integration of yin and yang but was synonymous with the Neo-Confucian's Principle (*li*) and the Way (*dao*). Moreover the term "qi" was used with a meaning different from that of "vital energy" current in medicine or taijiquan practice. This is generally thought of as an energy current circulating within the body and supporting life and health as well as body movement in taijiquan.

Qi was used here in the wider sense of basic energy (or "matter-energy") which makes up all things, opposed to Principle (*li*), the innate organization of all things, both animate and inanimate, and is generally opposed to Principle (*li*), the innate organization of all things. This classic Neo-Confucianist opposition suggested that one immediate philosophical frame of reference was the Neo-Confucianist synthesis of the Song Dynasty (960–1279): an attempt to integrate Daoist cosmological concepts within the socio-ethical Confucianist tradition.

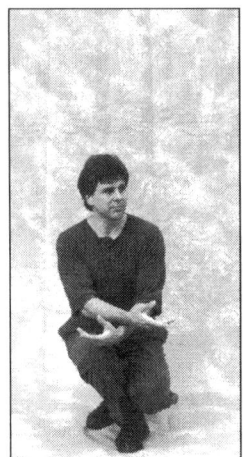 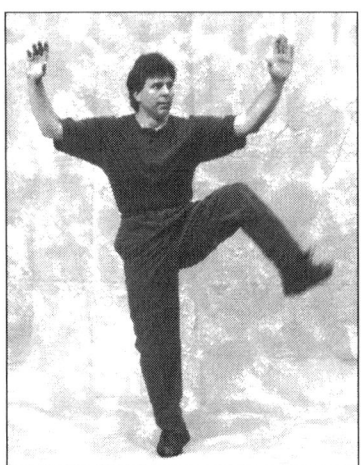 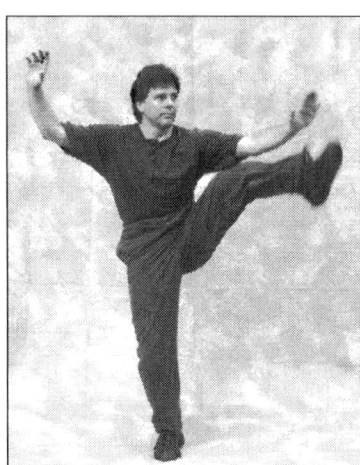

Chen Style left separate base.

The incongruity of this conceptual framework with my expectations of taijiquan as a "Daoist practice" only made sense once I realized that the texts in question did not deal with taijiquan at all, and were not, in fact, written by Chen Xin. Catherine Despeux had noted in her thesis (1976: 30–2) that the main spiral representation of the taiji in Chen Xin's book[9] occurs in a diagram in a late Ming Dynasty (1368–1644) edition of Shao Yong's (1011–77) *Huangji Jingshi Shu* (Book of Cosmological Chronology), and that in both cases the representation is attributed to Lai Zhide (1525–1604). However, when I consulted a copy of Lai Zhide's own *Lai Zhu Yijing Tujie* (Lai's Compilation of Illustrated Explanations of the Book of Changes), I discovered that Chen Xin owes a great deal more than a single diagram to Lai Zhide (Lai, 1969). The very seventy-page section of Chen's book that had most intrigued me is almost entirely taken directly from Lai's work, a book which according to Larry Schultz (1982) was an extremely popular, though never officially endorsed text for *Yijing* scholars throughout the Qing Dynasty (1644–1911). Moreover, these texts are duly attributed to Lai in Chen's book by the annotation "Lai Chu" (Lai's Compilation).

If the philosophical discussion in Chen Xin's book was not the author's, can it still be thought to contribute to an understanding of his martial art? To what extent does Lai's sixteenth-century explanation of taiji shed light on the twentieth-century practice of taijiquan? Such questions required a clarification of the different conceptual frameworks appealed to in the two cases.

Interpreting the Term Taiji

In Professor Robinet's survey of the meaning of the expression "taiji" in pre-Ming Daoist sources (1990: 373–411),[10] it appears that aside from references to the taiji as a high divinity or as the pole star (and thus the pivot and center of the universe), this concept often acts as hinge between the One and the Many, origin and unfolding, Non-Being (*wu*) and Being (*you*). These relationships are foreshad*owed in the classic formulation of the Great Appendix (Xici) to the* Book of Changes: "The *Yi* has its *Taiji*, and the Taiji gives birth to the two principles [Yin and Yang]."[11] The Taiji thus is set between the Absolute (of potential to change) of the Yi and Relativity (of change) of yin and yang. Similarly, the fourth-century BCE book *Zhuangzi* and the second-century BCE *Huainanzi* placed the Taiji after the absolute Dao which in Laozi gives birth to the One, which gives birth to Two, and thus the many (Henricks, 1989: 106).

Speculating on the mechanisms of the cosmos, the Daoists integrated the Taiji into their evolutionary series of Five Geneses (*wutai*, the Five Greats) from primary chaotic and indistinguishable unity to the universe of the differentiated myriad things. Both composite and origin of the Two (yin and yang), the Taiji encapsulates the concepts of burgeoning division and return to the One.

Because of this role as hinge between One and the Many, it is no surprise that the Daoist Taiji is often preceded (logically even if not temporally) by an absolute, the *Wuji* (Ultimateless) characterized as empty, spontaneous, tangible.

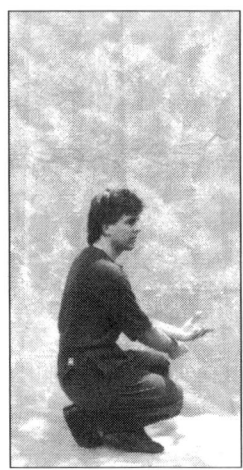 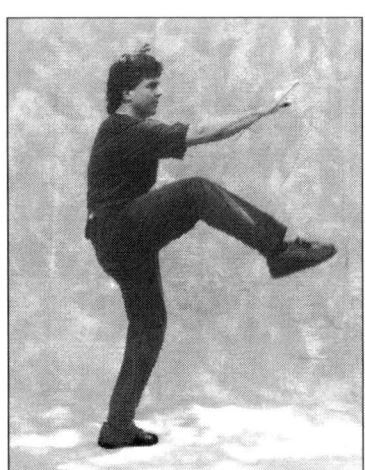 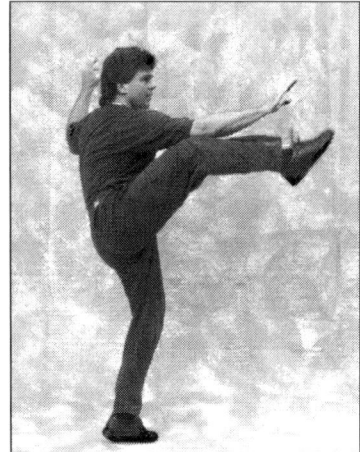

Chen Style right separate base.

Such Daoist interpretations of the Taiji and Wuji were no doubt enriched by the interest and metaphysical scope given these notions by some of the Song

Dynasty Neo-Confucianists,[12] if only by the controversy and reflection these authors stimulated. Later, the writings of Zhu Xi (1130–1200), which constituted the official orthodoxy studied by Chinese scholars for six hundred years, characterized the Taiji as identical to Principle, and elsewhere as identical to the *Wuji* (Ultimateless). Thus, the Taiji gradually took on the role of absolute for the Neo-Confucianists, giving them a totem as prestigious as the Dao of the Daoists.

In his re-evaluation of Zhu Xi orthodoxy, Lai Zhide reinstated the primacy of the *Wuji* (Ultimateless) over the *Taiji* (Supreme Ultimate): he represented the former by an empty circle, like some of his Daoist predecessors, and the Taiji by a black and white spiral with the same "empty circle" in its center. This is the relation between the two terms that is adopted by Chen Xin, who presents taijiquan as an intermediary and means of access from the ordinary world of the Myriad Things to the absolutes of Principle (*li*) and Wuji. Lai's symbol now frequently appears as a symbol for Chen Style taijiquan schools.[13]

Yijing Commentary in the Daoist and Confucianist Tradition and Relevance to Taijiquan Practice

Both Daoist and Confucian traditions see value in "a good life," but their goals are rather different. Daoists tend to take a high ethical standard as a necessary but not sufficient condition for harmonizing with the Universe or achieving personal immortality. For Confucianists (and Neo-Confucianists), personal moral development is both the duty and the destiny of humanity. One much quoted phrase from the *Book of Changes* summed up this challenge: "Exhaust Principle and plumb the depths of Nature in order to reach Heavenly Destiny" (Chen, 1991: 62).

The *Book of Changes* was popular in both Daoist and Confucianists circles. Daoism has tended to focus on the patterns of change to better understand and harmonize with the workings of the universe, while Confucianist commentary has interpreted the examples and images in the book as ethical teachings. Of course, in practice, these two, with Buddhism (the other main Chinese socio-religious tradition), have interpenetrated and enriched each other constantly.

The ideal of human development adopted by Lai Zhide, who spent some thirty years in solitary ascetic meditation on the *Book of Changes*, was self-alignment with Human Nature or Principle by dominating and eliminating self-centered desires. An illustrated analysis of the patterns of change in the stars, moon, and earth, matched with the cycle of sixty-four hexagrams in the *Book of Changes*, is presented as the heavenly model of non-egotistical conduct human beings should emulate to achieve their destiny.

While the Lai Zhide texts provide elements of an ethical and cosmological framework that includes Neo-Confucianist as well as Daoist references, these elements are compatible with rather than specific to the art of taijiquan, which aims at harmonious development of the physical, mental, and (for some) spiritual capacities of human beings. The links between Lai Zhide's vision and the taijiquan training system are superficially reinforced in Chen Xin's book by the similarities of terminology; such similarities conceal different conceptual frameworks. However, in the short texts I studied, two aspects did seem relevant to the taijiquan practitioner's moral and spiritual growth: 1) the idea of banishing a sense of self as separate from the Universe, and 2) the central role given to the human heart/mind (*ren-xin*) as the connecting agent between gross and subtle energies in the cosmos as well as in the individual.

Conclusion

Whereas Chen Xin's book is hardly satisfying as a coherent synthesis of metaphysical and martial art, his attempt to contribute to the literary tradition of taijiquan has certainly met with recognition and has helped establish the role of the Chen clan as central in the history of taijiquan. In the sixty-five years that separate us from the publication of this work, no other author in the field has made a more ambitious attempt.

Glossary

Chen Pai Taijiquan	陳氏太极拳
dao	道
li	理
taiji	太極
wuji	無極

Chinese Authors

Chen Xin	陳鑫
Chen Zhenglei	陳正雷
Lai Zhide	來知德
Qiao Biao	喬檦
Liu Ronggan	劉榮淦
Tang Hao	唐豪
Wang Xi'an	王西安
Wu Tunan	吳圖南

Notes

[1] This research was made within the academic structure of a master's program at the University of Aix-en-Provence, supervised by Professor Isabelle Robinet, a specialist in Daoism.

[2] Danny Vercammen (1994) has attempted to catalogue the variations of the Chinese texts in *Neiji Wushu: The Internal School of Chinese Martial Arts, Vol. 1*.

[3] The *Zhunguo Wushu Da Cidian* (Wu, 1990: 503) cites 1931 as the first publication date of Chen Xin's *Chenshi Taijiquan Tujie*. Dufresne and Nguyen (1994: 29) mention 1931 as the year when the Henan Martial Arts Academy director bought

the manuscript and give 1933 as the year of its first publication.
4. The *Zhunguo Wushu Da Cidian* lists it as "one of the most important works on taijiquan" (Wu, 1990: 503). Huang writes that Chen's book is "a secret ancient text preserved at Chen Chi Kou, Honan, ..." (Huang, 1973: 48).
5. Catherine Despeux's 1976 academic work was revised for the general reader and republished in 1981.
6. See Hu (1993 a-b; August 1993) for a translation of a hand-copied extract of the official family history and for a discussion of the unreliability of Chen Xin's and other's accounts.
7. Rivalry and conservation of family prestige are of course still current in the martial arts world. A recent edition of Chen Xin's work (*Chen Shi Taijiquan Tushou*, Xi'an, 1991), in a passage on page 380 dealing with Chen Changxing's numerous students, omits the sentence "Yang Fukui was the most famous of them" found in the Taipei edition (Chen, 1970: 214).
8. Apparently discovered in 1852, this text may be the oldest to use the term taijiquan, which appeared in the title. Within the text, "taiji" is found as a philosophical term.
9. This taiji diagram appears on pages 17, 20, 21, 63, 65, 70, 78, and 80 of Chen Xin's book.
10. The present paragraph and the following three paragraphs are based on Professor Robinet's article (1990).
11. This formulation is taken from the *Zhou Yi* (Book of Changes) (ch. III, section 10, p. 62), found in *Si Shu Wu Jing*, vol. 1.
12. Two authors in particular, Zhou Dunyi (1017-1073) and Shao Yong, both of whom had links with Daoism and indeed Buddhism, used the term Taiji to connect the One with the Myriad Things through the evolutions of yin and yang. In his *Illustrated Explanation of Taiji* (Taiji Tushou), Zhou integrated the Five Elements (*wuxing*) system; while in his *Book of Cosmological Chronology*, Shao Yong assimilated the Eight Trigrams (*bagua*) system.
13. I have not come across earlier uses of this symbol.

Bibliography – Works in English and French

Chen, B. (1995). A recollection of the book san san liu quan pu. *Journal of the Chenstyle Research Association*, 3: 19–21.

Cheng, M. (1982). *Master Cheng's thirteen chapters on tai chi ch'üan*. (Wile, D., Trans.). New York: Sweet Ch'i Press.

Despeux, C. (1981). *Taiji quan: Art martial, technique de longue vie*. Paris: Guy Trédaniel.

Despeux, C. (1976). *Tai-ki k'iuan: Technique de longue vie, technique de combat*. Paris: Mémoires de l'Institute des Hautes Etudes Chinoises, vol. III, Collége de France.

Dufresne, T., and Nguyen, J. (1994). *Taiji quan: Art martial de la famille Chen*. Paris: Editions Budostore.

Feng, Z. and Feng, D. (1984). *Chen Style Taijiquan*. Hong Kong: Hai Feng Publishing Co.

Fung, Y. (1983). *A history of Chinese philosophy*. (Bodde, D., Trans.). Princeton: Princeton University Press.

Henricks, R. (1989). *Lao-tzu te-dao ching*. New York: Ballantine Books.

Hu, W. (June 1993a). Ch'en-shih chia-p'u translated with commentaries. *Journal of the Chenstyle Taijiquan Research Association, 1*(3): 1–6.

Hu, W. (June 1993b). Ch'en Chung-sheng and the problem of sources, part 1. *Journal of the Chenstyle Taijiquan Research Association, 1*(3): 7–18.

Hu, W. (August 1993). Ch'en Chung-sheng and the problem of sources, part 2. *Journal of the Chenstyle Taijiquan Research Association, 1*(4): 4–16.

Huang, W. (1973). *Fundamentals of t'ai-chi ch'uan*. Hong Kong: South Sky Book Company.

Jacobs, A. (Dir.). (1990). *Encyclopédie philosophique universelle, vol. II*. Paris: Presses Universitaires de France.

Jou, T. (1980). *The tao of tai-chi chuan, way to rejuvenation*. Warwick, NY: Tai Chi Foundation.

Kelly, P. (1994). *Tai ji secrets*. (no location given): G&H Publications.

Kleinman, S. (Ed.). (1986). *Mind and body east meets west, big ten body of knowledge symposium series, vol. 15*. Champaign, IL: Human Kinetics Publishers.

Liao, W. (1990). *Tai Chi Classics*. Boston: Shambhala Publications Inc.

Lo, B., Inn, M., Amacker, R. and Foe, S. (1979). *Essence of t'ai chi ch'uan: The literary tradition*. Berkeley: North Atlantic Books.

Ly, A. (1990). *L'art du tai ji quan, le dao et le qi*. Paris: Lierre et Coudrier.

Ni, H. (1983). *The book of changes and the unchanging truth*. Malibu, CA: Shrine of the Eternal Breath of Tao.

Robinet, I. (1991). *Histoire du taoïsme des origines au xive siécle*. Paris: Editions du Cerf.

Robinet, I. (1990). The place and meaning of the notion of taiji in Taoist sources prior to the Ming dynasty. (Wissing, P., Trans.). *History of Religions, 29*(4): 373–411.

Schultz, L. (1982). Lai Chih-te (1525–1604) and the phenomenology of the "Classic of Change." Ann Arbor: University Microfilms International.

Seidel, A. (1970). A Taoist immortal of the Ming dynasty: Chang San-feng. In *Self and Society in Ming Thought*. (deBary, W., Ed.). New York: Columbia University Press.

Vercammen, D. (1994). *Neijia wushu: The internal school of Chinese martial arts, vol. 1*. Gent, Belgium: Rijksuniversiteit.

Wang, P. and Zheng, W. (1983). *Wu style taijiquan: A detailed course for health and self-defence and teaching of three masters in Beijing*. Hong Kong: Hai Feng Publishing Co.

Yang, J. (1991). *Advanced Yang style tai chi chuan, vol. 1*. Jamaica Plain, MA: Yang's Martial Arts Association Publication Centre.

Works in Chinese

Chen, X. (1970). *Chenshi taijiquan tujie* (Illustrated explanations of Chen Style Taijiquan). (Hua, Y., Ed.). Taipei: Hualianguan Chubanshe.

Chen, X. (1991). *Chenshi taijiquan tushuo* (Chen Style Taijiquan illustrated and explained). (Xiao, P., Ed.). Xi'an: Sanqin Chubanshe.

Chen, Z. (1991). *Chenshi taijiquan xiehui zong* (Chen Style Taijiquan association's ancestors). Xi'an: Gaodeng Jioyu Chubanshe.

Lai, Z. (1969). *Lai zhu Yijing tujie* (Lai's compilation of illustrated explanations of the Book of Changes). Taipei: Yiqun Chubanshe.

Matsuta, T. (1984). *Zhongguo wushu shilüe* (Chinese martial arts biographical sketch). Chongqing: Siquan Kexue Dixue Chubanshe.

Qiao, B., and Liu, R. (1990). *Jing gong Chenshi taijiquan* (Energy work in Chen Style Taijiquan). Beijing: Beijing Tiyu Xueyuan Chubanshe.

Tang, H. (1963). *Taijiquan genyuan*. (The origins of taijiquan). Hong Kong: Bailing Chubanshe.

Wang, X. (1993). *Chenshi taijiquan laojia*. (Chen Style Taijiquan old style). Zhengzhou: Henan Kexue Jishu Chubanshe.

Wu, T. (1986). *Taijiquan zhi yanjiu*. (Taijiquan research). Hong Kong: Shangwu Chubanshe.

Wu, T. (1990). *Zhongguo wushu da cidian*. (Great dictionary of Chinese martial arts). Beijing: Renmin Tiyu Chubanshe.

Yang Taiji Practice
Through the Eyes of Western Medical Health Guidelines
by Michael A. DeMarco, M.A.

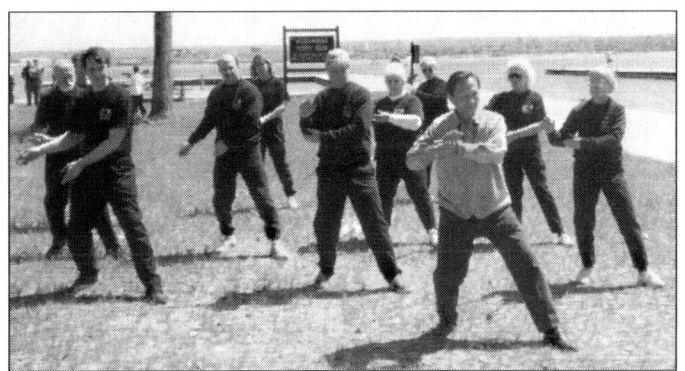 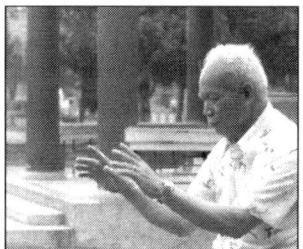

Right: Master Yang Qingyu lives in Puli, Taiwan, where he teaches the traditional Yang Taiji system. Left: Lin Shengxuan is one of Yang Qingyu's longtime students from Taipei. During a visit to Erie, Pennsylvania (April 1998), Mr. Lin taught my students a repetitive drill based on the "grasp sparrow's tail" sequence in eight directions. Photographs courtesy of M. DeMarco.
* Note: This paper was prepared for presentation at the International Council for Health, Physical Education, Recreation, Sport and Dance (ICHPER•SD) 8th European Congress July 14-19, 1998 London, England.

Introduction*

According to Chinese consumer packaging labels and research reports—green tea, beer, peanuts, qigong, acupuncture, taijiquan, and "Long Life" brand cigarettes—all have a strong commonality. Each promises the benefits of greater strength and vigor, improvement in mental faculties, deeper spiritual awareness, and (of course) increased sexual prowess. In short, many Chinese exercise and dietary programs claim to offer a healthy, happy life with the longevity of the pine, tortoise, and crane.

The tendency of the Chinese to claim such benefits from so many of their products and activities raises valid questions concerning their acceptability as being truly conducive assets for a healthier lifestyle. This paper will focus on the unique art of Yang Style taijiquan, usually referred to in abbreviated form simply as taiji. During the last few decades, there has been a rapid growth in taiji practice outside Asia, a growth largely linked to claims concerning its health nurturing qualities (Baer, 1997). To verify these claims, this paper will utilize the most recent health and fitness guidelines provided by leading research institutes. These guidelines can serve as criteria for analyzing and assessing Yang Style taiji as an activity that we may consider in our research concerning the relationship between lifestyle and well-being. Therefore, this paper:

1) defines and lists the established guidelines for health and fitness.
2) describes what taiji is and how it is practiced, and
3) ascertains the role taiji may take in our lives according to the ideals set by the world's leading authorities on health and fitness.

Guidelines for Health and Fitness

According to the World Health Organization, "Health is defined as a state of complete physical, mental, social, and spiritual well-being, and not merely the absence of disease and infirmity." Dr. Nieman adds that "Physical fitness is a condition in which an individual has sufficient energy and vitality to accomplish daily tasks and active recreational pursuits without undue fatigue" (1998: 4).

A review was made of some of the published literature that focuses on health and physical fitness. The general guidelines derived from these works permit practical, clear-cut conclusions helpful in the assessment of any exercise program, including taiji. A synopsis of their findings is given in the following eight guidelines for a successful approach to adopting and maintaining a physically active lifestyle (U.S., 1996: 46, 47; Nieman, 1998: 17):

1) Be active!
2) exercise at least 30-minutes daily (this can be accumulated time).
3) participate in an exercise program of moderate intensity.
4) consider behavioral and attitudinal factors in selecting a program.
5) have support from family and friends.
6) select an activity open to males and females of varied ages, which has appeal to all.
7) eliminate "high-risk" behaviors.
8) select an activity that can be done life long.

The importance of these eight guidelines are obscured by their simplicity. A closer look at the meaning of each guideline and how they interrelate with each other represents an enormous amount of medical knowledge in a concise format. Therefore, we should not dismiss the guidelines because of their simplicity but come to understand the implications of each and their importance in our lives.

The rational for adopting the above guidelines, including the social and medical factors influencing such a decision, will be described after the following section describing the Yang taiji curriculum. Thus, the significance of both the modern medical guidelines for health and Yang taiji as an activity can be simultaneously presented in the concluding section.

Overview of the Taiji Curriculum

Chen Wangting (cir. 1597–1664) is credited as being the founder of the original Chen Style taiji. As a garrison commander in Henan Province, Wangting absorbed many noted boxing styles of his day. He is said to have created boxing routines and associated exercises from which all other forms of taiji were derived (DeMarco, 1992: 14-15; Wallace, 1998; Gu, 1984: 1-12).

The Chen Style was passed on for numerous generations only within the Chen family clan and a direct lineage continues today (Huang, 1993: 51-54; Stubenbaum, 1994: 90-99). However, a Chen family servant named Yang Luchan (1799-1872) was taught by the 14th generation master, Chen Changxing (1771-1853). Yang was the first "outsider" to learn and popularize the system which is now associated with his family name and lineage (DeMarco, 1992: 20; Jou, 1988: 42-44; Wile, 1996: 3).

Like the evolution of painting styles, the original Chen Style taiji differs from the Yang Style for social and political reasons related to the history of Chinese boxing. As modern weaponry became common, the necessity for secrecy waned in the traditional boxing traditions. At the same time, the purpose and function of taiji changed to meet the times (Wile, 1996: 3-30).

The Yang Style was adapted to public needs and some of the original movements were eliminated or changed. The routines came to be practiced in a slow, even tempo, and relaxed manner. Once taiji was available to the public, rumors spread of how practicing the art helped many improve their health and the number of practitioners rapidly rose. As a result, Yang Style taiji soon spread across China. Its popularity and fame as an exercise system continues to spread throughout the world (DeMarco, 1992: 20-24).

As a pure fighting system, the original Chen Style was developed for facing life-and-death situations. This necessitated familiarity with assorted weaponry and open hand fighting skills. Leading masters attempted to take under consideration every aspect of the human condition which would help the boxer emerge victorious in any conflict. The truths they learned about the human body, mind, and spirit remains important today, even though the original intent of their research has been overshadowed by the emergence of taiji as an appropriate activity adaptable to modern health care (Koh, 1981a).

Taiji has a long history based on Chinese cultural traditions reaching back over a millennium (Koh, 1981b). However, it was not until the early twentieth century that Yang taiji became standardized under Yang Chengfu (1883-1936), the grandson of the founder Yang Luchan (Huang, 1993: 65-68; Wong, 1998: 204-205; Jou, 1988, 42-47). To this day, the leading representatives of the various taiji systems retain the traditional skills and knowledge associated with the original fighting arts, such as mastery of the straight sword, staff, and other weapons. But true masters of complete taiji systems are rare.

Today, many study taiji solely for health benefits and some dabble in self-defense aspects. As a result, Yang taiji is the most popular style and is often mistakenly looked upon only as an exercise for the elderly (Lim, 1996: 91). It appears this way because many teachers have only studied taiji for its health benefits and are unfamiliar with the complete system.

There are four aspects of taiji that should be noted. Taiji is a martial art, a holistic health exercise, an aesthetic dance-like art, and a form of moving meditation. Most students begin their taiji study because of an interest in one of these aspects. As a result, the traditional Yang Style taijiquan curriculum focus on the following practices:

1) a solo routine,
2) two-person routines, and
3) taiji sword routines.

The Traditional Yang Style Solo Routine

Most students, even many taiji teachers, only practice the taiji solo routine. Traditionally, this routine consists of 108 martial movements which are arranged in a flowing sequence from beginning to end as a river current. There are forward, backward, sideways, and turning movements. The body moves harmoniously in a continuously even tempo which is slow enough to finely focus on being relaxed and balanced with every gesture (Jou, 1988; Huang, 1993; Wong, 1996).

Some taiji movements look poetically inspired with names like: "wave hands like clouds," "snake creeps downward," "rooster stands on one leg," and "embrace moon." Other movements are clearly martial in application, such as "lotus kick," deflect, push, rollback, punch, and press.

For a beginning student, solo practice is characterized by tenseness, staccato movements, and off-balanced postures. To make the routine evolve into an exercise characterized by balance, smoothness, and relaxed grace can take many decades of continuous polishing through the forge of practice (DeMarco, 1997: 48–58).

In China, taiji practitioners usually meet daily at dawn amid the fresh air and tranquil surroundings of a lake, park, or riverbank (Reynolds, 1982: 104–110). They often chat and stretch while waiting for others to arrive. When the teacher arrives, students organize to do the solo routine together in synchronized fashion. The routine takes from twenty to thirty minutes to perform, depending upon the tempo and exact number of movements included in the style. After the routine, the teacher will instruct beginners in new movements or offer tips to advanced students on how to improve a movement or offer insights into the deeper aspects of taiji's underlying philosophy (Horwitz, et. al., 1976: 15–25; Lehrhaupt, 1993, 61–69; DeMarco, 1997).

After class, students may depart for breakfast, work, school, or remain to socialize for a short time. They usually discuss taiji in between more personal discussions concerning family, work, or other matters.

Some beginning students find taiji too boring and soon quit. Others, who have the patience to get through this initial stage, may continue the daily routine for years on end. Because of changing personal schedules, many practitioners quit the group after learning the solo exercise and practice on their own (U.S., 1996: 46; Horwitz, et., 1976: 15–25; Lehrhaupt, 1993, 61–69). The stability of the group rests primarily on the teacher's talents and knowledge which allows the teacher to provide continuous instruction, guidance, and inspiration for maintaining the interest of each student. Unfortunately, many so-called "taiji teachers" do not know the complete system and students may eventually quit the group and often taiji practice altogether.

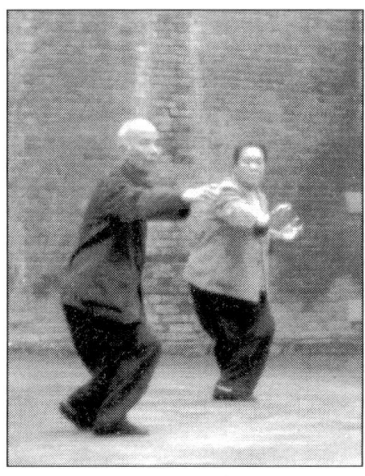

Part of the early morning
taiji routine in a park in Xi'an, China.
Photograph courtesy of M. DeMarco.

The solo routine can be practiced daily for one's entire life and there will always be more to learn within its subtle complexities. A perceptive practitioner will receive instruction indirectly from the solo routine itself by continuously discovering ways of moving, thinking, and sensing that results from dedicated practice. The solo routine was designed for the practitioner to learn about himself, i.e., how the body and mind function together holistically (DeMarco, 1994). Thus, taiji is not just physical exercise. It is considered an "internal art" because of the importance placed on cultivating one's mental, emotional, and spiritual aspects. Since it is a "person" who does taiji, it is necessary to cultivate the whole person to make progress in mastering taiji.

Two-Person Taiji Routines and Taiji Sword Routines

The true martial arts have always dealt with personal combat. If taiji's solo routine was designed to allow the individual to "know himself," two-person routines were designed to allow him to "know others." What this means can be ascertained by a description of the practices involved.

There are three main two-person exercises associated with Yang taiji. The first, called "push-hands" (*tuishou*), is a two-person exercise based on fundamental martial applications aligned in the four cardinal directions. The movements are ward off, rollback, press, and push (Chen, n.d.; Kuo, 1994: 33–42; Jou, 1988: 226–253; Davis and Mann, 1996: 55–56; Ma and Zee, 1990). Another duet practice is referred to as "four-corners" or "large rollback" (*dalu*) since it covers the four directions between the cardinal points with movements called: elbow, split, pull-down, and shoulder-strike. Duets are practiced in fixed stances or with active stepping (Chen, n.d.; Smith, 1997: 56–69; Jou, 1988: 253–256).

There is another rare duet routine called *sanshou*, often translated as "free hands" or "dispersing hands," which may refer to the self-defense goal of meeting any confrontation in a relaxed, easy manner to defeat the opponent. This is more complex than dalu and tuishou, containing a lengthy arrangement of attack and counter movements (Yiu, 1981).

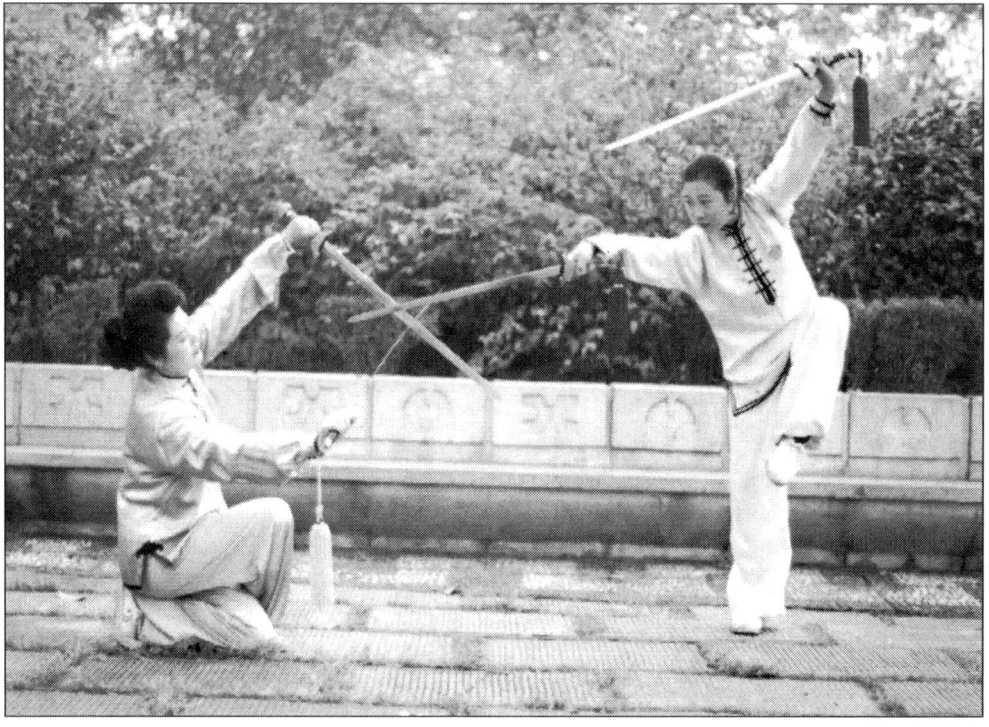

Wu Hangxin and Jin Huiying practicing two-person sword routines in Hangzhou, China. Photograph courtesy of D. Mainfort.

The taiji sword routines have similar movements as those found in the solo routine. In the traditional solo sword routine, the sword's weight and length allows the practitioner to sense how his own movements effect the sword. A duet routine allows each swordsman to extend his sensitivity through the blade to detect the movement of his partner.

The duet practices of tuishou, dalu, sanshou and the taiji sword are complementary to the solo routine. They enlarge the scope of taiji by bringing in a complex host of elements such as speed, movement, direction, and intention. All the routines should follow the fundamental taiji principles of relaxation, balanced movement, coupled with a developed sensitivity required to be aware of the "oneself" and "others" (Honda, 1995; Jacobson, 1997).

Two-person practices in action.

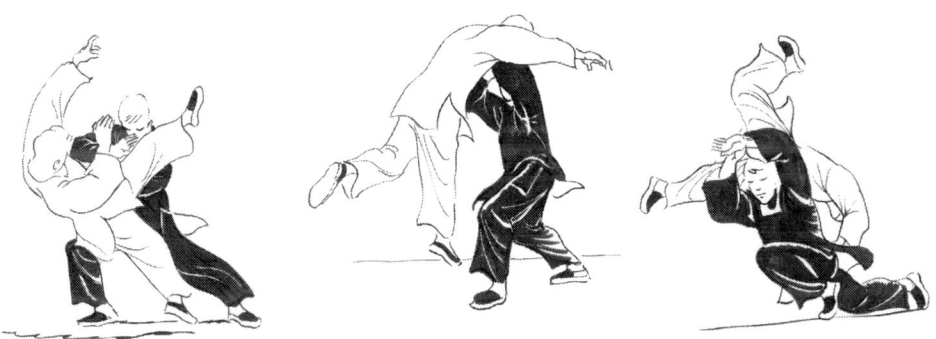

Left to right: Push-hands (*tuishou*). Four-corners (*dalu*). Free hands (*sanshou*).
Illustrations courtesy of Oscar Ratti.

Assessing Yang Taiji as an Activity for Health

Eight guidelines for a successful approach to adopting and maintaining a physically active lifestyle were presented earlier in this paper. We can gain a better understanding of the role taiji may take in our lives by looking at these guidelines as criteria for Yang taiji practice.

1) Be Active!

The National Institutes of Health concluded that "All ... should engage in regular physical activity at a level appropriate to their capacity, needs, and interest" (U.S., 1996: 41). They reached this conclusion in large part because inactivity is a major risk factor for cardiovascular disease (CVD), a leading cause of death. The activity chosen can greatly effect other CVD risk factors, including high blood pressure, lipid levels, and obesity. However, people who are not physically fit, such as those who are overweight, smoke, or have arthritic problems, may find many exercises to be too difficult or strenuous to do. The paradox is that they need to exercise but feel that exercise is too grueling to carry on regularly.

Taiji is highly adaptable to the practitioner's state of health and fitness. The movements can be done in high or low postures, in narrow or wide stances. Practicing the movements in a slow, relaxed manner ensures that anyone who can walk can learn the traditional solo routine. As one gradually learns the routine, he gains strength and flexibility (Lai, 1995). There is an awareness of becoming gradually more fit and taking satisfaction in the progress made.

2) Exercise at Least Thirty-Minutes Daily

Inactivity is not only a major cause of cardiovascular disease, but bears heavily on other diseases, such as diabetes, osteoporosis, hypertension, and even some cancers (U.S., 1996: 43). A minimum of thirty minutes exercise is considered ample for reducing such ill effects (ACSM, n.d.: 163).

The traditional Yang Style solo routine takes just about thirty minutes to perform. It can therefore be easily fit into a daily schedule with the practitioner knowing that the minimum exercise time is met.

The Yang taiji solo routine is a comprehensive approach to exercising, affecting the cardio-respiratory system, body composition, muscular strength, and joint flexibility (Koh, 1982; Lumsden, 1998; Powerful, 1996; Jacobson, et. al., 1997). Benefits can be measured even after a month or two of taiji practice. However, as the National Institutes of Health stresses, "... physical activity must be performed regularly to maintain these effects" (U.S., 1996: 43; Nieman, 1998: 46).

Physical fitness is health and skill related. With the daily practice of taiji, skills are acquired which inspire the practitioner to not miss the exercise. As one acquires greater insights into the art, one's state of health also continually improves.

3) Participate in an Exercise Program of Moderate Intensity

High-intensity and fast-moving sports are attractive to competitive athletes, but these activities pose dangerous to their health. Their motivating factors may be a quest for fame and excitement rather than for health and fitness. Those who are truly seeking an activity for their health should beware of any dangers associated with the sport or activity they may consider. Under proper instruction, taiji poses no risk to the practitioner.

"The majority of benefits of physical activity can be gained by performing moderate-intensity activities" (U.S., 1996: 43). Whether taiji's solo routine fits into the "moderate-intensity" range is questionable (Zhuo, et. at., 1984: 9). A cardio-respiratory rate at 50% VO_2max is recommended for general health (Nieman, 1998: 9; ACSM, n.d.: 158), but taiji's slow motion movements may not meet this criterion. More research is needed in this area to be certain. However, if the associated duet and swords routines are included in the assessment, then taiji would certainly meet this criterion as well. Because taiji practice falls in the low and moderately-intense category of exercise, there is little risk of injuring oneself during practice. There is also a stronger inclination for the individual to continue taiji practice on a regular basis.

4) Consider Behavioral and Attitudinal Factors in Selecting a Program

A big factor in selecting an activity for health and fitness is personality. The "behavioral and attitudinal factors that influence the motivation for and ability to sustain physical activity are strongly determined by social experiences, cultural background, and physical disability and health status. For example, perceptions of appropriate physical activity differ by gender, age, weight, marital status, family roles and responsibilities, disability, and social class" (U.S., 1996: 46). Although these barriers may be found in some degree in taiji practice, the most foreboding barrier is that taiji may be too exotic to be easily assimilated. First, one must be aware of what taiji is and what it has to offer. This may then motivate one to learn the art.

It is recommended that an activity should be enjoyable, easily fit into one's daily schedule, should be of low financial or social cost, and should present a minimum of negative consequences, such as injury, peer pressure, and self-identity problems (U.S., 1996: 46). All these recommendations concur with taiji practice, except that it is not easily accessible. Although there are more and more people claiming to teach taiji, most do not possess the appropriate experience or credentials. It is unfortunate that more competent teachers are not available; it is sad that charlatan posing as taiji instructors discredit the art and may harm their students through poor instruction.

5) Support from Family and Friends

The decision to start participating in a particular activity and the resolve to maintain a regular exercise schedule on a long-term basis greatly depends on the support, encouragement, and fellowship of others. This may be indirectly given by others who do not partake in the exercise itself, but direct support offered by fellow practitioners proves to be very significant for anyone who wishes to maintain a regular exercise activity.

Taiji is usually taught in pleasant natural surroundings conducive to the relaxed mode of the routine. The teacher-student relationship is important since the instructor serves as a example of a healthy lifestyle which should inspire and guide students in their own practice and lifestyle habits. This is further reinforced by like-minded individuals who have decided to make taiji part of their own lives (U.S., 1996: 46).

Taiji practitioners not only exercise together but discuss what they learn through their practice and incorporate it into their lives as much as possible. For example, taiji theory tells us to "go with the flow" and be in harmony with the movement of others, even when their movements are aggressive. When we are confronted with daily problems at home or at work, we can utilize the same principles: be calm, patient, balanced, and work with the situation without making the problem worse. A novice practitioner soon learns that taiji is more than just physical exercise. It demands the integration of one's whole being, tying-in the physical with the mental and spiritual aspects as well. Teacher and fellow students come to represent a "taiji family" which encourages regular practice and a commitment to a lifestyle conducive to the ultimate health goals of taiji.

6) Select an Activity Open to Males and Females of Varied Ages and Appeals to All

Many exercises and leisure activities attract individuals of a particular age or gender. Taiji is usually taught in groups, but the foundation of its practice rests on the individual regardless of gender or age. A dedicated teacher will instruct on a one-on-one basis to develop the student as an individual artist with a unique personal makeup. It has been shown that any comprehensive physical fitness program must be individualized (Yan, 1995: 62–63).

Taiji can be practiced by anyone, but does it appeal to all? It does not, primarily because it is too exotic, and its theory and practice is little understood by the general public (Honda, 1995). However, even without a clear understanding of what taiji is, people are attracted to it for one or more of its qualities as a martial art, a wholistic exercise, a moving meditation, and a dance-like art form. For anyone who has taken the time to watch taiji for a few hours, there is a good chance that they would be drawn into its practice for one of the reasons mentioned.

7) Eliminate "High-Risk" Behaviors

The fundamental objectives in practicing the taiji solo routine are to seek relaxation in every move and to execute the movements slowly in a steady flow of balanced form. When students begin to practice taiji seriously, they soon discover many tensions in their bodies. Often, even when performing the simplest movements, they feel tense and awkward. They find that it is not the movement itself, which is difficult to master, but dealing with underlying conditions that distort the movements. Taiji may bring an initial awareness of underlying problems and thus a desire in the individual to eliminate these problems.

Improvements in taiji practice can be felt by the practitioner and noticed by other students. To make continual progress requires the student to look inward, to modify any factors which cause the taiji movements to be too tense or the postures to fall off-balance. As a result, the student is encouraged by the presence of teacher, classmates and the art of taiji itself to modify any high-risk behaviors, such as smoking and poor diet. To reinforce such changes in behavior, involvement in taiji calls for an appropriate change in attitude which guarantees a better, healthier lifestyle than the present one. Taiji beckons one to be constantly aware to make continual improvements in lifestyle, for only in this way can one approach a masterful level in the art.

8) Select an Activity That Can Be Done Life Long

"A key ingredient to healthy aging, according to many gerontologists, is regular physical activity" (Nieman, 1998: 32). Taiji is noted for its suitability as an exercise for the elderly (Wolf, et. al. 1996, 1997b; Wolfson, et al., 1996; Schaller, K. 1996; Province, 1995). Its movements are slow and non-strenuous yet invigorating to mind and body.

Taiji's suitability for the elderly does not mean it is unsuitable for younger generations, but many younger persons fail to see the value in taiji as an activity. Their temperaments are often too unruly, and they usually do not have the patience to try taiji for a long enough time to actually feel the beneficial effects of the exercise.

Those attracted to taiji are usually adults in their thirties and older. The quest for relaxation is a primary motivation factor, but others come to taiji from other sports and activities that have caused them physical or mental injury. In general, taiji is looked at for its therapeutic benefits to mind, body, and spirit (Zhuo, 1982).

The desire to obtain such benefits can start at any age. A look at the graceful aging of many noted taiji instructors illustrates that they often started taiji because of an illness, benefited from it, and so dedicated themselves to daily practice for the rest of their lives. Some centenarians continue to teach taiji daily to "youngsters" in their 70's, 80's, and 90's.

Summary

There is a strong agreement between the National Institute of Health's guidelines and the Yang taiji curriculum indicating that taiji meets the criteria as an activity that we may consider in our research concerning the relationship between lifestyle and well-being. However, we should look a little closer before making any conclusion.

Guidelines numbered 1 thru 3 involve the participation in an activity of moderate intensity, hopefully daily. Regularity of practice is necessary to attain and/or maintain health. Through its own design and traditional method of instruction, taiji clearly meets these guidelines (Koh, 1981a: 15–17, 21).

Guideline number 4 considers behavioral and attitudinal factors in selecting an exercise or activity. Yang taiji is based on Daoist principles, which value spiritual and mental development along with the physical aspects. It is non-competitive and not as exciting as most mainstream sports. For these reasons, Yang taiji is fitting for some personalities, but certainly not all. Similarly, in respect to guideline 6, Yang taiji may be open to all, but it has a limited appeal because of its call for patient students who are able to find joy in the subtleties of the art.

The calming, relaxed practice of taiji attracts individuals who prefer or need this in their life. So, as encouraged in guideline number 5, taiji practitioners find an active support group from like-minded practitioners and others who may see the value in it but may not have the time or opportunity to be involved themselves.

> **"If you're one with the Dao,
> to the end of your days
> you'll suffer no harm."**
> — Laozi, in Henricks, 1989: 68

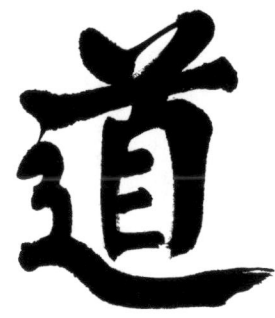

— Above character for Dao by taiji Master Yang Qingyu.

Activities conducive to a healthy lifestyle are given special attention in guideline 7. When we consider the theory and practice of Yang taiji, we find that, in addition to offering an encompassing system for health and fitness, its practice has a strong tendency to eliminate "high-risk" behaviors (U.S., 1996: 46). To make progress in doing taiji, it is necessary to look deeply into one's character development. Only when a practitioner does this can the movements reflect the tranquility, grace, and balance associated with the art. This concurs with an ancient Chinese proverb: "What is accomplished in the mind, is made known by the hand."

Guideline 8 requires that such an activity be suitable for long-term practice. Yang taiji body mechanics allow almost anyone to practice the art. The fact that it is noted for benefitting the elderly attests to its suitability for the aged as well as a therapeutic system (Nieman, 1998: 125; Yan, 1995: 61; Wolf, 1997a).

To assess Yang Style taiji as a physical activity we must be aware that it is based on the Daoist yin-yang principle. It seeks to harmonize the body and mind, the internal with the external. Yang taiji involves the total person, working on all the body's systems. Because of its focus on relaxation, even when practiced with moderate intensity, the movements gently exercise the joints, develop balance, and calm the nerves.

From research regarding Yang taiji, we see that this unique art offers "health" in the complete sense as defined by the World Health Organization "as a state of complete physical, mental, social, and spiritual well-being." It is unfortunate that such an artistic gem remains hidden behind cultural barriers which color our receptivity to the exotic.

Bibliography

American College of Sports Medicine [ACSM]. (n.d.). *ACSM's Guidelines.* pp. 153–176.

Baer, K. (1997, July). A movement toward t'ai chi. *Harvard Health Letter, 22*(9), 6.

Chen, Y. (n.d.). *T'ai-chi ch'uan: Its effects and practical applications.* Hong Kong: n.p.

Davis, D., and Mann, L. (1996). Conservator of the taiji classics: An interview with Benjamin Pang Jeng Lo. *Journal of Asian Martial Arts, 5*(4), 46–67.

DeMarco, M. (1992). The origin and evolution of taijiquan. *Journal of Asian Martial Arts, 1*(1), 8–25.

DeMarco, M. (1994). The necessity for softness in taijiquan. *Journal of Asian Martial Arts, 3*(3), 92–103.

DeMarco, M. (1997). Taijiquan as an experiential way for discovering Daoism. *Journal of Asian Martial Arts, 6*(3), 48–59.

Gu, L. (1984). The origin, evolution and development of shadow boxing. In Zhaohua Publishing House (Compilers), *Chen style taijiquan* (pp. 1–12). Hong Kong: Hai Feng Publishing Company.

Henricks, R., (Trans.). (1989). *Lao-tzu te-tao ching.* New York: Ballantine Books.

Honda, C. (1995 February). Cultural diversity: Tai chi chuan and Laban Movement Analysis. *Journal of Physical Education, 66*(2), 38.

Horwitz, T., Kimmelman, S., and Lui, H. (1976). *T'ai chi ch'uan: The techniques of power*. Chicago: Chicago Review Press.

Huang, A. (1993). *Complete tai-chi: The definitive guide to physical and emotional self-improvement*. Rutland, VT: Charles E. Tuttle Co.

Jacobson, B., Chen, H., et al. (1997 February). The effect of t'ai chi chuan training on balance, kinesthetic sense, and strength. *Perceptual & Motor Skills, 84*(1), 27.

Jou, T. (1981). *The tao of tai-chi chuan: Way to rejuvenation*. Warwick, NY: Tai Chi Foundation.

Koh, T. (1981a). Tai chi chuan. *American Journal of Chinese Medicine, 9*(1), 15–22.

Koh, T. (1981b). Chinese medicine and martial arts. *American Journal of Chinese Medicine, 9*(3), 181–186.

Koh, T. (1982). Tai chi and ankylosing spondylitis—A personal experience. *American Journal of Chinese Medicine, 10*(1–4), 59–61.

Koh, L. (1994). *The t'ai chi boxing chronicle.* (Guttmann, Trans.). Berkeley, CA: North Atlantic Books.

Lai, J., et. al, (1995 November). Two-year trends in cardiorespiratory function among older tai chi chuan practitioners and sedentary subjects. *Journal of the American Geriatric Society, 43*(11).

Lehrhaupt, L. (1992). Taijiquan: Learning how to learn. *Journal of Asian Martial Arts, 2*(1), 60–69.

Lim, P. (1992). The combative elements of Yang taijiquan. *Journal of Asian Martial Arts, 5*(3), 90–99.

Lumsden, D., (1998 February). T'ai chi for osteoarthritis: An introduction for primary care physicians. *Geriatrics, 53*(2).

Ma, Y., and Zee, W. (1990). *Wu style taijiquan push-hands (tuishou)*. Hong Kong: Shanghai Book Co.

Nieman, D. (1998). *The exercise-health connection*. Champaign, IL: Human Kinetics.

Powerful evidence that the martial art tai chi can help frail patients with osteoporosis. (1996 June). *Backletter, 11*(6), 63.

Reynolds, D. (1982). *The quiet therapies: Japanese pathways to personal growth*. Honolulu: University of Hawaii Press.

Schaller, K. (1996 October). Tai chi chih: An exercise option for older adults. *Journal of Gerontol Nursing, 22*(10), 12–17.

Smith, R. (1994). Dalu and some tigers. *Journal of Asian Martial Arts, 6*(2), 56–69.

Stubenbaum, D. (1994). An encounter with Chen Xiaowang: The continued growth of Chen taijiquan. *Journal of Asian Martial Arts, 3*(1), 90–99.

U.S. Department of Health and Human Services. (1996). Physical activity and health: A report of the Surgeon General. Atlanta: U.S. Department of Health and Human Services, Centers for Disease Control and Prevention, National Center for Chronic Disease Prevention and Health Promotion.

Wallace, A. (1998). Internal training: The foundation for Chen taiji's fighting skills and health promotion. *Journal of Asian Martial Arts, 7*(1), 58–89.

Wile, D. (1996). *Lost t'ai-chi classics from the late Ch'ing dynasty.* Albany, NY: State University of New York Press.

Wolf, S., et al. (1993, March). The Atlanta FICSIT study: Two exercise interventions to reduce frailty in elders. *Journal of the American Geriatric Society, 41*(3), 329–332.

Wolf, S., et al. (1996, May). Reducing frailty and falls in older persons: an investigation of tai chi and computerized balance training. Atlanta FICSIT Group. Frailty and Injuries: Cooperative Studies of Intervention Techniques. *Journal of the American Geriatric Society, 44*(5), 489–497.

Wolf, S., et al. (1997a). Exploring the basis for tai chi chuan as a therapeutic exercise approach. *Arch Physical Medical Rehabilitation, 78*(8), 886–892.

Wolf, S., et al. (1997b). The effect of tai chi quan and computerized balance training on postural stability in older subjects. Atlanta FICSIT Group. Frailty and Injuries: Cooperative Studies on Intervention Techniques. *Physical Therapy, 77,* 371–381.

Wolfson, L., et al. (1996, May). Balance and strength training in older adults: intervention gains and tai chi maintenance. *Journal of the American Geriatric Society, 44*(5), 498–506.

Wong, K. (1996). *The complete book of tai chi chuan: A comprehensive guide to the principles and practice.* Rockport, MA: Element Books, Inc.

Yan, J. (1995, November/December) The health and fitness benefits of tai chi. *JOPERD, 66*(9), 61.

Yiu, K. (1981). *Tui shou and san shou in t'ai chi ch'üan.* Hong Kong: Self Published.

Zhuo, D., Shephard, R., Plyley, M., and Davis, G. (1984). Cardiorespiratory and metabolic responses during tai chi chuan exercise. *Canadian Journal of Applied Sport Science, 9*(1), 7–10.

Zhuo, D. (1982). Preventive geriatrics: An overview from traditional Chinese medicine. *American Journal of Chinese Medicine, 10*(1–4), 32–39.

The Nature of Rooting in Taijiquan: A Survey
by Stuart Kohler, M.Ls.

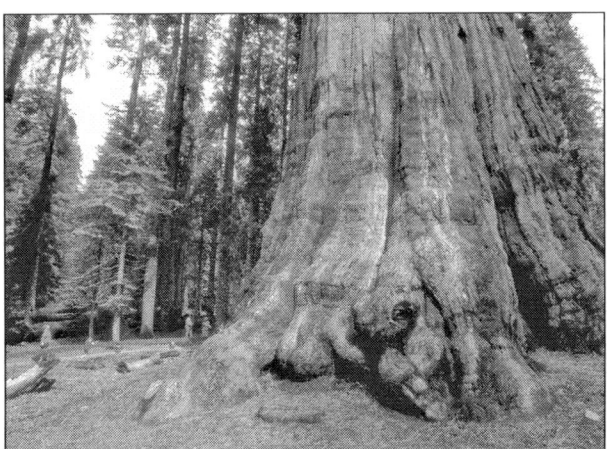

Introduction

As essential a concept as it is usually taken to be, the nature of root (*gen*) remains surprisingly undiscussed if not mysterious in the literature of taijiquan. From the perfectly simple description, "the root is at the feet," in the Yang tradition *Classic of Zhang Sanfeng* (Yang, 1991: 213) to the statement in the Chen tradition classic by Chen Xin, *Illustration of Taijiquan*, that one must "grip the ground with the toes" (Yan, 1997: 8), it would seem that the exact nature of discovering and developing root is either beyond words or so obvious that it need not be discussed.

Being unwilling to accept either position, the author intends in this chapter to report what may be found in the literature of taijiquan, with the goal of perhaps stimulating in-depth study by scholars and experts. Such study, arriving at a consensus, would be of great value to students of taijiquan, both novice and advanced.

Overview: The Relaxed Foot

At its most basic presentation, there appear to be two contradictory definitions or descriptions of root. The first, predominantly a Yang tradition concept, is that the root is formed at the *yongquan* or "bubbling well" point, also known as Kidney 1, located on the sole of the foot, just behind the ball of the foot. In this tradition, root is formed or enhanced by 'opening' this point to allow earth energy to rise into the body or to allow negative energy to drain from the body, particularly in traditional standing meditation posture (*zhanzhuang*). The activation of this point is accomplished by relaxation (*song*) and having the foot basically splay out as it relaxes into better and better contact with the ground. The weight is to be equally distributed around the sole of the foot (Diepersloot, 1995: 25). However, the *yongquan* points do not usually touch the ground due to the natural arch of a healthy foot. A minor variation of this view is to place the location of the specific point slightly further back, in the center of the arch of the foot (Wallace, 1998: 79).

Students are often told to employ the mental imagery of tree-like roots emanating from their feet as they relax and deepen their root for both martial and health purposes (e.g., Chuen, 1991: 31). A distinction is often made between these two, between being deeply sunk into the earth in a manner that is nearly immovable and being securely rooted in a manner that maintains a flexible martial position. Descriptions of rooting for health may seem to encourage a deep root that is unconcerned about the classical recommendation that in every movement "every part of the body is light and agile."

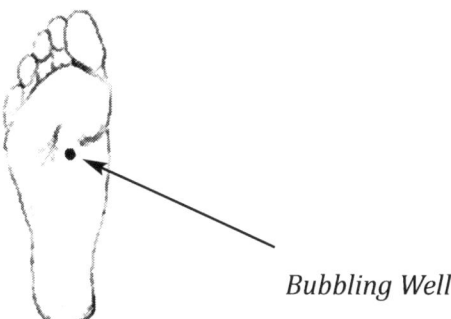

Bubbling Well

Gripping Toes

In contrast to the relaxed foot idea is the second concept, mostly found in Chen tradition (although there are occasionally references in the Yang tradition as well [Smalheiser, 1996, December: 10]), of achieving the root by gripping the ground with the toes. Within this tradition, there ranges a variety of opinion of exactly how this is to be done, from a slight but actual physical flexing of the muscles of the foot (Montaigue, 1995: 9) to a strictly mental flexing that does not activate foot musculature, but stresses relaxation (Ting, 1996; Smalheiser, 1996, December: 10).

Ting Kuopiao offers an interesting extension to the 'gripping' description. Applying this concept to movement, he writes:

> Every motion in [taiji] originates from the feet. By moving the feet, one can maintain optimum balance, allow the whole body to move together, and gain maximum force. Moving from the feet increases speed and flexibility; we call it cat walking.
>
> When a movement requires a step in another direction, most people simply push from the foot carrying their body's weight. But moving from the feet is a completely different concept. For example, in order to advance, as soon as the front foot contacts the earth, its toes grab the ground and pull forward. At the same time, the stationary foot pushes, moving the body's weight forward.

In other words, it is as if one pulls the body's weight forward with the lead foot, and at the same time the rear foot pushes the body in the same direction. It is important to emphasize that moving with the feet cannot be effective if all [taiji] principles are not used throughout the motion.

– Ting, 1995: 18

A more Western example of adding pulling to pushing to increase efficiency is found in bicyclists who add toe clips to the pedals. This enables them to create power strokes out of upstrokes as well as downstrokes.

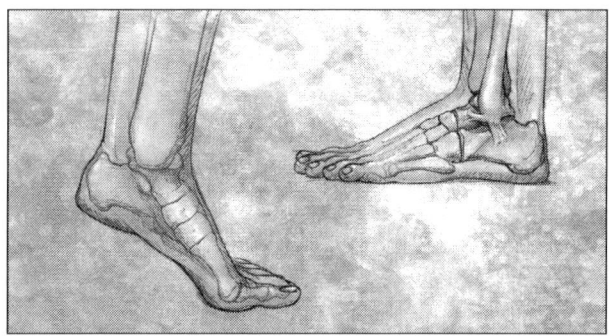

Note on the Body's Integration

It should be noted that root is not solely a matter of the foot. If the upper body is stiff or disconnected, a solid root is not possible regardless of how the feet are used. For example, the *Zhang Sanfeng Classic* says: "No part should be defective, no part should be deficient or excessive, no part should be disconnected" (Yang, 1991: 213). The classic continues: "The entire body and all the joints should be threaded together without the slightest break" (Yang, 1991: 215). Craven gives some common references on this point, writing that "The education of the foot is much more than just one point or just gripping or not gripping the ground. In the subject of health, the bubbling well is activated in different ways, but the overriding point is that the entire body must be relaxed, and the lock points and tensions of the body must be eliminated one by one to get the grand circulation of force" (Craven, 1997).

The reader is referred to Drill #2 in the list of rooting drills at the end of this chapter for an experiential exploration of this phenomena. Nonetheless, the aspect of root that is the focus of this chapter relates primarily to the use of the foot, hence the apparent disregard for the necessary integration of the rest of the body.

Another level of subtlety that merits note is further distinction of types of root. Some teachers distinguish between intrinsic root, which can be either static (*zhanzhuang*) or moving (as to remain rooted during an entire round of the form), and functional (sometimes referred to as 'responsive') root, which relates to remaining rooted while confronted by an external force (Gallagher, 1994).

Western Perspective

When viewed from a strictly Western perspective, root would be a matter of center of gravity, balance, and/or biomechanics. On the chance then that the literature of Western science (medicine, physiology, biomechanics) might yield some insight, a brief foray was made into that body of information. However, there does not appear to be an exact Western counterpart for either the concept of root or the structure or location known as the bubbling well in non-Western literature.

As related to what is called "quiet standing" in this literature, the useful information is somewhat limited in that the standard posture for such studies traditionally involves locked knees, used to apply the model of an inverse pendulum with the ankles as the pivot point (Horstmann, 1990: 165). A closer approximation to 'taiji' posture would be what is described as the "stance phase of gait" (Oatis, 1988: 1). The investigations of the biomechanics of walking and running offer some interesting insights, particularly as regards postural control systems invoked related to functional or responsive root (Rothwell, 1994: 280), but this extends beyond the scope of this survey. As an aside, it is interesting to note that the reverse may be truer: there are ever increasing numbers of references in Western journals investigating the medical benefits of taijiquan, particularly regarding the sense of balance in the elderly.

Analysis

Is it possible, then, to reconcile these various descriptions of root? Setting aside sectarian concerns, several authors have proposed interesting theories regarding the apparent differences in description of establishing a deep root. Jan Diepersloot advances the theory that the relaxed foot is the root for health and healing, while the 'gripping' foot is the root of issuing energy (*fajing*) (Diepersloot, 1996).

A second, perhaps more ecumenical view is that both descriptions describe the same practice and that the difference in terminology relates more to the difficulty of articulating an elusive construct. On the one hand, there is the instruction to relax, often accompanied by the instruction to remain "light and agile," i.e., to avoid a flat-footed root. Extending the relaxed foot instruction is "the weight of the feet should be evenly distributed over all the cells of the sole, as if the foot were spreading itself out and grabbing the floor slightly" (Diepersloot, 1995: 25). On the other hand is the description of "gripping the ground with the toes." However, in most instances, a statement accompanies this instruction that one does so more as a matter of intention rather than physical use of muscle contraction. There is frequent mention that while gripping the ground with the toes, it is critically important to maintain a relaxed state. Ting Kuopiao discusses this concept by saying:

> 'Gripping the ground with the toes' is a sentence from a classic Chinese book about [taiji]. However, this does not mean that the student is not

> relaxed while he roots himself solidly with his feet. This concept is not understood by a lot of people. They mistakenly feel that gripping the ground with your toes automatically means you are not relaxed. You must relax in order to feel deeply rooted with your feet. Your toes slightly grip the ground, body remains relaxed and if you are relaxed, you will be much more rooted.
> – Ting, 1996

In this sense, perhaps, it could be that the "gripping" advocates seek to avoid a misunderstanding of *song* that could lead to a flat-footed or 'dead' root (even more understandable when the metaphor of choice changes from tree-like roots to "visualizing the legs as two piles vertically inserted into the earth" (Dai, 1997: 32). Accordingly, "gripping the ground with toes" without activating musculature could be an alternative description of a *song* foot. It would therefore be possible to appreciate the commonality of these seemingly contradictory descriptions.

It should be noted that for this interpretation to hold, one would need to accept the recommendation for an actual, physical gripping (which involves the musculature of the foot) as a literalist, almost fundamentalist, view.

One additional view of forming the root and weighting the heel bears mentioning. When pressed for the exact location of root, Master Ha Fong replied that root at the bubbling well point is more for health and root at the heel is more for martial purposes (Ha, 1996).

Erle Montaigue further discusses rooting with the weight at the heel:

> The heels are very important in grounding. In pushing the heels down into the ground, we activate the "qi entering" point called Kidney 1. This point is where the ground qi comes into the body, and it is the heels that activate it. So, when we sink into the ground through the heels, we do not think about K1 point, but rather we simply push the heels into the ground by placing all of the body weight on them.
> – Montaigue, 1996: 33–34

Yang Zhenduo also mentions the heel in relation to root. Of particular interest is his mention of both heel and "gripping toes":

> "Your heel," Yang said, "is like the foundation of a building as you firmly plant the heel. Then as you grab with the toes, the energy goes down to the floor and also unites with the upper body movement the minute you stabilize your heel.
> – Smalheiser, 1996a: 10

In the final analysis, rather than attempting to divide variations in concepts of root into separate views, the larger view of Master Ha Fong may provide the most appropriate approach in seeking the nature of root. While he did provide the information referenced above relating to locating the root, he prefers to say root is not a matter of such effort. In fact, Master Ha counsels ignoring virtually all mental or theoretical constructs. He states, "Stand up. If you don't fall, you are rooted. The more you stand the better your root becomes" (Ha, 1996)!

A slightly more formal presentation of the same thought may be found in an interview with Master Ha:

> Fong Ha said that by putting yourself in a standing position such as Wuji, "You are activating your own automatic maintenance system. So it doesn't matter if you have bad posture. Every single cell in your body will want to maintain itself so you can stand up straight.
>
> Therefore it is self-correcting at all times, regardless of your state of health, regardless of the state of destruction going on in your body. Your body is automatically self-adjusting and self-ma*dantian*intaining.
>
> By simply doing the Wuji stance, you are activating it already. There is nothing else you have to do. In my theory, you don't have to be able to stand in any special way. Just stand up and already the work is done.
> – Smalheiser, 1996b: 16

A Call for Scholarship

The subtitle, "A Survey," was carefully chosen for this chapter in that the author is only able to draw upon references found in the contemporary and popular literature of taijiquan. As suggested in the introduction, it is hoped that scholarly contributions on this topic will lead toward a deeper and more definitive understanding about the nature of root in taijiquan and perhaps in Asian martial arts in general.

ROOT DRILLS — EXPLORING ROOT EXPERIENTIALLY

1) Horse Stance

Deliberately move the weight into the heel, feel the involvement of the quadricep muscles. Deliberately move the weight into the toes, feel the involvement of the calf muscles. Roll to the outside and inside of the feet. Then return to passing the weight directly through the bubbling well point. Feel the foot splay out. Notice the alignment of the knee does not extend beyond the toes when weight is passed through the bubbling well point (experiential confirmation of the "rule" to never extend the knee beyond the toe).

Variation: Use single-legged stances from the taiji form to explore the location of root.

2) Bow Stance/Ward0ff

Find the correct alignment of the spine so that a gentle push or pull is directed immediately down to the bubbling well point of the front foot. Deliberately 'break' the alignment at the waist by leaning forward just a fraction while receiving a gentle push or pull from a partner. Notice how small the amount of lean is required to completely disrupt the root. This may be taken as experiential confirmation of the line from the *Wang Zongyue Classic*, "No tilting, no leaning" (Yang, 1991: 218).

Variation: Deliberately distribute your weight 50/50 and notice how little force is required to break the root when applied to the centerline.

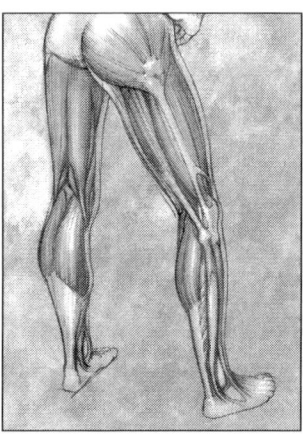

3) Bow Stance to Cat Stance

"Pour" the weight from the front foot (bow stance) into the rear foot (cat stance). Feel the bubbling well point in the rear foot, although do not ignore exploration of rooting from the heel in a rear-weighted stance. "Pour" the weight back into the front leg, directly down the shin, through the bubbling well point, into the ground. Deliberately move the weight into the heel or the toes of the front foot and notice the disruption of the root.

4) Alternating Bow Stance (as in twist step, brush knee sequence)

Pour the weight directly into the bubbling well point of the front foot with each step. Deliberately allow the weight to pour into the heel or toes and notice the disruption of the root.

Substitution of a forward shuffle step or forward triangle step may be more familiar to some martial traditions. The latter is particularly significant when exploring the idea of "pulling with the front foot" when moving forward as articulated by Ting Kuopiao (Ting, 1995: 18).

5) Wave Hands Like Clouds (one side, e.g., left)

Have a partner stand at approximately right angles to you and extend opposite arm (i.e., if you will be 'waving' your left arm, partner extends right arm, insides of wrist points toward you). Step out to the side and pour the weight into the bubbling well point; as the hand rotates across, lightly grip your partner's wrist and gently pull the partner's weight into your bubbling well point. Deliberately move your weight into the heel or toes and notice the inefficiency of your pull.

6) Bow Stance

Partner pushes gently into abdomen—keep the *dantian* soft. Staying soft permits redirection of energy into the root. Otherwise, one would be creating a false root at the *dantian* and would lose stability if the partner suddenly withdraws energy.

7) Facing Horse Stances

Each partner rests tips of fingers lightly on upper chest or shoulders of the other. Take turns applying gentle pressure to see where the pusher loses the root (i.e., is pushed back into instability).

Variation: Simultaneous gentle pushes, until one partner is pushed back into instability.

8) Dropping Into Root

Begin in horse stance, arms crossed against chest. Partner gently and steadily pushes on the crossed arms as energy is directed into the root of the feet. When the energy becomes too much for the root to withstand, drop back into bow stance, immediately "falling" into the root of the front foot.

Advanced variation: Once a bow stance is adopted, the partner continues to push until root of bow stance is broken and the root is moved into the rear foot.

9) "Receiving Energy"

An advanced drill: as your partner is just about to initiate a real push, advance slightly toward your partner while remaining completely 'sunk' (or "slid," as Paul Gallagher likes to describe it) in the energy-body and very rooted. If the timing is correct, the partner will be unbalanced backwards by the force of his or her own push.

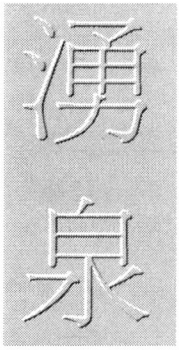

Bubbling Well.

Note: Paul B. Gallagher (1994) provided Drills 8 and 9.

Bibliography

Chue, L. (1991). *The way of energy*. New York: Simon and Schuster, Inc.

Craven, J. (1997, June 14). Letter to the author.

Dai, D. (1997, October). How to establish a good root. *T'ai Chi, 21*(5), 32–33.

Diepersloot, J. (1995). *Warriors of stillness: Meditative traditions in the Chinese martial arts, volume 1*. Walnut Creek, CA: Center for Healing and The Arts.

Diepersloot, J. (1996, November 15). Letter to the author.

Gallagher, P. (1994, July). *Seminar on rooting*. Guilford, VT: Deer Mountain Taoist Academy.

Ha Fong. (1996, July). *Seminar on Yiquan*. Northfield, VT.

Horstmann, G. and Dietz, V. (1990, August). A basic posture control mechanism: The stabilization of the centre of gravity. *Electroencephalography and Clinical Neurophysiology, 76*(2), 165–176.

Montaigue, E. and Babin, M. (1995). *Power taiji*. Boulder, CO: Paladin Press.

Montaigue, E. (1996). *Ultimate dim-mak*. Boulder, CO: Paladin Press.

Oatis, C. (December 1988). Biomechanics of the foot and ankle under static conditions. *Physical Therapy, 66*(12), 1815 to 1821.

Rothwell, J. (1994). *Control of human voluntary movement*, 2nd ed. New York: Chapman and Hall.

Smalheiser, M. (1996, December). Yang Zhenduo on unifying internal energy. *T'ai Chi, 20*(6), 6–11.

Smalheiser, M. (1996, June). Wuji qigong: Harvesting inner resources. *T'ai Chi, 20*(3), 14–17.

Ting, K. (William Ting). (1995, August). Fundamentals of correct t'ai chi practice, *T'ai Chi, 19*(4): 14–18.

Ting, K. (William Ting). (1996, October 16). Letter to the author.

Wallace, A. (1998). Internal training: The foundation for Chen taijiquan's fighting skills and health promotion. *Journal of Asian Martial Arts, 7*(1): 58–89.

Yan, G. and Cravens, J. (1997, April). Rooting: The secret of getting power from the earth. *Internal Martial Arts Research Newsletter*, pp. 5–9, 16–17.

Yang, J. (1991). *Advanced Yang style tai chi chuan, vol. one*. Boston: Yang's Martial Arts Association

• 29 •
The Pedagogy of Taijiquan in the University Setting
by Andy Peck, M.S.Ed.

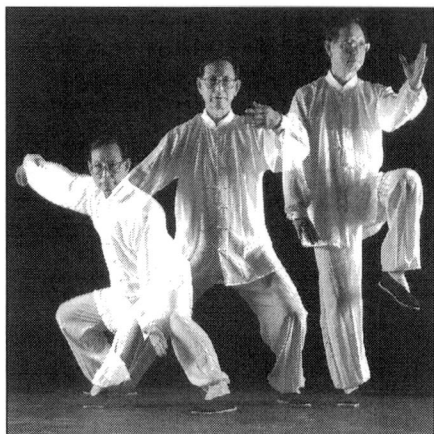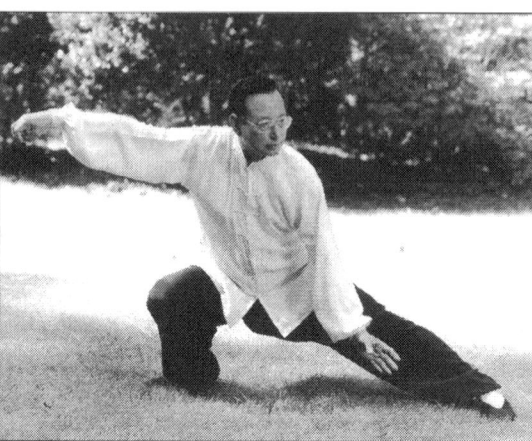

All photographs courtesy of Dr. Xu Tingsen.

Introduction

The landscape of universities in the United States is changing. According to the U.S. Department of Education, women will outnumber men in undergraduate and graduate programs by 9.2 million to 6.9 million by the year 2008. Not only are there changes in the make-up of gender on college campuses, but the number of students entering colleges for re-training is also on the rise. Changes in the demographics of college students also includes a higher average mean age (Koerner, 1999). These factors are coupled with a trend of decreasing physical education requirements in college curriculums.

The phenomenal growth of taijiquan (abbreviated below at taiji) during the past decade has occurred because it addresses the needs of a growing number of Americans, including college students. Taiji offers a low impact, life-long exercise, coupled with intellectual stimulation and effective stress management. This chapter will look at how one college presents taiji classes.

Background or Dr. Xu Tingsen

One taiji instructor addressing the needs of the modern college student is Dr. Xu Tingsen. Dr. Xu is eminently qualified as both an academician and martial artist. A native of Shanghai, China, Dr. Xu received his doctorate degree in biochemistry from the Academy of Medical Sciences in Moscow. He has accumulated over 43 years of experience in researching medical biochemistry, particularly in the areas of metabolism and cholesterol regulation. As an academic Dr. Xu has been quick to apply the scientific method to the effects of the practice of taiji. During his tenure at the Shanghai Academy of Sciences, Dr. Xu and his colleagues found that patients with high blood pressure who practiced taijiquan five times a week, while taking no medication, reduced their blood pressure by 35%. Patients who combined taiji practice with medication were able to reduce their blood pressure by 50% (Chase, 1995). As an associate professor of physical rehabilitation at the Emory University School of Medicine, Dr. Xu was awarded a grant by the National Institute of Aging (NIA) and the National Center for Nursing Research. This grant funded research to explore new ways of improving strength, mobility, balance, and endurance in people over 75 years of age. In this study, Dr. Xu and his associates found that the practice of taijiquan reduced the participant's risk of multiple falls by 47.5% (Barnhart, et al., 1996). Not only is Dr. Xu a seasoned academician but his martial arts background is equally extensive. He began his taiji training at the age of 15 and studied the Chen form of taiji under Gu Liuxin, a student of Chen Fake. He studied the Yang Style under the guidance of Po Bingru, senior student of Yang Chengfu, and pursued the Wu Style taiji under the guidance of Shen Renzhu, senior student of Wu Jianquan, founder of a Wu Style. Dr. Xu has taught taiji in the United States for over 18 years and has been a tireless promoter of taiji. Dr. Xu has been the Executive President of the World Taiji Research Association, Beijing, and a National Advisor to the United States of America Wushu Kung Fu Federation.

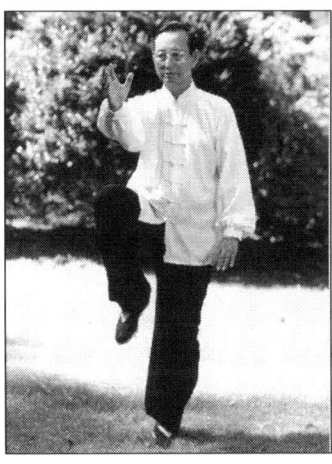 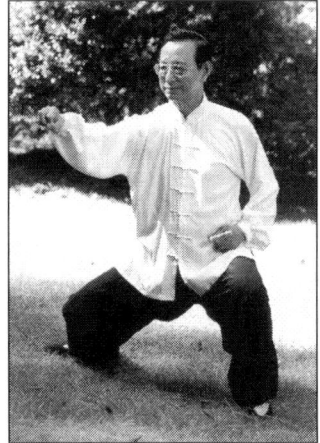

Eastern vs. Western Methodologies

Traditionally in China, teachers take an interest not only in the student's academic life but also in their social and moral development, viewing the student holistically. There is heavy emphasis on past tradition and memorization. Great importance is placed upon the absorption of pre-existing facts. In class "students present themselves as attentive, respectful, and above all passive" (Grove and Hu, 1991). Self-expression and self-assertiveness are discouraged. Western approaches to teaching, on the other hand, tend to attach importance to analysis and creativity rising from that analysis. More emphasis is placed upon processes than is placed on pre-existing fact. In many instances students are taught to question and challenge the status quo. Western teachers value and appreciate student comments and input. While western teachers do show concern for their students, it is considered "unprofessional" for the instructor to address areas of the student's life not directly related to the subject being taught.

Dr. Xu's Approach

Dr. Xu attempts to employ both Eastern and Western approaches to his teaching. Dr. Xu's class however is, without a doubt, a window into Chinese culture and ways of thinking. Dr. Xu states that "in China, loyalty to a master is almost devout. American students respect the instructor but not like Chinese students, but that is understandable. Chinese students would have the same problem trying to understand American football at first." He further states that "Their [the students'] mind should be like an empty vessel waiting for the knowledge of their instructor" (Smalheiser, 1992).

The Essence and Application of Dr. Xu's Teachings

The prevailing theme of Dr. Xu's taiji instruction is that of balance. Dr. Xu emphasizes balance in the physical practice of taiji, in social relationships (including martial confrontations), and in the mental/spiritual realm as well. Inherent in the concept of balance is the premise of paired opposites or yin and yang. These opposites may manifest themselves as attack and defense, giving and receiving, expansion and contraction, pride and humility, and so on. Taiji practitioners view these paired opposites as going through cyclical changes that, like the yin and yang symbol, are changes characterized by circular, spherical or spiraling patterns of motion. In all the practical taiji applications which Dr. Xu teaches, the principle of balance through cyclical change is evident. Movements from the traditional taiji practice of "push-hands" also embody the cyclical change of opposites.

Another characteristic of the yin-yang symbol is that a small part of one extreme is always found within the opposite extreme. Just as inhalation is about to reach its peak the potential for exhalation begins to arise. Therefore, according to Dr. Xu, even when retreating, the idea of advancing must be retained. The intermingling of the two opposites gives a unique quality to the motions of the taiji practitioner. This quality is summed up in such traditional sayings as: "resist without opposing", "yield without retreating", "relaxed but not limp" and "firm but not hard, soft but unyielding." While these sayings may sound paradoxical, there are practical applications. Occasionally Dr. Xu and his students will practice pressing on each other. In this practice those receiving the pressure learn to resist not with muscular tension but with a relaxed strength generated by specific skeletal alignment. This alignment creates a clear line of force through the body from the ground to the point of contact. Strength generated in this manner is referred to as "whole body power."

Dr. Xu's students learn to apply this principal of alignment with "whole body power" not only in static positions but in all their motions. Guided by this inner principle they can flexibly adapt to a myriad number of unique situations.

Interviews with Dr. Xu's Students

Interviews I conducted with students of Dr. Xu's taiji class reveal what happens when western students are given a glimpse into Chinese culture and teaching methodologies. All of the students interviewed were undergraduate students at Emory University located in Atlanta Georgia. When students were asked how their classroom experience differed from the expectations they had had before beginning the class, they stated how pleasantly surprised they were to have philosophy presented both as physical motion and as a lifestyle. Dr. Xu recognizes that the western mind set is geared toward immediate gratification. On the other hand, he knows that the art of taiji cannot be mastered in a matter of a few weeks or months.

While Dr. Xu transmits a tremendous amount of knowledge in a very short time span, he refuses to compromise the quality of what he teaches. The students interviewed said that the class was very detail oriented. Yet while the class seemed to move at a slow pace, it stayed precisely on schedule as the school term progressed. Dr. Xu was careful to monitor the progress of his students. The students said that the quantity of material covered by Dr. Xu was determined by their own progress.

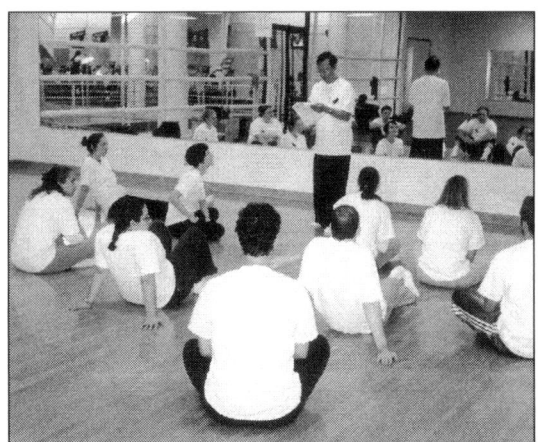
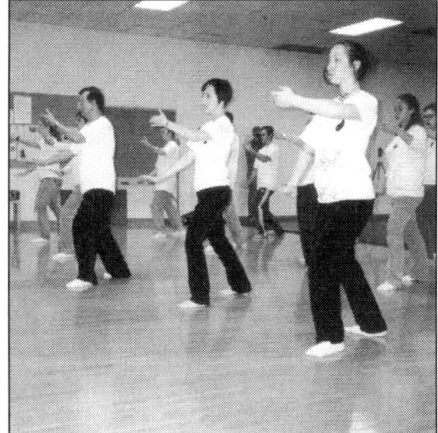
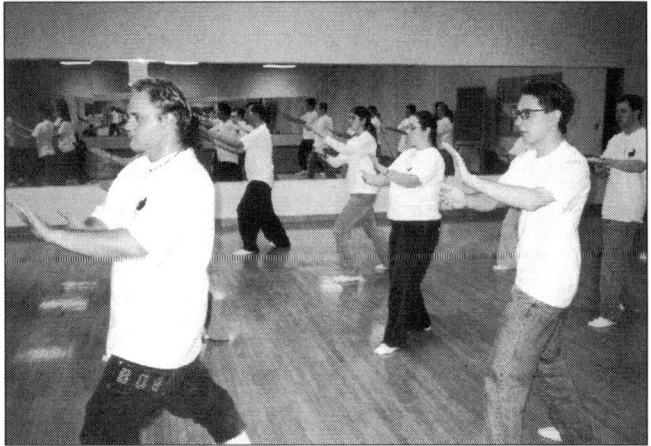
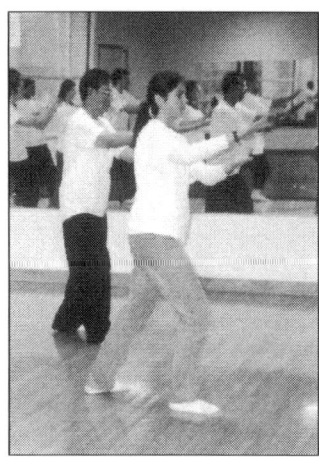

In terms of evaluation, the students indicated that they were critiqued and corrected in the process of learning, receiving immediate feedback on their performance. While final grades were based on the subjective opinion of Dr. Xu, all the students interviewed felt that his evaluations were fair and even-handed. This may be related to the fact that Dr. Xu had earned the respect of his students. They stated that they trusted his experience and background and that his instruction seemed in no way "franchised."

When asked about what insights or impressions they had gained into Chinese culture, the students indicated that having a "native" teacher was very helpful. They also found the philosophy presented by Dr. Xu to be "totally different from the book type of philosophy." Dr. Xu gave them further exposure to Chinese culture by presenting the histories of each of the different taiji styles.

Finally, the students interviewed were asked about the benefits they had received from the class. The students responded by citing the following benefits. Taiji practice provided an enhanced focus of mind. They found the practice of taiji to be a natural stimulant. They indicated that their inclination to use caffeine or cigarettes to stay awake while studying was decreased. One student indicated that when he tired of his studies, a few minutes spent going through some of the basic taiji movements invigorated him, enabling him to continue his studies. Taiji was a great form of stress management and relaxation. Regular practice improved both physical and mental balance. They learned that taiji was a healthy form of exercise.

Conclusion

It is apparent from the student responses that Dr. Xu does teach taiji in a very traditional manner. At the same time attempting to cover the diverse areas of taiji in a fourteen-week academic semester, Dr. Xu has certainly had to make some modifications and allowances for the western approach to learning. What is also evident from the interviews with Dr. Xu's students is that taiji does address the needs of the contemporary college student. While students find the eastern perspective to be intriguing and even perhaps refreshing, they also discover practical and healthy ways to combat stress. They learn to find balance both mentally and physically. They see how a philosophy can permeate a lifestyle. They are given concepts and practices which can benefit them for a lifetime. While there may be some depth lacking due to the brevity of a college semester, university students are given a glimpse into a world they had not previously known.

References

Barnhart, H., Coogler, C., Kutner, G., McNeely, E., Wolf, S., and Xu, T. (1996) Reducing frailty and falls in older persons: An investigation of tai chi and computerized balance training. *Journal of the American Geriatrics Society 44*, 489–497.

Chase, L. (1995–96, Winter). The art of balance. *Southern Lifestyles*, 18.

Grove, G., and Hu Wenzhong. (1991). *Encountering the Chinese*. Yarmouth, Maine: Intercultural Press, Inc.

Koerner, B. (1999, Feb. 8). Where the boys aren't. *U.S. News and World Report*, 47–50.

Smalheiser, M. (1992). Tai chi and life: A search for balance. *Tai Chi, 16*(6), 5.

Acknowledgments

Mr. Peck would like to acknowledge the collaborative effort of Dr. Xu Tingsen in the writing of this chapter. Dr. Xu and his students were most supportive in providing content specifics and editorial review for this chapter.

• 30 •
Reviving the Daoist Roots of Internal Martial Arts
by Mark Hawthorne

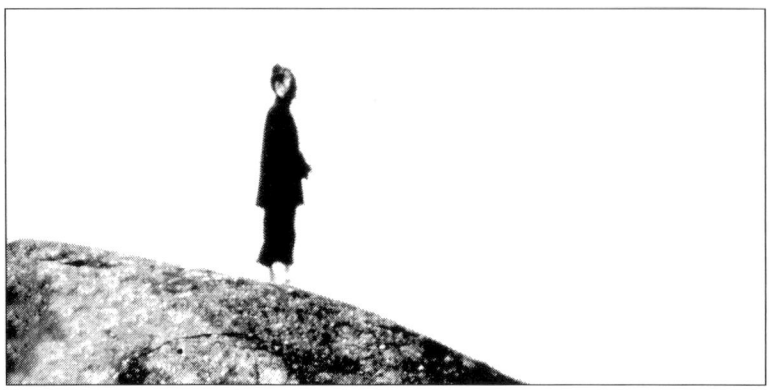

Monk of the orthodox Complete Reality Sect. Photograph by Kipling Swehla.
Photos courtesy of the Taoist Restoration Society.

When Zhang Sanfeng began developing taijiquan as a comprehensive system of martial arts in the thirteenth century, this Daoist monk ensured his place in history as the first patriarch of the art. Of course, history can get muddled with the passing centuries, but Zhang is generally credited with synthesizing the philosophical principles of Daoism with a martial art that could be used for both self-defense and a method to enhance one's internal energy (qi). Thus, Daoist monks used taijiquan to defend themselves and as an exercise for the mind and body (Liang, 1996: 8–9).

Seven centuries later, taijiquan is still a popular martial art, both in China and around the world. But while the art has flowered into a global practice, its roots have been nearly destroyed, and Daoism exists only as a fragile remnant of the past or more a vestigial tradition than the vigorous philosophy and religion that was once one of China's most important belief systems. Whether or not Daoism can be revived may well depend on the efforts of those in China now struggling to rebuild the monasteries and temples and to bring back the clergy who once populated them.

The threat to Daoism began in the last century as the power of the Qing Dynasty (1644–1912) began to decline. As China became weak enough to be invaded by Western powers, many suspected the Daoists of plotting against the emperor, and imperial support began to drop. China finally shed its imperial dynasties and founded a Nationalist Government in 1912; gone were the powerful emperors who had long supported the Daoist monasteries and temples. The new government, which believed Daoism to be based on superstition and folklore, allowed the system to struggle on its own, and monasteries and temples fell into disrepair.

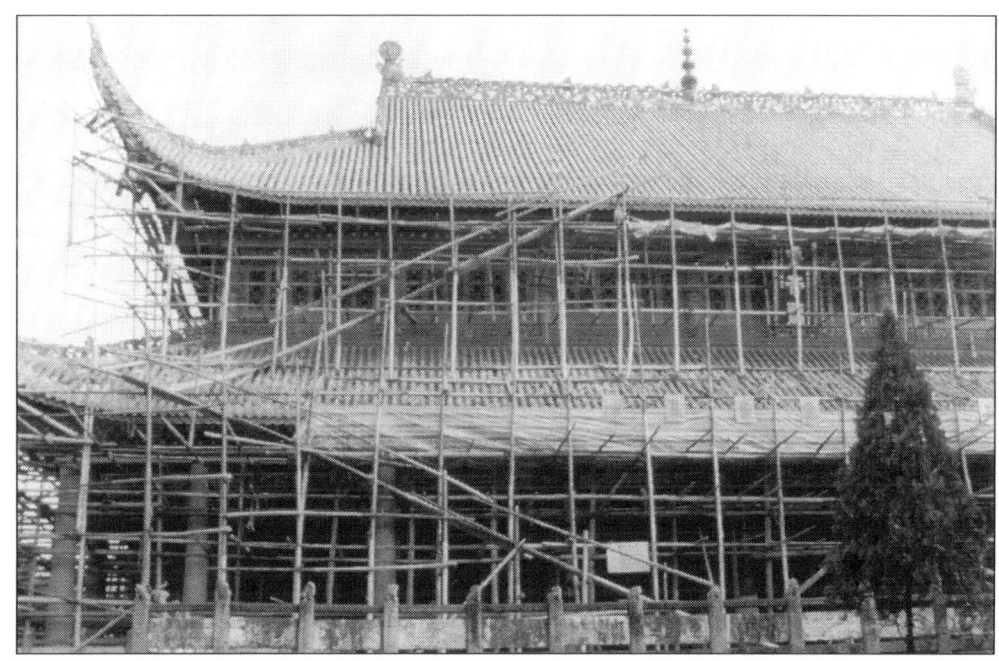

Photography by Kipling Swehla.

In 1949, Mao Zedong and his Communists toppled China's government and then outlawed Daoism altogether. They reasoned that an ideologically perfect state made religion unnecessary. Monasteries were destroyed or requisitioned as government buildings, and monks, nuns and Daoist officials were imprisoned in labor camps, reducing the clergy from several millions to about 50,000.

Today there is a new mind-set in China, a more liberal attitude that sees religious expression as an important part of traditional Chinese culture and a direct link to such martial arts as xingyiquan and taijiquan. Daoist sites must be restored, say supporters of this ancient tradition, and the clergy must be allowed to transmit their mystic teachings to the next generation. And thus, the race to save Daoism, China's oldest indigenous religion, is on.

One group leading the work to rescue Daoism is the Taoist Restoration Society (TRS) (Taoist, 1999). Brock Silvers founded the nonprofit organization nine years ago after visiting China and seeing for himself how Daoism was threatened with extinction. "By the early 1980's," he says, "most Western scholars believed that Daoism had been effectively stamped out by China's modern upheavals. We thought Daoism was a dead religion" (personal communication, 1999).

Although based in the U.S., the TRS works out of Beijing to support the restoration of monastic institutions and assist Daoist communities. The organization works to rebuild Daoist sites for their original purpose, not as museums or tourist attractions. It also supports the revival of organized Daoism and is especially involved in the restoration of temples, almost all of which somewhere in the tens of thousands—were requisitioned or destroyed by the government.

The Chinese leadership has joined the effort with its own organization, the National Daoist Association (NDA), which officially oversees all Daoist activity in China. Headquartered in Beijing, the NDA runs the entire national Daoist organization. Its new director is Min Zhiting, a well-respected Daoist monk. These two groups, combined with the work of Daoist monks, nuns and other supporters, are working within what Silvers sees as a "ten-year window of opportunity to save Daoism" (personal communication, 1999).

Dao of Daoism

Nature is the model that Daoists use as a guide for ideal behavior, including the practice of martial arts. By observing nature, we see that everything is in balance and governed by the same laws. By imitating nature, we learn to both survive and live in harmony. Hua Tuo (141–203 CE), a Chinese physician, introduced a system of renewing one's qi with a combination of mental, physical and breathing exercises called *daoyin*. He also created a system of exercises known as the Sport of the Five Animals, which seeks to imitate the speed, agility and power of such animals as the bear, crane, deer, monkey and tiger. From these exercises came Hua's Five Animal Games, regarded as the first system of martial arts in China (Breslow, 1995: 192–195).

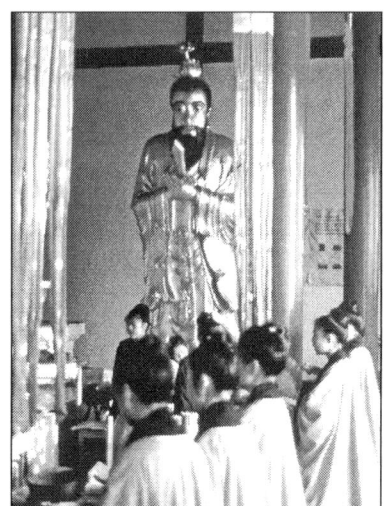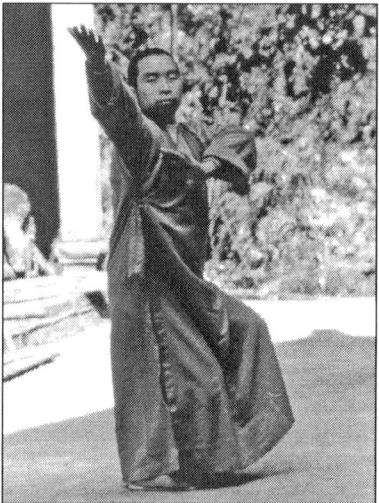

Photography: left, by Brock Silvers, and right, by Katherine McVety.

Daoism refers to both a philosophy (*Daojia*) and a religion (*Daojiao*) and is thought to have developed in China in the sixth and fifth centuries BCE. As a philosophy, Daoism stresses that one should not try to change the way things are—nature provides everything. Religious Daoism evolved from several philosophical and religious movements, and the first temple was founded in the second century CE. Religious Daoism incorporates the worship of many gods and a veneration of nature and simplicity. Because Daoists view the body and spirit as one, the goal is not to liberate the soul from the body but to nurture one's qi and attain the Dao by realizing the truth within you (Schumacher, 1996: 162–173).

Dao ("the Way") plays an important role in both religious and philosophical Daoism. It is concerned with the course of events and order of the universe. It is an intangible reality that gives rise to existence. All things, in time, return to the Dao. Dao may also be understood as "the Way things do what they do." There is a Way to do everything, and once you master that, you need not be concerned with it. For example, after learning the Way to ride a bicycle, the rider doesn't have to think about it; he simply does it. Practitioners of Daoism attempt to gain mystical union with the Dao through meditation and by following the nature of the Dao in thought and action (Schumacher, 1996: 163–166).

The Dao is a principal feature of two classic Daoist texts, the *Daodejing* (The Book of the Way and Its Power) and the *Zhuangzi*. Many scholars credit authorship of the *Daodejing* to Laozi, the Chinese philosopher believed to have lived in the sixth century BCE. Although the book's origin is in debate, it forms the basis of both religious and philosophical Daoism. The Daoist sage Zhuangzi (c. 369–286 BCE) is regarded as the author of the text by the same name. The *Zhuangzi's* views on Dao, *de* ("power") and *wuwei* ("non-doing" or "inaction") mirror those of the *Daodejing* (Schumacher, 1996: 210–211).

Wuwei is an important tenet in martial arts. Inaction finds its power within the individual and his understanding of the nature of all things. It is a natural law for all things to always be what they are—interfere with this law and you have failed. Challenges are to be ignored, says the *Daodejing*, and *wuwei* is the only means of achieving true success (Barrett, 1993: 28). Compare these principles with the efficacy of redirecting an opponent's attack, allowing him to be thrown off-guard and conquered by his own inertia.

Yin-yang is another central aspect of Daoism. These two contradictory yet complementary energies are said to be the cause of the universe and represent the duality of existence. Yin and yang are manifestations of the Dao of the supreme ultimate, or the Supreme One, which is known in Chinese as *taiji* (*taijiquan* translates as the "fist of the supreme ultimate"). Yin is feminine, receptive and soft. Yang is masculine, creative and hard. While *yin* symbolizes the moon, shadows, death and earth, *yang* represents the sky, light, life and fire. These two polarities are in constant fluctuation, with one side dominating and then yielding to the other. Nothing is ever purely yin or yang; all things are comprised of varying degrees of both. A cloud, for example, might be yin because it is soft and yang because it is white (Schumacher, 1996: 216–219).

Dao of Martial Arts

Although taijiquan might seem the most obvious connection, the Daoist tenets of yielding and softness have given birth to other martial arts, especially the "internal" styles. In Daoist spiritual training the internal martial arts are used for both spiritual development and external power. The four internal styles are bagua, xingyiquan, liuhebafa and taijiquan (Wong, 1997: 226).

"The differences between external and internal martial arts do not arise from specific techniques employed by the various styles," says Wai Lun Choi, who teaches internal martial arts in Chicago, Illinois. "The differences stem from the way the movements are produced. External styles emphasize speed and power, but this is also true of the internal arts. What really differentiates them are the training methods used to develop this speed and power. Internal styles require a precise unity of breathing, weight distribution, joint alignment, leverage, etc., any time a movement is executed" (personal communication, 1999).

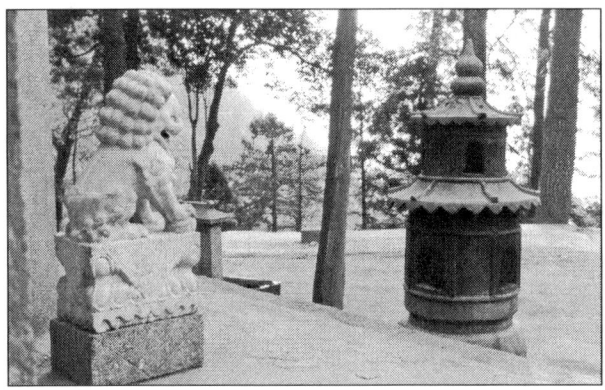

Photography by Kipling Swehla.

Bagua ("Eight Trigrams," refers to heaven, earth, water, fire, thunder, wind, mountain and lake) most likely grew from Daoism in the seventeenth century into a variety of systems practiced around the world today. The bagua boxing style uses fluid motions and swift footwork, moving in circles to confuse the opponent. The victor outflanks his rival, remaining safely behind or beside the source of danger. Bagua demands exceptional concentration (Wong, 1997: 226–227).

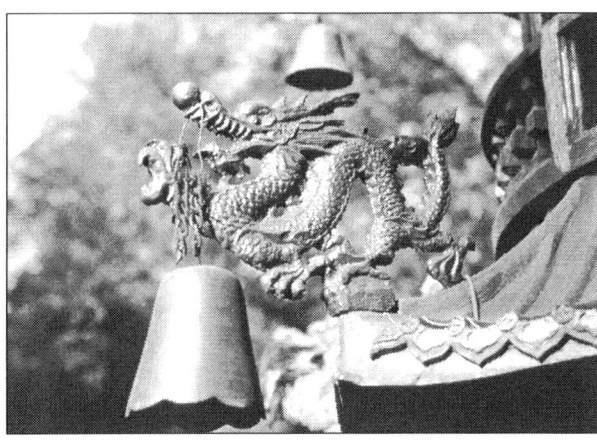

Photography by Kipling Swehla.

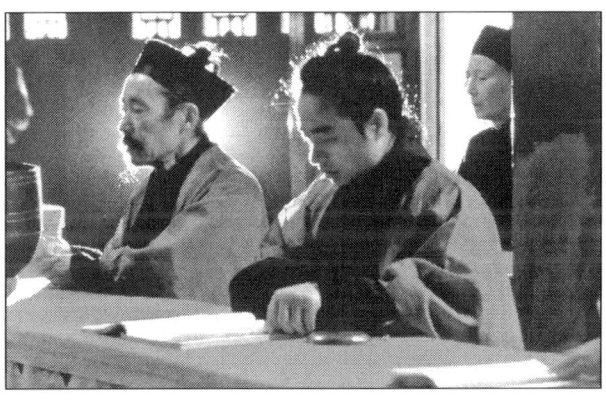

Photography by Kipling Swehla.

Xingyiquan ("Form and Intention Fist") is attributed to Yue Fei, a twelfth century Chinese general. Although he helped popularize it, Yue credited a wandering Daoist with teaching him the art. As with many legends, its accuracy is questionable (others date the art to the Shaolin Temple in the sixth century), but xingyiquan remains very martial in appearance, characterized by pounding, thrusting and hitting with bursts of movement. Xingyiquan is efficient in its expression of power, with the practitioner using a full range of body motions for grappling, locking, throwing and trapping techniques (Wong, 1997: 227).

Liuhebafa ("Six Harmonies and Eight Methods") is probably the least known of the internal martial arts, at least in the West. This art blends elements of taiji, bagua and xingyiquan. "Unlike the other three internal arts," says Wai Lun Choi, "liuhebafa uses over 700 different techniques. The art rests on a foundation of biology, physiology and anatomy, and the spirit enables its proper performance. Its theory, from every perspective, complies with what is practical and scientifically sound. To develop yourself, you must turn away from mysticism and the belief in secrets you imagine will transform you. Science and nature are your true teachers, and correct training is what will transform you" (personal communication, 1999).

Taijiquan, perhaps the most popular of the internal arts founded on Daoism, is a subtle system practiced today primarily for its health benefits. The style, which seeks to cultivate one's qi, finds maximum efficiency through integrating the mind and body in harmonious movement. *Qi* is described as that through which the Dao manifests itself and then differentiates into two forces—yin and yang. Taijiquan practitioners use the doctrine of yin and yang throughout their training. In push-hands practice, for example, it is only by achieving softness and yielding to the opponent's attack that he is effectively repelled (Kauz, 1997: 60). "Most of the traditional internal martial arts training is still underground in China and was so long before Mao," says Dr. Yang Jwing-ming, author and martial arts instructor for more than thirty years. "These arts have been considered top secret since ancient times when they were taught mainly in the monasteries. Even then, they were taught with the goal of spiritual enlightenment." All that changed in 1911.

"Beginning in the late Qing Dynasty, and continuing for some time afterward, the knowledge of internal martial arts was gradually revealed to people outside the monastic community. But then the Communist party took over and they started to control the martial arts community and kept the real martial arts suppressed, fearing the martial artists would unite against the party rule. Combat techniques in martial arts training have been gradually neglected in China ever since" (personal communication, 1999).

Dr. Yang, who was raised in Taiwan and has lived in the U.S. for 25 years, believes there is only one way to keep the internal martial arts alive. "I visited mainland China recently," he says, "and I was surprised to learn that no one under fifty even understands the relationship between qi and the *jin*—that is, internal power. There is still some traditional training in the Chinese countryside, but only a small number of traditional practitioners. I realized the only way to preserve the internal arts was to teach them outside of China" (personal communication, 1999).

Although Daoism's link to external martial arts is more difficult to establish, a case can be made that many of these arts are indebted to the central Daoist principle of the duality of opposites. Indeed, probably any style that advocates fluid motion, yielding responses and avoiding or redirecting an opponent's attack can claim Daoism as its inspiration. As the *Daodejing* says:

> **Rushing into action, you fail.**
> **Trying to grasp things, you lose them.**
> **Forcing a project to completion,**
> **You ruin what was almost ripe.**

– Mitchell. 1991: 64

Daoism Today

TRS and NDA would like to ensure that every major city in China has at least one major Daoist place of worship. Although there is no official restoration plan, major Daoist sites have been the first to be renovated, a task that often involves a construction company. Smaller projects are usually handled by Daoist clergy, often with the assistance of volunteers from the lay community. While the government pays for its own projects, funds for much of the other reconstruction come from supporters throughout Asia, Europe and the United States. The final cost of a restoration varies widely: anywhere from a few hundred U.S. dollars to several million, depending on the size of the site and extent of damage.

Silvers notes that it is difficult to control the use of Daoist iconography and symbols. "From what I have seen," he says, "the government doesn't really care about authenticity. And even those who do care—officials and monks alike—are often hampered by a combination of poverty and ignorance" (personal communication, 1999). Which is why TRS not only helps fund projects but puts pressure on the Chinese government to use greater care as sites are being rebuilt.

The government's National Daoist Association and local religious affairs bureaus across China are also working to save the tradition from extinction, with varying degrees of success. Last January, for example, the government opened a renovated temple dedicated to the god of Tai Shan. The ancient temple, one of the largest in Beijing, was a favorite of the Qing emperors and was rebuilt by a local tourist bureau. Thus, rather than being renovated as a place of worship, the temple now stands as a cultural museum and no Daoist clergy are allowed to engage in religious activity there.

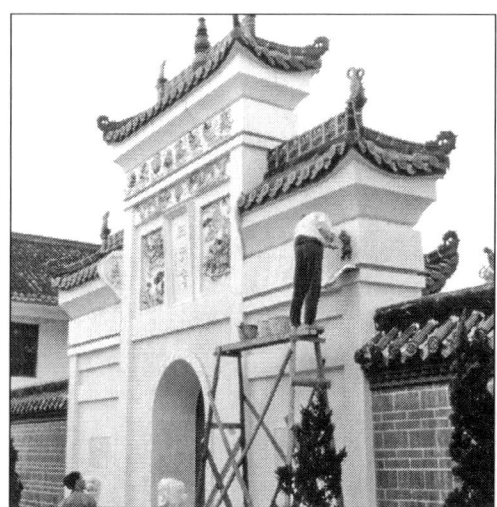 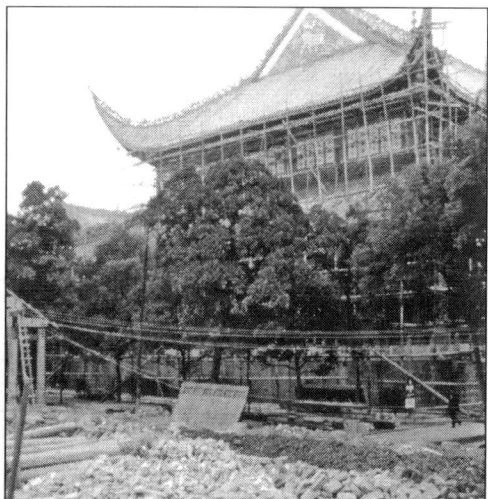

Photography by Katherine McVety.

Daoism Tomorrow

With so many people working on national and local levels toward a goal that is paramount to preserving China's culture, it is tempting to believe that the fight to save Daoism is won. After all, if it's something everyone wants, why the struggle? But turning the tide on a century of destruction is not a simple matter.

The good news is that the restoration of Daoism seems to be taking hold, with major temples crowded on holidays, new sites being constructed and the quality of renovations constantly improving. People throughout China have been very receptive to their reborn Daoist traditions, with more and more viewing themselves as Daoist. But it will take more than renovated temples and contented practitioners to ensure Daoism's survival. As Silvers explains:

> ... The real window of opportunity involves the expected life spans of the old, pre-Communist generation of clergy—the 'laodao' masters—who are generally seventy to one hundred years old. With each temple that is restored or reactivated, more *laodao* are recalled from the fields, the retired workers' hospitals or any kind of work unit to which they might have been assigned.

Although these *laodao* are not numerous, they have embraced the task of breeding a new generation of religious seekers and leaders. It is imperative that organized Daoism reclaims its heritage before the current supply of *laodao* passes away. When these adepts pass away, the previous Daoist age will go with them.

– personal communication, 1999

These *laodao* (elder Daoists) include China's many martial arts masters, whose teachings were suppressed under the threat of imprisonment and death during Mao's reign. The progressive decline of China's traditional martial arts is also a loss to the world, where the destruction of any cultural expression is disgraceful.

Adds Silvers (personal communication, 1999): "It would certainly be a tragedy to witness the functional extinction of the tradition which gave so much impetus and energy to the early development of the internal martial arts. The internal arts and Daoism will forever be linked; can one really be whole without the other?"

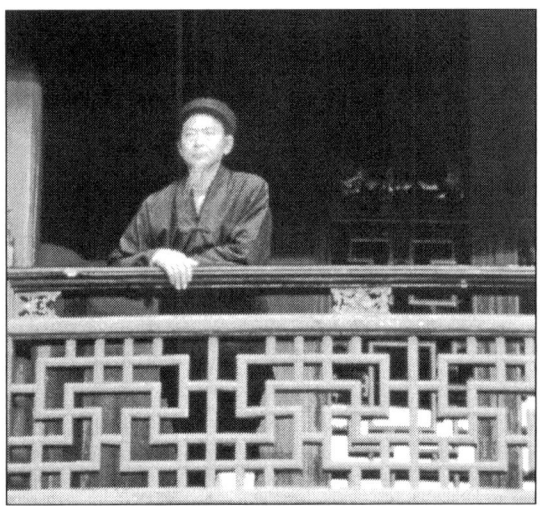
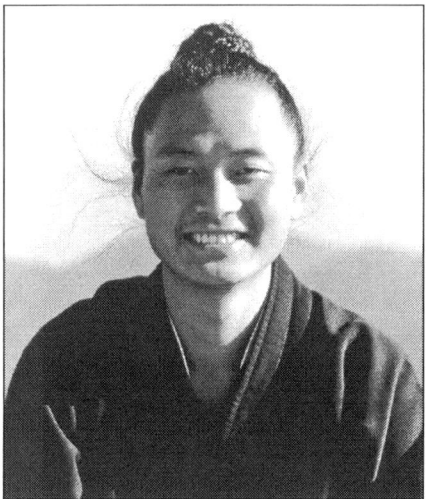

Photography by Kipling Swehla.

Mindful that Chinese President Jiang Zemin already has his hands full, Silvers remains hopeful. "Things are already so much better than they were ten or twenty years ago," he says. "Average Han Chinese people do have more religious freedom than their parents did. And the human soul abhors a vacuum. But traditions and places and rituals and songs and prayers and the like are being forgotten every day. Half a religion probably can't survive. But we might succeed yet" (personal communication, 1999).

▼●▼

Bibliography

Barred, T. (1993). *Dao: To know and not be knowing*. San Francisco, CA: Chronicle Books.

Breslow, A. (1995). *Beyond the closed door: Chinese culture and the creation of t'ai chi ch'uan*. Jerusalem, Israel: Almond Blossom Press.

Chuang-Tzu. (1998). *The essential Chuang-Tzu*. (S. Hamill and J.P. Seaton, Trans.). Boston, MA: Shambala Publications.

Frantiz, B. (1998). *The power of internal martial arts: Combat secrets of bagua, tai chi and hsing-i*. Berkeley, CA: North Atlantic Books.

Kauz, H. (1997). *Push hands: The handbook for noncompetitive tai chi practice with a partner*. Woodstock, NY: The Overlook Press.

Liang, S. (1996). *Tai chi chuan*. Rosindale, MA: YMAA Publication Center.

Mitchell, S. (1991). *Tao te ching*. New York, NY: HarperPerennial.

Schumacher, S., and Woerner, G. (1996). *Shambala dictionary of Daoism*. Boston, MA: Shambala Publications.

Taoist Restoration Society (1999). http://www.taorestore.com.

Wong, E. (1997). *The Shambala guide to Daoism*. Boston, MA: Shambala Publications.

• 31 •
The Nurturing Ways of Chen Taiji: An Interview with Yang Yang
by Michael A. DeMarco, M.A., and A. Edwin Matthews

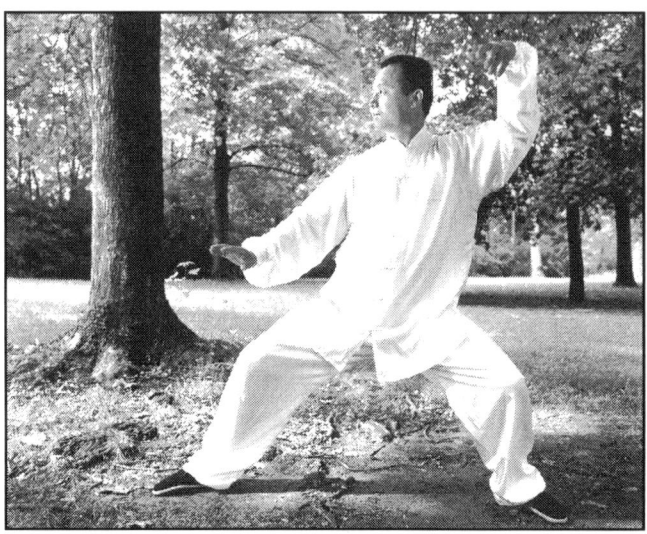

Photography courtesy of David Riecks.

Introduction

Taiji forms and styles are not all alike. There are different teaching and training methods involved. Plus, the overall reasons for practice may represent a wide range of particular goals. It seems that a style's uniqueness is greatly influenced from the leading instructor of that system. If we look at Chen Style taiji, we find an array of sub-styles that reflect the flavor of individuals who have developed their own branch from the lineage. One of the more notable branches come from Grandmaster Feng Zhiqiang, born in 1926, who teaches in Beijing. We were fortunate to conduct an interview with one of Feng's direct disciples, Mr. Yang Yang, who provided an in-depth perspective on this system of Chen taiji.

The following interview was derived from two meetings with Yang Yang which followed workshops he conducted in Erie, Pennsylvania. These were held at Ed Matthew's studio called Body Awareness on October 12–15, 1998, and October 12–15, 1999. Yang told of how he became involved with Chen taiji at an early age and eventually became a formal disciple of Feng Zhiqiang. Feng has developed a clear, comprehensive way of teaching his system. Since Yang arrived in the United States to complete a doctoral program at the University of Illinois-Urbana, he continues to teach Feng's system to students here. The system is a balanced blend of the standard Chen taiji routines, locking techniques (*qinna*), silk reeling (*chansijing*), push-hands (*tuishou*), and energy work (*qigong*).

Following the interview section is a technical section which illustrates some of silk reeling exercises and locking techniques. It is hoped that readers will closely compare the movements shown in both these sections to find how particular segments can be found in both the silk reeling and locking techniques. According to Feng and Yang, these same movements can also be found in the Chen Style routines, push-hands, and qigong since all work together for health as well as self-defense.

INTERVIEW
Yang Yang's Start in Taiji

■ *Where did you live in China and how did you learn about Chen taiji?*

I am from the city of Jiaozuo. It is about twenty-five miles from the Chen Village, and so Chen Style is popular there. Likewise, because the Shaolin Temple is just south of the Yellow River, Shaolin boxing is also very popular in my city. In the local parks you can see people play different martial arts. The interesting thing is that we can also see different versions of the Chen Style. There are specific areas in the park where people practice their version and push-hands. It's a small city where people are very friendly. It's a good environment to start taiji study.

■ *What attracted you to study Chen taiji?*

When I was very young, I had a health problem and got sick almost every week. I couldn't walk. I wanted to run, and my face would get pale. The doctor said, "Don't do any physical education class. It will kill you." I was born in 1961. That was a difficult time in China. There were a high percentage of kids who were born at that time with health problems. We were not allowed to do any physical activity like basketball or soccer. Then a relative from Xi'an said, "You're lucky you stay so close to Chen Village. Why don't you try Chen taiji?" So, when I was twelve years old, I went to meet two teachers at our main city park. Later, they introduced me to a third teacher Zhang Xitang. They are all friends. So, we just learned from each other.

■ *Who are these teachers and how did you meet?*

First, I went to Master Wu Xiubao, who was a high-ranking official in our city. My mother was his secretary. When my mom took me to him, I had to wear very clean clothes and be on my best behavior. Then he looked at me and asked, "Ok, what's the reason why you want to study taiji?" My mom spoke, "You know he has a heart defect, but we don't have the money to do the surgery. This may help, so I rather you could teach him." He said, "I'm busy, but I will let my student teach him first." So actually, I started with Master Yuan Shiming. Now Master Yuan Shiming is quite old. I think he is in his 80's.

■ *Plus, all these teachers are good friends?*

Yes, it's amazing, the city, the people—the human environment is so good. There's no hatred, there's no complications, because there's no money involved. Just pure people that love the art. Usually students stay with one primary teacher, but sometimes the teacher will tell you to go to a particular teacher to learn something he excels in, such as push-hands or qinna. They will tell you, "Ok, go learn from this teacher" and introduce you to that person.

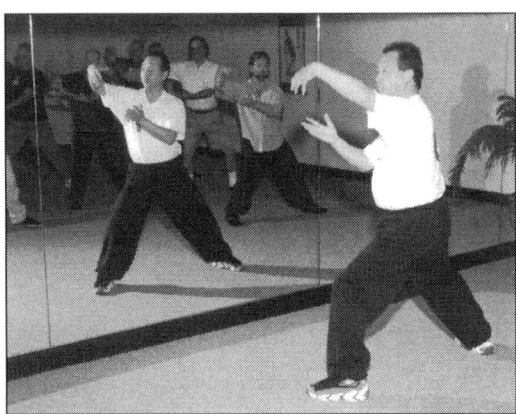

Photography courtesy of Larry Justinas.

■ *Of these three teachers, which one was most influential for you?*
The most influential was the first one: Master Yuan Shiming. He was the one I studied with most of the time. He was very kind, very generous, and kept no secrets. Whatever he knows, he teaches you.

■ *At the time of your introduction, did you have a concept of what taiji was?*
No, I just practiced. Every morning at 5:00 a.m. my dad got the stick "Get up, get out of bed, go to the park and play taiji." He said, "otherwise you're going to die. We don't have the money to send you to Shanghai to do the surgery. The only thing you can do is practice taiji." You must go to the park at least thirty minutes before the teacher. You cannot be later than the teacher. That's rude. I would usually go one hour before. You make sure you do the homework before the teacher comes. Otherwise, you would be embarrassed if you feel you cannot do what he assigned you.

■ *After studying with him, did you have a pretty good overview of the Chen Style?*
I studied with him seven years, but I cannot say I had a very good view of Chen taiji yet. I only got some basic idea of what to work on: the first and second routines, and some push-hands. The first couple of years we worked on the first routine before starting the second.

■ *Do most instructors teach the first routine to focus on relaxation?*
Relaxing is one aspect and obviously a starting point for beginners. Other

fundamental exercises, such as wuji practice, are just as important to teach relaxation. All of the Chen Style principles can be learned from practicing the first routine. If you do the first routine well, you can also do the second routine (*paochui*) and weapons forms well. If you have not learned the first routine well, your second routine and weapon forms will be just as lacking.

- *Who did you practice push-hands with?*

I practiced with my taiji classmates. Sometimes with my teacher or his friends, who were teaching in the same big park. Sometimes we play push-hands with other teachers' students, too.

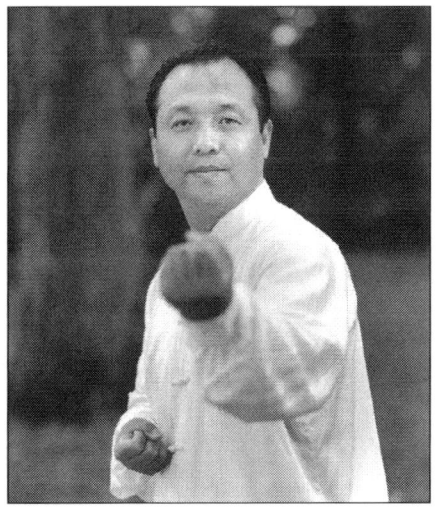

Photography courtesy of David Riecks.

- *Did you practice push-hands through the whole period?*

After I finished the first routine. The reason teachers want you to wait a little bit is because they know that before we start learning taiji we already have accumulated stiffness in our whole body. Why learn to relax? We want to go back to our original condition in terms of relaxation. For example, a one-year-old or six-month-old baby is difficult to hold. Why? Because he or she is very relaxed. There is no stiffness there. As we grow older, we get more and more tense, mentally and physically. So, we want to go to another extreme. But if you start push-hands at the very beginning it may make it worse. So, this is why teachers say you should work on the form first.

- *Are you usually left to practice by yourself?*

Most students go to the park every day to practice with a teacher. They just find a place near the teacher and practice by themselves. The teacher practices too. If students have a question, he will talk with them, show them a new movement, or make corrections.

■ *If you couldn't do a particular movement correctly, what would the teacher do?*

It really depends on the teacher. In most cases, if the teacher is not happy, you would feel it. The only thing to do is go back and practice. It's not that you come to the park and that's the only time you practice. Practice in the morning, evening, during the day—you've got to do it. If you feel you are learning and improving through practice, then you go to the park regularly, otherwise you don't go back. That's what happens in a very traditional setting. There is not too much encouragement. Teachers just let you practice, practice, practice. Maybe sometimes they are happy inside, but they won't show it. They think that if they say too many good words, you'll get a big head. They may say little so you will work harder.

■ *Did you have any testing, or was it just day-by-day practice?*

There is no testing. Teachers just look at you and that's the test. They see you. They touch you, especially when you start doing push-hands. They touch you and they know. You cannot cheat them. That's probably what we can call testing—and it is all the time.

■ *Do students practice for the first year or so mainly to learn all the basics regarding body movement and how the taiji movements should feel?*

Yes. First, you've got to learn how your own body works. Then the teacher will tell you where you've got tension, where your alignment is incorrect, how to adjust your feet, and how to coordinate your body. You try to make the form correct based on his standards.

■ *After studying with these teachers for seven years, you felt you didn't have a clear overview of Chen taiji yet. Did you finally feel more comfortable after meeting other teachers and seeing more practitioners?*

I would say there was a breakthrough after my teacher introduced me to Master Chen Zhaokui in 1980. That was a big turning point because Chen Zhaokui showed the applications, push-hands skill, and internal energy at a level of mastery I had never seen before.

■ *You then traveled to study more?*

I went to study engineering at a college in Shanghai. Because my dad is a musician, he believes if one wants to learn how to play music well it is always good to visit the best teachers. However, even though someone is a well-known or famous teacher that does not necessarily mean that he really understands the art. You should be able to recognize that. The more you visit, the more you can compare and learn. So, he always encourages me to visit teachers. So, I applied that idea to my taiji practice. Plus, I'm lucky I had good teachers to encourage and help me. They helped me a lot. For example, my first three teachers are all friends of Chen Zhaokui. They learned from him, so I also got the opportunity to learn from him. I did this whenever I went back to my hometown on my summer vacation from Shanghai.

■ *Did Chen Zhaokui study with Chen Fake in Beijing?*
Yes, Chen Zhaokui is Chen Fake's son. He lived in Beijing for most of his life. Later, he spent a lot of time traveling and teaching taiji in other cities. So, people from Chen Village invited him back to teach. And the younger generation from Chen Village studied from him. Unfortunately, he died when he was pretty young. I think the reason he passed away had a lot to do with the political stress.

■ *Your next teacher was Feng Zhiqiang. How did you meet him?*
In 1982, I attended a national taiji conference in Shanghai called "Famous Taiji Masters' Gathering," or something like that. I met Master Feng there. What happened was that one of my hometown teachers, Zhang Xitang, also went to Shanghai to see the gathering. He was a good friend of Chen Xiaowang and asked him to try to introduce us to Master Feng. We just wanted to see him. So, one day during the seminar, Chen Xiaowang called to say, "I talked to uncle (he called Master Feng "uncle," because Feng is one generation older), and he would like to meet you guys."

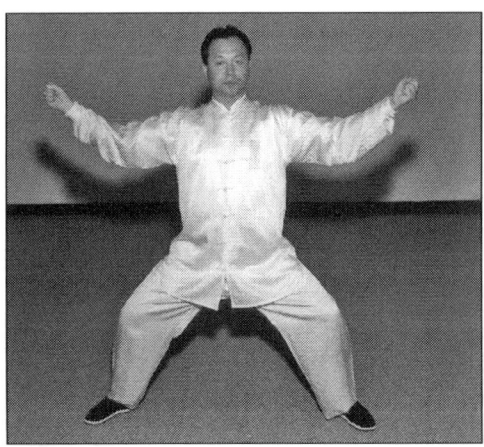

■ *You must have enjoyed this special gathering and seen many taiji styles?*
I loved it very much. That was the first and last biggest master's gathering in China to this day. That was the first time in my life to see so many top masters from the taiji community. Most of the best teachers of all taiji styles attended. It was hosted by Gu Liuxin because he held a good government position and had the power to arrange the gathering. People respected him because he was a scholar and was good in martial arts. For Chen Style, they had Master Feng, Hong Junsheng—another one of Chen Fake's recognized students—Gu Liuxin, and Chen Xiaowang.

For the Yang Style, they had Fu Zhongwen and Yang Zhengduo. For Wu Style, they had Ma Yueliang and his wife, Madam Wu, plus Wang Peisheng. For Sun Style, they had Madam Su Jianyun.

There were some others as well. With such masters giving presentations and demonstrations, this event offered people a very rare opportunity to see the different styles. I am not aware of any similar meeting taking place before or since then. Perhaps in the future there will be another.

■ *You left Shanghai to go to school in Beijing. How did you make time to study with Master Feng?*

During the last year of engineering school, in 1983, I was thinking about quitting college and just devoting my life to taiji training with Master Feng. I talked to him about it, and he said, "No, finish your degree. Just finish your work, and I'll try to get you a job here in Beijing." Getting a job is the easy part. In China, the problem is to change *hukou*, the local registration that everybody must have. Because my first job was in Shanghai, my huko was in Shanghai. There was almost no way for me to transfer my hukou from Shanghai to Beijing. That was a big problem. Master Feng did help me, and I tried very hard, but it didn't work out. The only way was to go to school, so I went to law school in Beijing. I skipped a lot of classes and instead went to the park to practice. But I did do well and passed the national bar examination in 1988.

■ *In which park does master Feng teach?*

It's called the Temple of Heaven. That park is unique because of the numerous evergreen trees—most of the Chinese martial artists believe you can get lots of energy from evergreen trees. So, we usually do qigong there.

■ *You practiced there early in the morning?*

Yes, early in the morning. I would usually get there about 6:00, sometimes 5:30. You must arrive there before the teacher does.

■ *It is interesting to hear you would go to class an hour to forty-five minutes before the teacher arrived.*

Even now in China for many social activities and even work, some people may be late. But as part of taiji training, it's a moral obligation to be on time. Especially in traditional training, you may find a knowledgeable teacher, but they don't have to tell you anything. They may want to see if you are always on time and make it regularly to class. They want to know if you are serious before accepting you as a student or not. What they teach is very valuable. You've got to treasure it.

■ *If someone wants to study with a particular teacher, how would a teacher establish the relationship?*

Before you begin studies, they may investigate you to see if you are a nice person, work hard, and whether you respect old people. The respect of old people is a primary criterion on their list. They say if you don't treat your parents well, you are not a person they want to be affiliated with. Teachers say, "If you do not treat your parents well, how can I teach you? How are you going to treat me?" It's very simple logic. So, they may investigate that, and investigate how you treat your friends. They may teach you some basic exercises and movements and, in the meantime, they test you.

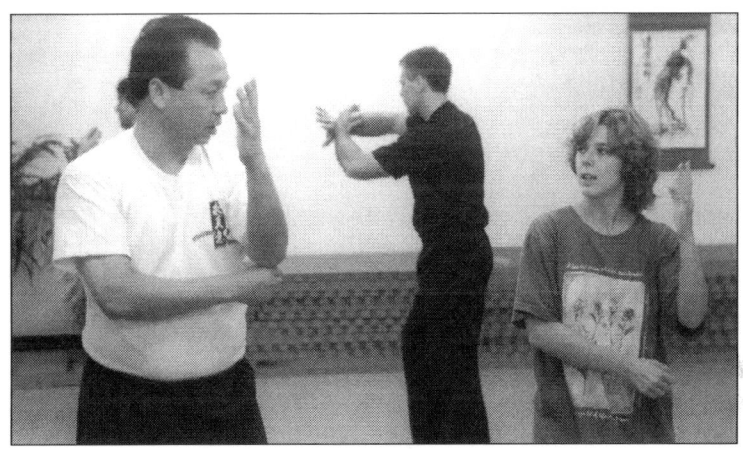

TEACHING THEORIES

■ *You studied at first for health. Why not Yang Style?*
There's no doubt Yang Style is more popular than Chen Style—than any style. But people can start with any style. Whether you have access to a teacher may determine the style you can study. If you can get access to all the different styles, then it's easier to choose which version you like. With Chen Style, you can start with any physical condition, background or age. I've been working with people who started in their 70's and they are doing very well. Some people have misunderstandings about Chen Style.

■ *Some say Chen Style is for fighting and Yang Style is for health and the elderly.*
Yes, I really want to talk about this. I'm not being critical of other styles, because any style may be good if taught by experts in that style. The key issue is whether you get the real stuff from your style or not. If I practice Chen Style but I couldn't get the real stuff I'd say, "Chen Style is not good" that's not fair, right? My point is that health and self-defense or fighting are one issue. Usually people separate the two—"I practice for health," or "I practice for fighting." I don't think that's the method for understanding taiji better. Such a division won't lead to a complete understanding of taiji practice. If you are not healthy, you can't fight well either.

Taiji is such a rich practice with so many benefits. Beginners cannot comprehend the wealth it contains. All aspects of the training system are related. You cannot say "I want this but not that." If you study only one part, then your returns will be considerably less than if you understand and practice the complete art. Why limit yourself from the beginning?

■ *So the primary thing is to work on being healthy?*

If you keep yourself healthy, then you can fight and you can defend yourself. That's about internal energy. That's taiji practice. Working on your internal energy and getting stronger is good both for your health and for your self-defense. You can use it for both.

■ *When you started teaching here, did you find that students wanted to progress faster, learn more and more movements, without giving the basics enough attention?*

Like taiji, Chinese martial arts, Beijing opera, music, you may have to follow their rules. You must start from the very beginning, otherwise nobody would teach you. You must follow their rules from the very beginning. That's good for you, because if you don't have the foundation you cannot go to a higher level. Yes, most of the students want to learn more and more forms, so they feel they are making progress. As teachers, we should point out to the students the importance of the quality of the form and the basics, which include qigong and theory.

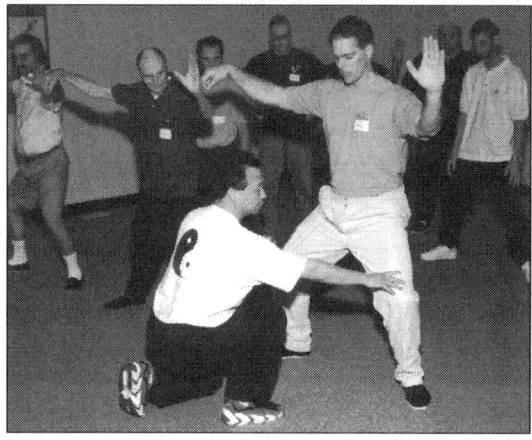

Photography courtesy of Larry Justinas.

■ *Can teaching be adjusted to the individual so they can progress according to their own abilities?*

Yes, in fact it should be that way in all aspects of training. We talk about the individual, their personal background, and physical and mental condition. In taiji, we talk about yin/yang: there should be some variations as we follow the principles. Going back to one of your other questions about the different versions of Chen Style... People have different understandings of the art.

The art is so rich; maybe you look at it from one angle and I look at it from another. As a result, we have a different understanding. It is more important to incorporate the principles. For example, it doesn't matter whether one practices taiji with a big frame or small one. The version may be different, but the principles should be the same.

There's an old saying in China, "First you copy, then you want to try to change."

At first, it's not easy to see how to do it—you make a copy. Like in the feeling of push-hands, even when you talk about hard/soft, you really must touch the teacher; you really must feel it. So, this is one of the subtle parts of taiji training. You cannot get this even on videotape. I really must touch to know what the teacher means. And even if you touch, you still must think very hard.

■ *Because you can still misunderstand the touch?*

Yes. Theory, form practice, and applications must be combined. We can get the feel of a movement or a technique, practicing it over and over so we can learn something and understand it better. Then we can talk about it. It is important to copy the movements. Even subconsciously, I can always learn from my teacher. Then we talk about including applications.

■ *Applications? Does this include all the variations?*

I think it's not good for beginning students to have too many choices. They should make a choice, and then consistently do the same thing so there's no confusion. Later, students start to see the other possibilities. "How about moving this way? If I'm going backwards, I could use my elbow instead of my fist?" But if you just start with one application, it is easier to build from there.

■ *How are the concepts of hardness and softness in Chen Style explained?*

There's one old saying from the classics: "Accumulation of softness will lead to hardness." We do need both, soft and hard, but we cannot start with hard. We need to accumulate softness and then transfer the softness to hardness.

■ *What is softness? Do you need to put your hands on an experienced teacher to know?*

To make it simple, softness is being relaxed. And here I want to make it very clear the differences between softness and collapse. The two are completely different. A lot of people make the mistake of collapsing when they try to be soft. You must feel it. You cannot learn it from a book, you cannot learn it from a video tape, or CD. Yes, you must feel it. Personal touch and feel.

■ *What does it mean to be double-weighted?*

There are two ways we can understand this. One is purely physical weight distribution. So, if we use this standard, it would be fifty percent on each leg, right? If we have a 50/50 percentage, we're double-weighted. But there's another way to understand this—it is whenever you lock yourself. If you can't move easily, you are double-weighted. Even if you have 60/40 percent distribution, you can still be double-weighted. If you cannot shift your energy from one point to another point, you have double-weightedness. That's my understanding.

■ *What do you mean exactly by "locking yourself"?*

Locking your energy flow within the whole body. If you feel it is difficult to move lightly and quickly, you are "locked." Even if my physical weight distribution is 50/50, but I can move my energy quickly with agility, I am not locked. Alternatively, if my weight is distributed 80/20 but I cannot move my energy from one point to another, I am locked.

■ *Some people have not completed copying a system from a competent teacher. Then they start to invent new movements or systems.*

I think this is why there are different styles such as Yang, Wu, and Sun. Of course, the safest way is to study a recognized style that has stood the test of time and/or was created by a recognized master in his initial art. Creative students have obtained the basics by copying; then they combine with their own personal experience from other martial arts. They create different styles. But they must study very hard for a long time. They have the ability and the knowledge. In America, most people don't have the patience to finish the first stage, so they probably won't be able to develop a new system.

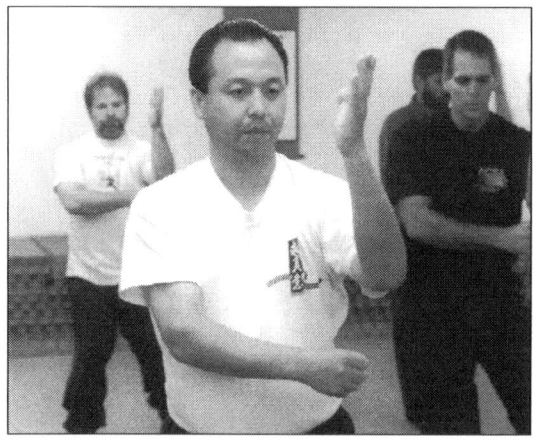

Photography courtesy of Larry Justinas.

■ *When compared with China, many teachers in the United States have a limited background in Asian martial arts. How can we progress?*

One of the advantages here in the U.S. is that there is more exposure to high quality Asian martial arts, especially now that people can come here from China. They also bring the culture and understanding with them. The good thing is that communication in America is very open. America is a rich country and people have the technology and means to learn. More and more, the top teachers of different styles are traveling to America to teach or give seminars. Communication and sharing of ideas are occurring at a much greater level than ever before. Most people work and have a family and don't have a lot of time to practice. The key is to make the practice as efficient as possible.

I want to be realistic. In China, in the old days, there was a saying that "you must be rich to study martial arts." The meaning was that most people didn't have the means to travel to see a teacher or spend time practicing. You don't have to be rich, but it is no easy task to reach a high level of gongfu, and it does require sacrifice. It depends upon how hard you try, how serious your practice is, how well you can truly understand and apply the principles in your daily practice. For any student, whether in Asia or America, there is also fate.

As long as we keep trying, we'll get the chance to meet some people who can really teach something worthwhile. For example, take my case. In 1980, Chen Zhaokui came to my hometown to teach. I was very lucky because my teacher knew him and introduced me. Unfortunately, I only had a short time with him before he passed away. I also had a chance to take private classes with Chen Xiaowang. He had to come to my city to take the train to Beijing. When he stopped here, he visited his "taiji uncle," Chen Zhaokui. Chen Zhaokui said, "This is my top student Chen Xiaowang," as he introduced me. Not long after that, Chen Zhaokui passed away.

In 1981 or 1982 at the National Taiji Gathering, Chen Xiaowang introduced me to Master Feng. In my hometown area, people talked about studying with Master Feng and Chen Zhaokui because they were the top 18th generation Chen Style representatives. My dream was just to meet them. I didn't think I could learn from them. It was just fate. When masters like Feng meet a new student, they check the student's personality as the training progresses—if they are respectful, whether they improve, whether they train hard—these kinds of things. Then they will decide whether they will take him or her as a formal student.

Shanghai is a good place for martial arts study. When I was in college there, I often went to visit Gu Liuxin. Master Gu was the president of the Shanghai Martial Arts Association. He was a very knowledgeable scholar, very kind and open. He would always say, "Master Feng's push-hands is the best." It's not easy to become his student because he is also very tough.

■ *In the United States, many think they can become "masters" in two or three years. Do you think this is possible?*

The "quick-learn masters" may be very smart, but nobody can be smarter than the accumulation of four or five hundred years of experience. You may be smarter than two generation's accumulation. Your technical experience may accumulate greatly in one generation and you may feel you have exceeded the skills of the old masters. But this is impossible because the members of the "family" lineage have devoted all their energy and lives to this art. I made similar mistakes too. In 1981, 1982, and 1983, I entered the Shanghai College martial art tournaments and took first place each year. However, after I met Master Feng, I realized that I knew nothing.

■ *One student was practicing a movement, and I asked her what she was doing. She said "pushing," but her body was moving backwards as her hand moved forwards. I stood in front of her and asked her to push me, and of course it didn't work.*

As a practitioner, I should know what my focus is and what I'm doing. You gave a perfect example of a very common misunderstanding of technique. Simple physics must be understood. For example, in movement my body may have twenty pounds, and my arms have five. If they move together in the same direction, I can get twenty-five pounds applied to the subject. If they are moving in opposite directions, I may get negative fifteen pounds. If my body moves backward, I may end up with only five pounds of pressure moving to the front. But if my body also moves in that direction, I end up with twenty-five pounds. It's simple physics. What happens to some people is maybe the teacher passes on misinformation or maybe the student's understanding is wrong.

■ *If someone has studied one martial art and watches another style, they think, "I know that technique." But perhaps they really do not.*

The technique should be essentially the same among different styles of taiji. Just make sure you really understand the style you are practicing. If possible, try the same technique from other styles. It will enhance your understanding. The technique is not fixed. Most people think, "I've learned one technique; it will keep me safe." One very good thing to find out about the whole training system is that it is limitless. For example, with qinna you can really make one technique after another. From one qinna, comes a counter qinna, then another qinna. If you become static, it does not work. Likewise with silk reeling exercises and the Chen routines. So, the silk reeling, the routines, the qinna, the counter qinna, and qigong—all work together all the time.

■ *Some people who are very busy with family or their work have only limited time to practice. Are there basic things that you never want to skip? Is there a priority?*

I would say, don't skip qigong. If you are busy, still do the qigong. If there is more time, then practice the routines and silk reeling.

■ *Silk reeling after the routines?*

The silk reeling and the routines are almost the same rank. After that, you learn push-hands. Push-hands is not only an exercise for you to consume energy. It can also be used to generate energy. That's a very important point. If we can make our practice more energy-oriented, no matter what we practice, we'll be okay. So why mention push-hands? Because lots of people think push-hands is just pure energy consumption. That's wrong. With push-hands, you should train in a gentle nurturing way. You can train to generate energy instead of purely wasting or consuming your energy.

■ *What type of qigong practices would you recommend? Standing pole?*

Yes, standing pole is one static part of qigong practice. There is also the dynamic or moving part. Start with the standing, and then later you can do some moving qigong exercises.

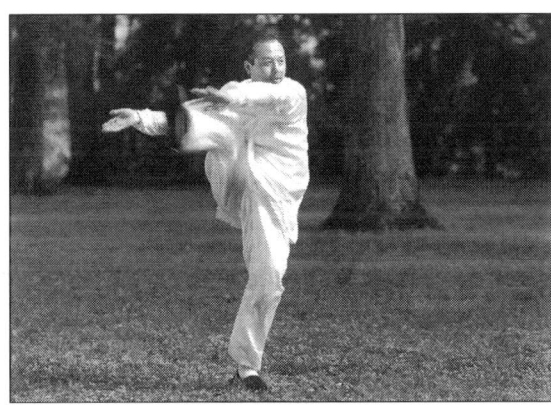

Photography courtesy of David Riecks.

■ *Is any particular type of qigong good for beginners? Are all the same?*

There are many styles of qigong. Like any other profession, you've got good and bad instructors, especially in qigong. People want quick results. Based on that demand, some people create strange exercises that are bogus. It has happened in China, and I expect it's going to happen in the United States, or already has happened here. So, I want to take this opportunity to say to the readers in your journal: be careful and make sure you're practicing correct qigong. Because this is something unlike the taiji routines. Practicing the routines incorrectly may hurt you, but not too bad. But, if you practice qigong the wrong way, you may cause great damage.

■ *How many different types of exercise are there in qigong?*

We do stationary qigong, including standing, sitting, and even lying down. Our routines, silk reeling and push-hands practice are dynamic qigong. If we can use it to generate more energy, it is qigong.

With push-hands there are a variety of exercises. You have two-person exercises with stationary feet, using a single-arm or a double-arm engagement. You have two-person exercises with moving steps.

■ *In qigong and silk reeling practice, what should we visualize? Should we look for a certain feeling or sensation? Or should we simply practice and wait to see what happens?*

Many different experiences come from qigong practice. It can be the feeling of becoming extremely small or huge. It can be very hot. It can make one side cold, or one side hot. It can cause trembling in the dantian. You may see some other person appearing huge. You may feel that your whole body becomes very light, or you become very happy. I would say, don't pursue this kind of thing or try to get this kind of experience. If you don't have this kind of feeling, it doesn't mean you are doing it wrong. You are okay. But if you pursue that kind of experience, you may have problems.

In my case, I had the feeling that my whole body was sinking into the ground. But my other taiji brothers and sisters had other experiences. There are a couple of criteria you can utilize: keep it simple and be natural. You can try the different versions of qigong, but don't fool yourself. Don't believe people who say they can send you energy, or you don't have to practice. You've got to do the work yourself to be your own healer. You are your own healer. We've got to do the work. Practice, but first try to make sure the things you get are correct. Improve with practice, and then keep working.

- *How does it benefit our taiji by having our inner energy flowing?*

In general, when we watch someone perform taiji, we usually ask if the taiji is "empty" or not. Is there energy there or is it just pure mechanical movement? An experienced teacher can check a student's energy flow in different ways, such as through push-hands, or just looking at the form. After you start practicing an internal art, it becomes very easy for you to see what energy is in the form.

- *Just like in calligraphy and other arts?*

Yes. It has content, feeling, and meaning. When you express yourself, you can really express it through the energy. I told my father, who is a musician: "Dad, people ask me, 'When you play taiji, why is it different every time?' And I tell them because it feels different." And I say, "That's from my music training." The art is yin/yang. Some part is high, some is low—one dynamic exchange between yin and yang. That's art. So, I would say, in order to understand taiji, if we have time, study other arts. And that will come back to help us understand taiji better. All arts are closely related.

- *Most think that qi will make them powerful. What is the role qi development has in improving one's taiji practice?*

According to Chinese medical theory, everybody has qi. It is one of our training goals to make our qi strong and balanced. It should come very naturally. A lot of people ask to see it. I really cannot let you see it, but when we try push-hands you can feel what that means. Here's another issue: Some people say that "The only people to fully develop their internal qi are special people, like monks on a misty mountain who train for fifty years." I would say no. Everybody can cultivate their qi. If you get the right form and practice the correct way with dedication, you can improve your qi. You can do it for your health, push-hands, and self-defense.

- *If somebody is very good in qigong, but never practiced push-hands, they probably would not do well in push-hands. They have to be healthy and also know the whole-body movement?*

Good qigong, form, and silk reeling will help you to know yourself better. Push-hands practice helps you to understand both yourself and your partner. You need both. It's a choice. You've got to do the routines, do the silk reeling, and you've got to apply your qi in these practices. That's true.

■ *Is qigong study one way to learn how the body works? And, how the qi circulates, opening meridians so that the qi flows naturally?*

Yes, qigong can also help us understand how our body works. The qi will flow naturally through the meridians by itself. The best way always is to be natural, letting it go by itself. Qigong generates more internal energy, making your qi stronger, and improves qi circulation in your taiji practice.

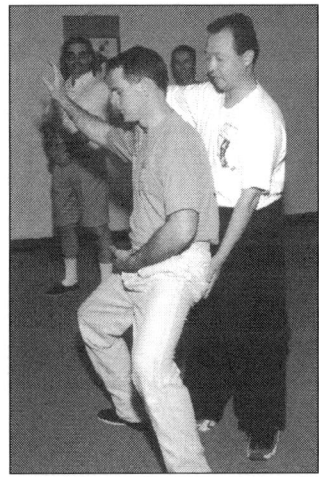 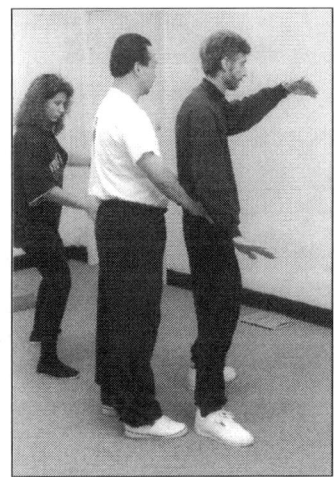 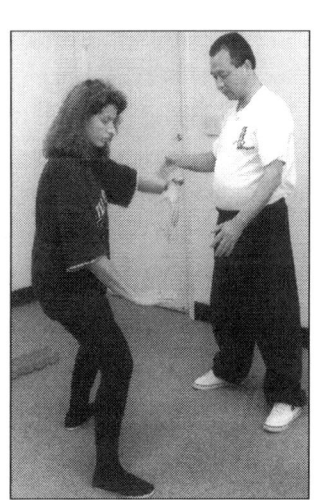

Photography courtesy of Larry Justinas.

■ *A beginner usually starts with qigong or the first routine?*

That depends on the teacher. Some like to start with qigong and others start with form. We must pay attention to cultural differences too, because generally people have an idea that taiji is a morning exercise for the elderly. They already have an image of taiji in their mind. So when I came to the United States and started teaching, I would ask, "So you guys think that is what taiji looks like? Let's try this."

After they got involved, they really enjoyed it. Then I'd say, "Here is the whole training system. Do you want to learn the real stuff?" After they practice qigong, they can easily tell the difference between only doing form and doing both (qigong and form). Then they can tell the difference between qigong and taiji and are happy to practice both. Recently, with the help of the media, people are getting a better understanding of taiji and qigong.

■ *How do you compare your teaching methods with Master Feng's?*

There are different levels of taiji training in terms of weight shifting, coordination, footwork, silk reeling, etc. It is difficult for beginning students to study, practice, and get the benefit if they start with the refined level. So, I first present the essential form and silk reeling. Gradually, based upon the student's progress, I will introduce the more subtle, refined movements and silk reeling. I refer to these levels as "essential" and "refined" forms. This method has been working very well. Every time I meet with Master Feng, I realize I still have so much more to learn. His system is so very rich. That's the biggest difference between us. There's also a small difference. I live in America, so I probably know American culture a little bit better than my teacher. So, in terms of how to present things, I needed to change the teaching method a little bit.

■ *What makes up the whole system as Feng teaches it?*

Master Feng's system is truly unique. It includes the Chen Style first and second routines, and many single forms repetition practices. For example, he teaches static qigong (standing and sitting qigong), dynamic qigong exercises called Hunyuan Gong, silk reeling exercises, push-hands drills, and sparring gong. There are about ten basic gong routines. I should say the thing his system focuses on most is being very natural. Second, it's scientific. What I mean by scientific is that the system always emphasizes nurturing. The whole process of practicing is to nurture yourself. That's his unique process. That is what makes his taiji so powerful. His techniques are unique.

To nurture, you must train in many aspects, like qigong and diet. Another important point is to pay attention to your emotional stability through spiritual training. Maybe you practice the first routine as training. So why practice qigong, and why have a moral standard for disciples? This is not only for moral reasons, but also for the art. Can you imagine a fighter, if he loses his temper all the time? If he always wants to hurt other people or doesn't have a peaceful mind? There's an old saying in China: "Ten thousand things come from quietness." Peacefulness comes from peace. By being quiet, we can accomplish ten thousand things in our life. We believe health and even fighting skills are highly related to one's moral, emotional and spiritual being. These are applied to taiji study. It's not pure technique or practice. Because Master Feng talks about spiritual nurturing, physical nurturing, and diet nurturing, I feel that his system is unique.

■ *He is very different from the other teachers you have trained with?*

Yes. You asked why I chose him as my teacher. Number one is fate. Also, the criteria I used to choose a teacher is by what he really knows. How I check this is by looking at his disciples to see if they're good. And I look at his practice to see if it's good or not. Another criterion is to see if he is willing to share his knowledge with me. Of course, you yourself should be good and pass his test. But assuming you pass his test, will he share his art with you or not? Because no matter how good the teacher is, if he doesn't want to share his knowledge with me, there is no reason to call myself his student. So, I think Master Feng is a very good person, plus he's knowledgeable, and he's willing to share with his students. So, I chose him.

■ *That is a valuable part of his system. How does Master Feng work with students' characters? Is it all indirect?*

He himself sets a good example for the student. He treats his teachers, taiji brothers, and even his neighbors very well. I was staying at his home when I traveled to Beijing, so I saw these relationships. Second, sometimes he would tell you some stories to teach you. I would say nobody is problem free. I have personal problems, sometimes very serious problems. I talk with him. He sometimes talked about applying taiji principles to our work, politics, and even personal crises. He is really a *shifu*—a teacher-father. He teaches you lots of moral values, instead of only, "here's the first routine, second routine, go ahead, do it," and then you graduate. Like the last time I went to Beijing, the first thing I must do is go see the teacher. It's what a son would do. For two years when I worked in Shanghai at the college, I traveled in the summer and winter to Beijing to train with him. The travel expenses took all my money, so he let me stay with him at his house. You have the feeling that if you don't practice hard, you feel guilty—you have that kind of feeling.

YANG'S TEACHING METHOD

■ *What is your reason for teaching Chen Style and what keeps you going?*
I feel a responsibility, an obligation to share my experience with the people here, and maybe some time back in my country. I started taiji practice because of poor health and it made me physically and spiritually strong. How these physical and spiritual aspects work together and how can we get more people to get the benefits—these are the big reasons I switched my academic major to the field of kinesiology.

A lot of people have skills that are much higher than mine. But not too many people felt as strongly as I did about taiji after it cured my health problems. So, I would like to share this. This is why I attempted to study kinesiology even though I didn't have any preparatory background. It is very hard for me to study this, but I think I can go forward. There's more research to be done in Chinese medicine. I need to study more of that, too. I need to study more physiology, biology, and anatomy to see whether we can really understand this art better.

■ *Your own personal research?*
Yes. I am very fortunate to conduct research under the guidance of my advisor Dr. Karl Rosengren, Dr. Eddie McCauley, and Dr. Rick Washburn leading professors in motor learning, exercise psychology, and exercise physiology. We are all excited about our preliminary research results and plans for future studies.

The other thing is the learning process. Everything moves together; it's one big thing. We can get many benefits from taiji training for the beginner, intermediate, and advanced practitioners. The more I study taiji, the deeper it seems. This includes how we apply taiji in our daily lives to handle our problems, such as financial, political, or whatever. It's very rich. More and more people also want to get the spiritual benefit from it.

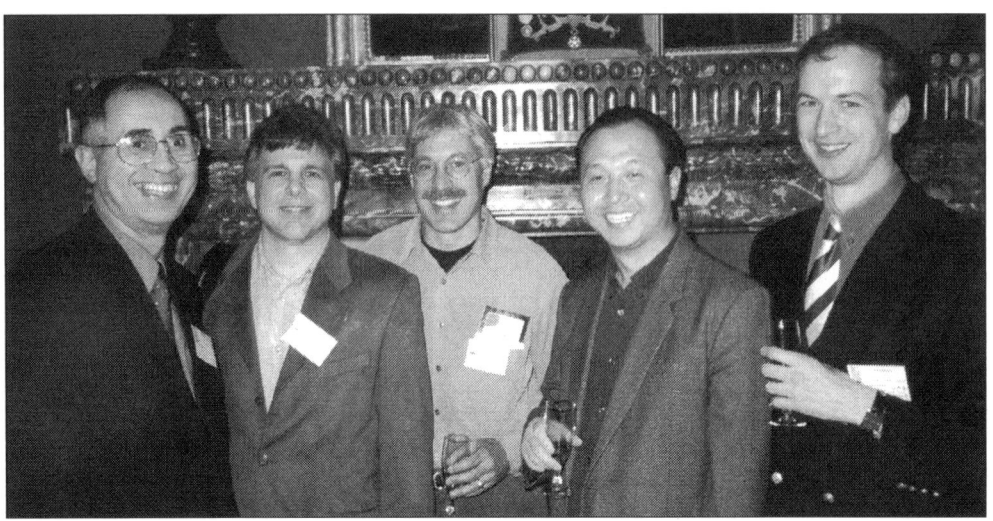

The first World Congress on Fighting Sports & Martial Arts was held from March 31 thru April 2, 2000, in Amiens, France. This photograph was taken during a reception held on April 1st at the mayor's office. Left to right: Dr. Willy Pieter, Michael DeMarco, Dr. Karl Rosengren (Yang's academic advisor), Yang Yang, and John Heijmans.

■ *What information and skills would you like a student to take home from your seminars?*

First, to understand that each part of the practice—the routines, qinna, qigong, push-hands, and silk reeling—are integral aspects of the whole system and are closely related to each other. These different parts are not isolated. Second, to focus on learning the twelve essential taiji principles as taught by Master Feng. The third thing is that I hope, by giving examples, that people can learn to apply the taiji principles to their daily life. This is the real benefit people sometimes don't recognize. Daily practice is important to gain benefits. For example, applying the principles can alleviate knee and shoulder problems which are common now. People can look at the Chen Style routines, applications, and silk reeling exercises to understand any martial art style better. And also, how we transfer our form and push-hands exercises to qigong exercises.

■ *Between an intermediate and an advanced student, is there a difference in emphasis, refinement, or in technique?*

Taiji is such a rich art, it is almost impossible for beginners to fully comprehend the potential benefits. Differences in level are relative—how can you draw the line between "intermediate" and "advanced"? There is a famous Chinese saying: *shan wai you shan, tian wai you tian*, which means after this mountain there is another mountain bigger and higher, after this world there is another, bigger world. So, how can you say what is "advanced"?

This said, I can answer your question in a general way. I would consider my "intermediate" students to be those who know the basic form and have begun practicing the refined movements, silk reeling, and push-hands and have reached a certain level in qigong. I can check their gong by touching them in push-hands and by looking to see the energy in their forms. I have been teaching in the U.S. for six years now. I would say that, in this time, I do not consider any of my students to have reached an "advanced" level. Beginners practice the first routine in a slower manner and higher postures than advanced students. Over time, when appropriate, they may increase speed and move into lower postures. At the beginning stage, it is important not to try to make the postures too low.

The beginner just builds the basic structure. On the side, we practice the silk reeling and even simple push-hand drills. Then, we proceed to bring these together. For example, through silk reeling we obtain more meaning in the form. We use silk reeling to generate more energy to supplement qigong practice, which also refines our form. Refining one aspect helps refine the others.

■ *Do you find push-hands practice is the best way of learning sensitivity?*
It's part of the training. We cannot say it is the best way, because the whole curriculum, the whole training, includes the routines, silk reeling, qigong, and push-hands. All of these should work together.

■ *Some say that all you need to practice is the routine. If you are ever attacked, you will automatically be able to defend yourself.*
There is a reason why all the different elements are included in the training system. The training curriculum was developed for some reason. Why do people practice the routines, qigong, qinna, and push-hands? There must be some reason. I would suggest that people will make better progress if they practice the complete system. It's better for us to try and see what happens. Some people practice twenty or thirty years and, when you touch them, they don't have the skills they should have. There must be some reason.

If you try just one year, or even six months—try the push-hands, silk reeling, and qigong exercises—see what happens. See whether that can make some difference for your progress.

■ *Do you feel it is important to learn the applications of each movement while you're learning the routines, or learn them later?*
Learn the applications along with the movements. Most of the movements have more than one application. But we should know the basic energy. For example, when we talk about the preparatory form, you have the *peng, lu, ji,* and *an* energies. Everything there is very clear. If you don't know the basic energies you can make some progress, but not as efficient as it's supposed to be. So, understanding the basic energies is a requisite for understanding the we should know the basic applications for of each movement.

■ *So if you teach the first routine, do you teach one application for each movement?*

Not for every movement, just for most of them. Basically, you should tell people what basic energy is there in terms of *peng, lu, ji,* and *an*. Because when we do push-hands, that's basically the application of *peng, lu, ji, an, cai, lie, zhou, kao*—especially during stationary push-hands. These are the main forces; therefore, we need to train these forces. So, when we do the routine, I think we should understand the *peng, lu, ji,* and *an* basic energies so it can make more sense for the practice. Like with the *an* energy, if you try it whenever you practice qinna, or push-hands, or whatever, you can apply it.

■ *Are there variations in the routines?*
Variations come for different reasons. Big variations arise because of differences in understanding the theory of the principles, and on personal training and experience. There may be some good or bad variations. It's difficult for people to judge which one is good or bad. My suggestion is to visit different teachers, then compare and see whether the thing you get is correct or should improve, because there's no way you can judge by yourself. If you cannot see the difference, how can you compare? So, I would say, read books, go to different seminars. That doesn't mean you do not respect your teacher, now. You really love the art; that means you love your teacher more.

■ *You have a variety of martial artists attending your workshops, but each seems to find something to help their own practice.*
Whatever you're practicing, see through the workshop whether you can get something maybe you missed, maybe your teacher missed, from the Chen system. Like the silk reeling. Any style has "white crane spreads wings." If you add silk reeling, see the energy there? Even that much makes a big difference. You don't have to change your style. You can get some things from the workshop. That's what I think—especially the silk reeling. Lots of people have knee problems. The problem happens because people have too low of a posture too early in their practice, or they hold an incorrect posture which may hurt their knees. Also, their alignment may not be correct. People twist a lot. The foot and the knee should be consistent with your body's direction. These two things help a lot of people in my workshops. I'm very happy with that. Some people just do the form the wrong way. They come from different styles, not only Chen Style. We do need to move the knee, but the range of motion should be reasonable. That's one big thing I like about Master Feng system: nurture!

PEOPLE				CITY
Chen Xiaowang	陳小旺	Hong Junsheng	洪均生	Jiaozuo 焦作
Chen Zhaokui	陳照奎	Wu Xiubao	吳秀寶	
Chen Zhaopei	陳照丕	Yang Yang	楊楊	
Feng Zhiqiang	馮志強	Yuan Shiming	原士明	
Gu Liuxin	顧留馨	Zhang Xitang	張喜堂	

TECHNICAL SECTION

SILK-REELING

The 1a-e series shows a single-hand exercise where the right wrist turns in a counterclockwise direction. This can be reversed in a clockwise direction with either hand.

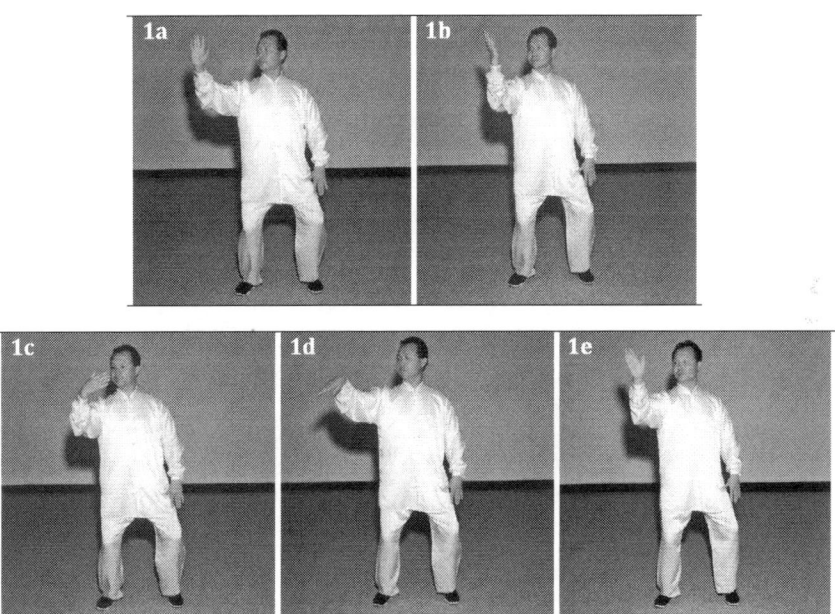

The 2a-c and 3a-c series are double-hand exercises with the wrists moving outward (2) and inward (3).

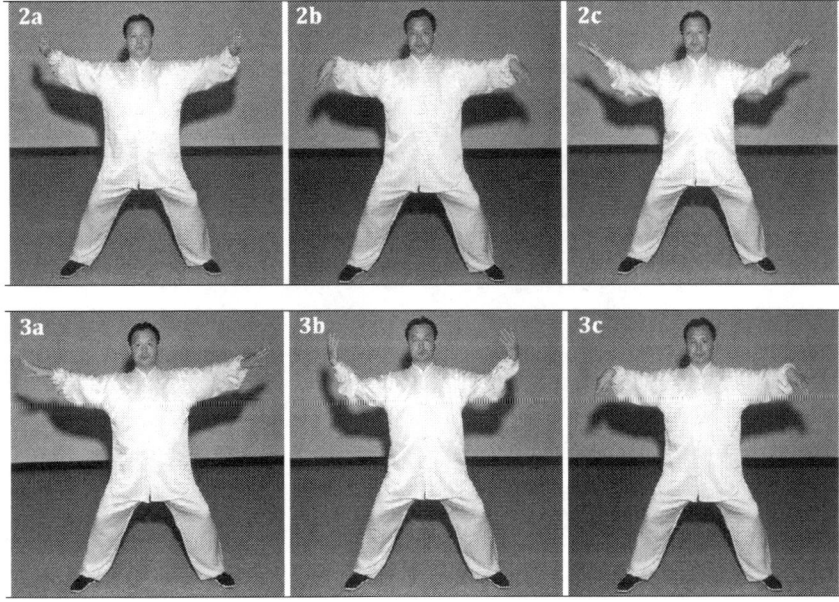

The 4a-f series involves moving the right arm in a circle while shifting the weight. From 4f. drop the right arm and shift into the 4a posture and repeat. Practice with the left side also.

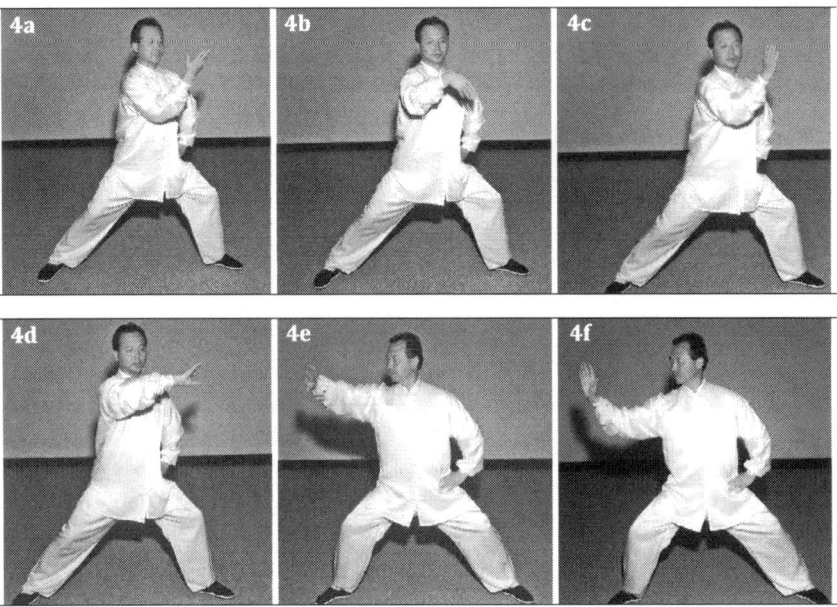

SILK REELING

The 5a-f series is like the preceding 4a-f series, except the rotation is done with the elbow circling.

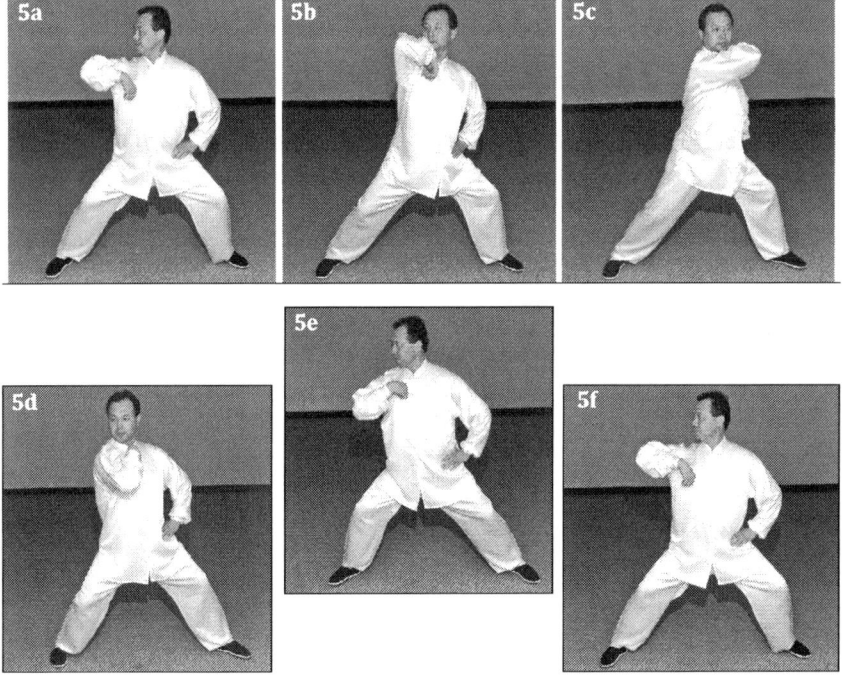

SILK REELING

The 6a-f series commences with both hands held in fists to the sides. They then cross in front of the navel and begin to circle upwards. You can see a rising of the waist as the legs slightly straighten. The arms continue to circle outward to the sides. The body sinks downward in unison with the arms' downward movement to their original position.

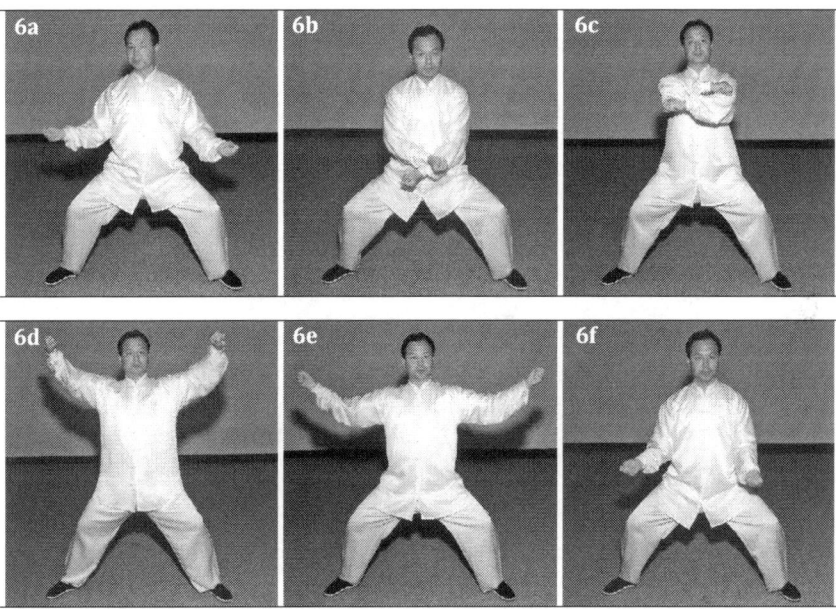

QINNA

In the following examples, two defensive locking techniques are shown. Yang's right wrist is grabbed from the same side in the 1a-d series. He moves his left hand over the top of the grabbing hand to hold it in place. As this is secured, he rotates his right hand over the opponent's to bring pressure on his wrist. The opponent sinks to relieve some of the pressure. If Yang continue to apply pressure in a downward motion, the opponent will go to the floor in submission.

x

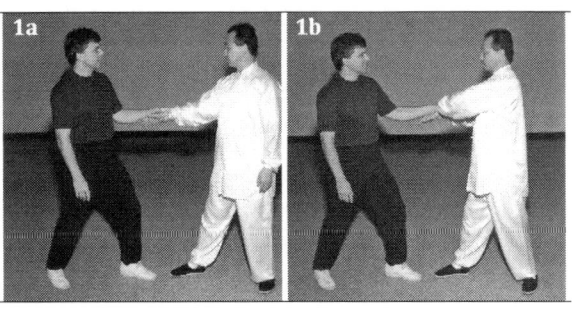

(1c and 1d on next page)

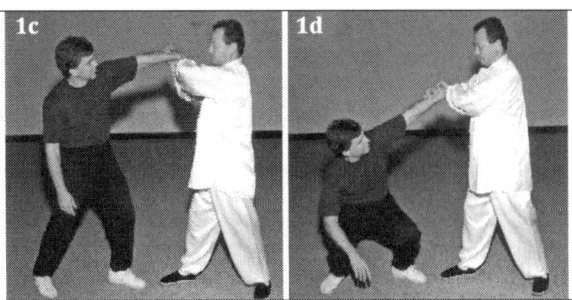

The 2a-d series is like the 1a-d series except the grab is done from the opposite side with the opponent reaching with his right hand for Yang's right wrist. Again, Yang secures the grabbing hand with his own left hand. This time, he circles his right hand clockwise around the opponent's wrist having the same result.

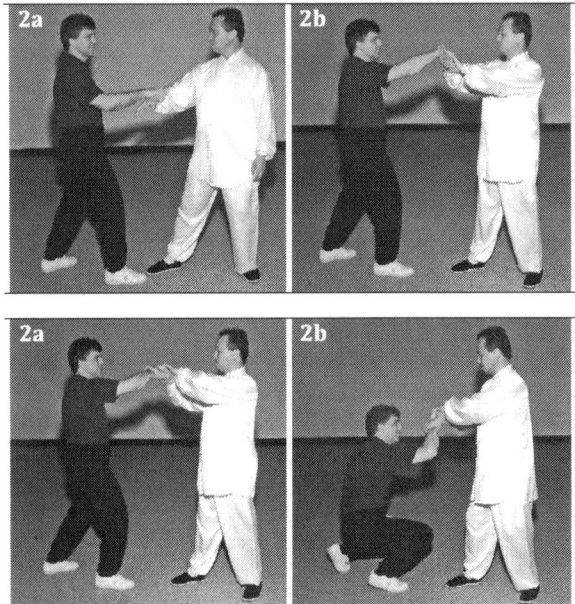

COUNTER-QINNA

Counter-qinna offers a way to respond to a locking technique with another locking technique. In the 1a-d series. Yang grabs his opponent's right wrist. The opponent moves into the wrist lock technique shown previously in the 2a-d series. With his left hand, Yang secures his opponent's hands while relieving the pressure on his own wrist by circling his right elbow upwards then onto his opponent's arms. As Yang sinks downward, his opponent is locked and placed off-balance. This makes it easy for Yang to shift into a shoulder-push.

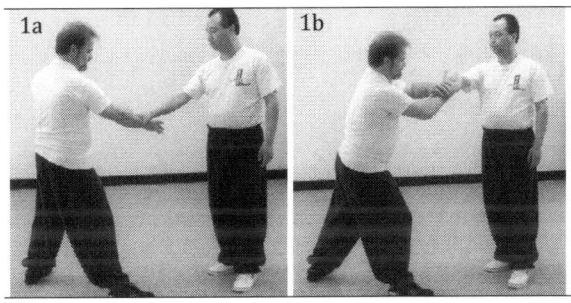

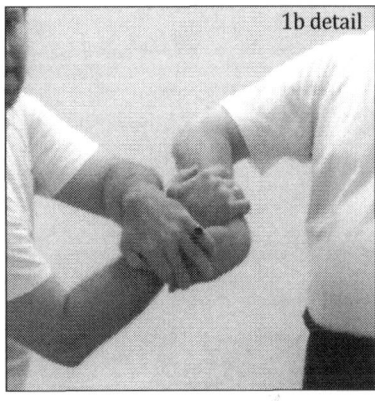

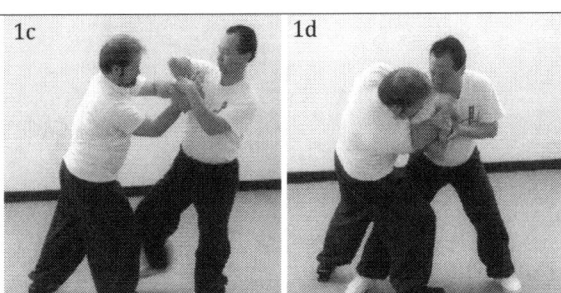

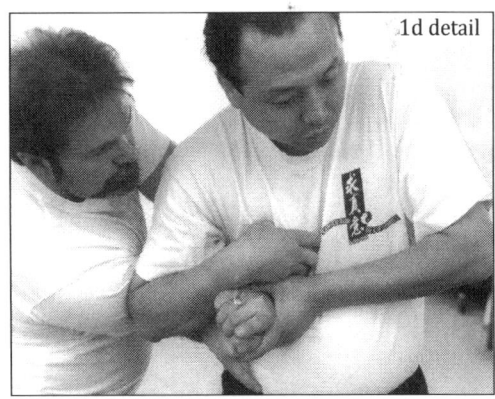

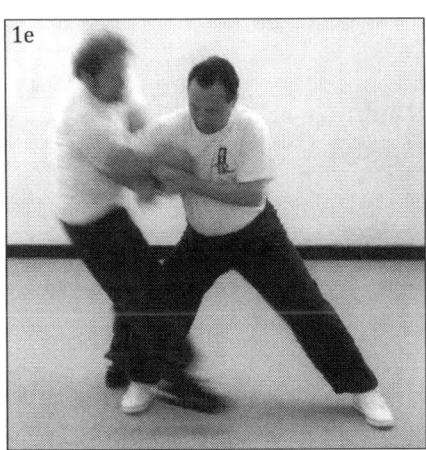

Photography courtesy of Larry Justinas.

Yang demonstrates three ways to counter a lock when pressure is applied to the wrist as the elbow is held (2A-B-C). According to what he senses, he first moves to render the lock ineffective and then throws the opponent either forward (A), past his right side (B), or downward (C).

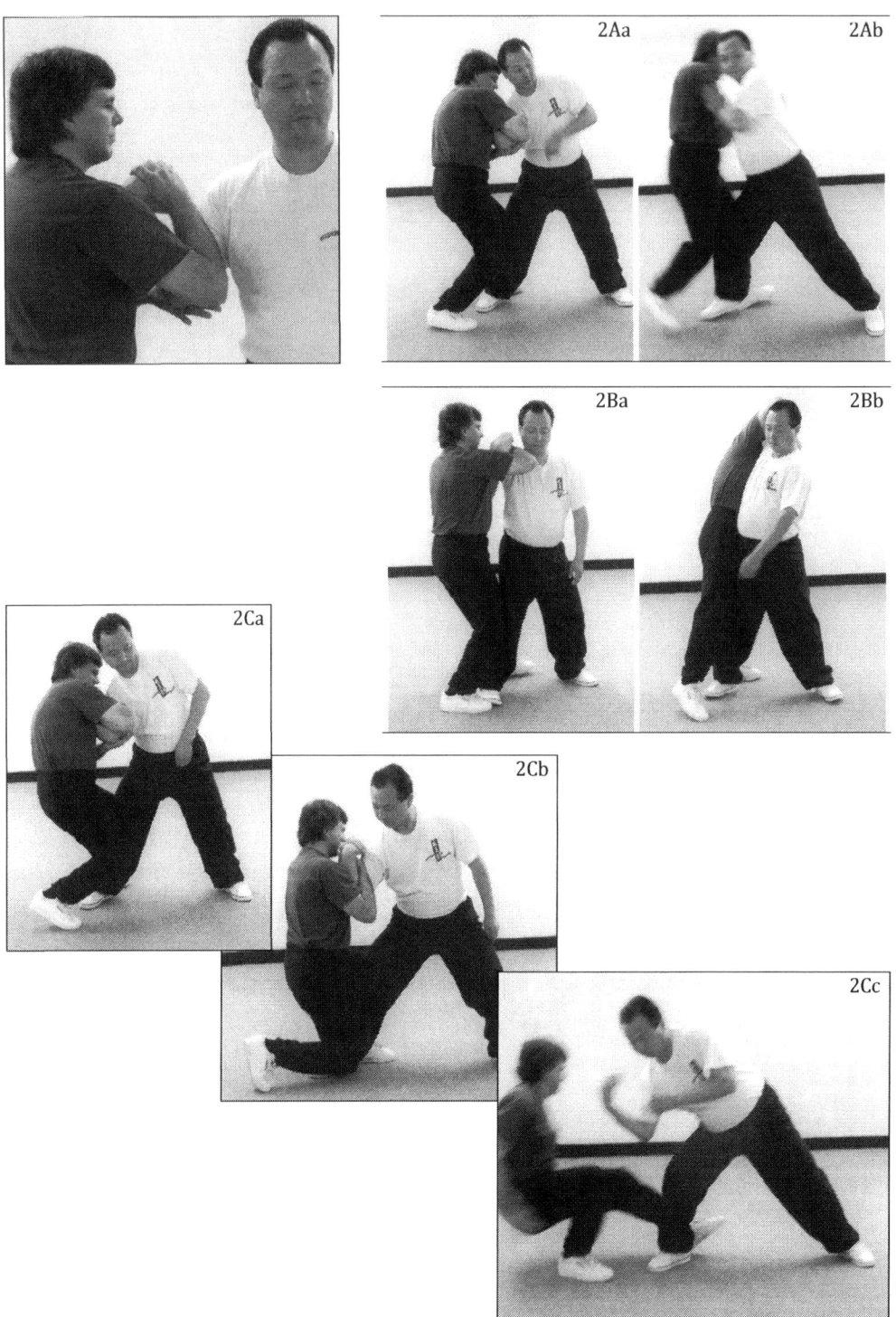

COUNTER-QINNA

Yang shows a simple counter to an upper-arm hold (3a-c). He turns his own arms outward which causes the opponent to lose the security of his grip. At the same time. Yang shifts forward to push his opponent off-balance.

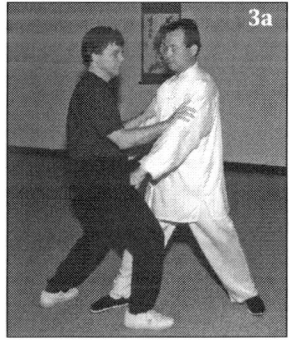
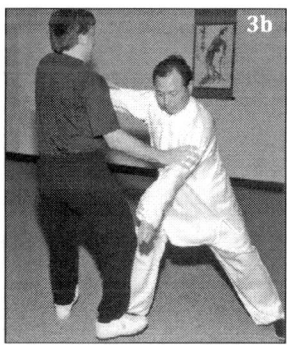
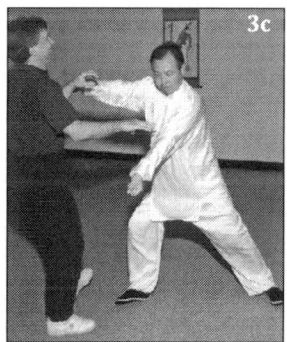

In series 4a-h, a grab is countered with a counter-qinna as shown previously in the 1a-e counter-qinna sequence. Yang follows the counter-qinna with another counter by sinking and moving into a forward push.

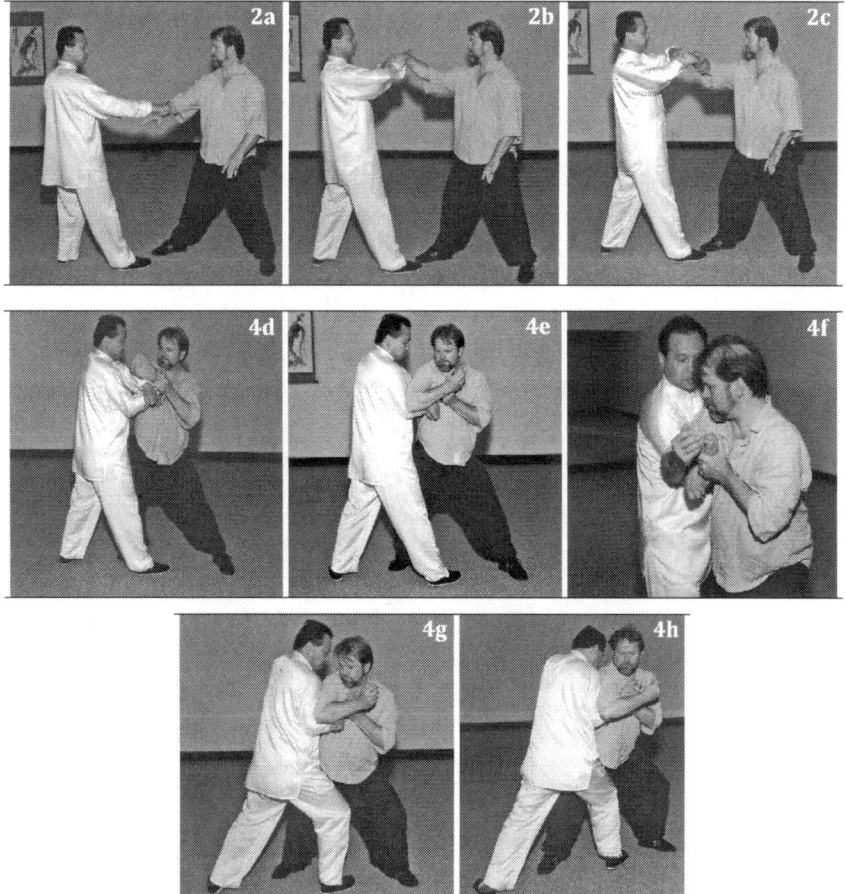

COUNTER-QINNA

Yang shows a defense against an upper arm grab or push in the 5a-d sequence. Rather than placing strength against strength. Yang counters by pushing his opponent's arms slightly outward to break the foundational source of his opponent's push. He then steps in to push the unbalanced opponent backwards.

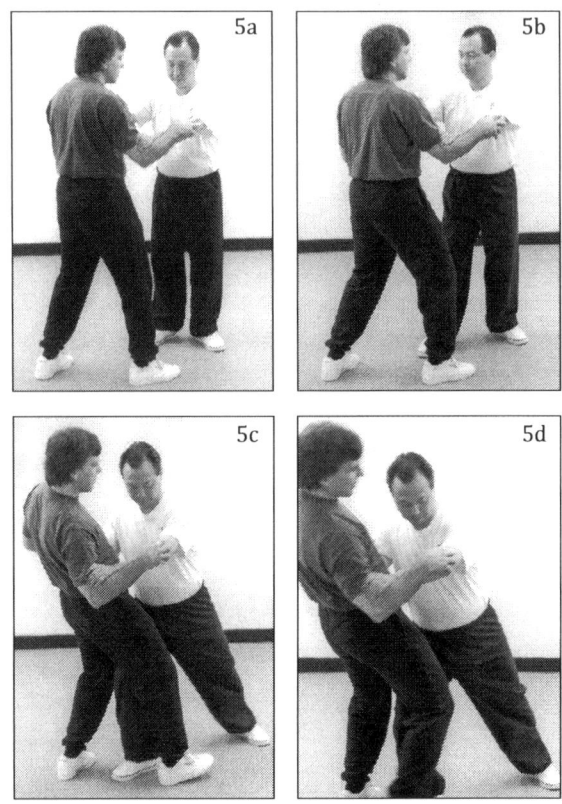

In the following sequences. Yang manipulates a one-hand push against his chest (6a-c) and against his stomach area (7a-c). Both are countered in a similar fashion by securing the opponent's elbow to secure the arm. This allows Yang to lock the opponent's forearm which applies pressure against his opponent's wrist. As the opponent withers in pain, it is easy for Yang to step forward to throw the opponent.

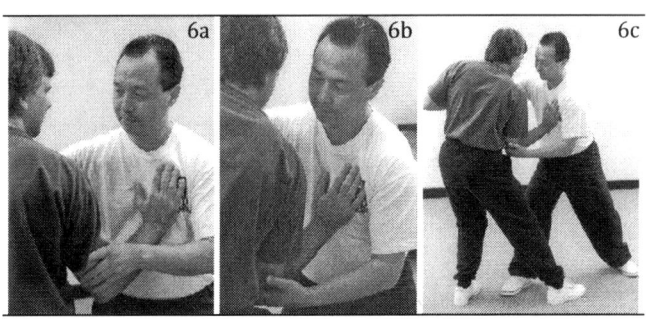

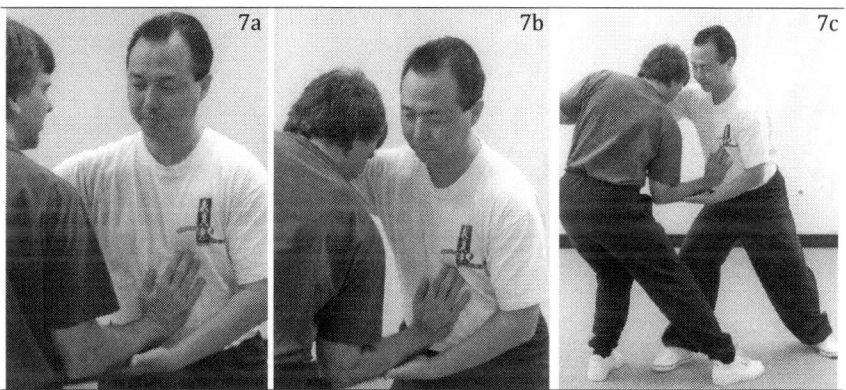

Concluding Remarks

The technical section provided on the previous pages is an attempt to illustrate how silk reeling and qinna practices are interrelated. The circular silk reeling movements can be found in locking techniques and counters, as well as in the Chen Style's solo routines and energy work (*qigong*).

• 32 •

Taiji's Chen Village Under the Influence of Chen Xiaoxing
by Stephan Berwick, M.A.*

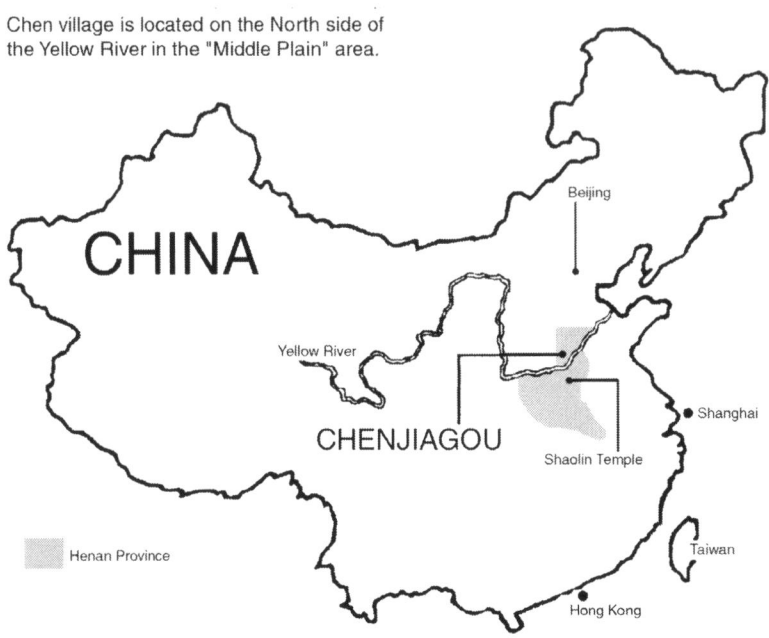

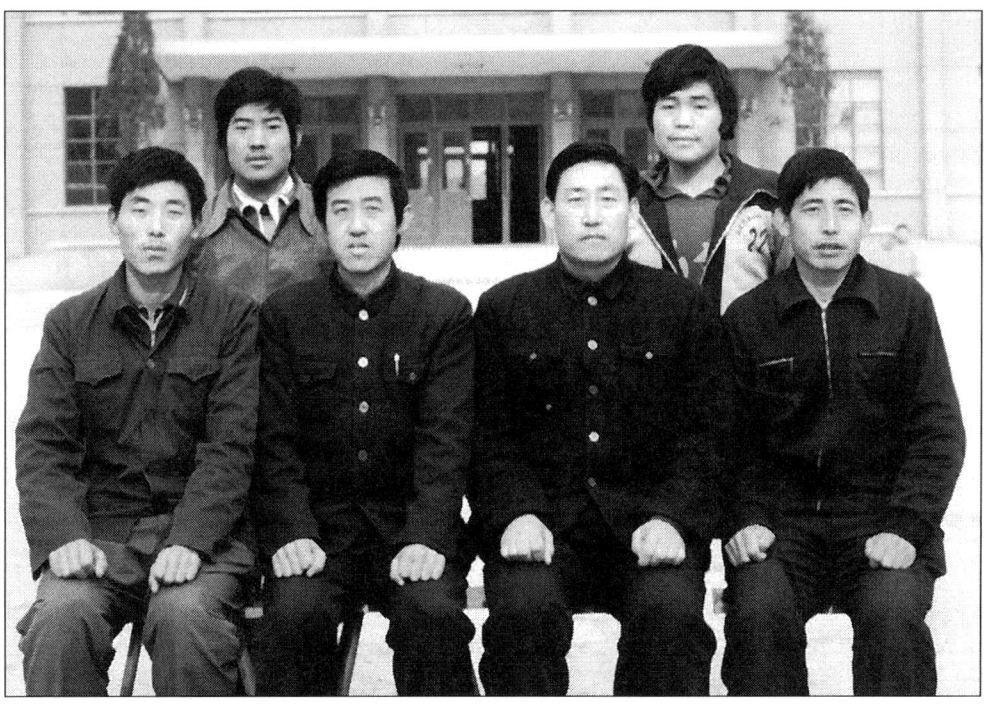

Rare photo from 1985 with (from right) Chen Xiaoxing, Chen Xiaowang, and Chen Zhenglei in front of the Chenjiagou Training Academy. Photos courtesy of Stephan Berwick, Chen Xiaoxing, and Ren Guangyi.

Introduction

Young athletes at the *Chenjiagou* (Chen Family Village) training academy usually begin their day with an "old-fashioned" breakfast of thick cornmeal soup, vegetables, and steamed bread. For hard-training boxers, their very large bowls of soup boast a clean, nourishing flavor that seems to fill the Chen Village boxing trainee with more than just breakfast. In this village of ancient boxers, the soup hints at the Chen Village saying, "If you drink the water in Chen Village, you will kick very well." In essence, this breakfast is a tradition that is a reminder of what fortified the early boxers of the renowned Chen Village.

The Chen Village gives the first-time visitor an infusion of both family and martial art spirit that is hard to find elsewhere. The village's houses and roads are virtually unchanged since its founding by the first Chen (nine generations ago), who settled in this gully area close to the Yellow River. Chen Village's untouched rural quality lends its boxing art a rare purity. Thus, what is usually only a memory in the world of Chinese martial tradition persists in Chen Village today.

Like all traditions, assimilating a martial arts tradition requires that one step back to move forward. Although the martial art standard bearers of traditions that breed combat mastery are becoming easier to find, training under them for an extended period remains difficult. In an age of high technology, economic opportunity, and firearms, committing to a quality teacher is often impractical for most contemporary martial artists. Regardless, today's traditional martial arts enthusiast continues to seek unbroken martial traditions. In the quest to find bearers of mature martial traditions, enthusiasts can seek out the best teachers they have access to or go to the source of their martial arts discipline—if the source still exists.

Be it by design or luck, the birthplace of taijiquan remains intact. The over 400-year-old village of the Chen family—in Wen County, Henan Province—is one of the few places in the world where one of the oldest and enormously influential martial traditions survives in purity. Even though some martial art researchers have questioned the exact origins of taiji, citing a lack of early martial art writings from Chen Village, its maturity and pervasiveness suggest otherwise (Wile, 1996: 117).

A normal day in Chen Village is built around farming and boxing. Boxing practice takes place everywhere: in the fields, at homes, and at the village school. However, the village school remains the nucleus of boxing training.

At the height of his teaching career, the eighteenth-generation grandmaster, Chen Zhaopei, organized classes for the villagers based out of his home. His promotion and organization of taiji instruction led to the evolution of Chen Village's formal training academy, built in 1982. This sleep-in, full-time training academy has its roots in Zhaopei's original ideas. Nineteenth generation exponents remember him as the Chen family boxing master responsible for the revival of taiji practice in the village amidst the political and social upheaval of China's contemporary history (Rich, 2000).

Chen Taijiquan Standard Bearer

Chen Zhaopei's example created a new standard of leadership for the modern masters of Chen Village. At Zhaopei's urging, Chen Zhaokui—son of Chen Fake—returned to Chen Village to train the best of the nineteenth generation masters that lead the art today. Of the small group that was mentored by Chen Zhaokui, Chen Xiaoxing was one of the youngest. With Chen Zhaopei's commitment to Chen Village as inspiration, along with intimate coaching from his older brother—Chen Xiaowang, protégé of Chen Zhaokui, and the current nineteenth generation style standard bearer—Chen Xiaoxing's early training prepared him to quietly emerge as the head teacher in Chen Village.

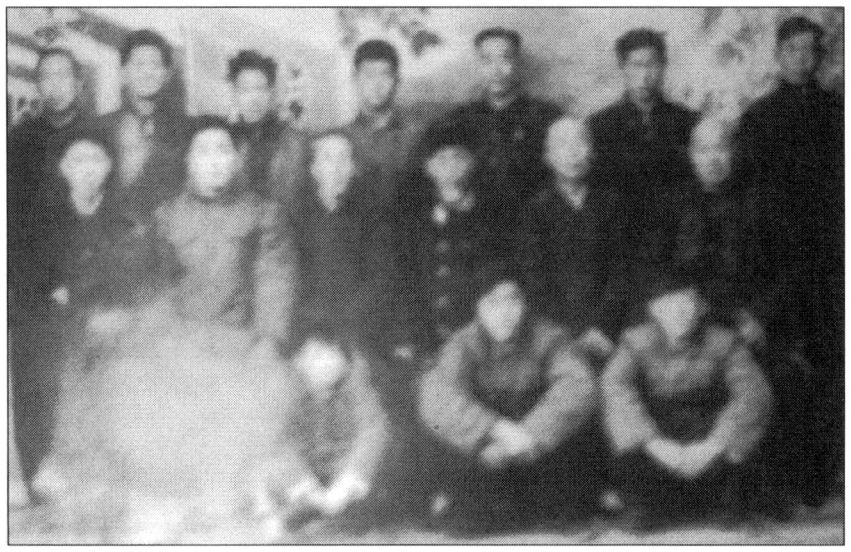

Extremely rare group photo from 1965. First seated teenager from right, Chen Xiaowang; third from right, Chen Xiaoxing. Second row: first from right, Chen Zhaopei; fifth from right, Chen Zhaokui. Grey spot on photo is from a camera flash.

As the head boxing teacher in Chen Village, Chen Xiaoxing is not only the senior boxing master in the village but is a community leader who commands respect. During morning and mid-day strolls with the grandmaster, the author witnessed the deference and affectionate respect accorded him. Villagers refer to him only as *shifu* (teacher) and *laoshi* (elder teacher) whenever they speak with him.

His early morning routine begins with tending to the affairs of the academy and teaching. He often ends the day with an occasional game of mahjong with village elders—often at a courtyard adjacent to the original training hall where fourteenth generation grandmaster and compiler of the old frame (*laojia*) forms, Chen Changxing, taught Yang Luchan.

Chen Xiaoxing's commitment to the village and its stable of boxers is unique in a martial arts era often dominated by legitimate masters, such as his world-renowned older brother, Chen Xiaowang, who work hard to spread their art by teaching seminars for students globally. In this vein, his older brother has done much to spread authentic Chen taijiquan. However, Chen Xiaoxing has chosen another, more traditional path to pass on the high standards of skill characteristic of Chen Style taiji boxers.

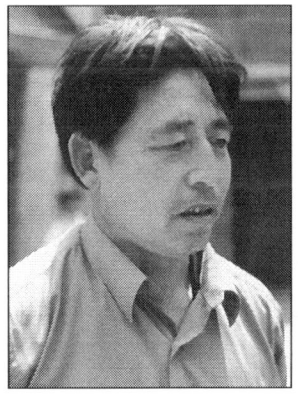 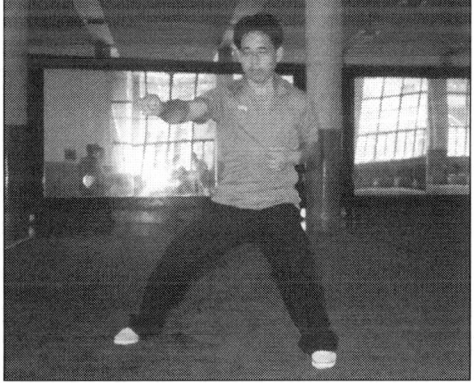

Left: Chen Xiaoxing in front of his family home.
Right: Chen Xiaoxing demonstrating punching skills.

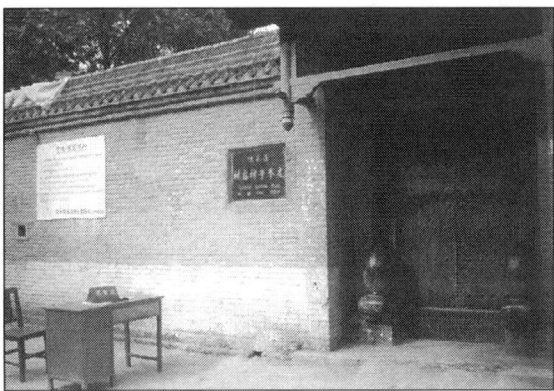

Above: The training hall in Chenjiagou, where Chen Changxing taught Yang Luchan.
Below: Chen Xiaoxing in front of the large Chen Family Taijiquan altar.

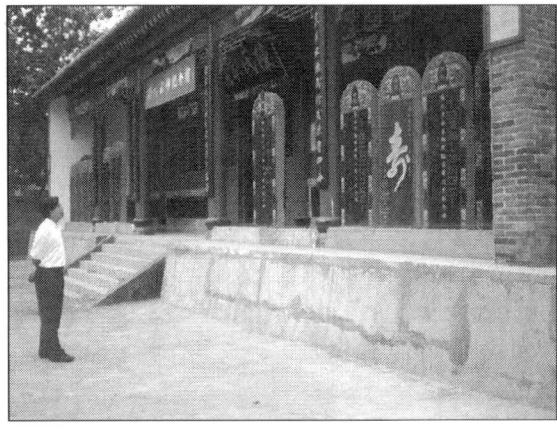

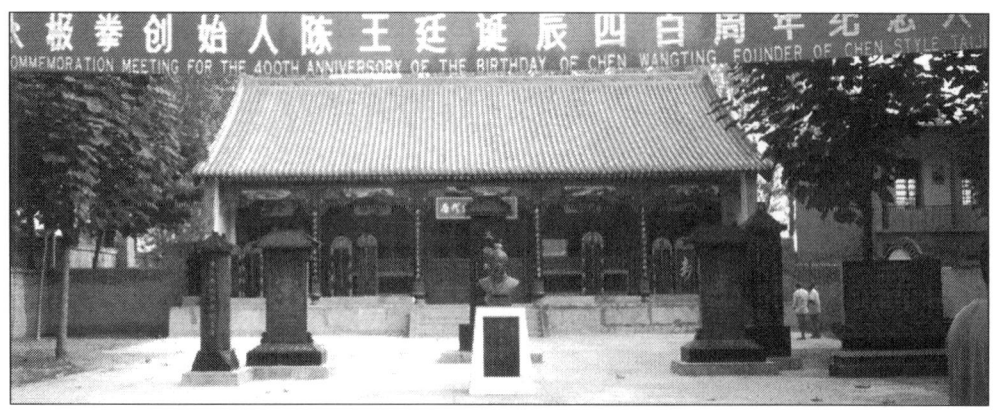

Wide view of the Chen family taijiquan altar with banner celebrating the 400th birthday of Chen taiji founder, Chen Wangting.

Continuing the tradition of high technical standards built around famous Chen taiji concepts, including the training of silk reeling energy (*chansijing*) and the application of the yin and yang theory, Chen Xiaoxing says: "I am inspired by my brother to pass on a high quality art." Chen Xiaoxing not only runs the village school, he also closely mentors the next generation of Chen taiji masters, including his nephew, Chen Xiaowang's youngest son and boxing prodigy, Chen Pengfei.

Like his elder, Chen Zhaopei, Chen Xiaoxing coaches aspiring village boxers and foreigners. Chen Xiaoxing asserts that "I am committed to remaining in Chen Village to teach and pass on the highest quality art possible to the next generation." His commitment to teaching in the village is an example of how traditions are preserved at the source.

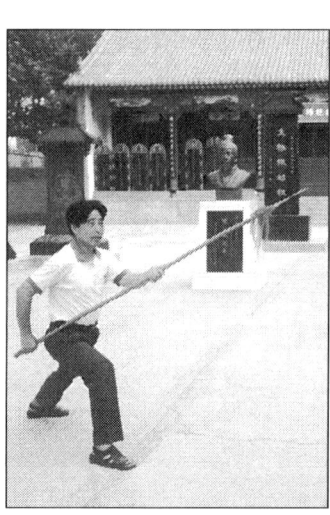 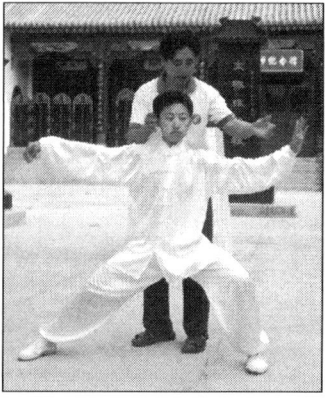 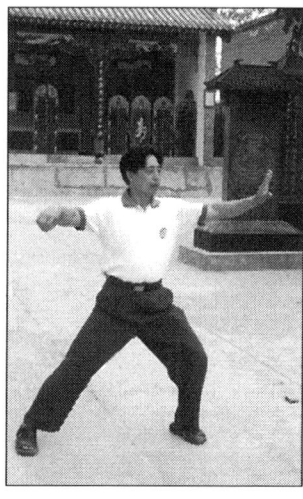

Left: Chen Xiaoxing demonstrating a spear form. Center and right: Chen Xiaoxing correcting and demonstrating for his nephew, Chen Pengfei, who is the youngest son of Chen Xiaowang.

The Making of a Traditional Boxing Master

Born in 1952, Chen Xiaoxing is one of only a handful of accomplished taiji masters alive today who were trained by the best of Chen taiji's legendary masters, including Chen Xiaowang, Chen Zhaopei, and his uncle, Chen Zhaokui. Chen Xiaoxing's martial arts training personifies an old Chen Village saying: "In Chen Village, by the time you're two, you can execute diamond pestle" [a classic Chen taiji technique].

Chen Xiaoxing began training at the age of six. He was first taught by his older brother, Chen Xiaowang, then Chen Zhaopei, and then again by his brother. Most of his early training was spent with just Chen Xiaowang. He describes this period, "as a peaceful, quiet time." He focused on the classic first form of Chen taiji, the old frame, first form (*laojia yilu*), averaging an astounding thirty repetitions of this long form per day. Later, weapons and push-hands training (*tuishou*) were added to his regimen. In 1972, he started training under Chen Zhaokui, who taught him Chen Fake's new frame (*xinjia*)—Chen Fake's more detailed version of the open-hand forms.

Chen Xiaoxing related that, "Chen Zhaokui's return to Chen Village in 1964 brought much change to the villagers' practice. Zhaokui corrected mistakes and elevated their skill." Xiaoxing studied under Chen Zhaokui until 1980. Because of his young age, he then resumed his training under his brother, who became Chen Zhaokui's protégé. When Chen Xiaoxing resumed training under his then highly advanced brother, his training "became especially intense."

His training history illustrates how traditions and standards are passed in Chen Village. Fathers, elder brothers, and uncles routinely mentor the best of the next generation in public and private classes. Now open to non-Chen family members, this type of family-shared training remains intact. This openness to teaching outsiders began when seventeenth-generation grandmaster Chen Changxing taught Yang Luchan in Chen Village.

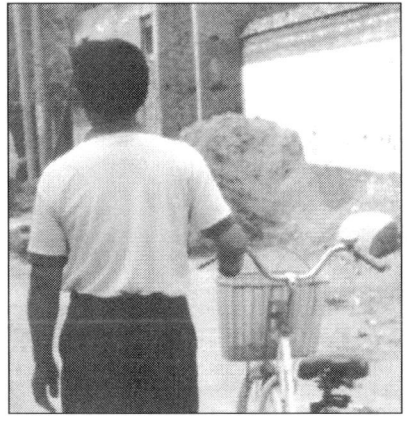
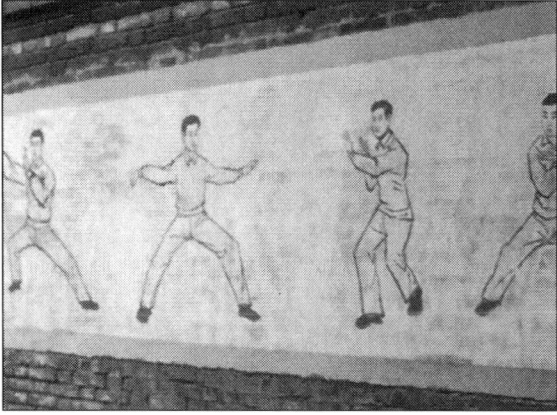

Chen Xiaoxing walking his bicycle next to an old Chenjiagou wall adorned with depictions of Chen taiji postures.

A Master Teacher Emerges

As standard practice among the Chen Village boxers, Chen Xiaoxing started teaching at age 18. In 1976, he traveled throughout China teaching taiji. By the mid-1980's, his teaching ideas began to change. Based on direct influence from his brother, he began to focus more on teaching core taijiquan principles such as standing exercises (*zhanzhuang*) and silk reeling. Chen Xiaoxing stated that because of this new approach, "by the 1990's, my teaching improved."

He now crafts his curriculum around the individual. He advises practitioners to focus on silk reeling and standing exercises for their foundation. Chen Xiaoxing reminds us that, "The serious Chen taiji student should seek to achieve a balance of yin and yang forces in the body." He also advises that students follow Chen Style's traditional five stages of training (Chen, 1990: Section 4; Berwick, 1999: 189–195).

In the late 1990's, he took over the management of the village training center. The school is very much "community oriented" according to Daniel Poon, an Englishman who has been living in Chen Xiaoxing's home to study full-time at the village school. The school is a center of local exhibitions, often for large groups of visiting government officials or foreigners. When visitors are expected, the young students go into action cleaning the grounds and assembling seating and snacks for the audience. Under Chen Xiaoxing's supervision, great care and spirit go into these often-last-minute performances.

Chen Xiaoxing says, "Taiji remains very popular in the village. The average Chen Village practitioner trains hard and possesses good skill. Most of the villagers are serious about taiji, but it is still hard to find protégés." Over the next few years, he hopes the school will offer regular academic subjects to the young live-in students, while remaining focused on taiji. He feels this will help attract and retain serious students.

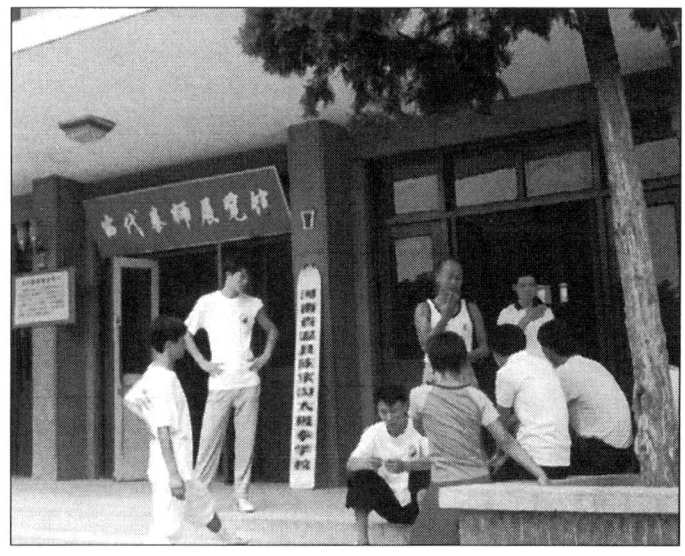

Students conversing on the footsteps of the Chenjiagou Training Academy.

Typical country hospitality belies his stature as the head boxing master in Chen Village. Very laid back and easy to talk to, Chen Xiaoxing treats foreign students as family guests. He remembers Chen Style starting to really become popular in 1979. He recalls, "In 1982, foreigners started to regularly visit the village, but in 1988, visits of foreigners decreased." Now he sees, "they are returning because China is becoming richer." He stated, "I invite all serious students—foreign and domestic—to come to Chen Village to train."

Training in Chen Village: The Foreign Student's Perspective

Short visits to Chen Village for specialized training have been the norm for a small but increasing number of foreign enthusiasts. But committing to stay in the village for extended periods of training can be daunting for even the hardiest. One such foreigner, thirty-three-year-old U.K. born, Daniel Poon, embarked on this trek with a willingness and freedom to leave behind his normal comforts and diversions to train classically in an isolated, highly rural environment.

With only an intermediate conversational skill in Mandarin, Poon took advantage of Chen Xiaoxing's offer to teach all those of good character and high commitment. He has been living at Chen Xiaoxing's home for almost a year studying boxing full-time. A taiji practitioner since 1995, Poon is a student of the UK's Michael Tse. Poon stated that he "came to Chen Village with an excellent foundation in Chen Style from Tse," a well-regarded qigong instructor who also teaches Chen taijiquan. Poon came to the village with training in the old frame form of Chen Style and experience with the application practice of sparring and push-hands. At Chen Village, he learned new frame, weapons, and continues his training in push-hands. His experience and observations reveal the unique pleasures and peculiarities of training in today's Chen Village—as both a village resident and a foreigner.

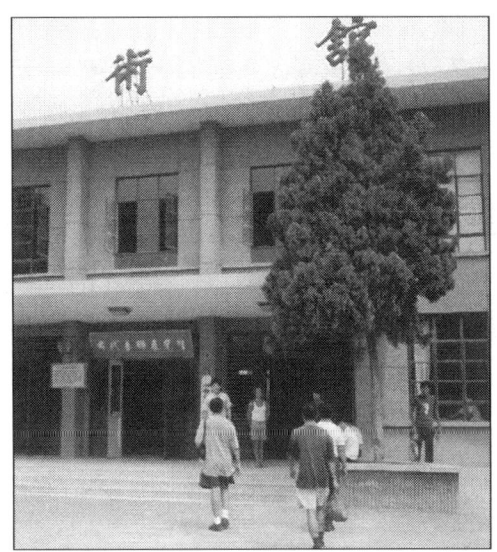 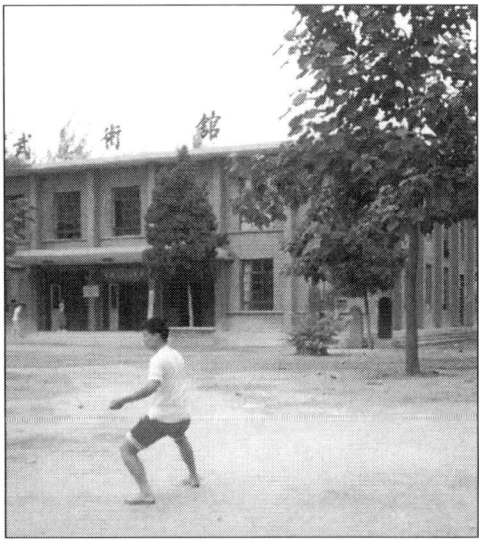

Left: Students entering the Chenjiagou Training Academy. Right: Training courtyard in front of the Chenjiagou Training Academy where people can be found practicing anytime.

At first, Poon studied under Chen Xiaoxing. He partly joked how "Chen Xiaoxing didn't want me to get trounced on by the locals [in training]. When you first get here, it can be overwhelming, so you need someone to hold your hand." After training with Chen Xiaoxing, Poon began to train at the village school. His learning then became "like osmosis." He describes the daily training as "very informal." Poon advises that, "One can learn forms easily from many in the village, but posture corrections are best had from the best instructors here." He says that in the village, "although there are many who practice, the best are the smartest ones."

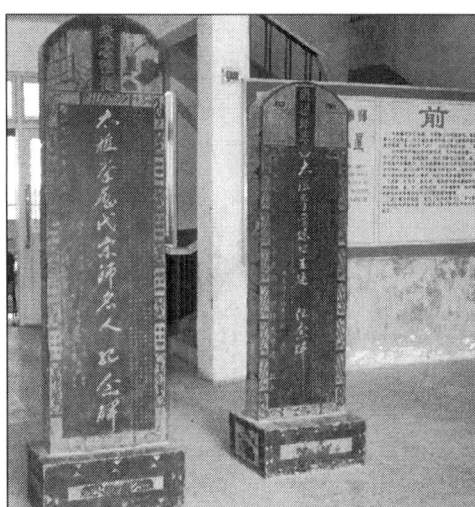 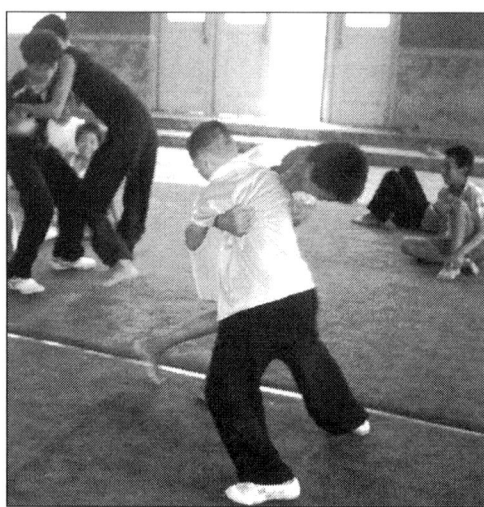

Left: Old Chen taiji lineage stone stile in the foyer of the Chenjiagou Training Academy.
Right: Youth sparring or "pushing" class in the Chenjiagou Training Academy.

In Chen Village, training remains highly traditional, yet accessible. This may very well be Chen Village's greatest gift to the contemporary taiji student seeking classical training. While training in Chen Village is arduous, it is not as rigid and fast-paced as the large government-sponsored wushu academies that exist in China's major cities. Coeducational training is standard, except for the push-hands training. Training at the village academy is intense before some national competitions and the recently established biannual international competition held in Wen County but is generally self-paced and progressive. Twice-per-day training sessions are the norm. Virtually all taiji students practice open-hand forms, weapons, and sparring daily. Poon observes, "Because of the physical hardship of the life here, along with the very young average starting age, training starts at a higher level. In the West, corrections are necessary for just learning how to stand properly, while in Chen Village posture corrections usually begin with the Single Whip posture."

From the beginning of training, the foundational old frame first form is emphasized without learning other material for long periods. In fact, the emphasis on perfecting the old frame first form continues for years, well into the advanced stages of proficiency that usually includes the new frame, weapons, and push-hands, plus plenty of wrestling and joint locking [*qinna*].

As a member of the village school, Poon is expected to participate in the demonstrations that occur frequently. Now considered a part of the Chen Village community, Poon insists, "I understand taiji's history and evolution much better." Unmistakably, his experience in Chen Village was, in essence, a step back in time, to move forward with his taijiquan.

* Translation assistance by Chen Pengfei and Ren Guangyi.

Bibliography

Berwick, S. (1997, October). Chen taijiquan combat training. *Inside Kung Fu, 24*(10), 189–195.

Chen, X. (1933). *Illustrated explanation of Chen family taijiquan*. No publisher given.

Chen, X. (1990). *Chen family transmission* (Chinese). Beijing: People's Sports Press.

Little, J. and Wong, C. (Eds.) (1999). *Ultimate tai chi*. Chicago: Contemporary Books.

Rich, H. (2000). Chen Style Taijiquan homepage. http://www.digidao.com.

Wallace, A. (1998). Internal training: The foundation for Chen taiji's fighting skills and health promotion. *Journal of Asian Martial Arts, 7*(1), 58–89.

Wile, D. (1996). *Lost tai chi classics from the late Ch'ing dynasty*. Albany, NY: State University of New York Press.

• 33 •
Chen Xiaowang on Learning, Practicing, and Teaching Chen Taiji
by Stephan Berwick

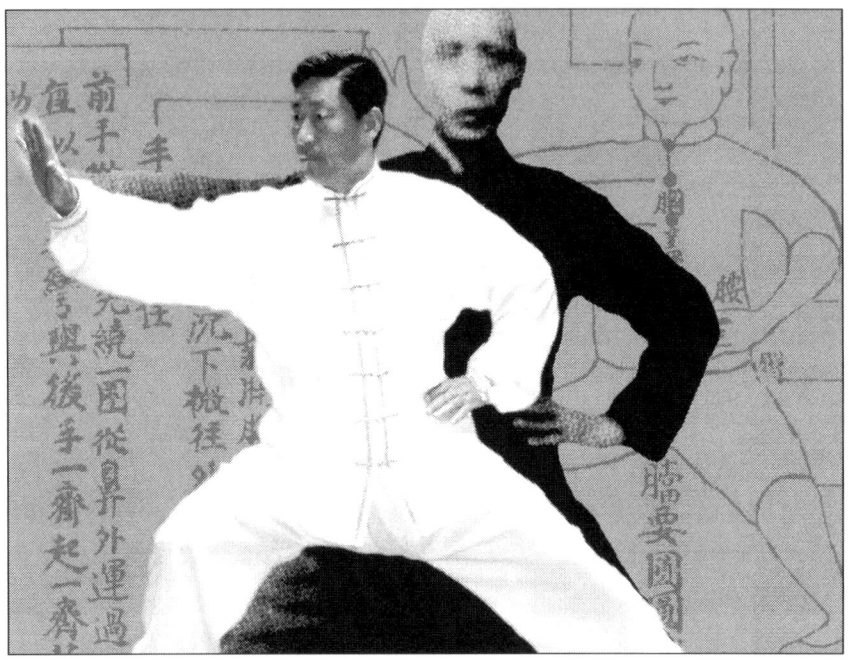

Chen Xiaowang demonstrating the laojia version of lazily tying coat.

The following is the only substantive interview Grandmaster Chen Xiaowang gave during his 2000 United States seminar tour. This is the first time Grandmaster Chen has shared the details of his early training and family history while offering profound insights into the practice and teaching of Chen taiji.

ON HISTORY

■ *What is your earliest martial arts memory?*
I remember waiting for my father, Chen Zhaoxu, to finish his morning practice before the family breakfast. Watching my father was like watching a movie. This gave me a sense or vision of what high-level taiji is. I didn't study his movements, I just watched him like a movie and retained the vision of what I saw.

■ *When did you begin training in taijiquan and what did you learn first? How serious was your training?*
I started training at the age of eight under my father. I practiced the old frame first form.

At thirteen, when I performed with a group of adult students, I caught the attention of the then senior village master teacher, Chen Zhaopei. When Chen Zhaopei saw me for the first time, he asked: "Whose kid is this?" So, I was very serious with my taiji—even at that young age.

■ *What and when exactly did you study specific aspects of the art?*
I focused on the old frame until 1964, when my uncle, Chen Zhaokui, returned to Chen Village after staying with his father—the famous Chen Fake, who was my paternal grandfather—in Beijing. I was 18 then and began studying Chen Fake's new frame along with qinna. From 1972, I began to focus on the new frame. From 1974 to 1984, I really emphasized new frame and the strength-building training with the [sixteen-posture] Chen Style "big pole" [heavy long staff] form.

■ *When did you first compete?*
I first competed nationally in 1979. I later competed at the first ever international martial arts competition held in Xi'an [Shaanxi Province] in 1985. I've been fortunate to win gold medals consistently during my competition days.

■ *You were a senior martial arts official in the Chinese Government. How did this happen?*
I represented Henan Province at China's 1986 National Congress. Because of my fame and reputation, I was elected to an important senior-level post as head of martial arts for the huge Henan Province—a region full of important martial arts history, including the founding of taiji in my birthplace, Chen Village, and the home of the Shaolin Temple.

■ *When did you first begin your active international teaching career?*
From 1981 to 1985, I was routinely invited overseas, but the Chinese Government was concerned that a martial artist of my standing would leave and not return. But by 1985, many foreigners were visiting Chen Village to learn taiji. So finally in 1985, I was allowed to visit Japan for a few weeks to teach.

ON TEACHING

■ *How do you approach teaching today—especially in light of your experiences teaching Westerners with the popular seminar format?*
I believe everybody can be good at taiji. So, I try to get students to understand taiji better. It is important to understand everybody—all people. I try to offer something individualized as much as possible. To best accomplish this with large groups, I approach each teaching session with a plan. I must be in an environment where I can control the room. Like a general, I speak very clearly while seeing and controlling the class. I never have a problem with the physical room in which a seminar is conducted. When I control the room, I control the students' minds.

■ *Your seminars routinely attract enthusiasts of diverse skill levels. How do you offer something for all, regardless of the material taught?*

There are three languages I use when teaching. They are the language of principles, the language of the body, and the language of corrections. I use different languages for different student levels. So, there is no need for me to separate students based on their skill levels. My seminars are like buffet dinners: I offer different choices of courses, or languages, for different palates on one table.

■ *But are there any real differences when teaching the beginner versus the advanced student?*

When a student is a beginner, I follow him. As he improves, he then follows me.

ON TRAINING

■ *How should the modern Chen taiji boxer train?*

The traditional curriculum is still the preferred route to foundational training, which can take years to perfect. First you focus on old frame first form. Later, weapons, push-hands, and qinna are added.

■ *What about practicing the seemingly more popular new frame?*

The new frame is more detailed and difficult than the traditional old frame. It features more issuing energy (*fajing*). So before practicing the new frame, I recommend the traditional plan of training, of which the old frame is the core. The traditional plan is like first learning to drive. You have no control of the car. As you progress, you will gain more control of the vehicle—in this case, your body and mind—so that you can do more with the car.

■ *What are the most important qualities you recommend to students seeking to gain greater mind/body control?*

You must emphasize an understanding of qi flowing or qi direction. When you understand the meaning of qi flow, you will not have to rely on much physical power. Chen taiji students must remember the movement principles, such as the spiraling characteristic of silk reeling energy. And always remember, the body follows the *dantian* (center).

■ *Can you elaborate on "following the dantian"?*

There are three basic principles: First when the dantian turns right, it also turns left. Second, when the dantian goes back, it also goes front. And third, principles one and two combine. My ancestor Chen Xin's important book on Chen taiji discusses these principles in detail.

■ *What about the much sought after fali or fajing skills?*

Fali [issuing power] should occur naturally. It all goes back to applying the concepts to correct movement.

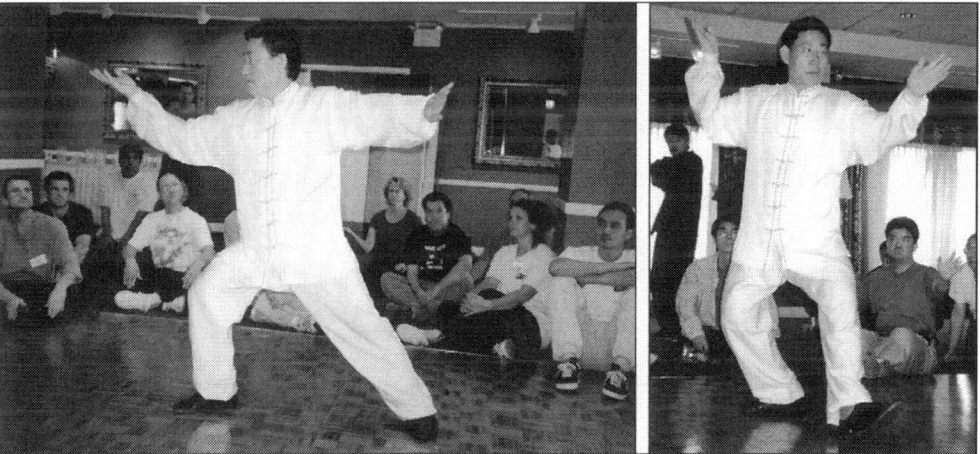

Chen Xiaowang demonstrating parting the horse's mane (left) and stepping at a recent seminar in New York City.

ON LEARNING

■ *What is your personal training like today?*
I remain focused on the details. Details are the most important things for me when seeking a higher level. Even though I teach so much now, I was never interested in making a living at this. I was always just concerned with the details.

■ *How are you still learning and improving?*
Even very recently there were some techniques that I only had a 50% understanding. For instance, in a 1997 seminar in Switzerland, a student tried to test my technique by suddenly and forcefully choking my neck from behind. I responded intuitively with fajing, using the rear elbow strike from the hidden hand punch technique, which hit him in his exposed xiphoid process. I was terrified to see that he immediately fell into cardiac arrest. To my relief, paramedics arrived in time to stabilize him. It was only after the incident that I fully understood that technique, because I never had to really use it before.

■ *What a story!*
I have many more. I love to tell stories, because I am still very much in love with taijiquan.

An Introduction to Seizing Techniques in Chen Style Taijiquan

by Yaron Seidman, L.Ac.

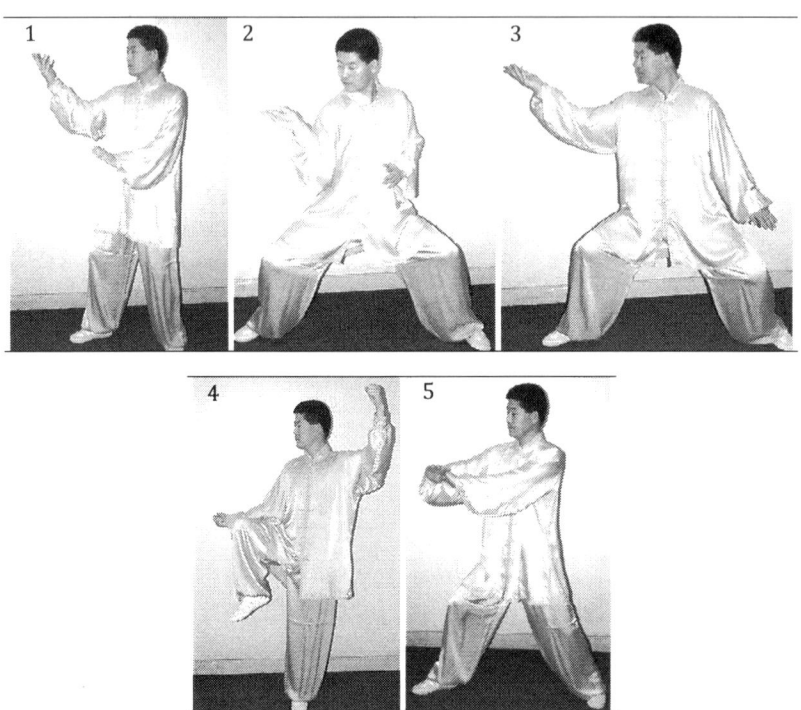

All photographs by Thomas Yeong.

Introduction

Chen taijiquan is the oldest of the taiji schools, dating back to the seventeenth century. This martial arts style is known for developing the fighting skills of its practitioners on various levels. The first and most basic skill is dealing with an incoming attack at the physical level. At this level, the practitioner learns to relax and adjust his body to the incoming power. By doing that, the attack is dissolved, and the practitioner changes his defense into attack. While at this phase, it is common to use seizing techniques. The practitioner locks his opponent's joints, thus ending the fight.

Qinna translates from Chinese Mandarin as "seizing and catching," however, it also means catching and putting somebody in a difficult position. It is an inseparable part of every Chinese martial artist's curriculum. Chen taijiquan is no different. As a martial art based on the principles of taiji and the so-called "thirteen postures," taijiquan utilizes qinna application within its frame of concept. The "thirteen postures" are thirteen arts of energy:

meet	follow	push	press
pluck	adverse	elbow	lean
advance	retreat	rightwards	leftwards
centering			

These energy arts are closely integrated in qinna techniques. Examples can be found on the following pages: "meeting" (A1), "following" (B4), "pressing" (E4).

Every single technique contains the whole thirteen postures. While applying qinna, the whole body is reacting as a one unified life energy (qi), which means that every part of the body is synchronizing with all other parts to work as one force. In one single technique, it is sometimes necessary for the hands to meet, the legs to follow, the anatomical center (*dantian*) to press, and the elbows to adverse all at the same time.

The taiji principle is "yin and yang." Yin and yang is "softness and hardness" and "slow and quick." In taijiquan's qinna techniques, the practitioner must clearly distinguish hardness and softness and moving slowly and quickly. When the opponent is hard, one must be very soft and follow. When the opponent yields, one must be very hard and penetrating. When the opponent is moving slowly, one must follow slowly and adhere. When the opponent is moving fast, one must respond quickly and reach first. As it is clearly stated in the *Taiji Classics*: "When you do not move, I do not move. When you move, I move first. When the opponent's internal energy reaches my skin, my internal energy reaches his bone marrow".

Keeping that in mind, the practitioner is primarily practicing taijiquan, as well as using qinna to supplement it. There are many steps on the path to mastering the vast field of taijiquan. Qinna is a building block on this path, which every practitioner should encounter and get familiar with.

TECHNICAL SECTION
Techniques demonstrated by Chen Zhonghua and Yaron Seidman.

1) WRIST LOCK — as in the form Buddha's warrior pounds the mortar.
- **1a)** Starting in the initial position for practicing all the different locking techniques (1 thru 5), two people face each other while standing about six feet apart.
- **1b)** When the attacker steps in and punches with his right fist, the defender steps in immediately with his right hand meeting the right wrist and his left hand meeting the attacker's right elbow.
- **1c)** The defender then pushes his right hand forward, causing the punching hand to bend backwards toward the attacker's face. At the same time, the defender's left hand controls the attacker's right elbow from moving. At this stage, it is important for the defender to have both his elbows close to each other to gain control over the attacker's arm.

See following page for 1a, 1b and 1c.

1d) The defender sinks and uses his body weight to press down on the attacker's right wrist. At the same time, the defender uses his left hand to push the attacker's right elbow upward.

1e) The defender turns his waist towards the left and sinks more, bringing the attacker down to the ground.

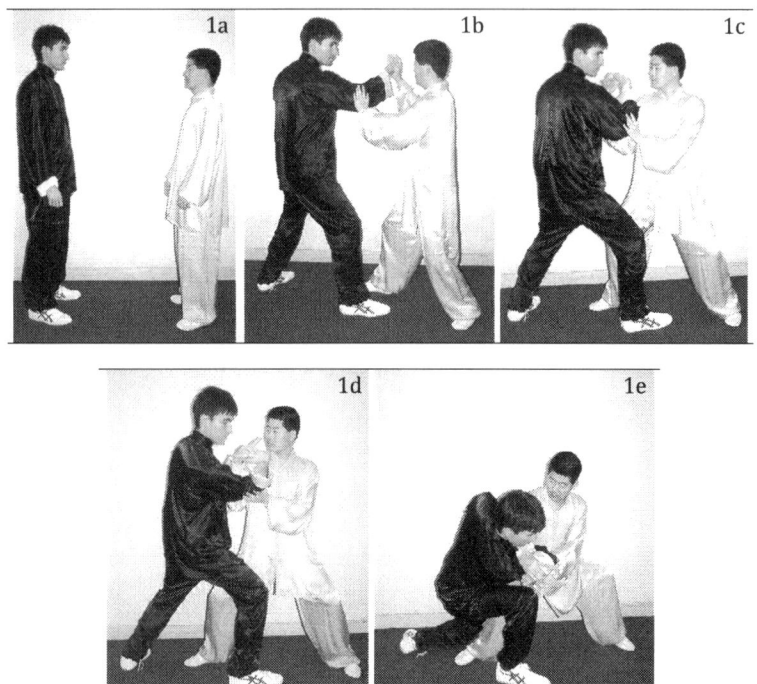

Points of attention:
In this technique, it is vital to synchronize the movements of the hands with the movements of the hips and legs. In addition, when pulling the opponent down, it is mandatory to keep oneself in an upright position, and not bend forward.

2) ELBOW LOCK — as in six sealing and four closing.

2a) When the attacker steps in and punches with his left fist, the defender meets the attacker's left wrist with his left hand.

2b) The defender continues to advance with his right foot and places his right wrist on the attacker's left elbow.

2c) The defender then uses his left hand to pull the attacker's left fist downward. At the same time, he presses with his right palm on the attacker's elbow.

2d) The defender then bends his right knee and presses down with his right forearm on the attacker's elbow while using his left hand to pull the attacker's forearm backward and upward.

2e) Following this last move, the defender can shift his weight on to the left foot, using the momentum to pull the attacker off his feet.

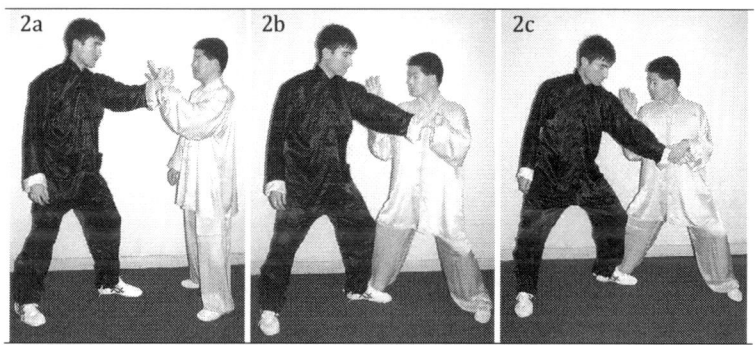

Points of attention:
The defender's right elbow must synchronize well with his left hand. Pulling, grabbing and twisting all must happen together. In addition, when shifting the weight onto the left foot, the right

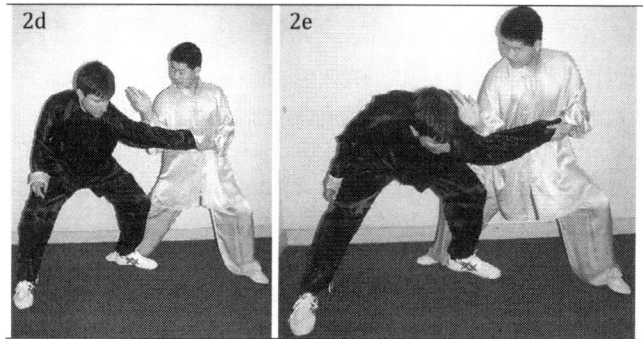

foot must keep rooted into the ground. The posture must stay upright and not lean forward or sideways.

3) SHOULDER LOCK — as in part the horse's mane.
  3a) When the attacker steps in and punches with his left fist, the defender takes a small step with his right foot and blocks the attack with his left hand.
  3b) Immediately after that, the defender steps in with his right foot, placing his right arm underneath the attacker's left upper arm.
  3c) He then pushes the attacker's left hand downward and his upper arm upward, so that the attacker's left shoulder and elbow are locked.
  3d) The defender then sinks and turns his waist to the right, pressing with his right elbow on the attacker's left ribs, causing him to lose balance.

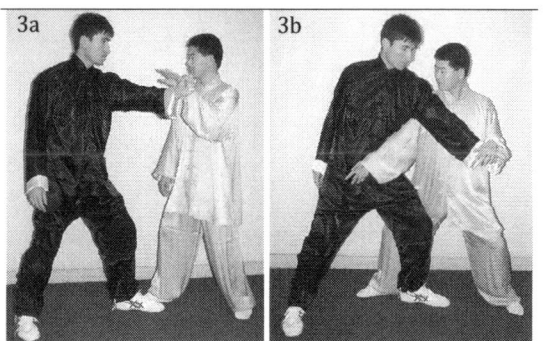

Points of attention:
While locking the attacker's shoulder and lifting him up, the defender must keep his feet rooted to the ground.

See following page for 3c and 3d.

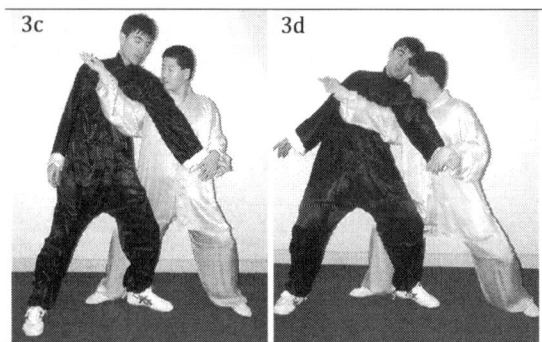

4) HIP LOCK — as in turn the flowers out of the bottom of the sea.
- **4a)** When the attacker steps in to strike with his left fist, the defender immediately steps in and uses his left hand to block the attack.
- **4b)** The defender steps behind the attacker's left foot and, at the same time, inserts his right forearm under the attacker's left upper arm.
- **4c)** The defender then moves his arm upward and his left hand downward which locks the attacker's left elbow while breaking the rooting of his right foot.
- **4d)** The defender then turns his hips to the right, raises his right knee pushing the attacker's left knee upward. At the same time, the defender presses down with his right elbow on the left side of the attacker's ribcage, causing him to lose his balance and fall backward.

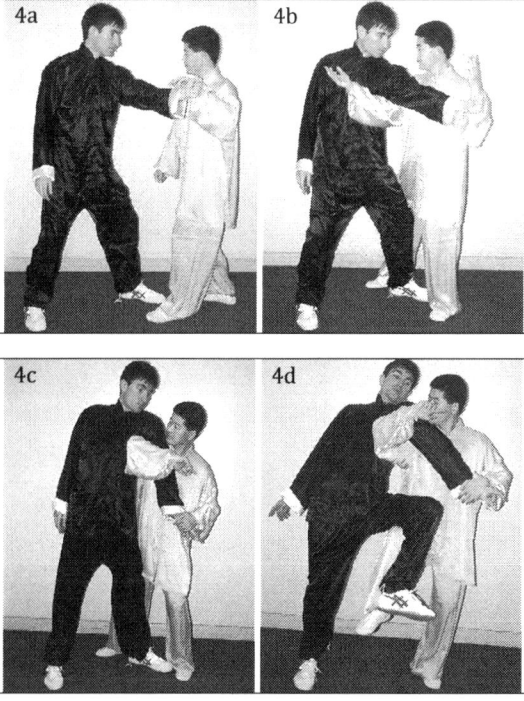

Points of attention:
In this technique, prior to locking the attacker's hip, it is necessary to lock his left elbow and sever his right foot rooting. This action causes the attacker to rely on his left foot for balance. As a result, when the defender raises his right knee, pushing the attacker's left knee upward, the attacker will lose balance and fall.

5) WHOLE BODY LOCK — as in the form wade forward and twist step.
- **5a)** When the attacker steps in with his right foot, using his right hand to grasp the defender's right hand, the defender immediately steps in with his right foot, and offers slight resistance to the grab.
- **5b)** The defender then places his left hand on top of the attacker's right hand. The defender holds the attacker's right hand to his own wrist, eliminating the possibility of the attacker escaping. The defender pushes his right hand upward, turns his hips and right hand to the right, locking the attacker's right elbow and shoulder.
- **5c)** Without pausing, the defender sinks his waist down, pushing the attacker's right forearm down, further locking the attacker's right hip.
- **5d)** The defender then pushes his own anatomical center (*dantian*) forward and downward, locking the attacker's right knee as well.

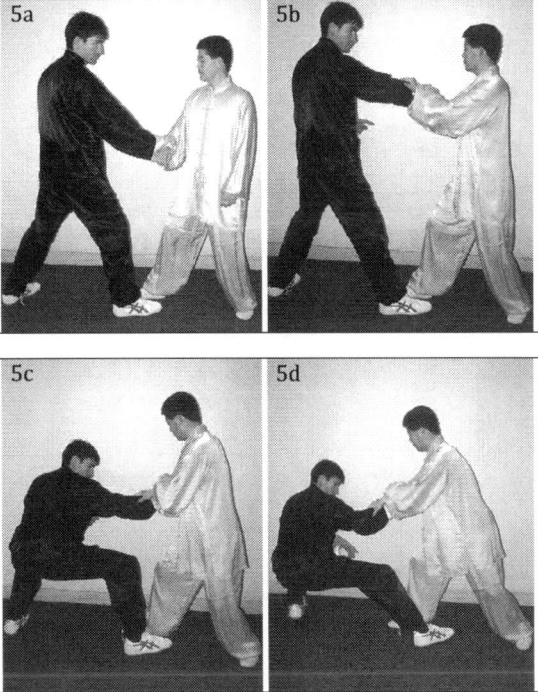

Points for attention:
In this technique, it is important to synchronize the movements of the defender's right hand and hips. At a beginner level, it is necessary for the defender to use both

his hands to lock the attacker's joints (as demonstrated above). However, at a more advanced level, the defender will use only his right hand to lock the attacker's whole body.

Conclusion

Taijiquan combat skills have several levels. The most basic one is using the muscles and joints to deal with an opponent. At a higher level, it is important to sense the opponent's energy and neutralize it with one's own energy. The highest skill is to know the opponent's intentions before they are initiated.

When learning taijiquan, the levels of progress are: 1) training the body (as in qinna techniques); 2) training the energy (qi); and 3) at the highest realm, training the mind/intentions (yi). However, knowledge of body mechanics and qinna are essential for one's progress and cannot be overlooked.

• 35 •
A Comparison of Yang Style Taijiquan's Large and Medium Frame Forms
by Joel Stein, M.S.

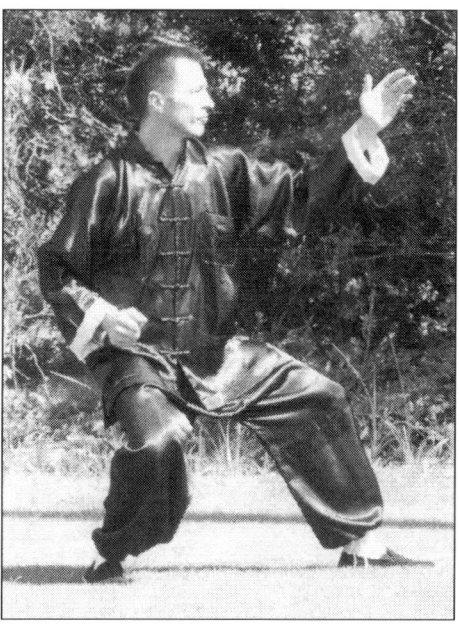

Illustrations courtesy of Joel Stein.

Introduction

Classical Yang Style taijiquan (or taiji) offers three variants or "frames" within its agenda of fixed forms: the small, medium, and large frames. It is important to understand that the term "frame" does not refer to the outward appearance of postures but rather the internal movement characteristic of taiji. However, there are external as well as internal differences in each of the three frames. While much of the information about the masters and their associated forms was handed down as oral tradition, we can realize their intentions from the historical and social context in which they developed.

Yang Jianhou's medium frame form was a modified version of the original Chen Family Style called old frame (*laojia*). The revised format helped Yang Taiji gain a considerable following. However, it was not until Yang Chengfu made additional changes that Yang taiji's popularity reached worldwide proportions.

This chapter investigates the medium frame form in its role as the basis for Yang Chengfu's large frame form by comparing the stances of both. Comparison of the large and medium frame forms should shed light on the necessity of Yang Chengfu's revisions. It should also give a better understanding of the body mechanics involved in both forms.

CHARACTERISTICS OF MEDIUM AND LARGE FRAME FORMS

Medium
- Focuses on energy discharge at point of contact and centering gravity
- Martial aspects more obvious in the executed form
- Medium circular movements
- Standard base (shoulder-width) and height constant (regular) throughout form
- Offense/defense directed at point of contact
- Coiled energy emphasized

Large
- Focus is on *song*, opening joints, stretching tendons and ligaments,
- Martial aspects not as obvious in the form
- Large circular movements
- Standard base (shoulder-width) and height constant (regular) throughout form
- Ward off (*peng*) energy at any point
- Relaxed (*song*) energy emphasized

Background

As Yang Luchan's reputation as a peerless fighter spread throughout China, more and more people wanted to learn the style he created. The style he practiced was called "cotton boxing" or "shadow boxing." Its strength was derived from internal power rather than external force. Yang Style became the "softest" of the internal styles. However, it presented a problem in that it was a very difficult style to learn.

Yang Zhenduo comments on the progression of Yang family taiji dating back to Yang Luchan (1799–1872; also known as Yang Fukui):

> To meet popular needs, Yang Luchan gradually deleted from the series of movements such difficult actions as jumps and leaps, explosion of strength and vigorous foot stamping. After revisions by his third son Yang Jianhou (1839–1917), this series of movements came to be known as *"zhongjia"* (medium frame). Later, it was again revised by Yang Chengfu (1883–1936), the third son of Yang Jianhou, which finally developed into the present *"dajia"* (big frame) style because of its extended and natural posture, slow and even movements. It was different from his uncle Yang Banhou's style which was known under the name *"xiaojia"* (small frame). – Yang, 1991: 5

Yang Luchan first practiced a form known as Chen family *"laojia"* or "old frame." Yang Zhenduo speaks about the origins of Yang taijiquan in his book, *Yang Style Taijiquan*:

> The Yang school of taijiquan was born out of the Chen school of taijiquan which was known as *"laojia"* ("old frame"). The movements are

relaxed, even and graceful like the drifting clouds and flowing stream, quite unlike the Chen Style (cannon fist) which alternates slow and quick movements, and vigorous with restrained and controlled actions.
– Yang, 1991: 5

Yang Luchan's third son, Yang Jianhou (1839–1917), revised the forms his father taught him. He omitted the hard stomps, leaps, and complex hand and foot movements. He also modified the small circular movements by making them larger and more obvious for his novice students. This revision was called the medium frame format. The form was somewhat easier to learn but still required the discipline and dedication of a talented student to master.

According to T. Y. Pang, Yang Luchan's third son Jianhou (1839–1917) created a medium form set and Jianhou's younger son Chengfu (1883–1936) created a new big form that became the most popular taiji style.

Yang Chengfu went on to revise the medium frame form by adding still larger circular movements and moving the body weight distribution further behind the front leg. He changed the weight ratio of 70/30 to 60/40 to shift the burden of the front leg and open the pelvic joints. These revisions, along with a viable instructive program, made Yang Style taiji popular throughout the world. Yang Zhenduo remarks about the Yang Chengfu's revisions:

> Yang Jianhou taught Yang Chengfu very seriously. . . . Yang Chengfu removed the vigorous *"fajing"* (release of power), energetic jumping, heavy stepping, and other difficult movements to create *"da jia"* (large frame style). *Da jia* has slow, steady, and soft movements suitable for general practitioners. The posture is neat and simple; the structure is elaborate and centrally balanced without leaning towards any sides...
> – Yang, 20 February 2001b

Yang Chengfu's large frame form became the most popular in the world. Master Vincent Chu, author of *Beginner's Tai Chi Chuan*, writes about Yang Chengfu's revisions to the form in his article, "Yang Style History":

> After Yeung Ching Po [Yang Chengfu] came to Southern China, he realized that [taijiquan] was also effective in treating chronic diseases, building up one's health, and bringing longevity. When he gave [taijiquan] exhibitions in "Zhiru Wushu Association" during his early days in Shanghai . . . he performed his kicks with speed and force. Later, however, to suit the needs of chronic disease, he changed them into slow movements with inner exertion of force. And in such movements as punching downward and punching the opponent's groin, he only made initiations instead of manifest exertions of force, thus making the movements continuous and with an even pace. . . . Creating a style all

his own, he had mastered extraordinary skill in *"tuishou"* or push-hands and was good in both attack and defense.

– Chu, 12 February 2001

Characteristics of the Medium Frame

At first glance the medium frame form bears a striking resemblance to the large frame form but there are major structural differences. Both form sets are executed at the same speed and timing and the same number of movements. The medium frame form appears more compressed and coiled than the large frame form. Both the large and medium frame forms have a shoulder-width standard for the base.

Overall, circular movements are smaller in the medium frame form. In the large frame form the torso is held upright and perpendicular to the ground and the rear leg is bent. In the medium frame form the torso is inclined forward placing more weight over the front leg. There is more emphasis on opening the joints in the large frame form.

Medium frame characteristics are more apparent when we compare photos of similar postures in large frame form. However, it is important to note that the most significant differences in the two forms are in the movements leading up to the stances.

There are no fixed or rigid applications for classic Yang taiji postures. Although certain postures are applicable to circumstances, they are not necessarily designed for only one specific attack or defense. The movements are flowing and flexible and they conform to the situation at hand. This holds true for both medium and large frame forms.

Analysis of Large and Medium Frame Postures

Dimitri Mougdis, a senior student of Grandmaster Chu Gin Soon, is the director of the Internal Arts Institute of Hobe Sound, Florida. He believes that teaching both the large and medium frame forms offers his students a more complete transmission of classic Yang taiji. The postures he demonstrates in this chapter are common to both the medium and large frame forms.

In the medium frame press (fig. 1), the body weight distribution is 70 percent over the front leg and 30 percent over the rear leg. The press is sensitive to tension and is issued the instant it is detected in an opponent. In the large frame press (fig. 2), the inclined torso is straightened to a 90-degree angle, redistributing the body weight to 60 percent on the front leg and 40 percent on the rear leg. The bent rear knee allows for opening pelvic socket joints (*kua*).

In the medium frame fair lady plays shuttles posture (fig. 3), the torso is tilted forward, and the body weight is over the front and rear legs in a 70/30 percent distribution. Energy is focused and issued through the right palm. The large frame shuttles posture (fig. 4) holds the torso upright with a 60/40 percent weight distribution. Striking energy is also issued through the palm at the point of contact.

Although the two postures seem to be the same in outward appearance, the movements leading up to the final stances are different. Large frame fair lady plays shuttles has large circular movements leading up to the demonstrated stance. The medium frame movements are compressed and coiled; the circular movements are not as obvious.

Medium frame ward off (fig. 5) is both an offensive and defensive posture. The pelvic girdle is inclined slightly forward with 70 percent of the body weight over the front leg. Energy is concentrated and then issued from the left forearm when contact with an opponent is made. The large frame ward off (fig. 6) sinks the center of gravity down to the coccyx and through the legs with 60 percent of the body weight on the front leg. Energy travels from the legs (including the feet) to the waist and up through the arms and hands. It can be issued at any point of contact.

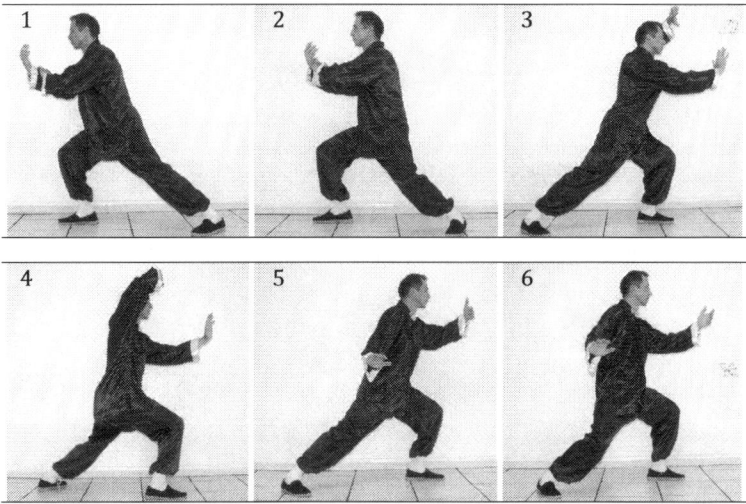

When applied, the rollback is used to pull an opponent off his center of gravity. In the medium frame rollback (fig. 7) stance, the head faces the direction of the forward leg with the waist at a 45-degree angle. Arms are held firmly in position and the upper body is tilted slightly forward. Although the application is the same in the large frame rollback stance (fig. 8), there is a more pronounced twisting of the torso at a 90-degree angle from the front foot. The upper body is held perpendicular to the ground and "sunk." This aids in opening the joints. Arms and hands are relaxed and keep the form's structure.

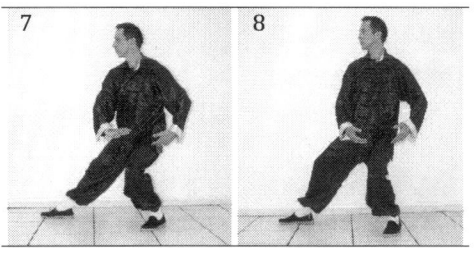

The snake creeps down posture is both evasive and offensive. Medium frame snake creeps down (fig. 9) is a noticeably coiled posture with the upper body leaning forward and with the front leg straight. Yang Chengfu modified this posture in the large frame form by setting the upper body at a 90-degree angle, by having the left elbow bent. In the large frame snake creeps down (fig. 10) the front leg is bent at the knee. This is another example of the emphasis Yang Chengfu placed on *song* or sinking the weight to open the body. In this case, the pelvic region (*kua*) and waist (*deng*) benefit.

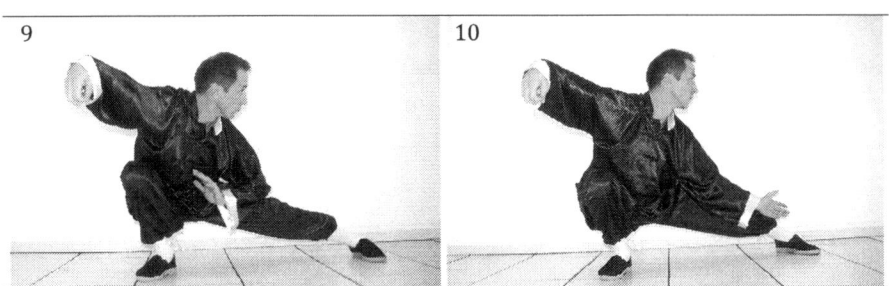

Body weight is distributed 70 percent on the front leg and 30 percent on the rear leg in the medium frame single whip (fig. 11). The left hand seems to move straight from the chest, but this is actually a circular movement, which is imperceptible if not pointed out. The same movement in the large frame single whip (fig. 12) is executed with a large circular movement of the striking hand. In the large frame single whip, the upper body is perpendicular to the ground. There is a slight sinking of weight (*song*) down through the coccyx/tailbone region. This sinking at the conclusion of this posture also enables the pelvic joint sockets to stretch or open.

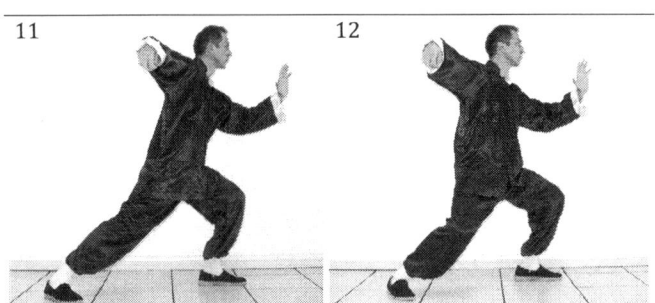

In the medium frame cross palm posture (fig. 13), the head faces in the direction of the front foot. Seventy percent of the body weight sinks down through the front leg and the rear leg is held straight. In the medium frame posture the back of the right hand touches the elbow and there is a slight bend in the striking arm.

Yang Chengfu modified the angle of the waist in the large frame cross palm posture (fig. 14). The upper body is at a 90-degree angle and the rear leg is bent. The right hand guards the rib cage. These revisions allow further sinking and opening of the joints.

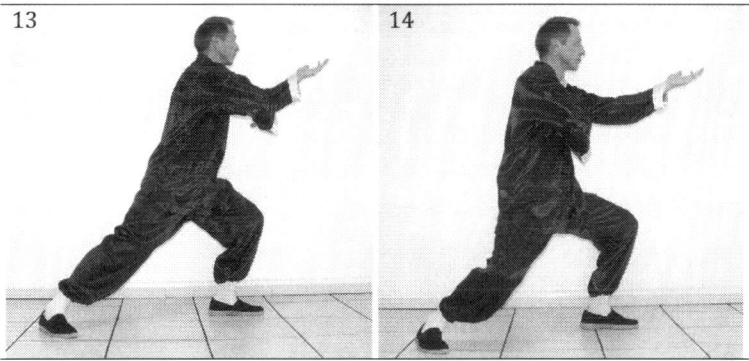

The medium frame play guitar posture (fig. 15) was modified to the large frame raise hands posture. In the raise hands posture, both palms face the opponent, and the body is held upright. The large frame includes raise hands (fig. 16) and play guitar as part of the form.

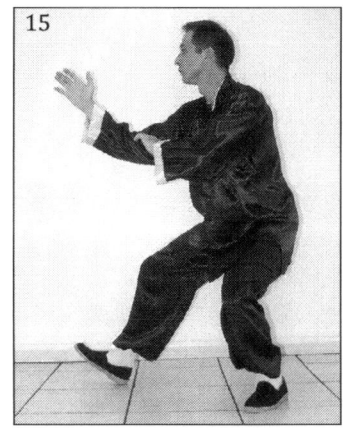

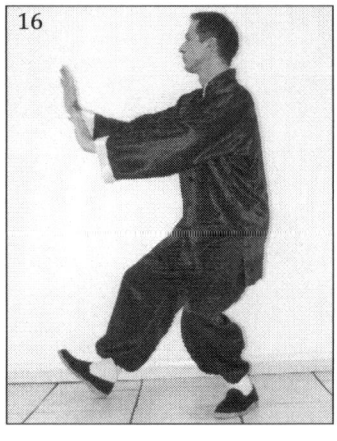

Conclusions

Yang Chengfu modified the medium frame form by shifting the center of gravity in its postures. He stressed large circular movements and the sinking of body weight through relaxation. This enables novice students to open their joints, stretch tendons and ligaments, and to become more aware of their center of gravity in a more facile manner compared with the medium frame form.

The importance of the Yang Style medium frame's role in the creation of the Yang Style large frame form cannot be overemphasized. It provided the infrastructure from which Yang Chengfu created his revised form. The brilliant innovations helped thousands of individuals to learn the mechanics of taijiquan.

However, the medium frame form is an integral part of classic Yang Style transmissions. Great masters such as Yang Sau Chung (1910–1985) practiced the medium frame form exclusively. And Yang Chengfu once commented that the Yang family transmissions are not complete without it.

Acknowledgment
Mr. Dimitri Mougdis deserves credit for
the medium and large frame poses
that appeared the chapter.

References

Chu, V. (1999). *Beginner's tai chi chuan*. Burbank, California: Multi-Media Books and CFW Enterprises.

Pang, T. (1987). *On tai chi chuan*. Bellingham, Washington: Azalea Press.

Yang, Z. (1991). *Yang style taijiquan*. Beijing: Morning Glory Publishers.

Zhang, L. (1992). *Wonderful taiji kungfu*. Henan, China: People's Physical Education Press.

Yang, Z. (20 February 2001b; download date). Introduction to grandmaster Yang Cheng-fu. http://www.yangstyletaichi.com/Home/History/Yang_Cheng-Fu/yang_cheng-fu.html.

Sources of Original Publication

Articles in this anthology were originally published in Via Media Publishing's *Journal of Asian Martial Arts,* and from the book titled *Asian Marital Arts: Constructive Thoughts and Practical Applications.* Listed according to the table of contents for this anthology:

DeMarco, M. (1992)	Vol. 1 No. 1, pp. 8–25
Wong J./DeMarco, M. (1992)	Vol. 1 No. 1, pp. 26–35
Delza, S. (1992)	Vol. 1 No. 4, pp. 80–89
Holcombe, C. (1993)	Vol. 2 No. 1, pp. 10–25
Lerhaupt, L. (1993)	Vol. 2 No. 1, pp. 60–69
Derrickson, C. (1993)	Vol. 2 No. 3, pp. 64–75
Sutton, N. (1994)	Vol. 3 No. 1, pp. 56–71
Stubenbaum, D. (1994)	Vol. 3 No. 1, pp. 90–99
DeMarco, M. (1994)	Vol. 3 No. 3, pp. 92–103
Smith, R. (1995)	Vol. 4 No. 1, pp. 50–65
Lim, T.K. (1995)	Vol. 4 No. 2, pp. 64–73
Kohler, S. (1995)	Vol. 4 No. 2, pp. 74–85
Smith, R. (1995)	Vol. 4 No. 3, pp. 46–59
Davis, B. (1996)	Vol. 5 No. 2, pp. 36–59
Tyrey, B., and Brinkman, M. (1996)	Vol. 5 No. 2, pp. 74–79
Lim, T.K. (1996)	Vol. 5 No. 3, pp. 90–99
Smith, R. (1997)	Vol. 5 No. 4, pp. 20–45
Davis, D. and Mann, L. (1996)	Vol. 5 No. 4, pp. 46–67
Willmont, D. (1997)	Vol. 6 No. 1, pp. 10–29
Smith, R. (1997)	Vol. 6 No. 1, pp. 50–61
Smith, R. (1997)	Vol. 6 No. 2, pp. 56–69
DeMarco, M. (1997)	Vol. 6 No. 3, pp. 8–17
Wallace, A. (1998)	Vol. 7 No. 1, pp. 58–89
Breslow, A. (1998)	Vol. 7 No. 2, pp. 10–25
Mainfort, D. (1998)	Vol. 7 No. 3, pp. 56–71
O'Conner, M. (1998)	Vol. 7 No. 4, pp. 10–21
DeMarco, M. (1998)	Vol. 7 No. 4, pp. 22–35
Kohler, S. (1999)	Vol. 8 No. 1, pp. 91–101
Peck, A. (1999)	Vol. 8 No. 3, pp. 76–83
Hawthorne, M. (2000)	Vol. 9 No. 1, pp. 70–81
DeMarco, M. and Matthews, A. (2000)	Vol. 9 No. 2, pp. 48–79
Berwick, S. (2001)	Vol. 10 No. 2, pp. 88–97

Berwick, S. (2001)	Vol. 10 No. 2, pp. 98–101
Seidman, A. (2001)	Vol. 10 No. 3, pp. 76–83
Stein, J. (2002)	Vol. 11 No. 1, pp. 58–67
Cordes, A. (2002)	Vol. 11 No. 2, pp. 64–79
DeMarco, M. (2002)	Vol. 11 No. 4, pp. 30–53
Berwick, S. (2003)	Vol. 12 No. 4, pp. 34–47
Gaffney, D. (2004)	Vol. 13 No. 2, pp. 32–43
Loupos, J. (2004),	Vol. 13 No. 4, pp. 52–55
Wong, Y.M. (2005)	Vol. 14 No. 2, pp. 44–51
Gaffney, D. (2005)	Vol. 14 No. 4, pp. 32–47
Cai, N. (2006)	Vol. 15 No. 1, pp. 76–85
Kucher, S., et al. (2007)	Vol. 16 No. 1, pp. 36–45
Wolfson, G. (2007)	Vol. 16 No. 2, pp. 34–47
Henning, S. (2007)	Vol. 16 No. 3, pp. 22–25
Kauz, H. (2007)	Vol. 16 No. 3, pp. 60–63
Wile, D. (2007)	Vol. 16 No. 4, pp. 8–45
Cohen, R. (2001)	Vol. 17 No. 1, pp. 8–27
Gaffney, D. (2008)	Vol. 17 No. 2, pp. 56–67
Mason, R. (2008)	Vol. 17 No. 3, pp. 22–39
Burroughs, J. (2008)	Vol. 17 No. 4, pp. 42–55
DeMarco, M. (2009)	Vol. 18 No. 3, pp. 18–39
Cartmell, T. (2009)	Vol. 18 No. 4, pp. 46–63
Mason, R. et al. (2010)	Vol. 19 No. 2, pp. 72–107
Graycar, M. and Tomlinson, R. (2010)	Vol. 19 No. 3, pp. 78–95
Mosher, H. (2011)	Vol. 20 No. 1, pp. 94–109
Brown, D. (2011)	Vol. 20 No. 2, pp. 8–21
Baek, S. (2011)	Vol. 20 No. 3, pp. 62–85
Rhoads, C.J. et al, M. (2011)	Vol. 21 No. 1, pp. 8–31
Brodsky, G. (2012)	Vol. 21 No. 1, pp. 82–101
Gaffney, D. (2012)	*Asian Martial Arts,* pp. 66–69
Mason, R. (2012)	*Asian Martial Arts,* pp. 106–109
Yun Zhang (2012)	*Asian Martial Arts,* pp. 148–153

INDEX

A

acupuncture, 50, 96, 270, 315, 329, 373, 383, 588, 644, 658, 679, 683, 686, 893
adhering, 677, 934
alchemy, 225, 258, 265, 269–270, 272, 274 note 6, 350, 617, 628, 635, 642, 645, 647, 654, 657, 659, 672, 675, 873, 883–884, 907
An Exposition of the Principles of Taijiquan, 650
Analects, 1, 174, 180, 718, 808
Anglo-Chinese War, 757
anxiety, 32, 363, 597–598, 861, 901
arm movement, 9, 106–108, 110–114, 147–148
awareness, 32, 60, 96, 388, 392, 547, 557–558, 571, 575, 607, 613–614, 621–623, 644–645
Art of Taijiquan, 278–279, 283, 287 note 1, 631, 637
Art of the Internal School's Boxing Methods, 628, 634, 643, 645
Art of War (Sunzi), 180, 356 note 6, 648
Attaining Softness Taijiquan Society (*zhi rou*), 169
automatic writing, 162

B

baguachang, 51
baguazhang, 314, 562, 678
bajiquan, 733
baihui acupoint, 328, 868, 877
balance, 32–33, 104–106, 303, 319, 324–325, 327, 398, 408, 525, 571
Baopuzi, 45, 49, 265, 348, 617–618
beginning posture, 147, 302–303, 765
Beijing, 2, 10–13, 15, 20, 278, 280–281, 287 notes 1 and 2, 359–360, 407, 419, 422, 427–428, 463, 560–561, 606, 635, 648, 652, 660, 673, 703, 709, 713, 734, 754, 759, 763, 863, 934
Beijing Physical Education Research Institute, 287 note 1, 631, 755, 757
Beijing Martial Arts Research Society, 679
Beijing University, 713–714, 720
Bian, Renjie, 636
blood pressure, 218, 232 note 12, 314, 389, 407, 660, 678, 890, 892, 894, 898–899, 901–903

Bodde, Derk, 42
Bodhidharma, 3, 213, 220, 252, 254 note 8, 628, 630, 632–633, 655
Book of Changes (*Yijing, I Ching*), 69, 79, 91, 169, 174, 176, 180, 192–194, 248, 259–264, 269, 325, 374–378, 528, 627, 633, 637–638, 640–641, 659, 672, 675, 718
Book of Odes, 308
bow stance, 263, 402–404, 613
Boxer Uprising, 10, 660, 757
breathing, 318–319, 349–350, 362, 414, 416, 548, 642, 644, 682, 692 note 8, 866–867, 869, 872–873, 884, 887–888, 894, 897
breathing "pre-natal" or "reverse," 134, 210, 215, 217–218, 223, 227, 230, 231 note 10, 353, 894
broadsword (*dao*), 89, 154, 486, 579–582, 606, 618, 770
bubbling spring accupoint, 683, 397–404
Buddhism, 45–46, 52 note 24, 157, 220, 342, 350, 637, 639–640, 661, 708, 805, 807, 814–815, 816 note 15, 818–819, 899

C

Cai, Yuanpei, 168, 713
cannon fist (*paochui*), 8, 26, 98, 240, 313, 316, 318, 325, 475, 544, 573, 575, 698, 700, 856, 883
Cao, Delin, 24, 28
cardio-respiratory, 390, 599
cardiovascular system, 389, 751, 898, 901, 904
cat stance, 403
central equilibrium, 611, 736–737, 800, 814, 832, 851–852, 925
Central Military Academy (Huangpu, Whampoa), 169, 716, 806
Cernuschi Museum of Chinese Art, 127, 172, 718
Chan, Bun-Piac, 673, 691
Chan, Hak Fu, 594
Chang, Naizhou, 627, 640, 643, 645, 653
Chen, Bing, 709, 869
Chen, Bu, 634, 695–697
Chen, Changxing, 9–10, 12, 26, 193, 313, 316–317, 375, 380 note 7, 385, 454–455, 457, 537, 542, 544, 561, 572–573, 576, 583, 630–632, 635–636, 660, 691 note 3, 700–701, 706, 754–755, 759
Chen, Chunyuan, 11
Chen, Fadou, 703

484

Chen, Fake, 10–11, 24, 97–99, 315, 407, 427, 454, 457, 463, 483, 542–543, 569, 573, 583, 633, 673–674, 679, 703, 708
Chen family biographies, 312, 648, 656
Chen, Gene, 11
Chen, Gengyun, 10, 759
Chen, "Tacky" Hanqiang, 153–154
Chen, Kesen, 704, 707
Chen, Liqing, 360, 703
Chen, Panling, 216–217, 717
Chen, Pengfei, 456
Chen, Qingping, 11–12, 122, 314, 630, 653–654
Chen Village (Chenjiagou), 5–7, 10, 23–27, 98, 122, 312, 315, 328, 423, 427, 453, 455, 457–460, 481, 527, 560, 566, 569–573, 577, 579, 581, 583, 633–636, 643, 647–648, 650, 660, 695–709, 754, 756, 759
Chen, Wangting, 7–9, 11, 253 note 2, 312–313, 316, 318–321, 325–326, 384, 456, 539, 542, 544, 751, 573, 575, 579, 581–583, 634, 648, 659–660, 691 note 3, 697–700, 705–706, 865–866, 929
Chen, Weiming, 118, 120, 123–125, 160, 169–170, 177, 179, 183 notes 17 and 20, 193–194, 214–215, 239, 242, 252 note 2, 253 note 5, 277–279, 287 note 5, 281–286, 287 note 1, 288 note 11, 631, 637, 659, 715, 722, 729 note 9, 730 note 11, 761
Chen, Xiaowang, 11, 93–102, 313–318, 322, 324, 337, 427, 433, 452, 454, 456–457, 462–465, 481, 507, 524
Chen, Xiaoxing, 452–460, 574, 576, 696, 704–705, 828, 836, 869, 929–931
Chen, Xin, 372–380, 397, 464, 508, 527–540, 569–570, 633–634, 636–637, 643, 646, 648, 650, 703, 923
Chen, Xiufeng, 13–14, 281
Chen, Xiyi, 640, 660, 672, 675–676, 680–681, 692 note 5
Chen, Yanxi, 10, 24, 26, 94, 703
Chen, Yu, 869
Chen, Yuben, 11–12
Chen, Yuheng, 11
Chen, Zhangxing, 192, 238, 241, 280
Chen, Zhaokui, 99, 426–427, 433, 454, 457, 463, 481, 483, 547, 551, 553, 578, 708
Chen, Zhaopei, 453–454, 456–457, 463, 481–483, 488, 703–705, 707
Chen, Zhaoquai, 11
Chen, Zhaoxu, 99, 462
Chen, Zhenglei, 452, 481, 545–456, 550, 579–580
Chen, Zhongshen, 374, 539, 702
Chen, Zichen (William C.C. Chen), 20, 80, 119, 214–116, 221, 229 note 3, 232 note 10, 719–720, 915, 918
Chen, Ziming, 11
Cheng, Jincai, 482, 484
Cheng, Man-ch'ing (see Zheng, Manjing)
Cheng, Tinghua, 733–734, 739
Chenjiagou (see Chen Village)
Chenjiagou Taijiquan School, 573, 706–707
Chiang, Kai-shek, 714, 716, 718, 758, 763–764
Chiang, Kai-shek, Madam, 80, 731 note 17
Chongqing, 151, 153, 155, 159, 163 note 3, 169, 285, 632
Choi, Wai Lun, 416–417
Choy, Hokpeng, 15
Choy, Kamman, 15
Chu, Gin Soon, 476
Chu, Vincent, 475
cinnabar, 47–48, 185 note 39, 348, 831
Classic of Taijiquan, 65–66
coiling energy, 143, 326, 338, 544, 674, 868
cold energy, 203, 435
College of Chinese Culture, 171, 255 note 12
Commentaries on Taijiquan, 633, 640
Complete Form and Practice of Taijiquan, 606
Complete Principles and Practices of Taijiquan, 631
Communist Party, 169–170, 413, 418, 758
Confucianism, 166, 184 note 28, 242, 258, 261–262, 270, 342, 348, 350, 617, 626, 639–640
Confucius, 122, 128, 162, 164 note 6, 166, 173–174, 176, 180, 185 note 42, 260, 262, 271, 296, 347–349, 376, 378, 640, 654, 711, 808, 814
contact, 42, 63, 133–134, 137, 204–205, 247, 319, 321, 326, 554, 605, 608, 613–614, 700, 771, 777–796, 925
Cultural Revolution, 173–174, 482–484

D

Dai, Peisu, 358–360, 363
dalü (see large rollback)
damai meridian, 873–874, 884
Danjiangkou Wudang Martial Arts Research Association, 652–653

dantian, 95–96, 133–134, 175, 185 note 39, 211–213, 216, 219, 223, 229 note 2, 232 note 10, 249, 255 note 21, 274 note 4, 318, 324, 326–334, 336, 353, 404, 435, 464, 467, 531, 548–550, 553, 572, 583, 611
dantian rotation, 553, 686, 865–884
Daoism, 2–3, 6–8, 29, 41–56, 67, 74, 98, 103, 116, 119–120, 125, 155, 166, 173, 176, 180, 185 note 43, 192, 218–220, 224–225, 232 note 14, 233 note 17, 234 notes 21 and 23, 238, 248, 252, 254 note 8, 355, 361, 363, 378, 380 note 12, 412, 418, 625–662, 672–673, 691 note 2, 708
Daodejing, 79, 169, 173, 180, 219, 248, 415, 688, 718, 892
daoyin, 44–45, 47, 50, 116, 219, 318, 414, 642, 672
"dead spot", 143, 146
Delza, Sophia, 14, 66
Deng, Huijian, 590
Despeux, Catherine, 373, 376
diabetes, 315, 389, 893, 897, 900
diagonal flying, 123, 284, 364, 925–926, 928
Ding, Yidu, 169, 714
dianxue (see vital points)
A Discussion of Taijiquan, 66
dispersing hands (see *sanshou*)
Dong, Haichuan, 248, 562, 658
Dong, Huling, 15
Dong, Yingjie, 15, 119, 121, 157, 163 note 4, 177, 286–287, 288 note 10, 299, 631–632, 637, 762
Dongtuhe Village, 696
Du, Yuanhua, 644, 653
Du, Yuze, 10, 23–31, 94
dumai meridian, 884
Dun Prince Palace, 561–562

E
educational institutes, 546
effort, 59, 63, 70, 137, 569, 739, 779–780, 798, 844, 847, 872, 915–916
eight gates, 565
Eight Harmonies Boxing, 761
Eight Immortals, 351, 353
eight methods/energies (*bafa*), 316, 328, 417, 490, 554, 576, 681, 736
eight techniques, 563–564, 605
eight trigrams (*bagua*), 51, 261, 325, 380 note 12, 638
elixir field (see *dantian*)

elixir of immortality, 265, 344, 349–350, 355
Emerick, Danny, 151, 721, 727
emitting energy (*fajing*), 209, 316–317, 321, 323, 325, 328, 360–362, 400, 464–465, 475, 485, 535, 544, 547, 575–576, 578, 583, 703, 830, 837–838, 865, 883
energy cultivation (see *qigong*)
energy flow, 142, 145, 148, 200, 208, 866, 872, 877, 879–880, 884, 923
Epitath for Wang Zhengnan, 628, 630, 633
essence (*jing*), 74, 193, 213, 265, 267–273, 350–351, 574, 646, 684, 687
Essence and Applications of Taijiquan, 714–715, 729 note 6, 797
The Essential Principles and Practice of Taijiquan, 632
Evidence-Based Taijiquan (EBT), 893
Explanation of the Taiji Diagram, 660
external school (*weijia*), 280, 416, 418, 485
extraordinary meridians, 866–871
eye function, 32–40, 267, 305, 575

F
falling split, 537–539
falls, 595–603, 901
Falun Gong, 661
famine, 586, 618, 696, 702, 756
fangshi (magicians), 46–49, 53 note 26, 261, 344
fangsong, 609–610, 614, 837–838, 874, 883
Farber, Dan, 673
fascia attacking, 207–208, 255 note 17
fast-twitch muscle, 895–898, 902, 902 notes 7 and 8
FAR Gallery, 127, 718
feet, 109, 132–133, 147–148, 263, 398–401, 506, 621, 683
Feng, Yuxiang (General), 154, 758
Feng, Zhiqiang, 422, 427, 481, 646, 671, 673–674, 679–680, 685–688, 692 note 5
first routine (*yilu*), 8, 30, 98, 314, 316–317, 322, 325, 374, 424–425, 437–439, 441, 484, 489, 543–544, 551, 572–575, 578, 700, 703, 833, 865–866, 883
five animal frolics, 414, 673, 678, 764, 768
five phases/elements (*wuxing*), 42, 68, 265–266, 271, 304–306, 308–309, 374, 380 note 12, 863
five steps (*wubu*), 563–565, 647
Fong Ha, 40, 673
force (*li*), 73–74, 120, 124–125, 136, 138,

151, 248, 283, 383, 914
four corners, 290, 296, 302, 736, 849
four directions, 306, 387–388, 513, 736, 846
four frames, 135
Four Important Points of Solo Practice, 564
Fu, Zhongwen, 215, 287, 299, 427, 716
Fu, Zhongquan, 561, 568 note 5
Fundamentals of Tai Chi Chuan, 650

G

gait, 337, 400, 596, 598
Gan, Fengchi, 630, 633, 761
Gao, Fu, 671, 674
Ge Hong, 46, 265, 341, 348–349, 353, 617–619, 642
Gibbs, Tam, 91 note 1, 124–125, 130 note 7, 150, 161, 162 note 1, 176, 185 note 41, 254 note 8, 255 note 11, 297–298, 355 note 3, 725
glucose, 896–897
God of War (see also Guan Gong, Xuanwu), 3
great rollback (see large rollback),
group practice, 386, 393, 556–559, 768–769
Gu, Liuxin, 407, 427, 433, 581, 634, 648–649, 629 note 7
Gu, Luxin, 372
Guan Gong, 655
Guangzhou city, 15, 287 note 3, 585–586, 619
Guo, Lianying, 763
Guo, Qinfang, 151–152, 154, 156–157, 162–163
Guo, Shaojiong, 587
Guo, Tiefeng, 644
Guo, Tingxian, 764, 768
Guo, Yunshen, 216, 733

H

halberd (*guandao*), 97, 579, 581–582, 618, 619 note 2
Hall of Happiness, 724–725
Han, Qingtang, 717
Hangzhou, 46, 65, 71, 132, 138, 167, 198, 207, 272, 287 note 3, 349, 352, 354, 358–360, 362, 388, 625, 713
Hangzhou Wushan Taijiquan Society, 358, 362
Hao, Weizhen, 11–12, 122, 630, 734, 736
Hao, Weizheng, 11–12
Hao, Yuehju, 12
hatha yoga, 218, 909
He, Hongming, 635

health, 314–315, 318, 320, 327, 351, 363, 383–386, 389–394, 886–903
Hebei Province, 2, 12, 15, 116, 278–279, 281, 560, 651, 733, 754
Henan Form, 563
Henan Province, 3–7, 10, 12, 14, 26–27, 80, 102, 122, 220, 238, 278, 280, 312, 379 note 3, 384, 453, 463, 483, 488, 691 note 4, 562, 631, 634, 659, 695–697, 702, 754, 759, 762, 764
herbology, 206, 268, 270, 355, 642, 643, 712, 714, 716–717, 734, 802
Hong, Junshen, 360
Hong Kong, 14–15, 123, 128 note 2, 158, 247, 585–586, 588, 590, 594 note 1, 650, 673, 802
Hong Kong Jin Wu Sports Association, 586
Hong Kong Taiji Main Association, 594 note 1
Hong Kong YMCA, 586
Hong, Shihao, 158
horizontal dantian rotation, 874–876
horse stance, 263, 402, 404
Hu, Puan, 636, 761–762, 771
Hu, Yaozhen, 231 note 7, 673–674, 678–679
Hua Tuo, 414, 630, 678, 764
Huainanzi, 260, 266–267, 377
Huaiqing Prefecture, 26, 649, 696–698, 701–702
Huang, Baijia, 628, 631, 634, 640–641, 645
Huang, Feihong, 82, 586
Huang-Lao, 46, 345
Huang, Wenshan, 650
Huang, Xingxian, 83–85, 91, 118–119, 124
Huang, Zhaohan, 655
Huang, Zongxi, 625, 628, 634, 640, 651, 654
Hudson River Museum, 127, 718
huiyin acupoint, 328, 867–868, 871, 877, 879, 884
Hunan Martial Arts Academy, 716, 806
Hundun myth, 260, 263
Hunyuan Gong, 438
Hunyuan Taiji, 674
Huo, Chengguang, 673

I

Illustrated Explanation of Chen Taijiquan, 569, 703
Illustration of Taijiquan, 397
immortal (*xian*), 3, 218, 341, 343–344, 348–349, 351, 353–355, 356 notes 10 and 11

immortal pounds mortar, 318
immortality, 46–50, 53 note 38, note 54 note 45, 225, 232 note 14, 261, 265, 270, 341–357, 378, 617, 619, 627–628, 630, 637, 642–644, 647, 649, 651, 654–655
in vivo exposure therapy, 595, 598–599, 602
incense, 47
inner circle training, 144, 146–147, 149
inner elixir (*neidan*), 48–49, 54 note 43, 265, 348, 350–352, 638, 643, 656
intention, 67–68, 72, 75, 374, 388, 400, 472, 530, 548, 554, 575, 579, 610, 613, 645, 887, 894, 900, 903 note 2, 904 note 11, 910, 925
internal school (*neijia*), 249, 252, 279, 387, 412, 415–420, 627–629, 631–632, 642, 645, 648, 652, 655
Internal School's Boxing Methods, 628, 634, 643, 645
internal strength (*jin, neigong*), 78–79, 248–249, 255 note 20, 286, 322, 338, 546
International Taijiquan Forum, 886
Introduction to Chen Family Taijiquan, 634, 636, 646
Brief Introduction to Chinese Martial Arts, 633
Introduction to Original Taijiquan, 653
Isle of Immortals, 344
issuing energy (*fajing*), 202, 316, 321, 323, 325, 328, 360–362, 400, 464–465, 475, 485, 535, 544, 575–576, 578, 583, 703, 830, 837–838, 865, 883

J
jade, 43–44, 219
jade lady at shuttles, 78, 80, 126
Japan, 14, 26, 52 note 24, 124, 151, 168–169, 177–178, 210, 221–123, 232 note 10, 234 note 22, 242, 285, 344, 463, 483, 488, 577, 585–586, 634, 637, 639, 641, 646, 698, 713, 716, 734, 756, 758, 810, 817, 822
Jiang Fa, 630, 632–633, 654, 660, 702
Jiangsu Province, 2, 12, 169, 183 note 19, 239, 760–761, 763
Jianquan Taiji Association, 586, 588
Jin Yong, 640
Jiu Hao, 193, 197
Jou, Tsung Hwa, 66
Ju, Hongbin, 720, 730 note 16, 806, 818
judo, 222, 225–226, 503–504, 636, 639, 734, 897
Jung, Carl, 308

K
KaiMai acupuncture style, 893
Kan, Guixiang, 11
Ke, Qihua, 720, 806, 813
kinship, 629, 695–696
knight-errant (*xia*), 628, 630, 641, 657
Koh, Ahtee, 87, 91 notes 6 and 9

L
lactate, 896
Lai, Zhide, 376, 378
lance, 193–196,
laogong accupoint, 679, 870–871, 880
Laozi, 46, 164, 173, 213, 219, 240, 273, 301, 377, 393, 415, 627, 631–632, 637–640, 644, 653–654, 656, 661–662, 672, 684, 688, 728 note 2, 729 note 9, 910
large frame (*dajia*), 314, 360, 473–480, 482, 834
large rollback (*dalü*), 137, 283, 290–296, 388, 395
Le, Huanzhi, 761–762
Leaning on a Board (*kao ban*), 681
li (see force)
Li, Houcheng, 24, 28
Li, Jiying, 562
Li, Kuiyuan, 733
Li, Pinfu, 14
Li, Ruidong, 561–565
Li, Shirong, 636, 659–660
Li, Shoujian, 291, 298, 300
Li, Shudong, 482, 487
Li, Xiheng, 117–118, 128 note 2, 151, 717–718, 721, 727, 797–825, 925
Li, Xiyue, 642, 655
Li, Yaxuan, 288 note 11, 635, 714–715, 730 note 10
Li, Yiyu, 299 note 1, 630, 645, 653–654, 659
Li, Zhaosheng, 649, 656–658
Liang (T.T.) Dongcai, (Liang, Tongcai), 20, 66, 74, 78, 291–292, 297, 763
Ling Shan, 561
listening energy (*ting jin*), 127, 134, 137, 200, 204, 319, 553, 605, 613, 813
Liu He, 761
liuhebafa, 416–417, 672
"Lively Pace" Style, 12, 299
Lo, Benjamin Pangjeng, 238–257, 284, 291, 300 note 4, 716–717, 720, 727, 729 notes 3 and 8, 730 note 12, 800, 802–803, 813, 821

local defense, 756
locking techniques (*qinna*), 9, 97, 207, 246, 312, 316–317, 319, 321, 338, 361, 417, 422–423, 445–446, 451, 461, 467, 469, 471, 484, 487, 490–495, 544, 573, 578, 583, 781
long energy, 202
Long Fist (Changquan), 7, 316
longevity, 21, 47, 219, 248, 255 note 19, 261, 270, 273, 314, 320, 345, 383, 475, 644, 646, 654, 676, 678, 684, 773, 862
Lowenthal, Wolfe, 63–64, 124, 184 note 26, 247, 509, 813
Lu, Botang, 588, 591
Lu, Dimin, 635, 659
Lu, Dongpin, 672
Lu, Tongbao, 83–84, 86–87, 89, 91, 120, 124
Luo, Banzhen (see Lo, Benjamin)
Luoyang city, 5–6

M
Ma, Hong, 553
Ma, Jiangxiong, 589
Ma, Yuehliang, 14
Ma, Yueliang, 427, 589, 633, 637
magic, 2, 42, 50, 86, 193, 195, 349, 354
magical practitioners (*fangshi*), 46–49, 53 note 26, 261, 344
Malaysia, 77–92, 115, 118, 124
Manran San Lun, 77, 167, 174, 184 note 23, 286
Mao, Zedong, 173–174, 413, 705, 758
Master Zheng Taijiquan Study Association, 719, 728, 800, 806
Master of Five Excellences, 166, 242, 711–712, 719
Mayer, Michael, 673
Medium Frame, 473–480
Mencius, 42, 166, 180, 637
mental focus, 139
meridians, 96, 139, 186 note 56, 208, 255 note 15, 373–374, 437, 548, 671, 682, 686–687, 865–884
Ming Dynasty, 3, 6, 66, 177, 312, 376–377
mingmen acupoint, 327, 867–869, 871, 873
Mongkok School, 591, 594 notes 1 and 2
monkey/repulse-retreats, 114, 298, 510, 736, 738

N
Nanjing, 2, 15, 43, 116, 162, 170, 287 note 3

National Association for Practitioners of Traditional Chinese Medicine, 243
National Chinese Medical Association, 169, 714, 802
National Martial Arts Exhibition, 652
National Palace Museum, 176, 185 note 36, 720, 731 note 17
National Physical Education Committee, 652
National Zhinan University, 168
Nationalist Party, 14, 169–171, 174, 176, 763
Needham, Joseph, 41, 219–220, 225, 232 note 14
neigong (internal work), 79, 84, 116–117, 119–120, 124, 546, 673
Ng, Kionghing, 82
Neo-Confucianism, 50, 640
neurotransmitters, 898–899, 902
new frame (*xinjia*), 11–12, 24, 26, 97–98, 314, 317, 374, 457, 459–460, 463–464, 483, 543 573, 708, 573, 833
New Method of Self-Study in Taijiquan, 213, 699
New York, 14–15, 20, 123–127, 150, 161, 162 note 1, 163 note 5, 165, 172–174, 176, 184 note 26, 214–215, 243, 322, 465, 691 note 2, 718–719, 730 note 13, 797, 804, 812
no tension (*song*), 78–79, 397, 401, 474, 478

O
old frame (*laojia*), 24, 26, 93, 95–98, 314, 317, 454, 457, 459–460, 462–464, 473–474, 542–543, 551, 573, 700, 703, 865–866, 880
Opium War, 756–757
outer elixir school (*waidan*), 48, 265, 348–351, 643

P
Paris, 127, 172–173, 373, 718
patience, 61, 78, 89, 118, 153, 242, 322, 347, 386, 393, 432, 543, 548, 916
Peng, Tingjun, 673–674
pill of immortality, 341, 348–349
Po, Bingru, 407
posture, 9, 63, 79, 95, 119–121, 269, 284–285, 324–325, 329, 351, 363, 386, 389, 392, 574, 576–579, 599–603, 609, 717, 833–834, 843, 846
prenatal qi, 671, 677, 682, 684–685
press (*ji*), 144–145, 247, 292, 476–477, 509, 736

primordial taijiquan (*xiantian taijiquan*), 656
push (*an*), 135, 145, 247, 433
push-hands (*tuishou*), 7, 62–64, 79, 85, 89–90, 97, 99, 117–119, 122, 125–127, 132, 137–138, 156–158, 160, 199, 201–203, 208, 246–249, 255 note 16, 277, 280, 283, 290–291, 309, 316, 320, 326, 337–338, 362–363, 387, 408, 417, 422–426, 431, 433–436, 438, 440–442, 457, 459–460, 464, 489, 507, 509, 526, 547, 551

Q

qi, 41–45, 47, 49, 53 note 38, 63, 67, 73–74, 95–96, 98–99, 139, 153, 159, 175, 183 note 15, 186 note 56, 193–194, 206, 208, 211–213, 215–216, 219–221, 227, 233 note 17, 248–249, 255 note 15, 262, 265–270, 272–273, 279, 307, 318, 320, 322, 324–325, 327–331, 333, 335–337, 348, 350–354, 356 note 8, 373, 422, 548–549, 557, 571–574, 607–608, 610–611, 638, 643–646, 658, 671, 679–680, 686–688, 692 note 6, 836–837, 866, 922–923
Qi, Jiguang, 8, 313, 508, 581, 645, 648–649, 654, 698–699, 866
Qian, Mingshan, 169, 183 note 19
qigong, 41–42, 45, 47–51, 52 note 13, 54 note 43, 90, 96, 98, 134, 220, 255 note 20, 231 note 7, 249, 265, 283, 315, 318, 320, 322, 341, 348–349, 351–352, 373, 383, 423, 428, 430, 434–438, 440–441, 451, 459, 627, 637, 643, 646, 651, 671–688, 865–884, 886–903
Qin Shi Huangdi, 344
Qin Xu, 673
Qing Dynasty, 6, 10, 13, 23, 26–27, 167, 177, 253 note 2, 278, 312, 376, 412, 418–419, 560, 582, 585, 606, 625, 630–631, 640–641, 649, 655, 702, 711, 756–757, 760, 772
qinna (see locking techniques)
Questions and Answers on Taiji Boxing, 120, 215, 239, 279, 285

R

receiving energy (*jiejing*), 204, 281
relaxation (*song*), 89, 96, 120, 132, 215, 227, 320, 323, 328, 338, 397, 401, 474, 478, 716, 814
relaxation exercise, 89, 107, 110, 220
Ren, Changchun, 653
Ren, Guangyi, 312, 314–315, 318–319, 323, 326, 337–338, 832–833, 837–838
renmai meridian, 884
Republic of China Cultural Renaissance, 174, 718
ROC Chinese Boxing Association, 717
rollback, 68, 70, 135, 137, 144, 148, 246–247, 291, 294–295, 477, 491, 614, 736, 740–741, 848, 852–853
rooster stands on one leg, 9, 212, 277, 303, 313, 572, 767
root, 117, 133, 319, 337, 361, 397–404, 469–471, 515, 556, 571, 582, 621, 719, 799, 843

S

San Francisco, 11, 15, 23, 239, 673, 800, 804
sanshou (see dispersing hands), 83, 89–90, 137, 199, 290–291, 388, 605–615, 763, 771, 773
scholar tree, 696–697
Scripture of the Yellow Court, 634
sealing accupoints, 206
second routine (*erlu, paochui*), 8, 93, 97–98, 313, 316–318, 325, 424–425, 438–439, 484–485, 489, 544, 573, 698, 700, 770, 865, 883
Secret Transmissions on Taiji Elixir Cultivation, 628, 653, 659
Secrets of Shaolin Boxing, 639
self-cultivation, 3, 42, 49, 177, 198, 363, 507, 638, 642–644, 647, 685, 812
Self-defense Applications of Taijiquan, 631
sensitivity (*tingjing*), 79, 133, 137, 200, 202, 207–208, 319, 321–322, 325–328, 347, 388, 441, 486, 489–491, 557–558, 575, 577, 607, 622–623, 648, 680–681, 700, 735, 843, 846, 848–854, 858
sexual cultivation, 47, 213, 234 note 22
Shaanxi Province, 2, 6, 463, 630, 702
Shandong Province, 10, 15, 151, 154, 157, 168–169, 312–313, 459–460, 582, 700, 702
Shanghai city, 14, 117, 182 note 10, 183 note 16, 194, 277–279, 285, 287 notes 1 and 2, 359, 406, 424, 426–428, 433, 439, 475, 585–586, 588–589, 713–714, 729 note 7, 755, 761
Shanghai School of Fine Arts, 255 note 11, 713
Shanxi Province, 6, 116–117, 119, 122, 124, 169, 481, 634, 648, 654, 660, 673, 678, 696–697, 702

Shaolin boxing, 52 note 24, 78, 83, 183 note 15, 220–221, 226, 232 note 10, 253 note 2, 313, 361, 363, 505, 626, 628, 630, 639, 642, 651, 691 note 2, 733, 754, 757, 760–761, 763, 933

Shaolin Temple, 3, 6, 98, 220, 417, 423, 463, 695, 698, 709, 933

Shen, Xianglin, 587

Shi, Diaomei, 763

Shi, Shufang, 153, 221, 232 note 10

Shizhong (*Shr Jung, Shih Chung*), 165, 171–173, 176, 184 note 22, 717–720, 724, 727, 730 notes 13 and 16, 797, 800, 804, 806, 809, 812, 817–819

short energy, 122, 487,

Short Introduction to Taijiquan, 630

shoulder stroke (*kao*), 70, 246, 317, 364, 719, 734

Sichuan Province, 2, 20, 46, 124, 169, 285, 359, 642, 655, 672, 716

silk reeling (*changsijing, chansigong*), 315–316, 319–320, 322–323, 325–328, 331–338, 360–361, 422–423, 434–438, 440–442, 444, 451, 456, 458, 464, 527, 529, 532–534, 544, 553, 831, 835–836, 866–876, 882–883

Singapore, 14, 83–84, 87–88, 119, 176, 588, 719

single whip, 38–39, 284, 286, 318, 323, 460, 478, 529, 532–533, 549, 552, 574, 649, 715, 720

Sino-French War, 757

Sino-Japanese War, 714–716, 757, 817

six seal, four close, 368, 551, 840

slow-twitch muscle, 895–898, 902, 904 notes 7 and 8

small frame (*xiaojia*), 8, 299 note 1, 314, 360, 474, 482, 564, 566, 703

Smith, Robert W., 81, 156–157, 171, 244, 292–296, 356 note 5, 717, 721, 729 note 4, 729 notes 8 and 10, 730 note 14, 813, 823, 925–926

solo practice, 556–558

Song, Jianzhi, 638

Song, Shuming, 287 note 1, 630, 632–633, 637, 650

Song, You'an, 168, 714

Song, Zhijian, 633

Song, Zijian, 79–80, 84

South China Sports Association, 586

spear (*qiang*), 26, 93, 97, 313, 456, 501, 506, 576, 579, 581

spirit (*shen*), 74, 213, 265–268, 27–273, 350–352, 548, 638, 646, 684

splitting energy, 70, 576

stability, 104, 134, 404, 438, 531, 574

standard meridians, 867, 869–871

standing post (*zhanzhuang*), 315, 319, 322, 329–331, 397, 399, 458, 570, 678, 831, 841, 867–868, 872–874

Steel, Kelvin, 590

sticking energy (*nianjing, zhan*), 73, 199–200, 282, 576, 613–615, 631, 639, 736, 777–796, 814, 848, 851, 925–926, 934, 936

stimulated energy (*jing*), 73, 197, 267–270, 272–273, 350–351, 374, 574, 576, 646, 684, 687

straight sword (*jian*), 79, 90, 244, 279, 313, 385–388, 390, 496, 576, 579–580, 590, 606, 651, 655–656, 661, 690 note 1, 722, 797, 812, 855

Studies on Wudang Boxing, 652–653

Study of Taijiquan, 630, 633, 643, 734

Su, Jianyun, 427, 644, 733–734, 738

Summary of Zhang Sanfeng's Inner Elixir Theory, 656

Sun, Lutang, 11–12, 122, 193, 195, 278–279, 299, 314, 630, 637, 642–644, 691 note 3, 733–734, 736, 738–739, 751, 762

Sutton, Nigel, 115–116, 120–121, 123–127, 130 notes 12 and 13

T

Tai Chi and Mind-Body Research Program/Harvard Medical School, 901

Taiji: A Scientific Approach, 817

Taiji as philosophic term, 66–67, 248, 261–263, 306, 324–325

Taiji Classics, 65, 110, 140, 238–240, 245, 253 notes 5 and 6, 262–264, 268–269, 272–273, 291, 351–352, 355, 467, 507, 549, 554

Taijiquan Academic Research Committee, 717

T'ai Chi Ch'uan for Health and Self-Defense, 66

Taijiquan for Health and Self-Defense, 171

Taijiquan Practical Methods, 606

Taijiquan Sticky Thirteen Spear, 631

Taiping Jing, 43, 46, 49

Taiping Rebellion, 539, 606, 701, 756

Tan, Chingngee, 87
Tan, Desmond, 199
Tang, Dianqing, 761
Tang Hao, 66, 312, 372, 581, 625, 634–636, 639, 648–649, 652, 660
Taoist Restoration Society, 412, 635
Tay, Guanleong, 90
teacher-student relationship, 173, 391, 773,
Ten Essential Points of Taijiquan, 143
tensegrity, 828–839
Thirteen Chapters on Taijiquan, 90, 119, 285, 291, 372, 632, 659
thirteen postures, 6, 71, 291, 466–467, 612, 735–736
thirteen stances, 65, 68, 71–73, 75
Thirty-Eight Style, 97–99, 317–318
three heights, 135
Three Important Points on Partner Practice, 564
three powers posture (*santi*), 265–266, 738
three treasures (*jing, qi, shen*), 265–266, 350–351, 684
Tian, Xiuchen, 11
Tian, Zhaolin, 359
Tien, Moer, 696
Traditional Shaolin and Secret Transmissions of Shaolin Boxing, 639
thrusting hand, 146, 148, 579, 926
toes, 12, 106, 114, 330–332, 334, 397, 398–401, 531
training, learning process, 57–64, 254 note 9, 428, 429–442, 563–564, 569–584, 729 note 9, 754, 811, 855–864, 913
Treatise on Taijiquan, 654
Treatise on the Origins and Branches of Taijiquan, 630, 632
The True Essence of the Martial Arts, 643
Tu, Zongren, 24, 28–29, 57
tuberculosis, 20, 79, 168, 212, 220, 241, 277, 315, 713–714
tuishou (see push-hands)
two-person practices, 83, 89, 136–137, 326, 386–388, 435, 507, 525, 575, 606, 763, 771, 848
Twelve Continuous Fists, 562

U

Ueshiba, Morihei, 356 note 8
United Nations, 14, 171–172
uprooting, 202–203, 211, 319, 719, 799, 851, 915–916, 926

V

vertical dantian rotation, 877
vital energy (see *qi*)
vital points, 90, 154, 160, 162 note 1, 374, 474, 578, 646

W

waist, 9, 72, 110–111, 122, 143, 147–148, 159, 240, 263, 303, 317, 327, 332–334, 336–338, 360, 362, 487, 519, 609, 610–611
Waley, Arthur, 42, 45
Wan Chun, 561
Wan, Laiping, 653
Wan, Laisheng, 116–117, 156, 163 note 3, 216, 653
Wanchai District, 586, 594 note 2
Wang, Haijun, 543, 554
Wang, Jiaxiang, 10, 23–24, 27–28, 30–31
Wang, Juexin, 636
Wang, Lanting, 14, 282, 561–563
Wang, Peisheng, 359, 427, 934
Wang, Xi'an, 481, 484, 486, 489, 496, 704, 706
Wang, Xianggen, 198, 359, 363
Wang, Xiling, 655
Wang, Xiuai, 151
Wang, Yangming, 180, 647
Wang, Yannian, 116–118, 128 note 2, 158, 227, 288 note 11, 717, 721, 798
Wang, Yongfu, 673
Wang, Zongyue, 6–8, 14, 65–66, 122, 146, 241, 253 notes 2 and 5, 375, 403, 612, 630–631, 633, 636, 648, 659–660
ward off (*peng*), 70, 126, 143–144, 477, 510, 516, 521, 736, 834, 840, 847, 925–926
Warlord Period, 585, 634, 702, 757–758, 816
water image, 44, 58, 69–70, 103–104, 197, 259–274, 485, 549, 778
Waterside Pavilion, Beijing, 713
Wave Hands Like Clouds, 258, 403, 862
wei-so garrison units, 7, 384, 606, 649, 698, 759, 761
Wenzhou, 83, 167, 182 note 5, 712
White Cloud Monastery, 2, 351, 394
White Crane, 83, 442, 594 note 4, 691 note 2, 833, 862
White Lotus Society, 50, 756
World Health Organization/health guidelines, 384
women, 172, 177, 179, 406

Wu-Chan fight, 588
Wu, Chaojie, 590
Wu, Dakui, 586–588, 590–591, 594 note 2
Wu, Daqi, 587, 590
Wu, Gongyi, 585–588, 590–591, 594 note 4
Wu, Gongzao, 119, 585, 588–590, 594 note 3, 633, 640
Wu, Guozhong, 80–82, 84–88, 91 note 6, 118–119, 123, 130 note 10, 255 note 20
Wu, Hoqing, 14
Wu, Jianquan, 14, 119, 123, 130 note 9, 240, 287 notes 1 and 2, 314, 407, 508, 568 notes 2 and 8, 585–588, 590, 592, 594 notes 1 and 4, 631, 633, 637, 762
Wu, Kangnian, 588, 590
Wu, Mengxia, 156, 163
Wu, Quanyou, 14, 123, 130 note 9, 561, 590, 691 note 3, 934
Wu, Ruqing, 560
Wu style, 12, 14, 240, 253 note 5, 255 note 16, 287 note 2, 314, 359–360, 407, 427, 509, 525, 568, note 8, 585, 592, 691 note 3
Wu, Tunan, 122, 240, 375, 560, 633, 637, 659, 676, 817
Wu, Wenbiao, 590
Wu, Yanxia, 587, 590
Wu, Yinghua, 589
Wu, Yuxiang, 11–12, 14, 120, 122, 241, 253 notes 5 and 6, 299 note 1, 509, 568 note 1, 630–631, 641, 654, 659, 701, 734
Wu, Xiubao, 423
Wu, Zhiqing, 630, 636
Wudang Martial Arts Research Association, 652–653
Wudang Mountain, 2–3, 238, 252, 279, 344, 625, 627, 635–636, 648, 651–652, 695
Wudang Taijiquan, 653
Wudang sword, 359
wuji, 66–69, 75, 263, 324–325, 377–378, 402, 425, 570, 737–738, 745, 830–831, 833–835, 830, 840–841
Wuqing Taijiquan, 562
wuwei (non-action), 258, 274, 309, 346, 415, 639

X

Xia Tao, 132, 207, 272
Xi'an city, 2, 341, 360, 374, 387, 423, 463, 481, 579
Xiao, Huilong, 592

xingyiquan, 157, 194–195, 216, 248, 278–279, 314, 629–630, 639, 644, 657, 677–678, 691 notes 2 and 3, 733–736, 638–639, 777–778, 788–791
xinjia (see new frame)
xinyiquan, 359–360, 413, 416–417, 562, 673, 691 note 4
Xiong, Yanghe, 717, 752–753, 760–773, 776
Xu, Chongming, 721
Xu, Tingsen, 406–407
Xu, Yizhong, 151, 156, 184 note 22, 717, 719
Xu, Yusheng, 11, 177, 283, 285, 287 note 1, 630, 632, 637
Xu, Yuxiang, 299 note 1, 568 note 1, 630–631, 641, 654, 659, 701, 734
Xu, Zhengmei, 797, 816–819
Xuanwu (god of war), 628, 642, 651, 661, 675

Y

Yang, Banhou, 13–15, 119, 121, 123, 130 note 9, 136, 195, 199, 238, 255 note 16, 280–282, 287 notes 2 and 4, 299 note 1, 359, 474, 561–562, 606, 633, 646, 730 notes 10 and 11, 755, 759–760
Yang, Chengfu, 15, 20, 77–79, 115–124, 128 note 2, 143, 157–158, 160, 163 note 4, 169–170, 177, 179, 183 notes 17, 314, 359–360, 385, 407, 473–475, 478–480, 606, 631–632, 635–637, 639, 653, 714–716, 729 notes 6, 7, 8, and 9, 730 note 10, 755, 759–760, 762–763, 773, 797, 807, 925
Yang, Hongling, 656
Yang, Jianhou, 13–15, 116, 121–122, 195, 238, 280, 282, 287 note 1, 359, 473–475, 606, 729 note 9, 755, 763, 771
Yang, Jwing-Ming, 417, 509, 525
Yang, Luchan, 9, 12–15, 116, 121–122, 177, 185 note 47, 192–193, 195, 198–199, 204, 206, 238, 240–241, 248–249, 252–253 notes 2 and 5, 254 note 7, 255 note 16, 278–282, 287 note 7, 359, 375, 385, 454–455, 457, 474–475, 537, 560–563, 565–566, 568 notes 1 and 3, 583, 606, 615, 630, 634–636, 649, 654, 660, 691 note 3, 701, 709, 752–756, 759, 760, 772–773, 934
Yang, Qingyu, 57, 383, 764
Yang, Sau Chung, 480
Yang, Shaohou, 15, 122, 193, 279–280, 287 notes 1 and 4, 631, 730, 755, 759–760, 762

Yang, Zhengduo, 427
Yang, Zhenduo, 288 note 10, 401, 474–475
Yao, Hanchen, 314
Ye, Shuliang, 591–592
Yellow Emperor (Huangdi), 46, 50, 52 note 13, 344–345, 354, 355 note 1, 356 note 11, 344–345, 354, 355 note 1, 356 note 11, 630, 632
Yijing (see Book of Changes)
Yin, Wanbang, 761
Yip Man, 586
Yongnian, 15, 560, 568 note 1, 635, 754
yongquan acupoint, 329, 397, 881
Yuan, Shikai, 10, 759
Yuan, Shiming, 423–424
Yuan, Weiming, 727, 797, 799 note 1, 808–815
Yue Fei (General), 630, 655, 658, 691 note 4
Yue, Shuting, 82–86, 88–89, 124 note 11
Yuwen University, 168, 255, 713

Z

Zhan, Deshen, 721
Zhang, Daoling, 46
Zhang, Fengqi, 560–561
Zhang, Guan, 167, 182 note 10
Zhang, Qinlin, 116–117, 119, 124, 158, 169, 231 note 7, 255 note 20, 287 note 3, 288 note 11, 730
Zhang, Qingling, 78–79
Zhang, Sanfeng, 2–3, 5–6, 8, 87, 147, 238, 240–241, 252 note 2, 253 note 5, 254 note 7, 258, 279, 287 note 5 343–344, 354, 397, 399, 412, 587, 590–591, 625, 627–637, 639–642, 647–661, 672, 725
Zhang Sanfeng Classic, 147
Zhang, Shaotang, 560
Zhang, Wansheng, 563
Zhang, Xitang, 423, 427
Zhang, Youquan, 358–360, 360
Zhang, Zhigang, 20
Zhao, Kuangyin, 672
Zhao, Youbin, 635, 659
Zhao, Zhongdao, 672–674, 676–678, 682–685, 691 note 2, 692 note 5
Zhaobao, 11, 630, 634, 650–651, 653–654, 702, 791, 794
Zheng, Manqing, 15, 20, 77, 80–81, 84, 88, 91 note 11, 115–118, 121–124, 126–127, 128 notes 1 and 2, 129 note 4, 150–152, 154–156, 158, 161–162, 164 notes 6 and 8, 165–171, 173–174, 175–181, 181 note 2, 183 notes 14 and 17, 184 note 28, 185 note 37, 202, 204, 211–212, 215–216, 220, 229 note 4, 231 notes 7, 8 and 9, 232 note 11, 235 note 28, 277–288, 291, 297, 299, 346, 372, 507–509, 524, 607, 611, 623–624, 631–633, 636–638, 641, 646, 711–731, 763, 797–798, 800–802, 806–807, 809–811, 817–818, 821–822, 850, 916, 918, 925 note 19
thirty-seven-posture form, 78, 120, 122, 169–170, 179, 239
Zheng Manqing Memorial Hall, 720–721, 725, 731 note
Zheng, Patrick, 160–163, 164 note 8, 244
Zhong, Yueping, 587–588, 594 note 1
Zhongshan Hall, 716, 801–802, 807, 817
Zhou, Dunyi, 380 note 12
Zhou, Jiannan, 636
Zhu, Tiancai, 548, 704
Zhu, Yuanzhang, 696, 698
Zhu Xi, 42, 262, 350, 378, 637
Zhuang Shen, 636
Zhuangzi, 44, 219, 233 note 16, 260, 273, 308, 343, 377, 415, 626, 637, 642, 662, 812
Zuo, Laipeng, 78, 80, 84, 116–119, 124, 249, 255 note 20

Other Titles by Via Media Publishing

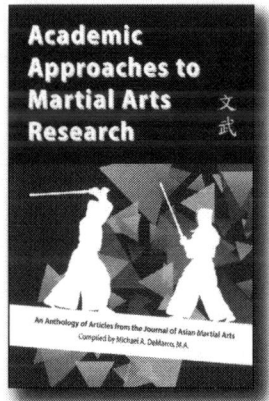

Academic Approaches
to Martial Art Research

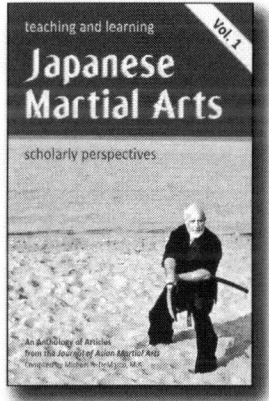

Teaching and Learning Japanese Martial Art Arts
Volume I and Volume II

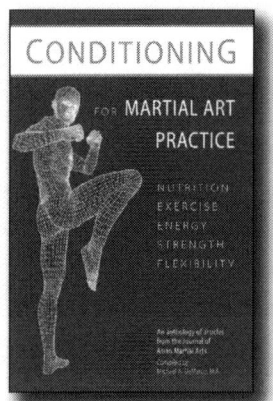

Conditioning for
Martial Art Practice

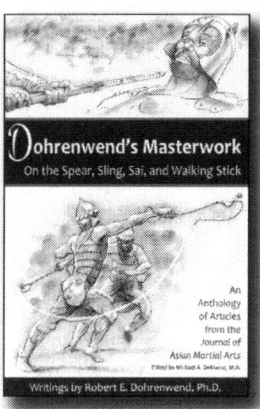

Dohrenwend's Masterwork
spear, sling, sai, walking stick

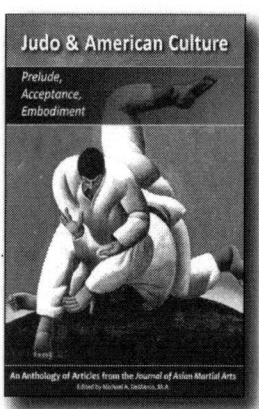

Judo and
American Culture

Fiction

Wuxia America - Emergence
of a Chinese American Hero

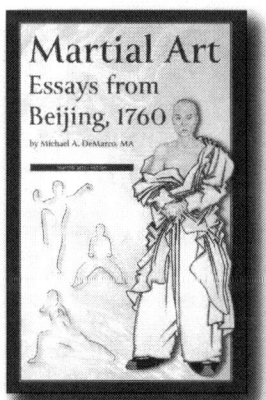

Martial Art Essays
from Beijing, 1760

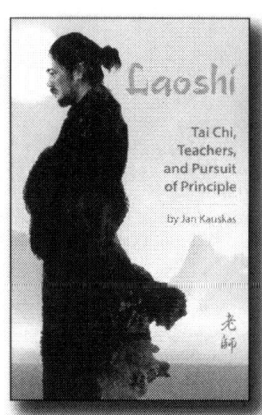

Laoshi: Tai Chi, Teachers,
and Pursuit of Principle

Printed in Great Britain
by Amazon

e5054514-7e4a-4893-9b98-c3b532ad2c81R01